T0237281

Medical Radiology

Diagnostic Imaging

Series Editors

Hans-Ulrich Kauczor
Paul M. Parizel
Wilfred C. G. Peh

The book series *Medical Radiology – Diagnostic Imaging* provides accurate and up-to-date overviews about the latest advances in the rapidly evolving field of diagnostic imaging and interventional radiology. Each volume is conceived as a practical and clinically useful reference book and is developed under the direction of an experienced editor, who is a world-renowned specialist in the field. Book chapters are written by expert authors in the field and are richly illustrated with high quality figures, tables and graphs. Editors and authors are committed to provide detailed and coherent information in a readily accessible and easy-to-understand format, directly applicable to daily practice.

Medical Radiology – Diagnostic Imaging covers all organ systems and addresses all modern imaging techniques and image-guided treatment modalities, as well as hot topics in management, workflow, and quality and safety issues in radiology and imaging. The judicious choice of relevant topics, the careful selection of expert editors and authors, and the emphasis on providing practically useful information, contribute to the wide appeal and ongoing success of the series. The series is indexed in Scopus.

More information about this series at https://link.springer.com/bookseries/174

Christoph Stippich

Editor

Clinical Functional MRI

Presurgical Functional Neuroimaging

Third Edition

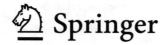 Springer

Editor
Christoph Stippich
Department of Neuroradiology and Radiology
Schmieder Clinic
Allensbach
Germany

ISSN 0942-5373   ISSN 2197-4187   (electronic)
Medical Radiology
ISSN 2731-4677   ISSN 2731-4685   (electronic)
Diagnostic Imaging
ISBN 978-3-030-83345-9   ISBN 978-3-030-83343-5   (eBook)
https://doi.org/10.1007/978-3-030-83343-5

© The Editor(s) (if applicable) and The Author(s), under exclusive license to Springer Nature
Switzerland AG 2007, 2015, 2022
This work is subject to copyright. All rights are solely and exclusively licensed by the Publisher,
whether the whole or part of the material is concerned, specifically the rights of translation,
reprinting, reuse of illustrations, recitation, broadcasting, reproduction on microfilms or in any
other physical way, and transmission or information storage and retrieval, electronic adaptation,
computer software, or by similar or dissimilar methodology now known or hereafter developed.
The use of general descriptive names, registered names, trademarks, service marks, etc. in this
publication does not imply, even in the absence of a specific statement, that such names are
exempt from the relevant protective laws and regulations and therefore free for general use.
The publisher, the authors, and the editors are safe to assume that the advice and information in
this book are believed to be true and accurate at the date of publication. Neither the publisher nor
the authors or the editors give a warranty, expressed or implied, with respect to the material
contained herein or for any errors or omissions that may have been made. The publisher remains
neutral with regard to jurisdictional claims in published maps and institutional affiliations.

This Springer imprint is published by the registered company Springer Nature Switzerland AG
The registered company address is: Gewerbestrasse 11, 6330 Cham, Switzerland

To my beloved family

Alexandra, Tim, Jan and Nils
home,
source of energy and contentment

Foreword to the First Edition

After functional mapping of the brain by magnetic resonance imaging (MRI) was found to be feasible in the early 1990s, many neuroscientists involved in research on brain function became interested in functional MRI (fMRI). In contrast to positron emission computed tomography (PET), which was used for many years to study brain function, fMRI is not based on ionizing radiation and thus can be repeated as often as necessary in patients or normal volunteers. The novel imaging method gained further in popularity when stronger magnets, stronger and faster gradients, and more advanced software for data analysis became available. Although many (neuro)radiologists had access to the hardware, relatively few also had the necessary background and drive to apply fMRI in a meaningful way. Not surprisingly, the new research field was therefore largely taken over by neuroscientists with time on their hands.

This dominance, which sometimes makes it hard for neuroradiologists to gain recognition for their (largely clinical) research on fMRI, still continues to this day. As long as the local MRI capacity is such that the clinical imaging demands are met and neuroradiologists are in a position to pursue their own research, no real problem occurs; in the ideal situation, there would be suitable MRI hardware reserved entirely for research. However, whenever neuroradiologists with their primary responsibilities to patient care compete with neuroscientists for MRI time, problems are guaranteed. Although under the pressure of a tight schedule resulting from clinical demands plus the "working in" of neurologic emergencies, neuroradiologists are generally blamed for the shrinking of research time. This seems unfair, as neuroradiologists alone can do little about this. The problem can only be reduced, and eventually perhaps solved, in an atmosphere of mutual respect and understanding, that is, under conditions where neuroscientists, neuroclinicians, and neuroradiologists work closely and amicably together.

Such is the atmosphere in which Christoph Stippich, a neuroradiologist with a background in magnetoencephalography, works and in which he conceived this book, at the Neurology, Neurosurgery and Neuroradiology department of the University of Heidelberg's "Kopfklinik" (which is also situated in close proximity to the EENT and Radiooncology departments). Stippich's idea was to clarify and then compile what is reliable and relayable current knowledge of presurgical neuroimaging, specifically fMRI. Given his experience of many years in this field, he is eminently suited for the editorship of such a book. The result of his endeavor and that of his collaborators, some of them world renowned, is so remarkable that I am convinced of the book having a significant clinical impact, primarily, but not exclusively, in neurosurgery. Christoph Stippich set out to show the scientific community what a determined neuroradiologist can do in an area dominated by "true" neuroscientists, and he has succeeded!

Heidelberg, Germany   Klaus Sartor

Foreword to the Second Edition

In the economic world, an inscription suggests that the book was considered by its publishers, after a close look at sales, to appeal to a large enough, possibly growing readership. In the scientific world, an inscription of a monograph suggests that the authors succeeded in finding readers for their special topic and keeping them. In the case of Clinical Functional MRI, I'm sure it is more than just keeping readers: it is making the entire clinical neuro-community aware of the increasing importance of this field. At the same time, the new edition provides a state-of-the-art summary, as it were, helpful to all those colleagues who are unable to closely follow the pertinent literature. As 7 years have passed since its first publication, Clinical Functional MRI was completely revised, and new chapters on emerging subtopics—e.g., on resting-state presurgical fMRI, presurgical fMRI in epilepsy, DTI tractography, and brain plasticity as seen in fMRI and DTI—were added. Christoph Stippich, now heading neuroradiology at the University of Basel/Switzerland, proved his excellence as editor by refining the book's concept, unifying the text, and strengthening his team of experts. My prediction? A third edition in less than 7 years.

Klaus Sartor
University of Heidelberg Medical Center
Heidelberg, Germany

Preface to the Third Edition

The third edition of this textbook accounts for the tremendous development of clinical functional MRI. All modalities employed for presurgical functional neuroimaging have seen a substantial evolution within the past years. Besides providing very detailed information on localization or lateralization of essential brain areas and functions in question for surgery, alterations in structural and functional brain connectivity can be assessed arising from the brains pathologies as well as from treatment.

Task-based functional MRI (TB-fMRI) is well established in many neuro-centers worldwide and plays an important role in the neuroimaging workup of functionally critical brain tumors or epilepsies. Resting-state functional MRI (RS-fMRI) has now proven clinical applicability, provides important complementary information, does not require active cooperation of the patient, and can even be used intraoperatively. In parallel, intensive research on neurovascular uncoupling (NVU) has been conducted, expanding our understanding of limitations, pitfalls, and possible solutions in BOLD-imaging. Moreover, ultra-high field MR-imagers achieved certification for clinical use and initial results on 7 T presurgical fMRI have been published. Diffusion tensor imaging (DTI) and -tractography (DDT) have undergone further refinement and represent an integral part of presurgical functional neuroimaging. While EEG-correlated fMRI and MEG are employed presurgically in highly specialized neurocenters, the role of PET and SPECT has shifted from imaging brain functions mostly to characterization of brain tumors and other brain pathologies.

To provide our readers with the latest information on presurgical functional neuroimaging, all chapters have been fully revised and updated, while keeping the text comprehensive and practical. "Multimodality in functional neuroimaging" was completely rewritten by a new author's team. It is now roughly 15 years of working together on this textbook with great pleasure. We hope that it will be of value for all working, or intending to work, in the field of clinical functional neuroimaging, and in particular with presurgical fMRI and DTI.

Allensbach, Germany   Christoph Stippich

Contents

Presurgical Functional MRI and Diffusion Tensor Imaging

Christoph Stippich

Contents

Abstract

Functional magnetic resonance imaging (fMRI) provides noninvasive localization and lateralization of specific brain functions by measuring local hemodynamic changes coupled to neuronal activation (neurovascular coupling) during active stimulation of the brain or in its resting state. Different magnetic properties of oxygenated (diamagnetic) and deoxygenated (paramagnetic) hemoglobin are exploited to generate the blood oxygen level-dependent (BOLD) contrast. Diffusion tensor magnetic resonance imaging (DTI) measures anisotropic (directional) diffusion of protons along myelinated fibers and thereby provides detailed information on the white matter architecture. Specific white matter tracts can be reconstructed using diffusion tensor tractography (DTT). During the last three decades both novel MR modalities have revolutionized the imaging research on human brain function and structure and its connectivity under physiological and pathological conditions.

Task-based (TB) presurgical fMRI in patients with brain tumors or epilepsies—with first clinical applications dating back to the mid-1990s—represents the best established and validated clinical application and has been integrated into the presurgical imaging workflow of leading neurocenters. Specific tasks need to be performed by the patient during the actual fMRI measurements activating the brain areas in question for surgery. Usually, essential cortical motor and language areas are localized and the language-dominant hemisphere is determined prior to treatment. Memory, auditory, somatosensory, visual, or

C. Stippich (✉)
Department of Neuroradiology and Radiology,
Schmieder Clinic, Allensbach, Germany

© The Author(s), under exclusive license to Springer Nature Switzerland AG 2022
C. Stippich (ed.), *Clinical Functional MRI*, Medical Radiology Diagnostic Imaging,
https://doi.org/10.1007/978-3-030-83343-5_1

other functions have also been investigated, but played a quantitatively minor role in presurgical fMRI.

Resting-state (RS) fMRI measures synchronized fluctuations in BOLD signals related to spontaneous brain activation. Besides localizing so-called eloquent functional brain areas various "resting-state networks" can be identified and analyzed for functional connectivity including changes related to the brain's disease. Since its introduction to presurgical functional neuroimaging arena—roughly a decade ago—RS-fMRI has seen a tremendous evolution, demonstrated promising results, and has relevant advantages for clinical application: Cooperation is not required and patients with severe functional deficits can be investigated. Time-consuming and demanding individual patient training prior to the fMRI exams is not necessary. Application is possible under sedation or anesthesia directly before or even during neurosurgery with ultrafast image processing at hand. However, the data available on validity, reliability, and potential patient benefit of presurgical RS-fMRI are still limited and require further investigation.

DTI and DTT provide complementary data on functionally important white matter connections to be spared during treatment, e.g., the pyramidal tract (motor function), the arcuate fascicle (language), the optic radiation (vision), and others. This imaging information is indispensable to establish the best possible treatment for each individual patient, and to achieve the ultimate goal of brain surgery: function-preserving complete or most radical removal of the pathology. To this end fMRI and DTI are integrated meaningfully into functional neuronavigation.

Meanwhile, relevant medical societies (e.g., the American Society for Functional Neuroradiology, ASFNR) have released guidelines and recommendations on imaging procedures and data evaluation for presurgical fMRI and DTI. However, all clinical functional neuroimaging modalities are far from being simple "push-button" techniques.

Responsible presurgical application requires profound knowledge of the imaging techniques employed, underlying functional neuroanatomy, physiology and pathology, neuroplastic alterations, influencing factors, artifacts, pitfalls, validity, and limitations. Finally, information on other—alternative or complementary—functional neuroimaging modalities and their multimodal integration is essential.

1 Introduction

Functional magnetic resonance imaging (fMRI) is a modern, noninvasive imaging technique to measure and localize specific functions of the human brain without the application of radiation (Bandettini et al. 1992; Kwong et al. 1992). Brain function is indirectly assessed with high spatial resolution via detection of local hemodynamic changes in capillaries (Menon et al. 1995) and draining veins (Frahm et al. 1994) of the so-called functional areas, e.g., regions of the human brain that govern motor, sensory, language, or memory functions. In *task-based fMRI (TB-fMRI)*, specific stimulation of the respective neurofunctional system is required (Belliveau et al. 1991). The stimuli are presented in a predefined manner during the fMRI measurement, which is called a stimulation *paradigm*. TB-fMRI is well established for the presurgical application in patients with brain tumors or epilepsies. It can be considered as the most commonly used and robust neuroimaging modality for motor and language function (Tyndall et al. 2017). The measurement of spontaneous brain activation is also possible, by using *resting-state fMRI (RS-fMRI)* techniques (Purdon and Weisskoff 1998). Here, low-frequency fluctuations in the hemodynamics of the brain are analyzed for synchrony to detect interconnected areas that constitute different functional systems. RS-fMRI is typically employed to study *functional brain connectivity* in neuroimaging research. Meanwhile, RS-fMRI has shown clinical applicability and can be considered as a powerful adjunct for presurgical functional neuroimaging (Lee et al. 2013; Rosazza et al. 2018; O'Connor and Zeffiro 2019; Seitzman et al. 2019).

The *blood oxygen level-dependent (BOLD)* fMRI technique makes use of blood as an intrinsic contrast (Ogawa et al. 1990, 1992, 1993), superseding the intravenous application of paramagnetic contrast agents (Belliveau et al. 1991) or radioactive substances (Mazziotta et al. 1982; Raichle 1983; Fox et al. 1986; Holman and Devous 1992). The different magnetic properties of oxygenated and deoxygenated hemoglobin are exploited to generate the BOLD contrast. Although the underlying physiological mechanisms of neurovascular coupling are not ultimately understood, there seems to be a very good correspondence of BOLD signals with actual neuronal activity (Logothetis et al. 2001; Logothetis 2002, 2003; Logothetis and Pfeuffer 2004; Logothetis and Wandell 2004). However, neurovascular uncoupling (NVU)—a phenomenon observed in some brain tumors and other pathologies affecting the brain's hemodynamic properties—represents a relevant limitation to the presurgical application of BOLD-fMRI (Agarwal et al. 2016, 2021; Pak et al. 2017). To assess possible NVU cerebrovascular reactivity mapping can be employed (Pillai and Mikulis 2015).

Powerful magnets, performant gradient systems, and ultrafast MR sequences enable examination of the entire brain in clinically feasible time frames. Furthermore, fMRI profits from high main magnetic field strength and multichannel head coils in terms of improved signal-to-noise ratio (SNR), higher spatial resolution, and/or shorter examination times. Novel multislice image acquisition helps to further reduce scanning times significantly (Kiss et al. 2018). While clinical fMRI studies of motor and language function can be conducted on well-equipped midfield MR imagers (1.0 T, 1.5 T), it is preferrable to employ 3 T MR machines for clinical BOLD functional neuroimaging (Tyndall et al. 2017). Recently, first installations of ultrahigh-field MR imagers (7 T) achieved certification for clinical use (Springer et al. 2016) and initial results on presurgical fMRI are available (Lima Cardoso et al. 2017). However, worldwide access to ultrahigh-field clinical MR imagers will stay very limited and as of today, higher patient benefit still awaits proof. Better functionality of data processing and immediate data analysis, as obtained with *real-time fMRI (RT-fMRI)*, facilitate the usability of fMRI in the clinical context (Fernandez et al. 2001; Weiskopf et al. 2003; Steger and Jackson 2004; Moller et al. 2005; Vakamudi et al. 2020). Today, most vendors offer some functionality with their MR imagers to analyze fMRI data at the scanners' console directly and stimulation devices designed for clinical fMRI are commercially available. In addition, various open-source data processing pipelines can be employed and automated workflows from image acquisition to medical reporting (Pernet et al. 2016). This technical evolution has facilitated the application of fMRI in the clinical environment, substantially.

Thus, fMRI not only offers a variety of novel options for clinical diagnostics and research but also has opened up a new diagnostic field of radiology and neuroradiology, by shifting paradigms from strictly morphological imaging to measurement and visualization of brain function (Stippich et al. 2002a; Thulborn 2006). Nonetheless, clinical fMRI has not become a simple "push-button" technique yet and requires profound expertise in the field of responsible physicians.

Presurgical TB-fMRI has demonstrated positive effects on patient mortality, morbidity, and clinical outcome (Vysotski et al. 2018); provides intraoperatively critical information in case of limited or infeasible electrocorticography (Rigolo et al. 2020); and can be adapted for pediatric patients (Jones et al. 2020). RS-fMRI has been introduced for presurgical application (Lee et al. 2013), validated (Qiu et al. 2014; Lemée et al. 2019), implemented into clinical routine (Lee et al. 2016; Leuthardt et al. 2018), and used in pediatric patients (Roland et al. 2019) and even intraoperatively (Qiu et al. 2017; Metwali et al. 2020a, b, 2021). Furthermore, resting-state networks enable us to study functional brain connectivity under physiological and pathological conditions.

The combination of fMRI with *diffusion tensor imaging (DTI)* has proven scientific and clinical relevance (Bick et al. 2012). By measuring the directed diffusion of protons along myelinated fibers, DTI provides complementary information on white matter architecture, i.e., on the course and integrity of functionally important white matter tracts. In neuroimaging research, DTI is mainly applied to study the human brain's *structural connectivity*, whereas *diffusion tensor tractography (DDT)* is often also employed for clinical applications (Leclercq et al. 2011; Vanderweyen et al. 2020). DTI measurements can be obtained together with fMRI in the same scanning session, which gives an even more complete picture of each patient's individual brain pathology. When integrated into neuronavigation patients may profit in functional outcome and extent of resection (Incekara et al. 2016).

With this textbook, we aim to provide the reader with thorough and comprehensive information on the abovementioned advanced MRI techniques, namely, task-based fMRI, resting-state fMRI, diffusion tensor imaging, and tractography in the presurgical context, which constitute their best established and validated clinical applications. A meaningful combination of these advanced MRI techniques with standard MR sequences (T2-FLAIR, T1-weighted sequences pre- and post-contrast administration) as well as with diffusion- and perfusion-weighted MRI is recommended to complete the state-of-the-art preoperative structural and functional neuroimaging in patients with brain tumors and drug-resistant epilepsy (Svolos et al. 2013) (Fig. 1). On current MR imagers with

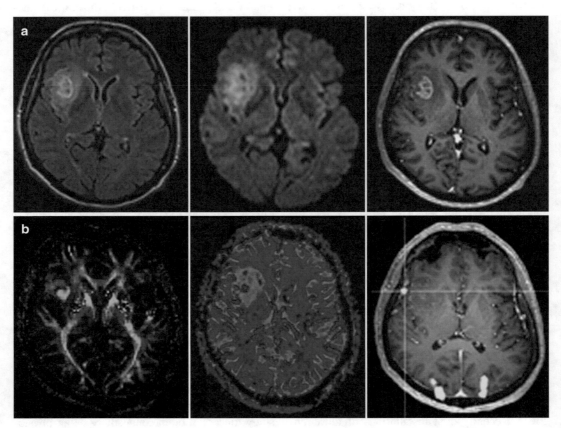

Fig. 1 The state-of-the-art preoperative multimodality MR imaging in a right glioblastoma affecting the basal ganglia, insula, and inferior frontal lobe as visualized on standard MR sequences (**a**, *upper row*). Advanced MR imaging (**b**, *lower row*) revealed disintegration of white matter architecture/alterations in fractional anisotropy on color-coded DTI maps (*left*), increased relative blood volume on dynamic susceptibility contrast-enhanced (DSCE) perfusion imaging (*middle*), and right language dominance on BOLD fMRI (*right*) in this left-handed male patient

main magnetic field strength of 1.5 T or above, equipped with powerful gradients and multichannel head coils, such protocols should not require more than 45 min of scanning time. To this end the MR protocol needs to be tailored to the different requirements in individual patients. As an approximation for TB-fMRI, a multiparadigm language mapping should require 10–20 min of scanning time and a somatotopic motor or somatosensory mapping of 5–10 min. RS-fMRI requires between 5 and 20 min as does DTI, depending on the imaging sequences used. It is recommended to acquire the complete MR protocol within the same scanning session in order to minimize coregistration inaccuracies and to include the T1-weighted 3D post-contrast data set—which will be used for the overlay of functional or structural images and for neuronavigation. When using strictly time-optimized image acquisition and the most relevant fMRI and DTI sequences only, both can be fit into a 30-min time frame, leaving enough time for the essential structural imaging, all within a typical routine neuroimaging time slot. Other meaningfully selected MR sequence may be added to such multimodal MR protocols, e.g., susceptibility-weighted imaging (SWI). MR-spectroscopy (MRS) and chemical-shift imaging (CSI) may require seperate scanning sessions

MR spectroscopy (MRS) and chemical shift imaging (CSI) are other MR modalities for advanced neuroimaging in oncology which may be added selectively and provide important complementary information on the brain's and the tumor's metabolism (Tsougos et al. 2012). Here, a second scanning session is recommended unless the patients are very cooperative.

2 Blood Oxygenation Level-Dependent Functional MRI (BOLD fMRI)

Enhanced synaptic activity resulting from stimulation of neurons leads to a local increase in energy and oxygen consumption in functional areas. The following local hemodynamic changes transmitted via neurovascular coupling are measured by fMRI with high spatial accuracy:

- Increase of regional cerebral blood volume (rCBV)
- Increase of regional cerebral blood flow (rCBF)
- Relative increase of oxyhemoglobin in capillaries and venous blood

In principle, fMRI measurements can be accomplished with different techniques; BOLD fMRI being the most frequently used in human brain is therefore often referred to as the *standard* technique (Thulborn et al. 1996; Thulborn 1998, 2006). Bolus tracking measures rCBV making use of external contrast agents (Belliveau et al. 1991), and spin tagging assesses rCBF using arterial blood for intrinsic contrast (Detre et al. 1992). In contrast, BOLD technique (Ogawa et al. 1990, 1992, 1993) takes advantage of the different magnetic properties of oxygenated (oxy-Hb) and deoxygenated (deoxy-Hb) hemoglobin to generate an image contrast. Paramagnetic deoxy-Hb produces local field inhomogeneities in a measurable range for MRI resulting in a signal decrease in susceptibility-weighted MR sequences (T2*), whereas diamagnetic oxy-Hb does not interfere with the external magnetic field. Specific neuronal stimulation augments local cerebral oxygen consumption, which initially results in a decrease of oxy-Hb and an increase in deoxy-Hb in the functional area. To provide the active neurons with oxygenated blood, perfusion (rCBF, rCBV) in capillaries and draining veins is increased within several seconds. This mechanism not only equalizes the initial decrease of local oxy-Hb concentration but even overcompensates it (Fox and Raichle 1986). Deoxy-Hb is progressively washed out which is reflected by a reduction of local field inhomogeneity and a raise of BOLD signal in T2*-weighted MR images (Turner et al. 1991).

BOLD measurements are currently exerted with ultrafast single-shot echo-planar-imaging (EPI) sequences as gradient echo (GRE) or spin echo (SE) (Stippich et al. 2002a, b). GRE sequences usually obtain higher BOLD signal predominantly from venous origin, whereas SE sequences also measure lower BOLD signals arising from the capillary bed in brain parenchyma (Hulvershorn et al. 2005a, b). Simultaneous multislice EPI significantly reduces scanning times (Kiss et al. 2018). Temporal resolution in paradigms with a blocked or parametric design corresponds to the chosen block duration but could be substantially improved (<100 ms) by the introduction of event-related measurements (Buckner et al. 1996). FMRI, however, cannot attain the temporal resolution of electroencephalography (EEG) (Berger 1929; Gevins 1995; Gevins et al. 1995) or magnetoencephalography (MEG) (Hari and Ilmoniemi 1986; Hämäläinen et al. 1993) but lacks the need for a complicated model-based calculation for source localization and offers higher spatial precision due to a direct correlation with the surface anatomy. Signal intensity and realizable spatial resolution vary with the magnetic field strength. MR scanners with magnetic field strengths below 1.0 Tesla (T) are not suitable for clinical functional BOLD imaging. The broadly available 1.5 T scanners allow reliable measurements of cortical activation provided that powerful gradient systems (possibly >30 mT/m) are on hand, while high-magnetic-field scanners with 3 T or above even permit functional imaging of subcortical structures and the brain stem (Thulborn 1999; Zambreanu et al. 2005). Despite excellent SNR and spatial resolution, the application of ultrahigh-field fMRI still has to be considered experimental (Goa et al. 2014; Hua et al. 2013; Huber et al. 2014). This is mainly due to technical and logistical difficulties as well as due to the very limited availability of ultrahigh-field MR imagers in a clinical setting. Recently, some vendors achieved certification for clinical use of their latest generation ultrahigh-field MR machines. Meanwhile, some leading medical imaging centers are equipped with clinical 7 T MR units (Lima Cardoso et al. 2017). Some methodological aspects have been addressed regarding presurgical 7 T-fMRI (Dymerska et al. 2019) and even integration with simultaneous EEG recordings is possible (Grouiller et al. 2016). Advantages of fMRI over positron-emission tomography (PET) (Mazziotta et al. 1982; Raichle 1983; Fox et al. 1986) or single-photon emission computer tomography

(SPECT) (Holman and Devous 1992)—other methods measuring brain activity indirectly with lower spatial/temporal resolution (glucose or oxygen metabolism, blood flow/perfusion changes)—are its noninvasiveness, lack of radiation, reproducibility, and broad availability of clinical scanners.

Task-based presurgical BOLD fMRI represents the best established and validated clinical application of fMRI. Due to the intrinsically low SNR, it is mandatory to perform multiple repeated stimulations during each task-based fMRI measurement in order to obtain robust BOLD signals. Statistical correlation of BOLD signal time courses with the chosen stimulation protocol (paradigm) enables the identification of those brain areas that show hemodynamic changes in synchrony with the task. A prerequisite for this is a further processing of fMRI data, which is normally done after the measurements with freely available open-source or commercial software (Cox 1996; Friston 1996; Gold et al. 1998; Roberts 2003; http://www.mriquestions.com/best-fmri-software.html 2020). However, only a few programs have been certified for medical use. Nowadays, most manufacturers of clinical high-magnetic-field scanners offer options for immediate *online* processing of fMRI data (Fernandez et al. 2001; Moller et al. 2005; Posse et al. 2013; Vakamudi et al. 2020). Since the functionality and the statistical calculations used vary considerably between the different software, the appropriate choice largely depends on individual criteria and preferences. Basically, any data processing software for fMRI should at least offer proper image alignment, motion correction, temporal and spatial data smoothing, multiple statistical tests to assess functional activation, and options for spatial normalization (Stippich et al. 2002a, b). Furthermore, each fMRI software used for neurosurgery or radiation treatment should provide precise and reliable tools for superimposing functional or morphological images, for the integration of fMRI with DTI data, and for data export (e.g., into neuronavigation systems).

This textbook has its traditional focus on presurgical functional neuroimaging. Today, presurgical TB-fMRI is the most widely used modality and is commonly combined with DTI and DTT to visualize both functionally important cortical areas and white matter tracts. As mentioned earlier, RS-fMRI has seen a tremendous evolution and is increasingly used for presurgical neuroimaging. Hence, we have now updated and substantially expanded the information available in this textbook on these complementary MR modalities TB-fMRI, RS-fMRI, DTI, and DTT, but keep the focus strictly on pre- and intraoperative applications in patients with brain tumors and epilepsy. A detailed methodological description of diffusion MRI and BOLD fMRI is beyond the scope of this book—for this purpose, we refer the reader to the extensive literature available.

3 Diffusion Tensor Imaging (DTI) and DTI Tractography (DTT)

Diffusion MR signal mainly originates from protons that move in the extracellular space of biological tissues (Brownian motion) (LeBihan 2006, 2013; LeBihan and Johansen-Berg 2012). Within a given voxel, the diffusion may be fully free and undirected (isotropic) or directed (anisotropic) due to barriers preventing proton movement (e.g., myelinated axons). DTI is capable to detect such anisotropic diffusion (Basser et al. 1994; LeBihan et al. 2001), but for this end diffusion must at least be measured in six different directions. Anisotropic diffusion can then be modeled mathematically using a 3D Gaussian probability function from which a 3×3 matrix is calculated, named *diffusion tensor*. The diffusion tensor is characterized by *eigenvalues* and *eigenvectors* and indicates the main orientation of diffusion within a voxel. The *fractional anisotropy* (FA) quantifies such directed diffusion. Isotropic (undirected) diffusion corresponds to an FA value of *0* which translates graphically to a sphere. In contrast, an FA value of *1* reflects the opposite extreme, i.e., a totally directed (anisotropic) diffusion which would graphically translate to a line but does not occur in biological tissues—thus, the typical shape of the FA is an ellipsoid.

Myelinated axons are lipophilic and represent diffusion barriers for hydrophilic protons that travel perpendicularly. In turn, this results in a preferred orientation and higher velocity of diffusion along such barriers. Thus, DTI reflects the white matter architecture and the course of functionally important fiber bundles rather indirectly by measuring the anisotropic diffusion of protons between and along axons. Basically, DTI fiber tracts are reconstructed by following and connecting the predominant directed diffusion across adjacent voxels. A well-established approach is to use anatomical regions as seed points for tractography. Standard DTI measurements and most mathematical algorithms employed for analyzing DTI data have limitations when different orientations of diffusion need to be differentiated within a voxel, when crossing fibers need to be reconstructed, or when diffusion anisotropy is affected by the brain's pathology, e.g., by tumor invasion or edema (Cortez-Conradis et al. 2013; Kallenberg et al. 2013; Kleiser et al. 2010; Stadlbauer et al. 2010). At the expense of scanning/processing time, more advanced MR techniques enable the assessment of the contribution of the differential intravoxel anisotropy (diffusion spectrum imaging, q-ball imaging, HARDI, etc.) or the employment of a more sophisticated (e.g., probabilistic or advanced deterministic) modeling for tractography (Bauer et al. 2013; Kuhnt et al. 2013a, b; O'Donell et al. 2012). In difficult cases such advanced DTI techniques in combination with fMRI-targeted tractography may provide clinically relevant results (Sanvito et al. 2020). In general, the *quality* of DTI images depends on the number of directions measured, the number of averages used, and the spatial resolution chosen, which are all inversely related to scanning time.

4 Presurgical fMRI and DTI

Presurgical fMRI and DTI measurements are carried out to facilitate function-preserving and safe treatment in patients with brain tumors and epilepsy by localizing and lateralizing specific brain functions, functionally important axonal connections, or epileptic activity, noninvasively (Bick et al. 2012; Dimou et al. 2013; Centeno and Carmichael 2014; Barras et al. 2016; Szaflarski et al. 2017; Black et al. 2019). This diagnostic information cannot be obtained from morphological brain imaging alone or from invasive measures prior to treatment.

Consequently, presurgical fMRI and DTI are always performed in individual patients to achieve a functional diagnosis. This differs fundamentally from applications in basic neuroscience research where normal or altered brain function is usually investigated in group studies to better understand physiological or pathological conditions in general. A direct contribution to the patient management is not required. In contrast, for clinical diagnostic applications, the experimental setup as well as the processing and evaluation of the data need to be adapted to the clinical environment so that patients—who may present with neurological or cognitive deficits—can be examined successfully in a standardized way. Still, in clinical fMRI and DTI, this is typically achieved via local experts, individual routines, and own validation (Pillai 2010). The novel applications of resting-state fMRI may have practical advantages, as an active cooperation of the patient is not required (Lang et al. 2014). Uncooperative, sedated, or anesthetized patients or children who are not able to perform task-based fMRI properly may profit from RS-fMRI. RS-fMRI can also be applied intraoperatively (Nimsky 2011; Qiu et al. 2017; Metwali et al. 2020a, b).

During the last years, more and more devices and software solutions have become commercially available that facilitate the clinical application of fMRI. These products are mainly dedicated to stimulation and data processing. Moreover, first attempts have been made to define robust clinical applications for task-based fMRI. To this end, paradigms have been proposed and published online by the American Society of Functional Neuroradiology (for details, please visit www.asfnr.org/paradigms. html). There is also instructive teaching material available online along with regular clinical fMRI case conferences. At least in the USA, CPT codes have been established for reimbursement of clinical fMRI examinations. It is important to note, however, that fMRI and DTI cannot be considered as fully standardized methods routinely used in clinical diagnostic neuroimaging. Hence, depending on the local situations, it may still be required to perform presurgical fMRI and DTI examinations in the framework of scientific studies until all hard- and software components used for medical application have been certified and official recommendations or guidelines have been issued by the relevant national medical association. Until then, individual routines and standards still need to be established for data acquisition, processing, and evaluation, as well as for the medical interpretation and documentation of clinical fMRI and DTI findings. For a meaningful clinical application, a profound knowledge of the specifications of the different software packages used, of possible sources of errors and imaging artifacts, and of relevant limitations of the techniques employed is indispensable. For presurgical mapping identification of reliable fMRI data sets, selection of optimal data postprocessing pipelines and determination of patient-specific statistical thresholds are crucial (Stevens et al. 2016). Furthermore a profound knowledge of limitations of the applied imaging techniques and of possible solutions is required. The same holds true for presurgical DTI and tractography (Vanderweyen et al. 2020). As a basic principle, presurgical fMRI and DTI examinations should still be performed, evaluated, and interpreted—or at least supervised—by trained and experienced physicians with particular expertise in this area, since careless use of this very promising technique could endanger patients.

There are numerous studies available suggesting a high reliability of fMRI to localize the different cortical representations of the human body within the primary motor and somatosensory cortices (Fig. 2) as well as the motor and sensory language areas (Fig. 3) prior to brain surgery, if indications and limits of the method are considered. The same holds true for the noninvasive determination of the dominant brain hemisphere for language function.

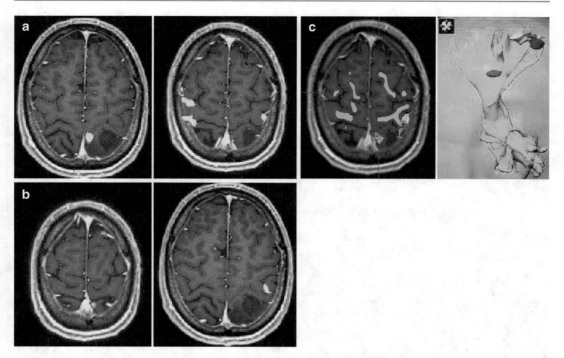

Fig. 2 Preoperative fMRI somatotopic mapping of the motor (**a**) and somatosensory (**b**) homunculus and DTI tractography of the corticospinal (pyramidal) tract in a symptomatic patient with a left parietal astrocytoma. Voluntary movements of the toes and fingers on the right side were used for motor mapping, and fully automated pneumatically driven tactile stimulation of digits 1 and 2 to the right foot and hand, respectively, was employed for somatosensory stimulation. Of note is the enhanced co-activation of the premotor and primary hand representa-tions in the right hemisphere during voluntary right-hand movements as an fMRI indicator for tumor-associated neuroplastic reorganization. Integration of the abovemen-tioned different functional body representations (foot motor (*dark blue*), foot somatosensory (*light blue*), hand motor (*yellow*), hand somatosensory (*orange*), tongue motor (*purple*)) and of the pyramidal tract (*green*) into a 3D data set for functional neuronavigation (**c**, *left*), 3D surface view (**c**, *right*)

Additional attention needs to be paid to technique-related inaccuracies due to the super-position of functional and morphological images, the referencing of fMRI data in neuronavigation systems, or the surgery-induced localization errors following removal of brain tissue or loss of cerebrospinal fluid (brain shift) (Reinges et al. 2004; Wittek et al. 2005). Safety of surgical pro-cedures in functional areas or their proximity can be improved by concomitant visualization of functional landmarks and important fiber tracts (e.g., pyramidal tract, arcuate fascicle) using dif-fusion tensor imaging (DTI) (Coenen et al. 2001; Holodny et al. 2001; Krings et al. 2001; Stippich et al. 2003a; Ulmer et al. 2004b; Holodny et al. 2005; Shinoura et al. 2005). The same holds true for the combined use of fMRI and EEG (Towle et al. 2003), MEG (Kober et al. 2001; Grummich et al. 2006), or PET (Baumann et al. 1995; Bittar et al. 1999). Tumor-induced hemodynamic changes can lead to erroneous fMRI localization and missing or artificial BOLD signals (Holodny et al. 1999, 2000; Schreiber et al. 2000; Krings et al. 2002; Ulmer et al. 2004a, b). Tumor-induced hemodynamic changes may arise from vascular compression, tumor neovasculature (Gould et al. 2018), and neurovascular uncoupling (Pak et al. 2017). Electrophysiological techniques are unsusceptible to these problems, since they directly measure electromagnetic fields resulting from synaptic activity (Berger 1929; Hari and Ilmoniemi 1986; Hämäläinen et al. 1993). However, localization of electromagnetic sources requires complicated modeling and calculations

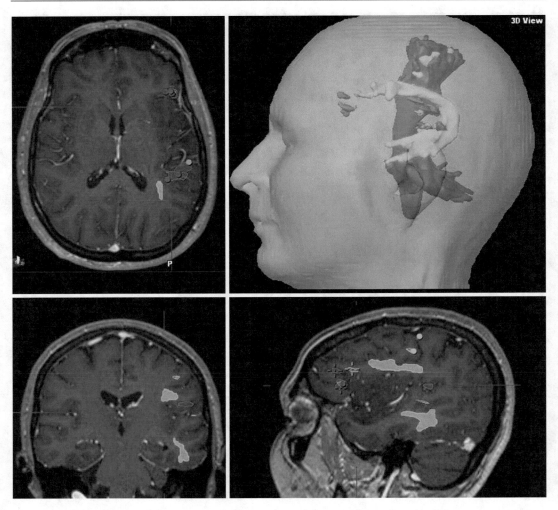

Fig. 3 Preoperative fMRI language mapping of the motor (Broca) and sensory (Wernicke) language areas and DTI tractographies of the arcuate fascicle (*green*) and pyramidal tract (*purple*) integrated into the T1-weighted post-contrast 3D MRI used for functional neuronavigation in a female patient with a symptomatic left astrocytoma involving the inferior frontal and superior temporal lobes and the insula; transverse, coronal, and sagittal views, 3D surface view. fMRI revealed a left language dominance and a good spatial agreement between the functional localizations obtained with four different language paradigms for both essential language areas

and is therefore limited in precision and accuracy. Furthermore, it should be borne in mind that fMRI and DTI results are generated by using mathematical correlations and therefore vary with the chosen statistical parameters or thresholds. Consequently, the size and extent of fMRI cortical activations or of reconstructed DTI fiber tracts do not reflect the *truth* and may confront the operator with an unfounded safety margin. Thus, resection borders cannot be determined reliably on the basis of fMRI or DTI data without standardization and validation. Of note, a retrospective analysis indicated that the lesion to activation distance and the degree of white matter involvement are predictive on preoperative, but not on postoperative, functional deficits (Bailey et al. 2015).

When applied in a standardized way, fMRI has the diagnostic potential to substantially contribute to the planning and implementation of function-preserving therapies in patients with brain tumors and epilepsy (Lee et al. 1999; Gaillard et al. 2000; Grabowski 2000; Hirsch et al. 2000; Sunaert and Yousry 2001; Baxendale 2002; Binder et al. 2002; Rutten et al. 2002; Stippich et al. 2003a, b, 2007; Van Westen et al. 2005; Thulborn 2006). Prior to and during neurosurgical interventions, fMRI can help to reduce the need for invasive diagnostic procedures, as intra-arterial Wada test (Wada and Rasmussen 1960; Rausch et al. 1993; Benbadis et al. 1998; Abou-khalil and Schlaggar 2002) or intraoperative electrocorticography (Penfield 1937; Cedzich et al. 1996; Duffau et al. 2002, 2003). Moreover, intraoperative fMRI supports surgical decision-making after limited or infeasible ECoG (Rigolo et al. 2020). Multimodal functional mapping with fMRI, DTI, and direct cortical stimulation/electrocorticography facilitates precision surgery (Flouty et al. 2017) and improves extent of resection in gliomas (Incekara et al. 2016). Whether the embedding of fMRI and DTI in presurgical diagnostics can indeed reduce surgery-related morbidity and mortality was addressed in prospective clinical trials. Meanwhile, positive evidence has been provided (Zacharaki et al. 2012; Castellano et al. 2017; Vysotski et al. 2018). Prerequisites are a consensus on measuring techniques, analysis procedures, and medical evaluation of clinical fMRI as well as the establishment of official recommendations and guidelines by the assigned medical association. As stated earlier, first attempts in that direction have been made.

5 Content Overview

Chapter "Revealing Brain Activity and White Matter Structure Using Functional and Diffusion-Weighted Magnetic Resonance Imaging" provides an easy, but in-depth, access to the techniques and underlying physiology of the abovementioned different *fMRI* and *DTI techniques* (Bandettini et al. 1992; Kwong et al. 1992; Ogawa et al. 1993; Basser et al. 1994; Purdon and Weisskoff 1998). The principles and basics of MRI, fMRI, and DTI, as well as the different established experimental designs for task-based fMRI, are presented along with the options for specific data analysis. The resting-state fMRI technique is explained in detail and what methods can be implemented to study functional connectivity in different resting-state networks. Finally, diffusion tensor imaging and tractography are addressed (LeBihan and Johansen-Berg 2012). On a solid methodological basis, the capabilities to study structural connectivity and to employ presurgical tractography are demonstrated.

Chapter "Functional Neuroanatomy" extensively deals with the relevant morphological and functional *neuroanatomy* to facilitate the reader's access to presurgical fMRI and DTI. In addition to a detailed systematic description of the surface anatomy and cytoarchitecture of the human brain, important morphological criteria for a straightforward identification of different anatomical structures are discussed. Comprehensive information on the functional neuroanatomy of the motor and language systems is provided. Here, it cannot be sufficiently stressed that a profound knowledge of the relevant neuroanatomy is indispensable for a correct medical interpretation of clinical fMRI and DTI data. In any case, the *precentral knob* is the only reliable anatomical landmark for a functional area, namely, the motor hand representation (Yousry et al. 1997; Fesl et al. 2003). There are no morphological landmarks for areas related to cognitive brain functions such as language or memory (Ojemann et al. 1989; Ojemann 1991). Due to the vast physiological interindividual anatomical variability (Amunts et al. 1999, 2000) and the dependence on various individual factors, functional areas are traditionally mapped intraoperatively by means of electrophysiological methods (Penfield 1937, 1950; Woolsey et al. 1979; Ojemann et al. 1989; Ojemann 1991; Uematsu et al. 1992; Cedzich et al. 1996; Duffau et al. 1999). However, this information is preoperatively inaccessible, and the time needed for surgery is therefore significantly prolonged. FMRI and DTI, on the other hand, yield relevant diagnostic information on anatomy, pathology, and function prior to surgery in one single examination. Thus, the indication for presurgical fMRI and DTI results from:

- Clinical signs and symptoms
- The limitations of morphological imaging
- The necessity to measure and visualize normal, modified neuroplastic, and pathological (e.g., epileptic) brain activity

Chapter "Task-Based Presurgical Functional MRI in Patients with Brain Tumors" covers *presurgical task-based BOLD fMRI* (*TB-fMRI*), which represents fMRI's best established, validated, and most widely used clinical application. Particular notice is given to practical and methodological-technical aspects (Sect. 3) as well as to specific requirements of fMRI diagnostics in patients with rolandic brain tumors (Sect. 4) or lesions with critical spatial relationship to language areas (Sect. 5). Diagnostic aims and selection criteria for patients are discussed, clinically tested examination protocols are proposed (Stippich et al. 1999, 2000, 2002b, 2003b, 2004, 2005, 2007; Stippich 2010), and their applications are illustrated with example cases. Presurgical TB-fMRI has positive effects on patient mortality, morbidity, and clinical outcome (Vysotski et al. 2018); provides intraoperatively critical information in case of limited or infeasible electrocorticography (Rigolo et al. 2020); and can be adapted for pediatric patients (Jones et al. 2020). Further, potentials and limits of presurgical TB-fMRI are depicted (Sect. 4.6 of chapter "Task-Based Presurgical Functional MRI in Patients with Brain Tumors").

Chapter "Presurgical Resting-State fMRI" highlights the clinical application of *resting-state fMRI* (*RS-fMRI*) as a novel functional neuroimaging modality in the presurgical workup of patients with brain tumors (Mitchell et al. 2013). Here, no stimulation or active cooperation of the patients is required to assess important functional systems, which is potentially of great value to further facilitate the clinical application of fMRI (Posse et al. 2013). RS-fMRI has been introduced for presurgical application (Lee et al. 2013), validated (Qiu et al. 2014; Lemée et al. 2019), implemented into clinical routine (Lee et al. 2016; Leuthardt et al. 2018), and used in pediatric patients (Roland et al. 2019) and even intraoperatively (Qiu et al. 2017; Metwali et al. 2020a, b). RS-fMRI provides additional information on the *connectivity* between different functionally important brain areas, which may be exploited in the future to study the effects of lesions, treatment, and medication on brain function (Niu et al. 2014; Smucny et al. 2014; Otten et al. 2012; Martino et al. 2011). Such neuroplastic alterations in brain function may be compensatory or pathological in nature.

Chapter "Simultaneous EEG-fMRI in Epilepsy" refers to the highly specific application of presurgical fMRI in patients with *epilepsy* which requires fundamentally different data acquisition and processing techniques as compared to both task-based and resting-state fMRI, such as EEG-correlated fMRI for the localization of epileptogenic foci (Centeno and Carmichael 2014: Chiang et al. 2014). To this end, major technical and methodological problems had to be solved, which now enables us to use electrical devices (EEG) inside MR scanners to correct for interferences and related artifacts and thereby precisely detect and localize the sources of epileptic activity in the human brain. EEG-correlated fMRI is by no means a standard application (Pittau et al. 2014). It should be considered as a valuable additional investigation tool in the field of epilepsy imaging which is available in some leading medical centers worldwide.

Chapter "Diffusion Imaging with MR Tractography for Brain Tumor Surgery" accounts for *DTI* and *DTT* with their proven value for functional brain tumor and epilepsy surgery with respect to both preoperative neuroimaging and intraoperative navigation (Potgieser et al. 2014; Shahar et al. 2014; Sternberg et al. 2014; Kuhnt et al. 2012b, 2013a, b). In this setting, DTI is fully complementary to fMRI, by providing additional relevant information on the course and integrity of important white matter tracts in relation to a surgical target. Hence, these techniques should be applied in combination whenever possible. Specific attention is given to the corticospinal tract and sensorimotor system; the arcuate, uncinate, inferior fronto-occipital fascicles and language systems; as well as the superior longitudinal fascicle, optic radiation, and visuospatial attention network.

Chapter "Functional Neuronavigation" addresses the specific aspects of functional neuronavigation (Orringer et al. 2012; Risholm et al. 2011). With the help of the functional landmarks provided by fMRI and DTI, the spatial relationship between the brain tumor or epileptogenic zone, functional brain areas, and essential white matter tracts can be evaluated preoperatively, which facilitates the selection of the most cautious therapy. Functional neuronavigation permits planning and implementation of radical and, at the same time, function-preserving operations. This goal is rarely achieved with morphological information alone, especially in the presence of brain malformations, anatomical variants, or a disturbed or destroyed anatomy due to tumor growth or pathology-related neuroplastic changes of brain function. Technical inaccuracies and corrections for brain shift due to intraoperative loss of cerebrospinal fluid and tissue removal have to be taken into account (Kuhnt et al. 2012a).

Chapter "Presurgical Functional Localization Possibilities, Limitations, and Validity" is dedicated to the *validation* of presurgical fMRI and DTI with established reference procedures such as intraoperative electrocorticography (ECoG) or intra-arterial administration of barbiturates (Wada test) (Leclercq et al. 2011). For a thorough understanding of the topic, these reference procedures are presented in detail together with a repetition of the relevant methodological aspects and limitations of fMRI. Today, it can be assumed that presurgical task-based fMRI is a robust and valid tool to localize different representations of the human body in the primary motor and somatosensory cortices, to localize essential language centers—namely, Broca's and Wernicke's areas—and to lateralize the brain's dominant hemisphere for language function. There is also substantial evidence that DTT is reliable to visualize the pyramidal tract, the arcuate fascicle, the optic radiation, and other large white matter bundles both pre- and intraoperatively (Shahar et al. 2014). fMRI and DTI have the potential to help

to reduce the number of invasive measures needed, to better select those patients who require such interventions, and to facilitate the planning and targeted intraoperative positioning of electrodes. If and to what extent a substitution of invasive measures may be appropriate is not fully clear, yet.

This topic is inherently related to chapter "Multimodal Functional Neuroimaging"—which has been completely rewritten—and provides the reader with an overview on *multimodal investigations* using multiparametric functional and structural MRI including volumetric/quantitative measures, DTI, DTT, MR spectroscopy, as well as other non-MR-based functional neuroimaging techniques (Wehner 2013). These methods include positron-emission tomography (PET) and single-photon emission computed tomography (SPECT)—the latter two techniques are from the domain of nuclear medicine that utilize radioactive substances/tracers and can be employed together with CT or MR scanners for hybrid imaging (Nensa et al. 2014)—just as the electrophysiological methods electroencephalography (EEG) and magnetoencephalography (MEG) that noninvasively measure electromagnetic fields as a direct correlate of neuronal (synaptic) activity with a very high temporal resolution (Grummich et al. 2006). These techniques are therefore not susceptible to hemodynamic or metabolic influencing factors.

Chapter "Brain Plasticity in fMRI and DTI" covers neuroplasticity from its definition to its implications for diagnosis, treatment, and prognosis in the clinical context from a neuroimaging's perspective (Niu et al. 2014; Tozakidou et al. 2013; Partovi et al. 2012). The measurable neuroplastic changes are also discussed on the basis of the underlying pathophysiology down to the cellular and molecular levels. The current understanding of neuroplasticity imaging is condensed from an extensive literature research on patients with stroke, epilepsy, brain tumors, multiple sclerosis, and peripheral nervous system disorders used to interpret neuroplastic imaging findings. Clinical examples are provided with a focus on neuroplasticity of the motor system, which in turn is helpful to better understand phenomena that may be observed in preoperative functional neuroimaging. Clear and valuable considerations are provided for a practical imaging of neuroplasticity.

Chapter "Clinical BOLD fMRI and DTI: Artifacts, Tips, and Tricks" accounts for pitfalls, drawbacks, and diagnostic errors in clinical BOLD fMRI and DTI. Important imaging artifacts, influencing factors of brain lesions, and pharmaceutical effects on the measurable BOLD response and DTI data are presented and discussed in detail. Practical suggestions to overcome these problems are provided for a successful application of presurgical diagnostic fMRI and DTI.

References

Abou-Khalil B, Schlaggar BL (2002) Is it time to replace the Wada test? Neurology 59(2):160–161

Agarwal S, Sair HI, Yahyavi-Firouz-Abadi N, Airan R, Pillai JJ (2016) Neurovascular uncoupling in resting state fMRI demonstrated in patients with primary brain gliomas. J Magn Reson Imaging 43(3):620–626. https://doi.org/10.1002/jmri.25012. Epub 2015 Jul 22

Agarwal S, Sair HI, Pillai JJ (2021) The problem of neurovascular uncoupling. Neuroimaging Clin N Am 31(1):53–67. Review. https://doi.org/10.1016/j.nic.2020.09.003. Epub 2020 Oct 29

Amunts K, Schleicher A et al (1999) Broca's region revisited: cytoarchitecture and intersubject variability. J Comp Neurol 412(2):319–341

Amunts K, Malikovic A et al (2000) Brodmann's areas 17 and 18 brought into stereotaxic space-where and how variable? Neuroimage 11(1):66–84

Bailey PD, Zacà D, Basha MM, Agarwal S, Gujar SK, Sair HI, Eng J, Pillai JJ (2015) Presurgical fMRI and DTI for the prediction of perioperative motor and language deficits in primary or metastatic brain lesions. J Neuroimaging 25(5):776–784. https://doi.org/10.1111/jon.12273. Epub 2015 Jul 14

Bandettini PA, Wong EC et al (1992) Time course EPI of human brain function during task activation. Magn Reson Med 25(2):390–397

Barras CD, Asadi H, Baldeweg T, Mancini L, Yousry TA, Bisdas S (2016) Functional magnetic resonance imaging in clinical practice: state of the art and science. Aust Fam Physician 45(11):798–803

Basser PJ, Mattiello J, LeBihan D (1994) Estimation of the effective self-diffusion tensor from the NMR spin echo. J Magn Reson B 103(3):247–254

Bauer MH, Kuhnt D et al (2013) Reconstruction of white matter tracts via repeated deterministic streamline tracking—initial experience. PLoS One 8(5):e63082, Print 2013. https://doi.org/10.1371/journal.pone.0063082

Baumann SB, Noll DC et al (1995) Comparison of functional magnetic resonance imaging with positron emission tomography and magnetoencephalography to identify the motor cortex in a patient with an arteriovenous malformation. J Image Guid Surg 1(4):191–197

Baxendale S (2002) The role of functional MRI in the presurgical investigation of temporal lobe epilepsy patients: a clinical perspective and review. J Clin Exp Neuropsychol 24(5):664–676

Belliveau JW, Kennedy DN Jr et al (1991) Functional mapping of the human visual cortex by magnetic resonance imaging. Science 254(5032):716–719

Benbadis SR, Binder JR et al (1998) Is speech arrest during Wada testing a valid method for determining hemispheric representation of language? Brain Lang 65(3):441–446

Berger H (1929) Über das Elektroenzephalogramm des Menschen. Arch Psychiatr Nervenk 87:527–570

Bick AS, Mayer A, Levin N (2012) From research to clinical practice: implementation of functional magnetic imaging and white matter tractography in the clinical environment. J Neurol Sci 312(1–2):158–165. https://doi.org/10.1016/j.jns.2011.07.040. Epub 2011 Aug 23

Binder JR, Achten E et al (2002) Functional MRI in epilepsy. Epilepsia 43(Suppl 1):51–63

Bittar RG, Olivier A et al (1999) Presurgical motor and somatosensory cortex mapping with functional magnetic resonance imaging and positron emission tomography. J Neurosurg 91(6):915–921

Black DF, Little JT, Johnson DR (2019) Neuroanatomical considerations in preoperative functional brain mapping. Top Magn Reson Imaging 28(4):213–224. Review. https://doi.org/10.1097/RMR.0000000000000213

Buckner RL, Bandettini PA et al (1996) Detection of cortical activation during averaged single trials of a cognitive task using functional magnetic resonance imaging. Proc Natl Acad Sci U S A 93(25): 14878–14883

Castellano A, Cirillo S, Bello L, Riva M, Falini A (2017) Functional MRI for surgery of gliomas. Curr Treat Options Neurol 19(10):34. Review. https://doi.org/10.1007/s11940-017-0469-y

Cedzich C, Taniguchi M et al (1996) Somatosensory evoked potential phase reversal and direct motor cortex stimulation during surgery in and around the central region. Neurosurgery 38(5):962–970

Centeno M, Carmichael DW (2014) Network connectivity in epilepsy: resting state fMRI and EEG-fMRI contributions. Front Neurol 5:93, eCollection 2014. https://doi.org/10.3389/fneur.2014.00093

Chiang S, Levin HS, Haneef Z (2014) Computer-automated focus lateralization of temporal lobe epilepsy using fMRI. J Magn Reson Imaging. https://doi.org/10.1002/jmri.24696

Coenen VA, Krings T, Mayfrank L, Polin RS, Reinges MH, Thron A, Gilsbach JM (2001) Three-dimensional visualization of the pyramidal tract in a neuronavigation system during brain tumor surgery: first experiences and technical note. Neurosurg 49(1):86–92; discussion 92–3. https://doi.org/10.1097/00006123-200107000-00013. PMID: 11440464

Cortez-Conradis D, Favila R et al (2013) Diagnostic performance of regional DTI-derived tensor metrics in glioblastoma multiforme: simultaneous evaluation of p, q, L, Cl, Cp, Cs, RA, RD, AD, mean diffusivity and fractional anisotropy. Eur Radiol 23(4):1112–1121. https://doi.org/10.1007/s00330-012-2688-7. Epub 2012 Oct 21

Cox RW (1996) AFNI: software for analysis and visualization of functional magnetic resonance neuroimages. Comput Biomed Res 29(3):162–173

Detre JA, Leigh JS et al (1992) Perfusion imaging. Magn Reson Med 23(1):37–45

Dimou S, Battisti RA et al (2013) A systematic review of functional magnetic resonance imaging and diffusion tensor imaging modalities used in presurgical planning of brain tumour resection. Neurosurg Rev 36(2):205–214; discussion 214. https://doi.org/10.1007/s10143-012-0436-8. Epub 2012 Nov 29

Duffau H, Capelle L et al (1999) Intra-operative direct electrical stimulations of the central nervous system: the Salpetriere experience with 60 patients. Acta Neurochir (Wien) 141(11):1157–1167

Duffau H, Capelle L et al (2002) Intraoperative mapping of the subcortical language pathways using direct stimulations. An anatomo-functional study. Brain 125(Pt 1):199–214

Duffau H, Capelle L et al (2003) Usefulness of intraoperative electrical subcortical mapping during surgery for low-grade gliomas located within eloquent brain regions: functional results in a consecutive series of 103 patients. J Neurosurg 98(4):764–778

Dymerska B, De Lima CP, Bachrata B, Fischmeister F, Matt E, Beisteiner R, Trattnig S, Robinson SD (2019) The impact of echo time shifts and temporal signal fluctuations on BOLD sensitivity in presurgical planning at 7 T. Invest Radiol 54(6):340–348. https://doi.org/10.1097/RLI.0000000000000546

Fernandez G, de Greiff A et al (2001) Language mapping in less than 15 minutes: real-time functional MRI during routine clinical investigation. Neuroimage 14(3):585–594

Fesl G, Moriggl B et al (2003) Inferior central sulcus: variations of anatomy and function on the example of the motor tongue area. Neuroimage 20(1):601–610

Flouty O, Reddy C, Holland M, Kovach C, Kawasaki H, Oya H, Greenlee J, Hitchon P, Howard M (2017) Precision surgery of rolandic glioma and insights from extended functional mapping. Clin Neurol Neurosurg 163:60–66. https://doi.org/10.1016/j.clineuro.2017.10.008. Epub 2017 Oct 10

Fox PT, Raichle ME (1986) Focal physiological uncoupling of cerebral blood flow and oxidative metabolism during somatosensory stimulation in human subjects. Proc Natl Acad Sci U S A 83(4):1140–1444

Fox PT, Mintun MA et al (1986) Mapping human visual cortex with positron emission tomography. Nature 323(6091):806–809

Frahm J, Merboldt KD et al (1994) Brain or vein—oxygenation or flow? On signal physiology in functional MRI of human brain activation. NMR Biomed 7(1–2):45–53

Friston K (1996) Statistical parametric mapping and other analyses of functional imaging data. In: John M, Toga AW (eds) Brain mapping: the methods. Academic Press, New York, pp 363–386

Gaillard WD, Bookheimer SY, Cohen M (2000) The use of fMRI in neocortical epilepsy. Adv Neurol 84: 391–404

Gevins A (1995) High-resolution electroencephalographic studies of cognition. Adv Neurol 66:181–195; discussion 195–198

Gevins A, Leong H et al (1995) Mapping cognitive brain function with modern high-resolution electroencephalography. Trends Neurosci 18(10):429–436

Goa PE, Koopmans PJ et al (2014) BOLD fMRI signal characteristics of S1 and S2-SSFP at 7 Tesla. Front Neurosci 8:49. https://doi.org/10.3389/fnins.2014.00049

Gold S, Christian B et al (1998) Functional MRI statistical software packages: a comparative analysis. Hum Brain Mapp 6(2):73–84

Gould L, Ekstrand C, Fourney DR, Mickleborough MJS, Ellchuk T, Borowsky R (2018) The effect of tumor neovasculature on functional magnetic resonance imaging blood oxygen level-dependent activation. World Neurosurg 115:373–383. https://doi.org/10.1016/j.wneu.2018.04.200. Epub 2018 May 5

Grabowski TJ (2000) Investigating language with functional neuroimaging. In: John M, Toga AW (eds) Brain mapping: the systems. Academic Press, San Diego, pp 425–461

Grouiller F, Jorge J, Pittau F, van der Zwaag W, Iannotti GR, Michel CM, Vulliémoz S, Vargas MI, Lazeyras F (2016) Presurgical brain mapping in epilepsy using simultaneous EEG and functional MRI at ultra-high field: feasibility and first results. MAGMA 29(3):605–616. https://doi.org/10.1007/s10334-016-0536-5. Epub 2016 Mar 5

Grummich P, Nimsky C et al (2006) Combining fMRI and MEG increases the reliability of presurgical language localization: a clinical study on the difference between and congruence of both modalities. Neuroimage 32(4):1793–1803

Hämäläinen M, Ilmoniemi RJ et al (1993) Magnetoencephalography—theory, instrumentation and applications to noninvasive studies of the working human brain. Rev Mod Phys 65:413–487

Hari R, Ilmoniemi RJ (1986) Cerebral magnetic fields. Crit Rev Biomed Eng 14(2):93–126

Hirsch J, Ruge MI et al (2000) An integrated functional magnetic resonance imaging procedure for preoperative mapping of cortical areas associated with tactile, motor, language, and visual functions. Neurosurgery 47(3):711–721; discussion 721–722

Holman BL, Devous MD Sr (1992) Functional brain SPECT: the emergence of a powerful clinical method. J Nucl Med 33(10):1888–1904

Holodny AI, Schulder M et al (1999) Decreased BOLD functional MR activation of the motor and sensory cortices adjacent to a glioblastoma multiforme: implications for image-guided neurosurgery. AJNR Am J Neuroradiol 20(4):609–612

Holodny AI, Schulder M et al (2000) The effect of brain tumors on BOLD functional MR imaging activation in the adjacent motor cortex: implications for image-guided neurosurgery. AJNR Am J Neuroradiol 21(8):1415–1422

Holodny AI, Schwartz TH et al (2001) Tumor involvement of the corticospinal tract: diffusion magnetic resonance tractography with intraoperative correlation. J Neurosurg 95(6):1082

Holodny AI, Gor DM et al (2005) Diffusion-tensor MR tractography of somatotopic organization of corticospinal tracts in the internal capsule: initial anatomic results in contradistinction to prior reports. Radiology 234(3):649–653

Hua J, Qin Q et al (2013) Whole-brain three-dimensional T2-weighted BOLD functional magnetic resonance imaging at 7 Tesla. Magn Reson Med. https://doi.org/10.1002/mrm.25055

Huber L, Goense J et al (2014) Investigation of the neurovascular coupling in positive and negative BOLD responses in human brain at 7T. Neuroimage 97:349–362

Hulvershorn J, Bloy L et al (2005a) Spatial sensitivity and temporal response of spin echo and gradient echo bold contrast at 3 T using peak hemodynamic activation time. Neuroimage 24(1):216–223

Hulvershorn J, Bloy L et al (2005b) Temporal resolving power of spin echo and gradient echo fMRI at 3T with apparent diffusion coefficient compartmentalization. Hum Brain Mapp 25(2):247–258

Incekara F, Olubiyi O, Ozdemir A, Lee T, Rigolo L, Golby A (2016) The value of pre- and intraoperative adjuncts on the extent of resection of hemispheric low-grade gliomas: a retrospective analysis. J Neurol Surg A Cent Eur Neurosurg 77(2):79–87. https://doi.org/10.1055/s-0035-1551830. Epub 2015 Jul 27

Jones JY, Selvaraj B, Ho ML (2020) Pediatric functional neuroimaging: practical tips and pearls. AJR Am J Roentgenol 214(5):995–1007. Review. https://doi.org/10.2214/AJR.19.22178. Epub 2020 Mar 31

Kallenberg K, Goldmann T et al (2013) Glioma infiltration of the corpus callosum: early signs detected by DTI. J Neurooncol 112(2):217–222. https://doi.org/10.1007/s11060-013-1049-y. Epub 2013 Jan 24

Kiss M, Hermann P, Vidnyánszky Z, Gál V (2018) Reducing task-based fMRI scanning time using simultaneous multislice echo planar imaging. Neuroradiology 60(3):293–302. https://doi.org/10.1007/s00234-017-1962-4. Epub 2018 Jan 4

Kleiser R, Staempfli P et al (2010) Impact of fMRI-guided advanced DTI fiber tracking techniques on their clinical applications in patients with brain tumors. Neuroradiology 52(1):37–46. https://doi.org/10.1007/s00234-009-0539-2. Epub 2009 May 29

Kober H, Nimsky C et al (2001) Correlation of sensorimotor activation with functional magnetic resonance imaging and magnetoencephalography in presurgical functional imaging: a spatial analysis. Neuroimage 14(5):1214–1228

Krings T, Reinges MH et al (2001) Functional and diffusion-weighted magnetic resonance images of space-occupying lesions affecting the motor system: imaging the motor cortex and pyramidal tracts. J Neurosurg 95(5):816–824

Krings T, Reinges MH et al (2002) Factors related to the magnitude of T2* MR signal changes during functional imaging. Neuroradiology 44(6):459–466

Kuhnt D, Bauer MH, Nimsky C (2012a) Brain shift compensation and neurosurgical image fusion using intraoperative MRI: current status and future challenges. Crit Rev Biomed Eng 40(3):175–185

Kuhnt D, Bauer MH et al (2012b) Intraoperative visualization of fiber tracking based reconstruction of language pathways in glioma surgery. Neurosurgery 70(4):911–919; discussion 919–920. https://doi.org/10.1227/NEU.0b013e318237a807

Kuhnt D, Bauer MH et al (2013a) Optic radiation fiber tractography in glioma patients based on high angular resolution diffusion imaging with compressed sensing compared with diffusion tensor imaging—initial experience. PLoS One 8(7):e70973, Print 2013. https://doi.org/10.1371/journal.pone.0070973

Kuhnt D, Bauer MH et al (2013b) Functional imaging: where do we go from here? J Neurosurg Sci 57(1):1–11

Kwong KK, Belliveau JW et al (1992) Dynamic magnetic resonance imaging of human brain activity during primary sensory stimulation. Proc Natl Acad Sci U S A 89(12):675–679

Lang S, Duncan N, Northoff G (2014) Resting-state functional magnetic resonance imaging: review of neurosurgical applications. Neurosurgery 74(5):453–464; discussion 464–465. https://doi.org/10.1227/NEU.0000000000000307

LeBihan D (2006) From Brownian motion to mind imaging: diffusion MRI. Bull Acad Natl Med 190(8):1605–1627; discussion 1627

LeBihan D (2013) Apparent diffusion coefficient and beyond: what diffusion MR imaging can tell us about tissue structure. Radiology 268(2):318–322. https://doi.org/10.1148/radiol.13130420

LeBihan D, Johansen-Berg H (2012) Diffusion MRI at 25: exploring brain tissue structure and function. Neuroimage 61(2):324–341. https://doi.org/10.1016/j.neuroimage.2011.11.006. Epub 2011 Nov 20

LeBihan D, Mangin JF et al (2001) Diffusion tensor imaging: concepts and applications. J Magn Reson Imaging 13(4):534–546

Leclercq D, Delmaire C et al (2011) Diffusion tractography: methods, validation and applications in patients with neurosurgical lesions. Neurosurg Clin N Am 22(2):253–268, ix. https://doi.org/10.1016/j.nec.2010.11.004

Lee CC, Ward HA et al (1999) Assessment of functional MR imaging in neurosurgical planning. AJNR Am J Neuroradiol 20(8):1511–1519

Lee MH, Smyser CD, Shimony JS (2013) Resting-state fMRI: a review of methods and clinical applications. AJNR Am J Neuroradiol 34(10):1866–1872. https://doi.org/10.3174/ajnr.A3263. Epub 2012 Aug 30

Lee MH, Miller-Thomas MM, Benzinger TL, Marcus DS, Hacker CD, Leuthardt EC, Shimony JS (2016) Clinical resting-state fMRI in the preoperative setting: are we ready for prime time? Top Magn Reson Imaging. 25(1):11–18. https://doi.org/10.1097/RMR.0000000000000075

Lemée JM, Berro DH, Bernard F, Chinier E, Leiber LM, Menei P, Ter Minassian A (2019) Resting-state functional magnetic resonance imaging versus task-based activity for language mapping and correlation with perioperative cortical mapping. Brain Behav 9(10):e01362. https://doi.org/10.1002/brb3.1362. Epub 2019 Sep 30

Leuthardt EC, Guzman G, Bandt SK, Hacker C, Vellimana AK, Limbrick D, Milchenko M, Lamontagne P, Speidel B, Roland J, Miller-Thomas M, Snyder AZ, Marcus D, Shimony J, Benzinger TLS (2018) Integration of resting state functional MRI into clinical practice—A large single institution experience. PLoS One. 13(6):e0198349, eCollection 2018. https://doi.org/10.1371/journal.pone.0198349

Lima Cardoso P, Fischmeister FPS, Dymerska B, Geißler A, Wurnig M, Trattnig S, Beisteiner R, Robinson SD (2017) Robust presurgical functional MRI at 7 T using response consistency. Hum Brain Mapp 38(6):3163–3174. https://doi.org/10.1002/hbm.23582. Epub 2017 Mar 21

Logothetis NK (2002) The neural basis of the blood-oxygen-level-dependent functional magnetic resonance imaging signal. Philos Trans R Soc Lond B Biol Sci 357(1424):1003–1037

Logothetis NK (2003) The underpinnings of the BOLD functional magnetic resonance imaging signal. J Neurosci 23(10):3963–3971

Logothetis NK, Pfeuffer J (2004) On the nature of the BOLD fMRI contrast mechanism. Magn Reson Imaging 22(10):1517–1531

Logothetis NK, Wandell BA (2004) Interpreting the BOLD signal. Annu Rev Physiol 66:735–769

Logothetis NK, Pauls J et al (2001) Neurophysiological investigation of the basis of the fMRI signal. Nature 412(6843):150–157

Martino J, Honma SM et al (2011) Resting functional connectivity in patients with brain tumors in eloquent areas. Ann Neurol 69(3):521–532. https://doi.org/10.1002/ana.22167. Epub 2011 Mar 11

Mazziotta JC, Phelps ME et al (1982) Tomographic mapping of human cerebral metabolism: auditory stimulation. Neurology 32(9):921–937

Menon RS, Ogawa S et al (1995) BOLD based functional MRI at 4 Tesla includes a capillary bed contribution: echoplanar imaging correlates with previous optical imaging using intrinsic signals. Magn Reson Med 33(3):453–459

Metwali H, Raemaekers M, Ibrahim T, Samii A (2020a) Inter-network functional connectivity changes in patients with brain tumors: a resting-state functional magnetic resonance imaging study. World Neurosurg 138:e66–e71. https://doi.org/10.1016/j.wneu.2020.01.177. Epub 2020 Jan 31

Metwali H, Raemaekers M, Kniese K, Samii A (2020b) Intraoperative resting-state functional connectivity and resting-state networks in patients with intracerebral lesions: detectability and variations between sessions. World Neurosurg 133:e197–e204. https://doi.org/10.1016/j.wneu.2019.08.188. Epub 2019 Sep 3

Metwali H, Ibrahim T, Raemaekers M (2021) Changes in intranetwork functional connectivity of resting state networks between sessions under anesthesia in neurosurgical patients. World Neurosurg 146:e351–e358. https://doi.org/10.1016/j.wneu.2020.10.102. Epub 2020 Oct 24

Mitchell TJ, Hacker CD et al (2013) A novel data-driven approach to preoperative mapping of functional cortex using resting-state functional magnetic resonance imaging. Neurosurgery 73(6):969–982; discussion 982–983. https://doi.org/10.1227/NEU.0000000000000141

Moller M, Freund M et al (2005) Real time fMRI: a tool for the routine presurgical localisation of the motor cortex. Eur Radiol 15(2):292–295

Nensa F, Beiderwellen K et al (2014) Clinical applications of PET/MR: current status and future perspectives. Diagn Interv Radiol. https://doi.org/10.5152/dir.14008. [Epub ahead of print]

Nimsky C (2011) Intraoperative acquisition of fMRI and DTI. Neurosurg Clin N Am 22(2):269–277, ix. https://doi.org/10.1016/j.nec.2010.11.005

Niu C, Zhang M et al (2014) Motor network plasticity and low-frequency oscillations abnormalities in patients with brain gliomas: a functional MRI study. PLoS One 9(5):e96850, eCollection 2014. https://doi.org/10.1371/journal.pone.0096850

O'Connor EE, Zeffiro TA (2019) Why is clinical fMRI in a resting state? Front Neurol 10:420, eCollection 2019. https://doi.org/10.3389/fneur.2019.00420

O'Donell LJ, Rigolo L et al (2012) fMRI-DTI modeling via landmark distance atlases for prediction and detection of fiber tracts. Neuroimage 60(1):456–470. https://doi.org/10.1016/j.neuroimage.2011.11.014. Epub 2011 Dec 2

Ogawa S, Lee TM et al (1990) Brain magnetic resonance imaging with contrast dependent on blood oxygenation. Proc Natl Acad Sci U S A 87(24):9868–8972

Ogawa S, Tank DW et al (1992) Intrinsic signal changes accompanying sensory stimulation: functional brain mapping with magnetic resonance imaging. Proc Natl Acad Sci U S A 89(13):5951–5955

Ogawa S, Menon RS et al (1993) Functional brain mapping by blood oxygenation level-dependent contrast magnetic resonance imaging. A comparison of signal characteristics with a biophysical model. Biophys J 64(3):803–812

Ojemann GA (1991) Cortical organization of language. J Neurosci 11(8):2281–2287

Ojemann G, Ojemann J et al (1989) Cortical language localization in left, dominant hemisphere. An electrical stimulation mapping investigation in 117 patients. J Neurosurg 71(3):316–326

Orringer DA, Golby A, Jolesz F (2012) Neuronavigation in the surgical management of brain tumors: current and future trends. Expert Rev Med Devices 9(5):491–500. https://doi.org/10.1586/erd.12.42

Otten ML, Mikell CB et al (2012) Motor deficits correlate with resting state motor network connectivity in patients with brain tumours. Brain 135(Pt 4):1017–1026. https://doi.org/10.1093/brain/aws041. Epub 2012 Mar 8

Pak RW, Hadjiabadi DH, Senarathna J, Agarwal S, Thakor NV, Pillai JJ, Pathak AP (2017) Implications of neurovascular uncoupling in functional magnetic resonance imaging (fMRI) of brain tumors. J Cereb Blood Flow Metab 37(11):3475–3487. https://doi.org/10.1177/0271678X17707398. Epub 2017 May 11

Partovi S, Jacobi B et al (2012) Clinical standardized fMRI reveals altered language lateralization in patients with brain tumor. AJNR Am J Neuroradiol 33(11):2151–2157. https://doi.org/10.3174/ajnr.A3137. Epub 2012 May 17

Penfield W (1937) Somatic motor and sensory representation in the cerebral cortex of man as studied by electrical stimulation. Brain 60:389–443

Penfield W (1950) The cerebral cortex of man. MacMillan, New York, 57 ff

Pernet CR, Gorgolewski KJ, Job D, Rodriguez D, Storkey A, Whittle I, Wardlaw J (2016) Evaluation of a presurgical functional MRI workflow: from data acquisition to reporting. Int J Med Inform 86:37–42. https://doi.org/10.1016/j.ijmedinf.2015.11.014. Epub 2015 Nov 30

Pillai JJ (2010) The evolution of clinical functional imaging during the past 2 decades and its current impact on neurosurgical planning. AJNR Am J Neuroradiol 31(2):219–225. https://doi.org/10.3174/ajnr.A1845

Pillai JJ, Mikulis DJ (2015) Cerebrovascular reactivity mapping: an evolving standard for clinical functional imaging. AJNR Am J Neuroradiol 36(1):7–13. Review. https://doi.org/10.3174/ajnr.A3941. Epub 2014 Apr 30

Pittau F, Groullier F et al (2014) The role of functional neuroimaging in pre-surgical epilepsy evaluation. Front Neurol 5:31, eCollection 2014. https://doi.org/10.3389/fneur.2014.00031

Posse S, Ackley E et al (2013) High-speed real-time resting-state FMRI using multi-slab echo-volumar imaging. Front Hum Neurosci 7:479, eCollection 2013. https://doi.org/10.3389/fnhum.2013.00479

Potgieser AR, Wagemakers M et al (2014) The role of diffusion tensor imaging in brain tumor surgery: a review of the literature. Clin Neurol Neurosurg 124C:51–58. https://doi.org/10.1016/j.clineuro.2014.06.009. [Epub ahead of print]

Purdon PL, Weisskoff RM (1998) Effect of temporal autocorrelation due to physiological noise and stimulus paradigm on voxel-level false-positive rates in fMRI. Hum Brain Mapp 6:239–249

Qiu TM, Yan CG, Tang WJ, Wu JS, Zhuang DX, Yao CJ, Lu JF, Zhu FP, Mao Y, Zhou LF (2014) Localizing hand motor area using resting-state fMRI: validated with direct cortical stimulation. Acta Neurochir (Wien) 156(12):2295–2302. https://doi.org/10.1007/s00701-014-2236-0. Epub 2014 Sep 24

Qiu TM, Gong FY, Gong X, Wu JS, Lin CP, Biswal BB, Zhuang DX, Yao CJ, Zhang XL, Lu JF, Zhu FP, Mao Y, Zhou LF (2017) Real-time motor cortex mapping for the safe resection of glioma: an intraoperative resting-state fMRI study. AJNR Am J Neuroradiol. 38(11):2146–2152. https://doi.org/10.3174/ajnr.A5369. Epub 2017 Sep 7

Raichle ME (1983) Positron emission tomography. Annu Rev Neurosci 6:249–267

Rausch R, Silfvenious H et al (1993) Intra-arterial amobarbital procedures. In: Engel JJ (ed) Surgical treatment of the epilepsies. Raven Press, New York, pp 341–357

Reinges MH, Nguyen HH et al (2004) Course of brain shift during microsurgical resection of supratentorial cerebral lesions: limits of conventional neuronavigation. Acta Neurochir (Wien) 146(4):369–377; discussion 377

Rigolo L, Essayed W, Tie Y, Norton I, Mukundan S Jr, Golby A (2020) Intraoperative use of functional MRI for surgical decision making after limited or infeasible electrocortical stimulation mapping. J Neuroimaging 30(2):184–191. https://doi.org/10.1111/jon.12683. Epub 2019 Dec 22

Risholm P, Golby AJ, Wells W 3rd (2011) Multimodal image registration for preoperative planning and image-guided neurosurgical procedures. Neurosurg Clin N Am 22(2):197–206, viii. https://doi.org/10.1016/j.nec.2010.12.001

Roberts TP (2003) Functional magnetic resonance imaging (fMRI) processing and analysis. ASNR Electronic Learning Center Syllabus, pp 1–23

Roland JL, Hacker CD, Snyder AZ, Shimony JS, Zempel JM, Limbrick DD, Smyth MD, Leuthardt EC (2019) A comparison of resting state functional magnetic resonance imaging to invasive electrocortical stimulation for sensorimotor mapping in pediatric patients. Neuroimage Clin 23:101850. https://doi.org/10.1016/j.nicl.2019.101850. Epub 2019 May 4

Rosazza C, Zacà D, Bruzzone MG (2018) Pre-surgical brain mapping: to rest or not to rest? Front Neurol 9:520, eCollection 2018. https://doi.org/10.3389/fneur.2018.00520

Rutten GJ, Ramsey NF et al (2002) Development of a functional magnetic resonance imaging protocol for intraoperative localization of critical temporoparietal language areas. Ann Neurol 51(3):350–360

Sanvito F, Caverzasi E, Riva M, Jordan KM, Blasi V, Scifo P, Iadanza A, Crespi SA, Cirillo S, Casarotti A, Leonetti A, Puglisi G, Grimaldi M, Bello L, Gorno-Tempini ML, Henry RG, Falini A, Castellano A (2020) fMRI-targeted high-angular resolution diffusion MR tractography to identify functional language tracts in healthy controls and glioma patients. Front Neurosci 14:225, eCollection 2020. https://doi.org/10.3389/fnins.2020.00225

Schreiber A, Hubbe U et al (2000) The influence of gliomas and nonglial space-occupying lesions on blood-oxygen-level-dependent contrast enhancement. AJNR Am J Neuroradiol 21(6):1055–1063

Seitzman BA, Snyder AZ, Leuthardt EC, Shimony JS (2019) The state of resting state networks. Top Magn Reson Imaging. 28(4):189–196. https://doi.org/10.1097/RMR.0000000000000214

Shahar T, Rozovski U et al (2014) Preoperative imaging to predict intraoperative changes in tumor-to-corticospinal tract distance: an analysis of 45 cases using high-field intraoperative magnetic resonance imaging. Neurosurgery 75(1):23–30

Shinoura N, Yamada R et al (2005) Preoperative fMRI, tractography and continuous task during awake surgery for maintenance of motor function following surgical resection of metastatic tumor spread to the primary motor area. Minim Invasive Neurosurg 48(2):85–90

Smucny J, Wylie KP, Tregellas JR (2014) Functional magnetic resonance imaging of intrinsic brain networks for translational drug discovery. Trends Pharmacol Sci. https://doi.org/10.1016/j.tips.2014.05.001. [Epub ahead of print]

Springer E, Dymerska B, Cardoso PL, Robinson SD, Weisstanner C, Wiest R, Schmitt B, Trattnig S (2016) Comparison of routine brain imaging at 3 T and 7 T. Invest Radiol 51(8):469–482. https://doi.org/10.1097/RLI.0000000000000256

Stadlbauer A, Buchfelder M et al (2010) Fiber density mapping of gliomas: histopathologic evaluation of a diffusion-tensor imaging data processing method. Radiology 257(3):846–853. https://doi.org/10.1148/radiol.10100343. Epub 2010 Sep 30

Steger TR, Jackson EF (2004) Real-time motion detection of functional MRI data. J Appl Clin Med Phys 5(2):64–70

Sternberg EJ, Lipton ML, Burns J (2014) Utility of diffusion tensor imaging in evaluation of the peritumoral region in patients with primary and metastatic brain tumors. AJNR Am J Neuroradiol 35(3):439–444. https://doi.org/10.3174/ajnr.A3702. Epub 2013 Sep 19

Stevens MT, Clarke DB, Stroink G, Beyea SD, D'Arcy RC (2016) Improving fMRI reliability in presurgical mapping for brain tumours. J Neurol Neurosurg Psychiatry 87(3):267–274. https://doi.org/10.1136/jnnp-2015-310307. Epub 2015 Mar 26

Stippich C (2010) Presurgical functional magnetic resonance imaging. Radiologe 50(2):110–122

Stippich C, Hofmann R et al (1999) Somatotopic mapping of the human primary somatosensory cortex by fully automated tactile stimulation using functional magnetic resonance imaging. Neurosci Lett 277(1):25–28

Stippich C, Kapfer D et al (2000) Robust localization of the contralateral precentral gyrus in hemiparetic patients using the unimpaired ipsilateral hand: a clinical functional magnetic resonance imaging protocol. Neurosci Lett 285(2):155–159

Stippich C, Heiland S et al (2002a) Functional magnetic resonance imaging: physiological background, technical aspects and prerequisites for clinical use. Röfo 174(1):43–49

Stippich C, Ochmann H, Sartor K (2002b) Somatotopic mapping of the human primary sensorimotor cortex during motor imagery and motor execution by functional magnetic resonance imaging. Neurosci Lett 331(1):50–54

Stippich C, Kress B et al (2003a) Preoperative functional magnetic resonance tomography (FMRI) in patients with rolandic brain tumors: indication, investigation strategy, possibilities and limitations of clinical application. Röfo 175(8):1042–1050

Stippich C, Mohammed J et al (2003b) Robust localization and lateralization of human language function: an optimized clinical functional magnetic resonance imaging protocol. Neurosci Lett 346(1–2):109–113

Stippich C, Romanowski A et al (2004) Fully automated localization of the human primary somatosensory cortex in one minute by functional magnetic resonance imaging. Neurosci Lett 364(2):90–93

Stippich C, Romanowski A et al (2005) Time-efficient localization of the human secondary somatosensory cortex by functional magnetic resonance imaging. Neurosci Lett 381(3):264–268

Stippich C, Rapps N et al (2007) Localizing and lateralizing language in patients with brain tumors: feasibility of routine preoperative functional MR imaging in 81 consecutive patients. Radiology 243(3):828–836

Sunaert S, Yousry TA (2001) Clinical applications of functional magnetic resonance imaging. Neuroimaging Clin N Am 11(2):221–236, viii

Svolos P, Tsolaki E et al (2013) Investigating brain tumor differentiation with diffusion and perfusion metrics at 3T MRI using pattern recognition techniques. Magn Reson Imaging 31(9):1567–1577

Szaflarski JP, Gloss D, Binder JR, Gaillard WD, Golby AJ, Holland SK, Ojemann J, Spencer DC, Swanson SJ, French JA, Theodore WH (2017) Practice guideline summary: use of fMRI in the presurgical evaluation of patients with epilepsy: report of the guideline development, dissemination, and implementation subcommittee of the American Academy of Neurology. Neurology 88(4):395–402. https://doi.org/10.1212/WNL.0000000000003532. Epub 2017 Jan 11

Thulborn KR (1998) A BOLD move for fMRI. Nat Med 4(2):155–156

Thulborn KR (1999) Clinical rationale for very-high-field (3.0 Tesla) functional magnetic resonance imaging. Top Magn Reson Imaging 10(1):37–50

Thulborn K (2006) Clinical functional magnetic resonance imaging. In: Haacke EM (ed) Current protocols in magnetic resonance imaging. Wiley, New York

Thulborn KR, Davis D et al (1996) Clinical fMRI: implementation and experience. Neuroimage 4(3 Pt 3):S101–S107

Towle VL, Khorasani L et al (2003) Noninvasive identification of human central sulcus: a comparison of gyral morphology, functional MRI, dipole localization, and direct cortical mapping. Neuroimage 19(3):684–697

Tozakidou M, Wenz H et al (2013) Primary motor cortex activation and lateralization in patients with tumors of the central region. Neuroimage Clin 2:221–228, eCollection 2013. https://doi.org/10.1016/j.nicl.2013.01.002

Tsougos I, Svolos P et al (2012) Differentiation of glioblastoma multiforme from metastatic brain tumor using proton magnetic resonance spectroscopy, diffusion and perfusion metrics at 3 T. Cancer Imaging 12:423–436. https://doi.org/10.1102/1470-7330.2012.0038

Turner R, Le Bihan D et al (1991) Echo-planar time course MRI of cat brain oxygenation changes. Magn Reson Med 22(1):159–166

Tyndall AJ, Reinhardt J, Tronnier V, Mariani L, Stippich C (2017) Presurgical motor, somatosensory and language fMRI: technical feasibility and limitations in 491 patients over 13 years. Eur Radiol 27(1):267–278. https://doi.org/10.1007/s00330-016-4369-4. Epub 2016 May 19

Uematsu S, Lesser R et al (1992) Motor and sensory cortex in humans: topography studied with chronic subdural stimulation. Neurosurgery 31(1):59–71; discussion 71–72

Ulmer JL, Hacein-Bey L et al (2004a) Lesion-induced pseudodominance at functional magnetic resonance imaging: implications for preoperative assessments. Neurosurgery 55(3):569–579; discussion 580–581

Ulmer JL, Salvan CV et al (2004b) The role of diffusion tensor imaging in establishing the proximity of tumor borders to functional brain systems: implications for preoperative risk assessments and postoperative outcomes. Technol Cancer Res Treat 3(6):567–576

Vakamudi K, Posse S, Jung R, Cushnyr B, Chohan MO (2020) Real-time presurgical resting-state fMRI in patients with brain tumors: quality control and comparison with task-fMRI and intraoperative mapping. Hum Brain Mapp 41(3):797–814. https://doi.org/10.1002/hbm.24840. Epub 2019 Nov 6

Van Westen D, Skagerberg G et al (2005) Functional magnetic resonance imaging at 3T as a clinical tool in patients with intracranial tumors. Acta Radiol 46(6):599–609

Vanderweyen DC, Theaud G, Sidhu J, Rheault F, Sarubbo S, Descoteaux M, Fortin D (2020) The role of diffusion tractography in refining glial tumor resection. Brain Struct Funct 225(4):1413–1436. Review. https://doi.org/10.1007/s00429-020-02056-z. Epub 2020 Mar 16

Vysotski S, Madura C, Swan B, Holdsworth R, Lin Y, Rio AMD, Wood J, Kundu B, Penwarden A, Voss J, Gallagher T, Nair VA, Field A, Garcia-Ramos C, Meyerand EM, Baskaya M, Prabhakaran V, Kuo JS (2018) Preoperative FMRI associated with decreased mortality and morbidity in brain tumor patients. Interdiscip Neurosurg 13:40–45. https://doi.org/10.1016/j.inat.2018.02.001. Epub 2018 Feb 14

Wada J, Rasmussen T (1960) Intracarotid injection of sodium amytal for the lateralization of cerebral speech dominance. Experimental and clinical observations. J Neurosurg 17:266–282

Wehner T (2013) The role of functional imaging in the tumor patient. Epilepsia 54(Suppl 9):44–49. https://doi.org/10.1111/epi.12443

Weiskopf N, Veit R et al (2003) Physiological self-regulation of regional brain activity using real-time functional magnetic resonance imaging (fMRI): methodology and exemplary data. Neuroimage 19(3):577–586

Wittek A, Kikinis R et al (2005) Brain shift computation using a fully nonlinear biomechanical model. Med Image Comput Comput Assist Interv 8(Pt 2):583–590

Woolsey CN, Erickson TC, Gilson WE (1979) Localization in somatic sensory and motor areas of human cerebral cortex as determined by direct recording of evoked potentials and electrical stimulation. J Neurosurg 51(4):476–506

Yousry TA, Schmid UD et al (1997) Localization of the motor hand area to a knob on the precentral gyrus. A new landmark. Brain 120(Pt 1):141–157

Zacharaki EI, Morita N, Bhatt P, O'Rourke DM, Melhem ER, Davatzikos C (2012) Survival analysis of patients with high-grade gliomas based on data mining of imaging variables. AJNR Am J Neuroradiol 33(6):1065–1071. https://doi.org/10.3174/ajnr.A2939. Epub 2012 Feb 9

Zambreanu L, Wise RG et al (2005) A role for the brainstem in central sensitisation in humans. Evidence from functional magnetic resonance imaging. Pain 114(3):397–407

Revealing Brain Activity and White Matter Structure Using Functional and Diffusion-Weighted Magnetic Resonance Imaging

Rainer Goebel

Contents

Abstract

Magnetic resonance imaging (MRI) is based on the magnetic *excitation* of body tissue and the reception of returned electromagnetic signals from the body. Excitation induces phase-locked *precession* of protons with a frequency

R. Goebel (✉)
Department of Cognitive Neuroscience, Maastricht University, Maastricht, The Netherlands
e-mail: r.goebel@maastrichtuniversity.nl

© The Author(s), under exclusive license to Springer Nature Switzerland AG 2022
C. Stippich (ed.), *Clinical Functional MRI*, Medical Radiology Diagnostic Imaging,
https://doi.org/10.1007/978-3-030-83343-5_2

proportional to the strength of the surrounding magnetic field as described by the *Larmor equation*. This fact can be exploited for *spatial encoding* by applying magnetic field *gradients* along spatial dimensions on top of the strong static magnetic field of the scanner. The obtained frequency-encoded information for each slice is accumulated in two-dimensional *k space*. The *k* space data can be transformed into *image space* by *Fourier analysis*.

Functional MRI (fMRI) allows *localizing brain function* since increased local neuronal activity leads to a surprisingly strong increase in local blood flow, which itself results in measurable increases in local magnetic field homogeneity. Increased local blood flow delivers chemical energy (glucose and oxygen) to the neurons. The temporary increase and decrease of local blood flow, triggered by increased neuronal activity, are called the *hemodynamic response* starting 2–4 s after stimulus onset. Increased local blood flow results in an *oversupply* of *oxygenated hemoglobin* in the vicinity of increased neuronal activity. The oversupply flushes *deoxygenated hemoglobin* from the capillaries and the downstream venules. Deoxygenated hemoglobin is paramagnetic reducing the homogeneity of the local magnetic field resulting in a weaker MRI signal than would be measurable without it. Oxygenated hemoglobin is diamagnetic and does not strongly reduce field homogeneity. Since the increased local blood flow replaces deoxygenated hemoglobin with oxygenated hemoglobin, local field homogeneity increases, leading to a stronger MRI signal as compared to a nonactivated state. Measured functional brain images thus reflect neuronal activity changes as blood oxygenation level-dependent (*BOLD*) contrast.

Functional images are acquired using the fast *echo planar imaging* (EPI) pulse sequence allowing acquisition of a 64×64 image matrix in less than 100 ms. To sample signal changes over time, a set of slices typically covering the whole brain is *measured repeatedly*. Activation

of neurons results in a BOLD signal increase of only about 1–5% and it lies buried within strong physical and physiological noise fluctuations of similar size. Proper *preprocessing* steps, including 3D motion correction and removal of drifts, reduce the effect of artifacts increasing the *signal-to-noise ratio* (SNR). In order to reliably *detect* stimulus-related effects, proper *statistical data analysis* is performed. In order to *estimate* response profiles condition-related time course episodes may be averaged in various *regions of interest* (ROIs). The core statistical tool in fMRI data analysis is the *general linear model* (GLM) allowing to analyze *blocked* and *event-related experimental designs*. To run a GLM, a *design matrix* (model) has to be constructed containing reference functions (*predictors*, model time courses) for all effects of interest (conditions) as well as confounds. The GLM fits the created model to the data independently for each voxel's data (time course) providing a set of beta values estimating the effects of each condition. These beta values are compared with each other using *contrasts* resulting in a statistical value at each voxel. The statistical values of all voxels form a three-dimensional *statistical map*. To protect against wrongly declaring voxels as significant, statistical maps are *thresholded* properly by taking into account the *multiple comparison problem*. This problem is caused by the large number of independently performed statistical tests (one for each voxel).

In recent years, *parallel imaging techniques* have been developed, which allow acquiring MRI data simultaneously with two or more receiver coils. Parallel imaging can be used to increase temporal or spatial resolution. It also helps to reduce EPI imaging artifacts, such as geometrical distortions and signal dropouts in regions of different neighboring tissue types.

MRI has not only revolutionized functional brain imaging targeting grey matter neuronal activity but also enabled insights into human white matter structure using diffusion-weighted magnetic resonance imaging. With proper measurement and modeling schemes including diffusion tensor imaging (DTI), major fiber tracts can be reconstructed using computational tractography providing important information to guide neurosurgical procedures potentially reducing the risk of lesioning important fiber bundles.

Since its invention in the early 1990s, functional magnetic resonance imaging (fMRI) has rapidly assumed a leading role among the techniques used to localize brain activity. The spatial and temporal resolution provided by state-of-the-art MR technology and its noninvasive character, which allows multiple studies of the same subject, are some of the main advantages of fMRI over the other functional neuroimaging techniques that are based on changes in blood flow and cortical metabolism (e.g., positron-emission tomography, PET). fMRI is based on the discovery of Ogawa et al. (1990) that *magnetic resonance imaging* (MRI, also called nuclear magnetic resonance imaging) can be used in a way that allows obtaining signals depending on the level of blood oxygenation. The measured signal is therefore also called "BOLD" signal (BOLD = *b*lood *o*xygenation *l*evel-*d*ependent). Since locally increased neuronal activity leads to increased local blood flow, which again changes local blood oxygenation, fMRI allows indirect measurements of neuronal activity changes. With appropriate data analysis and visualization methods, these BOLD measurements allow drawing conclusions about the localization and dynamics of brain function.

This chapter describes the basic principles and methodology of functional and diffusion-weighted MRI. After a description of the physical principles of MRI at a conceptual level, the physiology of the blood oxygenation level-dependent (BOLD) contrast mechanism is described. The subsequent, major part of the chapter provides an introduction to the current strategies of statistical image analysis techniques with a focus on the analysis of single-subject data because of its relevance for presurgical mapping of human brain function. This is followed by a description of functional connectivity focusing on the analysis of resting-state fMRI data. Finally, principles of diffusion-weighted MRI measurements are described including diffusion tensor imaging, which is the most common acquisition and modeling approach in clinical MRI.

1 Physical Principles of MRI

Magnetic resonance imaging makes it possible to visualize both anatomical and functional data of the human brain. This section shortly describes the main concepts of the physical principles of MRI. More detailed descriptions of the physical basis of MRI are available in several introductory texts, e.g., Huettel et al. (2004), Bandettini et al. (2000), Brown and Semelka (1999), NessAiver (1997), Schild (1990), and Uludağ et al. (2015).

A typical whole-body MR scanner has a hollow bore (tube) about 1 m across. Inside of that bore a cylinder is placed containing the primary magnet producing a very strong *static, homogeneous magnetic field* ($\mathbf{B_0}$). Today, nearly all scanners create the magnetic field with superconducting electromagnets whose wires are cooled by cryogens (e.g., liquid helium). Most standard clinical scanners used to image the human brain possess a magnetic field strength of 1.5 and 3.0 T; 1.5 T is 30,000 times the strength of the earth magnetic field (1 T = 10,000 Gauss). In some research labs, the human brain is imaged at the ultrahigh field at 7 T and beyond. In 2017, the first 7 T model was cleared for clinical use in both Europe and the United States. The stronger the magnetic field, the greater the signal-to-noise ratio, which can be used to image the brain at a higher spatial resolution. At higher field strengths it gets, however, increasingly difficult to create a homogeneous magnetic field, which is necessary for accurate spatial decoding of the raw measurement data. Since homogeneous fields are easier to create for scanners with small bores, scanners with higher magnetic fields (10–20 T) are currently only available for animal use, but human MRI scanners of up to 14 T are emerging (Nowogrodzki 2018). Besides the main magnet, additional coils are located inside the cylinder including shimming coils, gradient coils, and a radio-frequency (RF) coil. The shimming coils are used to shape the magnetic field increasing its homogeneity. The gradient coils are used to temporarily change the magnetic field linearly along any direction which is essential for spatial localization (see below). The RF coil is used to send radio-frequency pulses into the subject.

In a typical brain scanning session, a subject or patient in supine position is slowly moved into the scanner bore using a maneuverable table. Scanning of anatomical and functional images is managed from a terminal in a control room by specifying slice positions and by running appropriate MRI *pulse sequences*. The control room usually has a window behind the computer terminal, which allows looking into the scanner room. Before the subject is moved into the scanner, the head is placed in a small replaceable coil, called the *head coil*. This coil surrounds the head and is used to send radio-frequency pulses into the subject as well as to receive electromagnetic echos. When receive-only head coils are used, the radio-frequency pulses are provided by the RF coil in the cylinder of the scanner. The head coil is an example of a *volume coil*, which is designed such that the sensitive volume (e.g., brain) experiences a fairly uniform RF field. Surface coils are receive-only RF coils that are placed directly upon the surface of the anatomy to be imaged. They provide very high signal to noise in their immediate vicinity but recorded images suffer from extreme nonuniformity because the obtained signal intensity drops rapidly with distance and approaches zero about one coil diameter away from the coil. Phased-array coils are an attempt to combine the positive properties of volume and surface coils by combining images from two or more surface coils to produce a single image (see Sect. 1.2.6).

The physical principles of MRI are the same for anatomical and functional imaging. What makes functional imaging special is described in Sect. 2. The operation of MRI can be described in two major themes. The first theme refers to the excitation and recording of electromagnetic signals reflecting the properties of the measured object. The second theme refers to the construction of two- and three-dimensional images visualizing how the measured object properties vary across space.

1.1 Spin Excitation and Signal Reception

Magnetic resonance imaging is based on the magnetic excitation of body tissue and the recording of returned electromagnetic signals from the body. All nuclei with an odd number of protons are magnetically excitable. The atom of choice for MRI is ^1H, the most common isotope of hydrogen having a nucleus with only 1 proton. Hydrogen protons are ideally suited for MRI because they are abundant in human tissue and possess particularly favorable magnetic properties. Water is the largest source of protons in the body, followed by fat. Protons have magnetic properties because they possess a *spin*: they rotate like a spin top around their own axes inducing a small directed magnetic field. In a normal environment, the magnetic fields of the spins in the human body are oriented randomly and, thus, cancel each other out. If, however, the body of a subject is placed in the strong static magnetic field of an MRI tomography (called $\mathbf{B_0}$), the spins orient themselves in line with that field, either parallel or antiparallel (Fig. 1). Since a slightly larger proportion of spins aligns parallel to the scanner magnetic field, the body gets magnetized. The excess number of spins aligned with the external magnetic field is proportional to the strength of the external magnetic field and is in the order of 10^{15} spins at 1.5 T in a $2 \times 2 \times 2$ mm

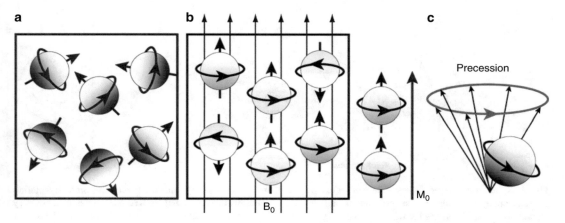

Fig. 1 Spinning protons are little magnets because of the spin property. (**a**) Without an external magnetic field, the directions of the spins are randomly distributed. (**b**) When placed within a large magnetic field, the spins align either with the field (parallel) or against the field (antiparallel). A slight excess of spins aligns with the external magnetic field resulting in a net magnetic field parallel to the external magnetic field. (**c**) A spin is actually not aligning its axis of rotation with the external magnetic field as shown in a and b, but rotates around the direction of the field. This motion is called precession

volume of water. The total magnetic field of the excess spins is called M_0. Just as a spinning top wobbles, the spinning protons wobble, or *precess*, about the axis of the external B_0 field (Fig. 1c). The precession frequency of the protons depends on the strength of the surrounding magnetic field. More precisely, the precession frequency ω is directly proportional to the strength of the external magnetic field and is defined by the *Larmor equation*:

$$\omega_0 = \gamma B_0$$

The symbol ω_0 is known as the precessional, Larmor, or *resonance* frequency. The symbol γ refers to the *gyromagnetic ratio*, which is a constant unique to every atom. For hydrogen protons, $\gamma = 42.56$ MHz/T. At the magnetic field strength of a 3 T scanner, the precession frequency of hydrogen protons is thus 128 MHz.

If an applied electromagnetic pulse has the same frequency as the proton's precession frequency, then the protons get "excited" by absorbing the transmitted energy. This important principle is called *resonance* and gives the method "magnetic *resonance* imaging" its name. Since the precession frequency is in the range of radio-frequency waves, the applied electromagnetic pulse is also called a radio-frequency (RF) pulse. As an effect of excitation, spins flip from the parallel (lower energy) state to the antiparallel (higher energy) state. The RF pulse furthermore lets the excited protons precess *in phase*. As a result, the magnetization vector M_0 moves down towards the x–y plane (Fig. 2). The x–y plane is perpendicular to the static magnetic field and is also referred to as the *transverse plane*. The angle, α, of rotation towards the xy plane is a function of the strength and duration of the RF pulse. If $\alpha = 90°$, the magnetization vector is completely moved into the x–y plane with an equal amount of spins aligned parallel and antiparallel (Fig. 2b). Since the protons precess in phase, i.e., they point in the same direction within the x–y plane, the magnetic fields of the spins add up to form a net magnetic field M_{XY} in the x–y plane. This *transversal component* of the rotating electromagnetic field can be measured (received) in the receiver coil (antenna) because it induces a detectable current flow.

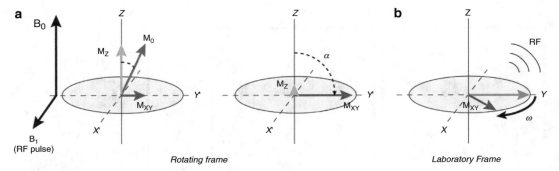

Fig. 2 Spins in the lower energy state can be excited by an electromagnetic pulse at the resonance frequency ω_0 forcing the spins absorbing the transmitted energy to precess in phase. (**a**) As an effect of excitation, the net magnetic field $\mathbf{M_0}$ (blue vector) smoothly tips down towards the x–y plane. The longitudinal component $\mathbf{M_z}$ (green vector) decreases over time while the transverse component $\mathbf{M_{xy}}$ (red vector) increases. This view assumes that the observer is moving with the precessing protons (rotating frame of reference). (**b**) Viewed from outside (laboratory frame of reference), the net magnetization vector rotates with angular velocity ω_0 given by the Larmor equation. The rotating magnetic field in the x–y plane emits radiofrequency waves, which can be measured by a receiver coil

The established in-phase precession is, however, not stable after the RF transmitter is turned off. Because of interactions between the magnetic fields of the protons, the transverse magnetization decays within a few tenth of milliseconds. These spin-spin interactions lead to slightly different local magnetic field strengths and, thus, to slightly different precession frequencies leading to phase shifts between the precessing spins (*dephasing*). The dephasing process is also called *transversal relaxation*. It progresses initially rapidly but slows down over time following an exponential function with time constant T_2 with values in the range of 30–150 ms. Due to magnetic field inhomogeneities in the static magnetic field and in physiological tissue, the spins get out of phase actually faster than T_2 and therefore the measured raw signal in the receiver coil, the *free induction decay* (FID), decays with the shorter time constant T_2* (Fig. 3):

$$\mathbf{M_{XY}} = \mathbf{M_0} e^{-t/T_2 *}$$

The fact that local field inhomogeneities lead to different precession frequencies increasing the speed of dephasing is an important observation for functional MRI because local field inhomogeneities also depend on the local physiological state, especially the state of local blood oxygen-ation, which itself depends on the state of local neuronal activity. Measurements of changing local magnetic field inhomogeneities (T_2* parameter), thus, provide indirect measurements of local neuronal activity.

The speed of spin dephasing is determined by random effects as well as by fixed effects due to magnetic field inhomogeneities. The dephasing effect of constant magnetic field inhomogeneities can be reversed by application of a 180° RF pulse. During a time duration of $t = \tau$ spins go out of phase. Then a 180° RF pulse is applied flipping the dephased spin vectors about the X' or Y' axis in the rotating frame of reference. As an effect of the pulse, the order of the spins is reversed (Fig. 4). At the *echo time* TE = 2τ, the vectors are back in phase producing a large signal, the *spin echo*. This process is similar to a race situation in which participants run with different (but constant) speed. At time τ they get a signal ("180° pulse") to turn around and go back; assuming that they continue in the same speed, they will all arrive at the starting line at the same time (2τ).

The amplitude of the obtained spin echo will be smaller than the amplitude during the FID because part of the signal is inevitably lost due to random spin-spin interactions (T_2 decay). As soon as the spins are all back in phase at the echo

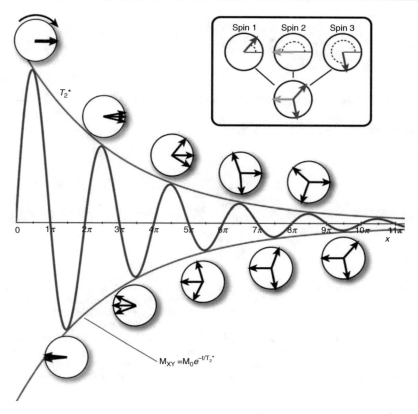

Fig. 3 The signal amplitude (red curve) of the measured raw MR signal, the free induction decay (FID), decays exponentially with time constant T_2^*. The raw signal itself is oscillating at the resonance frequency (blue curve). The signal is lost due to dephasing as indicated by the phase coherency plots (circles) with three representative, super-imposed spins (see inset). The amplitude of the signal at any moment in time is determined by the sum of the spin vectors. When the spins are all in phase (left side), the maximum signal is obtained; that is, the vector sum equals $\mathbf{M_0}$. When the spins are completely out of phase (right side), the signal is completely lost; that is, the sum of the spin vectors equals zero

time, they immediately start to go out of phase again. An additional 180° RF pulse will generate a second echo (Fig. 4). This process can be continued as long as enough signal is available. By setting the time of the 180° pulse, the amplitude of the T_2 signal can, thus, be assessed at any moment in time.

Besides dephasing, the spins reorient themselves with the direction of the strong static magnetic field of the scanner since the excited spins slowly go back into the low-energy state realigning with the external magnetic field. This reorientation process is called *longitudinal relaxation* and progresses slower as the dephasing process. The increase (recovery) of the longitudinal component $\mathbf{M_z}$ follows an exponential function with time constant T_1 with values in the range of 300–2000 ms:

$$\mathbf{M_z} = \mathbf{M_0}\left(1 - e^{-t/T_1}\right)$$

Note that the absorbed RF energy is not only released in a way that it can be detected outside the body as RF waves; part of the energy is given to the surrounding tissue, called the *lattice*. The spin-lattice interactions determine the speed of T_1 recovery, which is unique to every tissue. Tissue-specific T_1 and T_2 values enable MRI to differentiate between different types of tissue when using properly designed MRI pulse sequences.

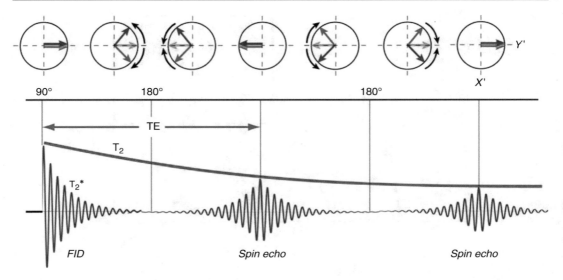

Fig. 4 The effect of constant magnetic field inhomogeneities can be reversed by application of a 180° RF pulse, which flips the dephased vectors about the X'-axis. This is indicated in the upper row with three spin vectors, one precessing at the resonance frequency (green vector), one precessing slightly faster (violet vector), and one precessing slightly slower (blue vector) leading to dephasing. The 180° RF pulse reverses the order of the spins, but not the direction of rotation. The faster spin now runs behind catching up over time, while the slower spin runs ahead slowly falling back. At time TE (echo time), the vectors are back in phase producing a large signal, the spin echo. A second 180° RF pulse will generate a second echo (right side). The maximum amplitude of the echos gets smaller over time because signal is inevitably lost due to random spin-spin interactions (T_2 decay, red curve)

1.2 Image Reconstruction

The described principles of magnetic resonance do not explain how one can obtain images of the brain. This requires attributing components of the signal to those positions in space from which they originated. Although not identical for all measurement sequences, the principles for localizing signal sources typically contain the combined application of three fundamental techniques, *selective excitation of a slice*, *frequency encoding*, and *phase encoding*. Each of these steps allows localizing the source of the signal with respect to one spatial dimension. Paul C. Lauterbur and Peter Mansfield were awarded the 2003 Nobel Prize in Medicine for their discovery that *magnetic field gradients* can be used for spatial encoding. The gradient coils of the MRI scanner allow adding a magnetic field to the static magnetic field, which causes the field strength to vary linearly with distance from the center of the magnet. According to the Larmor equation, spins on one side are exposed to a higher magnetic field and precess faster while spins on the other side are exposed to a lower magnetic field and precess slower than spins in the center (Fig. 5b).

1.2.1 Selective Slice Excitation

A magnetic field gradient is used to select a slice of the imaged object (*slice selection gradient*). Since spins precess with different frequencies along a gradient, protons can be excited selectively: an applied electromagnetic pulse of a certain frequency band will excite only those protons along the gradient precessing at the same frequency band. Spins outside that range will precess at different frequencies and will, thus, not absorb the transmitted RF energy. The selectively excited protons are located in a slice oriented perpendicular to the gradient direction. A gradient along the z-axis will result in an axial slice, a gradient along the x-axis in a sagittal slice, and a gradient along the y-axis in a coronal slice. Oblique slices can be obtained by applying two or three gradients simultaneously. The position and

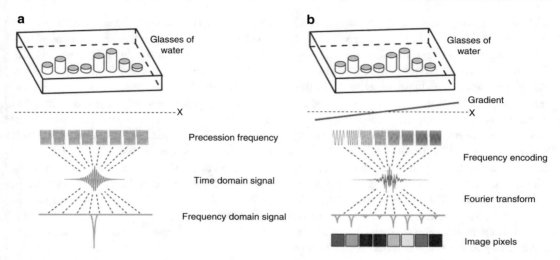

Fig. 5 Assume that eight glasses with different amounts of water are placed in the MRI scanner along the *x*-axis and that a single, thick slice containing all glasses has been excited. (**a**) In the absence of any gradients, all of the excited protons from all glasses are spinning at the same frequency. The received signal also oscillates at that frequency and its amplitude reflects the sum of excited water protons of all glasses. Since all protons precess at the same frequency, the Fourier transform cannot be used to identify signals from different spatial positions along the *x*-axis. (**b**) If a gradient is applied in the *x* direction, the spins will precess at frequencies that depend upon their position along the gradient. Spatial information is now frequency encoded: The strength of the signal at each frequency is directly related to the number of excited protons from the respective glass of water. The obtained composite time domain signal is the sum of these frequencies. The Fourier transform can now be used to determine the strength of the signal at each frequency. Since frequencies encode different spatial positions, an "image" of eight pixels can be formed. The grey values of these pixels reflect the relative amount of water in the different glasses

thickness of the selected slice depend on the slope of the applied gradient and the frequency band of the applied RF pulse. After selective slice excitation, the measured echo will be restricted to a compound signal from the excited protons within the slice. For subsequent spatial encoding, the slice selection gradient is turned off.

1.2.2 Frequency Encoding

While receiving the signal (FID or echo) from the excited slice, a magnetic field gradient can be applied along one of the two remaining spatial dimensions. This second gradient, running along one dimension of the excited slice, is called *frequency encoding gradient*. Note that this gradient is not used to selectively excite protons, but to encode a spatial dimension for those protons already excited in the slice. Due to the applied gradient, the protons within the slice precess with different frequencies along the respective dimension allowing differentiating spatial positions in the received signal (Fig. 5). The frequency encod-

ing gradient is also called *read-out gradient* since it is turned on during reception of the signal from the protons. The strength of the signal at each frequency is directly related to the strength of the signal at the encoded spatial position. The measured composite time domain signal consists of the sum of all frequency responses. The Fourier transform (FT) can be used to get from the composite signal the strength of the signal at each frequency (amplitude and phase information). Since space has been frequency encoded, the strength of the signal at different frequencies corresponds to the strength of the signal at different spatial positions. The obtained frequency-specific information can thus be used to form a spatial image (Fig. 5b). In such an image, the grey level is used to represent the strength of the signal at each picture element (pixel).

1.2.3 Phase Encoding

A further encoding step is required to be able to also separate signal components originating from different positions along the second dimension in the imaging plane. This is achieved by briefly adding another gradient to the static magnetic field oriented along the remaining (third) spatial dimension before receiving an echo. This third magnetic field gradient is called *phase encoding gradient*. While the frequency encoding gradient is turned on during reception of the signal, the phase encoding (PE) gradient is *turned off* just before receiving the echo and, thus, does not (permanently) change the frequency at different spatial positions. This is necessary since frequency encoding gradients in two dimensions would result in ambiguous spatial encoding in a similar way as the same number (e.g., 6) can be obtained in many different ways by the sum of two numbers (e.g., 2 + 4, 3 + 3, 5 + 1). Prior to read-out, the brief duration of the phase encoding gradient results in a short moment of different precession frequencies within each row of the slice. After turning off the phase encoding gradient, the protons within each row precess again with the same frequency but they will now precess with a systematic *phase shift* along the positions within each row. The amount of phase shift depends on the position of a proton along the encoded second image dimension. Through proper combination of frequency encoding in one dimension and phase encoding in the other dimension, all positions within a 2D image can be uniquely encoded with a desired resolution. Unfortunately, a single application of the phase encoding gradient is not sufficient to encode the second image dimension. The process of excitation and phase encoding must be repeated many times for a single slice. At each repetition, the strength of the phase encoding gradient is slightly changed in order to ultimately obtain a complete frequency × phase encoding of the slice.

1.2.4   Two-Dimensional *k* Space

The data obtained from a series of excitation-recording cycles can be arranged in a two-dimensional space called *k space*. Each row of *k* space corresponds to the data of one excitation-recording cycle with a different phase encoding step. As described above, the echo signal of one line in *k* space contains a frequency-encoded representation of one dimension of the selected slice. While the slice selection and frequency encoding gradients are the same from cycle to cycle, the slope of the phase encoding gradient is changed by a constant value across cycles and, thus, from line to line in *k* space. The imposed phase shift for a specific proton depends on the strength of the phase encoding gradient and on the proton's position along the second image dimension. A series of phase encoding steps "fill" *k* space in such a way that the second slice dimension ultimately also gets *frequency* encoded. The *k* space thus contains two-dimensional frequency-encoded information of the slice, which can be transformed into two-dimensional *image space* by application of the two-dimensional Fourier transform (2D FT).

1.2.5   Echo Planar Imaging

The described procedure is applied for each slice of a scanned volume. A properly specified series of electromagnetic pulses allowing to construct one or more 2D images from electromagnetic echos is called a *MRI pulse sequence*. The most often used sequence for functional MRI is *gradient echo-echo planar imaging* (GE-EPI). This sequence enables very rapid imaging of a slice by performing all phase encoding steps after a single 90° excitation pulse. This sequence requires switching the read-out gradient rapidly on and off to fill *k* space line by line resulting in a series of (e.g., 64) small *gradient echos* within the duration of a single T_2^* decay. A complete image can thus be obtained in about 50–100 ms as opposed to several seconds with standard (functional) imaging sequences. GE-EPI is very sensitive to field inhomogeneities influencing the speed of dephasing (T_2^* contrast). This is essential for functional imaging (see below) but also produces image distortions, called susceptibility artifacts, which occur especially at tissue boundaries. Running EPI sequences requires a high-performance gradient system to enable very rapid gradient switching.

1.2.6 Parallel Imaging and Parallel Excitation

In the last 20 years, *parallel imaging* (e.g., Pruessmann et al. 1999) has become a standard technique that has been introduced with different names by scanner manufacturers such as "SENSE," "IPAT," or "SMASH." The basic idea of parallel imaging is the simultaneous acquisition of MRI data with at least two (typically 32 or more) receiver coils, each having a different spatial sensitivity. During image reconstruction, complementary information from the different receiver coils can be combined to fill k space in parallel reducing the number of time-consuming phase encoding steps. Besides appropriate coils (phased-array coils), parallel imaging requires that MRI scanners are equipped with multiple processing channels operating in parallel. Note that parallel imaging may be used either to increase temporal resolution when using a standard matrix size or to increase spatial resolution using a larger matrix with a conventional image acquisition time. Using parallel imaging to reduce scan time without sacrificing image quality is especially relevant for patient scans. Furthermore, parallel imaging may also reduce GE-EPI imaging artifacts because it allows acquiring standard image matrices with shorter echo times; typical EPI artifacts, such as signal dropouts in regions of neighboring tissue types and geometrical distortions, increase with increasing echo times.

In the last 10 years, *parallel excitation* techniques have been increasingly employed that are able to excite more than once slice in parallel: If, for example, 8 slices are excited simultaneously, a whole-brain scan with 64 slices would be completed in the same time as 8 non-simultaneously recorded slices. To enable such powerful "simultaneous multi-slice" (SMS) or "multiband" techniques, advanced excitation hardware is required including multiple transmit channels. Furthermore, special MRI pulse sequences are needed (Moeller et al. 2010; Setsompop et al.

2012). Since multiple slices are acquired truly in parallel, imaging time is substantially reduced as compared to standard single-slice excitation techniques. This is especially beneficial for real-time fMRI neurofeedback studies (e.g., Goebel et al. 2010) since more time points (albeit temporally correlated) can help to calculate more stable feedback values in a given time window. Note, however, that the data received simultaneously from multiple slices need to be separated which becomes increasingly difficult with an increasing number of simultaneously excited slices. In order to avoid loss in image quality, the multiband factor (number of simultaneously excited slices) recommended for neuroscience applications is, thus, in the range of 2–8 depending on the targeted brain region (Todd et al. 2017).

2 Physiological Principles of fMRI

Neuronal activity consumes energy, which is produced by chemical processes requiring glucose and oxygen. The vascular system supplies these substances by a complex network of large and small vessels. The arterial part of the vascular system transports oxygenated blood through an increasingly fine-grained network of blood vessels until it reaches the capillary bed where the chemically stored energy (oxygen) is transferred to the neurons. If the brain is in resting state 30–40% of the oxygen is extracted from the blood in the capillary bed. The venous system transports the less oxygenated blood away from the capillary bed. Oxygen is transported in the blood via the hemoglobin molecule. If hemoglobin carries oxygen, it is called oxygenated hemoglobin (HbO_2), while it is called deoxygenated hemoglobin (Hb) when it is devoid of oxygen. While the arterial network contains almost only oxygenated hemoglobin, the capillary bed and the venous network contain a mixture of oxygenated and deoxygenated hemoglobin.

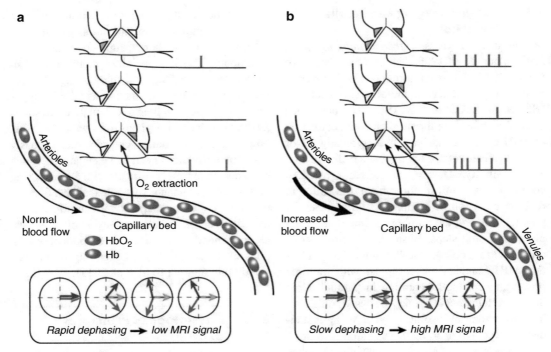

Fig. 6 From neural activity to BOLD MRI responses. (**a**) If a cortical region is in baseline mode, neural activity— including synaptic signal integration and spike generation—is low (upper part). Cerebral blood flow (CBF) is at a basal level. A constant oxygen extraction rate fueling neural activity leads to a fixed deoxygenated hemoglobin (Hb)-to-oxygenated hemoglobin (HbO₂) ratio in the capillary bed and venules. Since Hb is paramagnetic, it distorts the magnetic field. The Hb-related magnetic field inhomogeneities lead to rapid dephasing of excited spins resulting in a low MRI signal level (lower part). (**b**) If the cortical region is in activated state, synaptic signal integration and spiking activity increase, leading to an increased oxygen extraction rate (upper part). CBF strongly increases delivering oxygen beyond local need, which essentially flushes Hb away from the capillary bed (middle part). Since HbO₂ does not substantially distort the homogeneity of the local magnetic field, excited spins dephase slower than in the baseline state (lower part) resulting in an enhanced MRI signal (BOLD effect)

2.1 Neurovascular Coupling

A local increase of neuronal activity immediately leads to an increased oxygen extraction rate in the capillary bed and, thus, an increase in the relative concentration of deoxygenated hemoglobin. This fast response to increased neuronal activity is described as the "initial dip" (Fig. 7). After a short time of about 3 s the increased local neuronal activity also leads to a strong increase in local blood flow. This response of the vascular system to the increased energy demand is called the *hemodynamic response*. Simultaneous electrical recording and fMRI animal studies indicate that synaptic signal integration (measured by the local field potential, LFP) is a better predictor of the strength of the hemodynamic response than

spiking activity (Logothetis et al. 2001; Mathiesen et al. 2000). It thus seems likely that the hemodynamic response primarily reflects the input and local processing of neuronal information rather than the output signals (Logothetis and Wandell 2004). Note that it is not yet completely known how the neurons "inform" the vascular system about their increased energy demand. Important theories about this *neurovascular coupling* are described, among many others, by Fox et al. (1988), Buxton et al. (1998), Magistretti et al. (1999), and Uludağ et al. (2015). It appears likely that astrocytes play an important role because these special glial cells are massively connected with both neurons and vascular system. The hemodynamic response consists of increased local cerebral blood flow (CBF) as well as

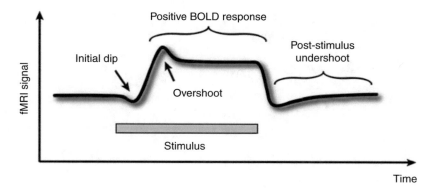

Fig. 7 Idealized time course of the hemodynamic response following a long (about 20 s) stimulation event. The theoretically expected initial dip is not reliably measured in human fMRI studies. For long stimulation events, the signal rises initially to a higher value (overshoot) than the subsequently reached plateau. When the stimulus is turned off, the signal often falls below the baseline signal level (undershoot), which is then approached slowly

increased cerebral blood volume (CBV), probably as a mechanical consequence of increased blood flow. The increased blood flow not only compensates quickly for the slightly increased oxygen extraction rate of activated neurons, but also results in a substantial local *oversupply* of oxygenated hemoglobin (Figs. 6 and 7). Note that it is not yet clear why the vascular system responds with a much stronger increase in cerebral blood flow than appears to be necessary. The increased CBV may help to explain the poststimulus undershoot (Fig. 7) observed in typical fMRI responses (balloon model, Buxton et al. 1998). While CBF and oxygen extraction rate may quickly return to baseline, the elastic properties of the dilated venules will require many seconds until baseline size is reached. In the expanded space of the dilated vessels more deoxygenated hemoglobin will accumulate reducing the MRI signal below the pre-stimulus baseline level.

2.2 The BOLD Effect

The most common method of functional MRI is based on the BOLD effect (Ogawa et al. 1990). This exploits the fact that oxygenated hemoglobin has different magnetic properties than deoxygenated hemoglobin. More specifically, while oxygenated hemoglobin is diamagnetic, deoxygenated hemoglobin is paramagnetic altering the local magnetic susceptibility, creating magnetic field distortions within and around the blood vessels in the capillary bed and venules. During the hemodynamic response (oversupply phase), the oxygenated-to-deoxygenated hemoglobin ratio increases resulting in a more homogeneous local magnetic field. As follows from the description in Sect. 1, excited spins dephase slower in a more homogeneous magnetic field leading to a stronger measured MRI signal in the activated state when compared to a resting state (Fig. 6). The BOLD effect, thus, measures increased neuronal activity indirectly via a change in local magnetic field (in)homogeneity, which is caused by an oversupply of oxygenated blood (Fig. 6). Note that these field inhomogeneities are detectable with MRI because of the different magnetic properties of oxy- and deoxygenated hemoglobin. The change in the local HbO_2/Hb ratio and its associated change in magnetic field homogeneity, thus, act as endogenous markers of neural activity.

2.3 The Hemodynamic Response

The time course of evoked fMRI signals, reflecting the BOLD hemodynamic response, is well studied for primary visual cortex (V1). After application of a short visual stimulus of 100 ms, the observed (positive) signal response starts to rise after 2–3 s (oversupply phase) and reaches a maximum level after 5–6 s. About 10 s later, the

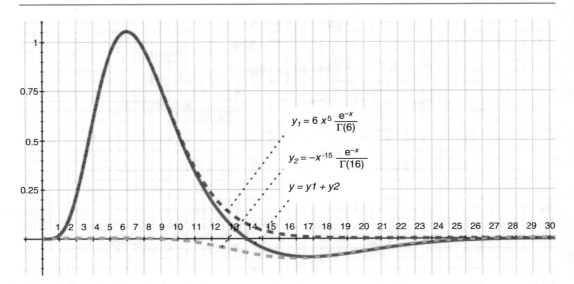

$$y_1 = 6\, x^5\, \frac{e^{-x}}{\Gamma(6)}$$

$$y_2 = -x^{-15}\, \frac{e^{-x}}{\Gamma(16)}$$

$$y = y1 + y2$$

Fig. 8 The two-gamma function allows to model typical hemodynamic impulse responses. One gamma function models the peak (τ) and dispersion (σ) of the positive BOLD response while the second gamma function models the peak and dispersion of the undershoot response. Parameter A scales the amplitudes of the individual gamma functions

signal reaches again the baseline level. As compared to the neuronal response of about 100 ms duration, the corresponding fMRI response is characterized by a delayed, gradual response profile extending as long as 20 s. Despite this sluggish response, the latency of response onset appears to reflect quite precisely neuronal onset times (see Sect. 2.4).

Assuming a linear time invariant (LTI) system, one can predict the expected time course of arbitrary long stimulation periods from the known response to a short stimulus. The response to a very short stimulus is called the *impulse response function* or, in the context of fMRI, the BOLD *hemodynamic response function* (HRF). The output (expected fMRI response) of a LTI system is the *convolution* of the input time course (e.g., stimulation "box-car" time course) with the system's response to an impulse function (Fig. 9). For primary visual cortex (V1), Boynton et al. (1996) showed that the measured responses to stimuli with varying amplitudes and durations could be indeed predicted well from the response profile obtained from a short visual stimulus. A well-suited function to model the hemodynamic impulse function is the probability density func-

tion (pdf) of the gamma distribution scaled by parameter A:

$$y\left(x;,A,\tau,\sigma\right) = Ax^{\tau/\sigma-1}\, \frac{e^{-x/\sigma}}{\sigma^{\tau/\sigma}\Gamma\left(\tau/\sigma\right)}$$

Parameters τ and σ define the onset and dispersion of the response peak, respectively. While Boynton et al. (1996) used a single gamma function to characterize the impulse response function, the sum of two gamma functions (Friston et al. 1998) also captures the undershoot of fMRI responses. The first gamma function typically peaks 5 s after stimulus onset ($\tau = 6$), while the second gamma function peaks 15 s after stimulus onset ($\tau = 16$, see Fig. 8). After convolution of a stimulus time course with the impulse function (Fig. 9), the calculated time course can be directly used as a reference function in a general linear model for statistical data analysis (see Sect. 3.3).

Note that the linear system assumption is reasonably valid only for stimuli of sufficiently long duration separated by long enough baseline periods. For a series of short stimuli separated by intervals shorter than 2–4 s, nonlinear interaction effects have to be expected (e.g., Robson

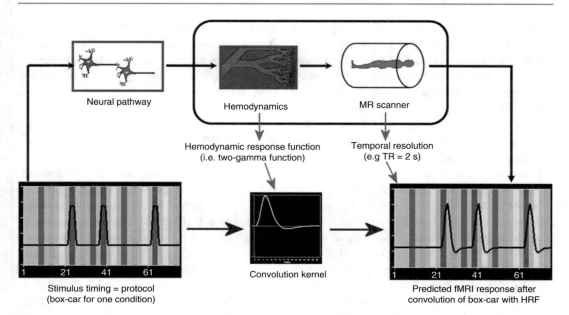

Neural pathway

Hemodynamics

MR scanner

Hemodynamic response function
(i.e. two-gamma function)

Temporal resolution
(e.g TR = 2 s)

Convolution kernel

Stimulus timing = protocol
(box-car for one condition)

Predicted fMRI response after
convolution of box-car with HRF

Fig. 9 Calculation of expected fMRI signal response for one condition of a protocol using convolution. The calculated response depends on the chosen model for the BOLD hemodynamic response function (HRF), e.g., two-gamma function (middle part). The expected response is obtained by convolution of the box-car time course (left) with the chosen HRF. The convolved time course is downsampled to the temporal resolution (sampling intervals) of the fMRI measurements given by the volume TR value (right)

et al. 1998). Note further that the calculation (convolution) of expected time courses requires as input the valid specification of the time course of assumed neuronal response profiles, which is often not simply a copy of stimulus timing. A simple box-car time course, for example, assumes that neurons in a stimulated cortical area are active with constant amplitude in prolonged "on" periods. It is, however, well known that this assumption is too simplistic for neurons in early sensory areas. For higher cortical areas, e.g., frontal areas involved in working memory, the neuronal response profile might differ substantially with respect to stimulus timing. Assuming that neuronal responses are correctly specified, it appears reasonable to use the same generic hemodynamic response function for all brain regions and participants to predict expected BOLD signal time courses. It has been, however, shown that the hemodynamic response varies substantially enough across subjects to justify creation of empirically derived individual HRFs when using event-related designs (Handwerker et al. 2004).

While fMRI responses clearly reflect the oversupply phase of the hemodynamic response, the theoretically expected initial dip (Fig. 7) has not been reliably detected in standard human fMRI measurements (for animal studies, see, e.g., Kim et al. 2000). This component of the idealized hemodynamic response is thus not included in the standard single- or two-gamma convolution kernels (Fig. 8). Data analysis of almost all fMRI studies is therefore based on the signals coming from the much stronger and sustained positive BOLD response.

2.4 Limits of Spatial and Temporal Resolution

The ultimate spatial and temporal resolution of fMRI is not primarily limited by technical constraints but by properties of the vascular system. The spatial resolution of the vascular system, and hence fMRI, seems to be in the order of 0.5–1 mm since relevant blood vessels run vertically through cortex in roughly that distance (Duvernoy et al.

1981). An achievable resolution of 0.5–1 mm might be just enough to resolve *cortical columns*. A cortical column contains thousands of neurons possessing similar response specificity. A conventional brain area, such as the fusiform face area, could contain a set of cortical columns, each coding a different basic (e.g., face) feature. Cortical columns could, thus, form the basic building blocks ("alphabet") of complex representations (Fujita et al. 1992). Since neurons within a column code for roughly the same feature, measuring the brain at the level of cortical columns promises to provide a relevant level for describing brain functioning. In cat visual cortex, for example, orientation columns could be measured with fMRI at ultrahigh magnetic fields (4 and 9 T, Kim et al. 2000). The observed pattern of active orientation columns systematically changed when showing cats gratings of different orientations. Using ultrahigh magnetic fields (7 T and higher), columnar resolution has also been achieved in the human brain (e.g., Cheng et al. 2001; Yacoub et al. 2008; Zimmermann et al. 2011; De Martino et al. 2015; Gentile et al. 2017; Schneider et al. 2019).

Despite the sluggishness of the fMRI signal, it has been shown that the obtained responses may reflect timing information with very high temporal precision. The signal of the left and right visual cortex, for example, reliably reflects temporal differences between stimulation of the left and right visual field as short as 100 ms (Menon and Kim 1999). When properly taking care of different hemodynamic delays in different brain areas, the analysis of BOLD onset latencies may also be very useful in revealing the sequential order of activity across brain areas within trials of complex cognitive tasks (fMRI mental chronometry, e.g., Formisano and Goebel 2003). In order to measure the brain with a temporal resolution in the order of milliseconds, other methods such as electroencephalography (EEG) and magnetoencephalography (MEG) must be used. If one succeeds in performing a proper combined analysis of EEG/MEG and fMRI data (Scherg et al. 1999; Dale and Halgren 2001; Bledowski et al. 2006), it becomes possible to describe brain function with respect to both its topographic distribution and its precise timing. While EEG/MEG data and fMRI data are conventionally obtained in different sessions, it is possible to measure EEG data directly during fMRI recording sessions (e.g., Mulert et al. 2004).

3 fMRI Data Analysis

A major goal of functional MRI measurements is the localization of the neural correlates of sensory, motor, and cognitive processes. Another major goal of fMRI studies is the detailed characterization of the response profile for known regions of interest (ROIs) across experimental conditions. In this context, the aim of conducted studies is often not to map new functional brain regions (whole-brain analysis) but to characterize further how known specialized brain areas respond to (subtle) differences in experimental conditions (ROI-based analysis). Furthermore, it is often of interest to estimate the shape of the response and how it varies across different conditions and brain areas. Inspection of the shape of (averaged) time courses may also help to separate signal fluctuations due to measurement artifacts from stimulus-related hemodynamic responses. In order to obtain fMRI data with relatively high temporal resolution, functional time series are acquired using fast MR sequences sensitive to BOLD contrast. As described above most fMRI experiments use the gradient echo EPI sequence, which allows acquisition of a 64×64 matrix in 50–100 ms. Using simultaneous multi-slice acquisition schemes (Sect. 1.2.6), more slices and/or larger matrix sizes can be used in the same time. A typical functional scan of the whole brain with a voxel size of 2 mm lasts only 1–2 s on state-of-the-art MRI scanners. The data obtained from scanning all slices once at different positions is subsequently referred to as a *functional volume* or a *functional 3D image*. The measurement of an uninterrupted series of functional volumes is referred to as a functional scan or *run*. A run, thus, consists of the repeated measurement of a functional volume and, hence, the repeated measurement of the individual slices. The sampling interval—the time until the same brain region is measured again—is called *volume TR*. The volume TR specifies the temporal resolution of the functional measurements since all slices comprising one functional volume are obtained once during that time. Note, however, that the slices of a functional volume are not (all) recorded simultaneously, which implies that data from different regions of the brain are recorded at different moments in time (see Sect. 3.2.2.3). During a functional experiment, a subject performs tasks typically involving several experimental conditions. A short experiment can be completed in a single run, which typically consists of 100–1000 functional volumes. Assuming a run with 500 volumes each consisting of 64 slices of 128×128 pixels and that 2 bytes are needed to store each pixel, the amount of raw data acquired per run would be $500 \times 64 \times 128 \times 128 \times 2 = 1{,}048{,}576{,}000$ bytes or roughly 1 giga byte (GB). In more complex experiments, a subject typically performs multiple runs in one scanning session resulting in several GB of functional data per subject per session.

Given the small amplitude of task-related BOLD signal changes of typically 1–5%, and the presence of many confounding effects, such as signal drifts and head motion, the localization and characterization of brain regions responding to experimental conditions of the stimulation protocol are a nontrivial task. The major analysis steps of functional and associated anatomical data will be described in the following paragraphs including spatial and temporal *preprocessing, statistical data analysis, coregistration* of functional and anatomical datasets, and *spatial normalization*. Although these essential data analysis steps are performed in a rather standardized way in all major software packages, including AFNI (http://afni.nimh.nih.gov/afni/), BrainVoyager (http://www.brainvoyager.com/), FSL (http://www.fmrib.ox.ac.uk/fsl/), and SPM (http://www.fil.ion.ucl.ac.uk/spm/), there is still room for improvements as will be discussed below. For the visualization of functional data, high-resolution anatomical datasets with a resolution of (or close to) 1 mm in all three dimensions are often collected in a recording session. In most cases, these anatomical volumes are

scanned using slow T_1-weighted MR sequences that are optimized to produce high-quality images with very good contrast between grey and white matter. In some analysis packages, anatomical datasets not only do serve as a structural reference for the visualization of functional information but are often also used to improve the functional analysis itself, for example, by restricting statistical data analysis to grey matter voxels or to analyze topological representations on extracted cortex meshes. The preprocessing of high-resolution anatomical datasets and their role in functional data analysis will be described in Sect. 3.4. Since some data analysis steps depend on the details of the experimental paradigm, the next section shortly describes the two most frequently used experimental designs.

3.1 Block and Event-Related Designs

In the first years of fMRI measurements, experimental designs were adapted from positron-emission tomography (PET) studies. In the typical PET design, several *trials* (individual stimuli or, more generally, cognitive events) were clustered in *blocks*, each of which contained trials of the same condition (Fig. 10). As an example, one block may consist of a series of different pictures showing happy faces and another block may consist of pictures showing sad faces. The statistical analysis of such *block designs* compares the mean activity obtained in the different experimental blocks. Block designs were necessary in PET studies because of the limited temporal resolution of this imaging technique requiring about a minute to obtain a single whole-brain functional image. Since the temporal resolution of fMRI is much higher than PET, it has been proposed to use *event-related designs* (Blamire et al. 1992; Buckner et al. 1996; Dale and Buckner 1997). The characteristics of these designs (Fig. 10) follow closely those used in event-related potential (ERP) studies. In event-related designs, individual trials of different conditions are not clustered in blocks but are presented in a random sequence with sufficient

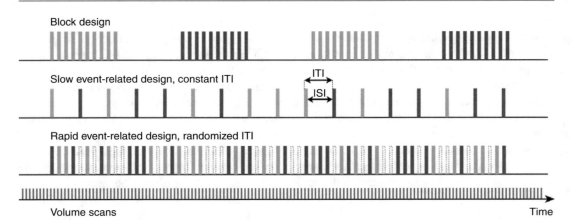

Fig. 10 In a block design (upper row), trials (events) belonging to the same condition are grouped together and are separated by a baseline block. In this example, two blocks of two main conditions (green—condition 1, violet—condition 2) are depicted. In slow event-related designs, trials of different conditions appear in randomized order and are spaced sufficiently far apart to avoid largely overlapping BOLD responses. Optimal intertrial intervals (ITIs) are about 12 s

time between trials to separate successive responses. Responses to trials belonging to the same condition are selectively averaged and the calculated mean responses are statistically compared with each other. While block designs are well suited for many experiments, event-related designs offer several advantages over block designs, especially for cognitive tasks. An important advantage of event-related designs is the possibility to present stimuli in a randomized order (Fig. 10) avoiding cognitive adaptation or expectation strategies of the subjects. Such cognitive adaptations are likely to occur in block designs since a subject knows what type of stimuli to expect within a block after having experienced the first few trials. Another important advantage of event-related designs is that the *response profile* for different trial types (and even single trials) can be *estimated* by event-related averaging. Furthermore, event-related designs allow *post hoc sorting* of individual brain responses. One important example of post hoc sorting is the separation of brain responses for correctly vs. incorrectly performed trials.

The possibilities of event-related fMRI designs are comparable to standard behavioral and ERP analyses. Note, however, that the hemodynamic response extends over about 20–30 s

(Fig. 8) after presentation of a short stimulus; if only the positive BOLD response is considered, the signal extends over 10–15 s. The easiest way to conduct event-related fMRI designs is to temporally separate individual trials far enough to avoid overlapping responses of successive trials. Event-related designs with long temporal intervals between individual trials are termed *slow event-related designs* (Fig. 10). For stimuli of duration of 1–2 s, the optimal *intertrial interval* (ITI) for statistical analysis is about 12 s (Bandettini and Cox 2000; Maus et al. 2010a). Since it has been shown that the fMRI signals of closely spaced trials add up approximately linearly (Boynton et al. 1996, Dale and Buckner 1997, see Sect. 2.3), it is also possible to run experiments with intertrial intervals of 2–6 s. Designs with short temporal intervals between trials are called *rapid event-related designs* (Fig. 10). While the measured response of rapid event-related designs will contain a combination of overlapping responses from closely spaced trials, condition-specific event-related time courses can be isolated using deconvolution analysis. Deconvolution analysis works correctly only under the assumption of a linear system (see Sect. 3.2) and requires randomized intertrial intervals ("jitter"), which can be easily obtained by adding "null" (baseline) trials when trial sequences are created for an experiment. Note, however, that single-trial analyses are only possible when using a slow event-related design. While adding null trials and simple permutations of trial types produce already good event sequences for rapid event-related designs, statistical power can be maximized by using more advanced randomization procedures (Wager and Nichols 2003; Maus et al. 2010b). In general, block and event-related designs can be statistically analyzed using the same mathematical principles (see Sect. 3.3.3).

It is important to note that conventional fMRI data does not provide an absolute signal of brain activity limiting the quantitative interpretation of results. The major part of the signal amplitude is related to proton density and T_2 tissue contrast varying across brain regions within and between subjects. Small BOLD-related signal fluctuations, thus, do neither have a defined origin nor a unit. In light of these considerations, signal strengths in main experimental conditions cannot be interpreted absolutely but have to be assessed relative to the signal strength in other main or control conditions within voxels. As a general control condition, many fMRI experiments contain a baseline ("rest," "fixation") condition with "no task" for the subject. Such simple control conditions allow analyzing brain activity that is common in multiple main conditions that would not be detectable when only comparisons between main conditions could be performed. More complex experimental (control) conditions are designed to differ from the main condition(s) only in a specific cognitive component allowing isolating brain responses specific to that component.

Responses to main conditions are often expressed as percent signal change relative to the mean of a time course or to a baseline condition. Furthermore, it is recommended to vary conditions within subjects—and even within runs—since the lack of an absolute signal level increases variability when comparing effects across runs, sessions, or subjects. Some experiments require a *between-subjects* design, including comparisons of responses between different subject groups, e.g., males vs. females or treatment group vs. control group. Note that the BOLD signal measured with conventional fMRI may be affected by medication that modifies the neurovascular coupling, e.g., by increasing or decreasing baseline cerebral blood flow (CBF). To obtain more quantitative evaluation of activation responses it is, thus, recommended for patient studies to combine standard BOLD measurements with CBF measurements using arterial spin labeling (ASL) techniques (e.g., Buxton et al. 2004).

3.2 Data Preprocessing

3.2.1 Two Views on fMRI Datasets

In order to better understand different fMRI data analysis steps, two different views on the recorded four-dimensional datasets are helpful. In one view (Fig. 11a), the 4D data is conceptualized as a *sequence of functional volumes* (3D images). This view is very useful to understand spatial analysis steps. During 3D motion correction, for example, each functional volume of a run is aligned to a selected reference volume by adjusting rotation and translation parameters. The second view focuses on time courses of individual voxels ("voxel" = "volume element" analogous to "pixel" = picture element). This second view (Fig. 11b) helps to understand those preprocessing and statistical procedures, which process *time courses of individual voxels*. Most standard statistical analysis procedures including the general linear model (GLM) operate in this way. In a GLM analysis, for example, the data is processed "voxel-wise" (univariate) by fitting a model to the time course of each voxel independently.

3.2.2 Preprocessing of Functional Data

To reduce artifact and noise-related signal components, a series of *preprocessing* operations are typically performed prior to statistical data analysis. The most essential preprocessing steps are (1) correction of EPI image distortions, (2) head motion detection and correction, (3) slice scan timing correction, (4) removal of linear and

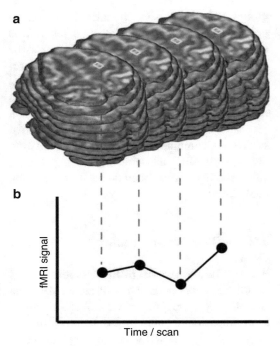

Fig. 11 During functional MRI measurements, a set of slices, often covering the whole brain, are scanned repeatedly over time. Although the repeated slice measurements look almost identical, small task-related signal fluctuations may occur at different brain regions at different moments in time (**a**). To visualize these subtle fluctuations, the time course of any desired brain region (region of interest, ROI) may be depicted (**b**). The smallest separate brain region one can select to display a time course in a two-dimensional image (slice) is called pixel (picture element) while the smallest region in a three-dimensional "image" is called voxel (volume element)

nonlinear trends in voxel time courses, and (5) spatial and temporal smoothing of the data.

3.2.2.1 Distortion Correction of Functional Images

The BOLD-sensitive GE-EPI sequence is used for most fMRI studies because of its speed and relatively high signal-to-noise ratio but it has the disadvantage that images suffer from signal dropouts and geometric distortions, especially in brain regions close to other tissue types such as air and liquor (susceptibility artifacts). These artifacts can be reduced substantially by using optimized EPI sequence parameters (e.g., Weiskopf et al. 2006) and parallel imaging techniques (see Sect. 1.2.6). A complete removal of

dropouts and geometric distortions is, however, not possible during scanning requiring further postprocessing using additional measurements. In one approach distortion correction routines use special *field map* scans measuring magnetic field distortions (Jezzard and Balaban 1995). Another approach exploits the fact that field inhomogeneities caused by susceptibility artifacts disrupt mainly the phase encoding dimension, which can be corrected by acquiring data in the opposite phase encoding direction producing pixel shifts of the same amount in opposite direction (Andersson et al. 2003; Breman et al. 2020). The distortion-corrected images may improve coregistration results between functional and anatomical datasets enabling a more precise localization of brain function.

3.2.2.2 Detection and Correction of Head Motion

The quality of fMRI data is strongly hampered in the presence of substantial head movements. Datasets are usually rejected for further analysis if head motion exceeds 5 mm. Although head motion can be corrected in image space, displacements of the head reduce the homogeneity of the magnetic field, which is fine-tuned ("shimmed") prior to functional scans for the head position at that time. If head movements are small, 3D motion correction is an important step to improve data quality for subsequent statistical data analysis. Motion correction operates by selecting a functional volume of a run (or a volume from another run of the same scanning session) as a reference to which all other functional volumes are aligned. Most head motion algorithms describe head movements by six parameters assessing translation (displacement) and rotation at each time point with respect to the reference volume. These six parameters are appropriate to characterize the motion of *rigid bodies*, since any spatial displacement of rigid bodies can be described by translation along the *x*-, *y*-, and *z*-axes and rotation around these axes. The values of these six parameters are estimated iteratively by analyzing how a source volume should be translated and rotated in order to better align with the reference volume; after applying a first estimate of the parameters, the procedure is repeated to improve the "fit" between the transformed (motion-corrected) and target (reference) volume. A similarity or error measure serves as a *cost function* to quantify how good the transformed volume fits the reference volume. An often-used cost function is the sum of squared intensity differences at corresponding positions in the reference volume and the transformed volume. The iterative adjustment of the parameter estimates stops if no further improvement can be achieved, i.e., when the cost function reaches a minimum. After the final motion parameters have been *detected* by the iterative procedure, they can be applied to the source volume to produce a *motion-corrected* volume replacing the original volume in the output (motion corrected) dataset. For visual inspection, fMRI software packages are usually presenting line plots of the three translation and three rotation parameters across time showing how the estimated values change from volume to volume. The obtained parameter time courses may also be integrated in subsequent statistical data analysis with the aim to remove residual motion artifacts (for details, see Sect. 3.3).

Note that the assumption of a rigid body is not strictly valid for fMRI data since the slices of a functional volume are not scanned all in parallel when using 2D GE-EPI sequences. Since abrupt head motions may occur at any moment in time, the assumption of a rigid body is, thus, violated. Imagine, for example, that a subject does not move while the first five slices of a functional volume are scanned, and then moves 2 mm along the *y*-axis and then lies still until scanning of that volume has been completed. The six parameters of a rigid body approach are not sufficient to capture such "within-volume" motion correctly. Fortunately, head movements from volume to volume are typically small and the assumption of a moving rigid body is, thus, largely valid.

To reduce artifacts from head motion it is important to start reducing it already during scanning. It has been shown that visual or tactile feedback may substantially reduce motion of participants. A strip of medical tape applied from one side of the magnetic resonance head coil, via the participant's forehead, to the other side, provides already useful feedback for participants resulting in substantially reduced head motion (Krause et al. 2019). Another approach to minimize motion artifacts is to detect and correct motion online during scanning. This technique is referred to as *prospective motion correction*. After detecting motion parameters during acquisition using recorded images (Thesen et al. 2000) or external optical tracking (Zaitsev et al. 2006), pulse sequence parameters are updated in real time in such a way that the imaging volume "follows" the moving head of the participant. While prospective motion correction techniques are arguably the best possible solution, errors during motion detection may lead to wrong adjustments, which in the worst case might even produce non-real motion artifacts. Prospective motion correction techniques need thus to be carefully evaluated and used with care.

3.2.2.3 Slice Scan Time Correction

For statistical analysis, a functional volume is usually considered as measured at the same time point. Individual slices (or a few slices when using state-of-the-art "multiband" sequences) of a functional volume are, however, scanned sequentially in standard 2D functional (EPI) measurements, i.e., each slice (or set of slices in multiband sequences) is obtained at a different time point within a functional volume measurement. For a functional volume of 30 slices, ascending scanning order of single slices, and a volume TR of 3 s, for example, the data of the last slice will be measured almost 3 s later than the data of the first slice. Despite the sluggishness of the hemodynamic response (Fig. 8), an imprecise specification of time in the order of 3 s will lead to suboptimal statistical analysis, especially in event-related designs. It is, thus, desirable to preprocess the data in such a way that after processing the data appears as if all slices of a functional volume were measured at the same moment in time. Only then would it be, for example, possible to compare and integrate event-related responses from different brain regions correctly with respect to temporal parameters such as onset latency. In order to correct for different slice scan

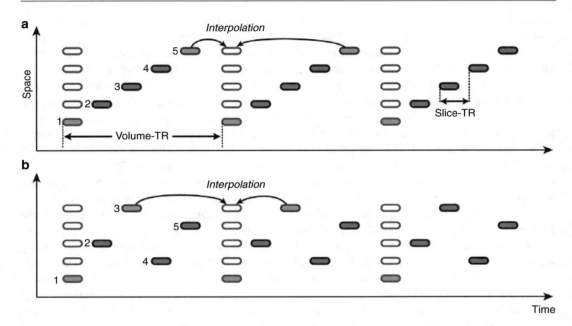

Fig. 12 During slice scan time correction, slices within each functional volume (black rectangles) are "shifted in time" resulting in a new time series (violet rectangles) in which all slices of a functional volume are virtually measured at the same moment in time. To calculate intensity values at time points falling in between measured time points, past and future values have to be integrated typically using sinc or linear interpolation. For correct interpolation, the volume TR, slice TR, and slice scanning order must be known. (**a**) Five slices are scanned in ascending order. (**b**) Five slices are scanned in interleaved order

timings, the time series of individual slices are temporally "shifted" to match a reference time point, e.g., the first or middle slice of a functional volume. The appropriate temporal shift of the time courses of the other slices is then performed by resampling the original data accordingly. Since this process involves sampling at time points that fall between measurement time points, the new values need to be estimated by interpolation of values from past and future time points (Fig. 12). The most often used interpolation methods are linear, cubic spline, and sinc interpolation. Note that the time points of slice scanning depend also on the *acquisition order* specified at the scanner console. Besides an ascending or descending order, slices are often scanned in an interleaved mode; that is, the odd slice numbers are recorded first followed by the even slice numbers. After appropriate temporal resampling, all slices within a functional volume of the new dataset represent the same time point (Fig. 12) and can, thus, be statistically analyzed with the same

hemodynamic response function; if slice scan time correction is not performed, hemodynamic response functions should be adjusted (shifted) on a per-slice basis.

3.2.2.4 Removal of Drifts and Temporal Smoothing of Voxel Time Series

Due to physical and physiological noise, voxel time courses are often nonstationary exhibiting signal drifts over time. If the signal rises or falls with a constant slope from beginning to end of a run, the drift is described as a *linear trend*. If the signal level slowly varies over time with a non-constant slope, the drift is described a nonlinear trend. Since drifts describe slow signal changes they can be removed by Fourier analysis using a *temporal high-pass filter*. The original signal in the time domain is transformed in frequency space using the Fourier transform (FT). In the frequency domain drifts can be easily removed because low-frequency components, underlying drifts, are isolated from higher frequency

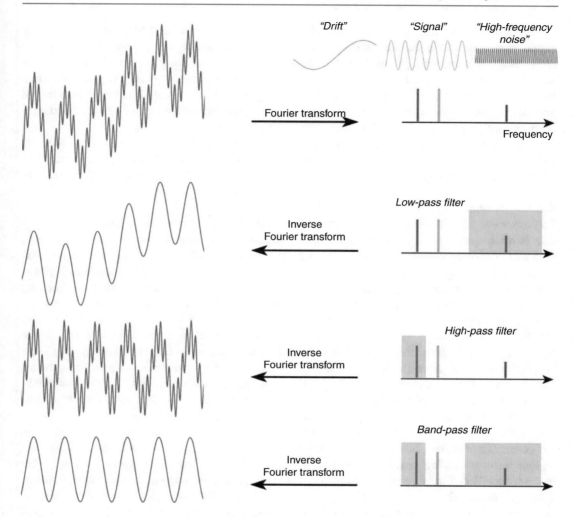

Fig. 13 Principle of temporal filtering using Fourier analysis. The time-domain signal can be converted in an equivalent frequency-domain signal using the Fourier transform (upper row). In this simplified example, the composite signal (upper row, left) consists only of three frequencies representing a drift, signal, and high-frequency noise component (upper row, right). In the fre-quency domain, frequencies can be filtered to remove unwanted signal components. The filtered signal can then be converted back into the time domain using the inverse Fourier transform. In the second row, a low-pass filter is applied, in the third row a high-pass filter, and in the fourth row a band-pass filter

components reflecting task-related signal changes and high-frequency noise. After applying a high-pass filter in the frequency domain (removing low frequencies), the data is transformed back into the time domain by the inverse Fourier trans-form (Fig. 13). As an alternative approach, drifts can be modeled and removed in the time domain using appropriate basis sets in a general linear model analysis. This approach can be performed either as a preprocessing step or as part of statisti-cal data analysis (for details, see Sect. 3.3.3). Removal of drifts is recommended as a prepro-cessing step since it is relevant not only for statistical data analysis but also for the calcula-tion of event-related time courses.

While less important, another temporal pre-processing step is *temporal smoothing* of voxel time courses removing *high-frequency signal fluctuations*, which are considered as noise. While this step increases the signal-to-noise ratio, temporal smoothing is not recommended when analyzing event-related designs since it may distort estimates of temporally relevant parameters, such as the onset or width of average event-related responses. Temporal smoothing also increases serial correlations between values of successive time points that need to be corrected (see Sect. 3.3.3.6).

3.2.2.5 Spatial Smoothing

To further enhance the signal-to-noise ratio, the data is often spatially smoothed by convolution with a 3D Gaussian kernel. In this process, each voxel is replaced by a weighted average value calculated across neighboring voxels. The shape and width of the Gaussian kernel determine the weights used to multiply the values of voxels in the neighborhood; that is, weights decrease with increasing distance from the considered voxel; voxels further apart from the center will, thus, contribute less to the weighted average than voxels close to the center of the considered voxel. Note that smoothing reduces the spatial resolution of the data and should be therefore applied with care. Many studies, however, aim to detect regions larger than a few voxels, i.e., brain areas in the order of 1 cm^3 or larger. Under these conditions, spatial smoothing with an appropriate kernel width of 4–8 mm is useful since it suppresses noise and enhances task-related signals. Spatial smoothing also increases the extent of activated brain regions, which is exploited in the context of group analyses (see Sect. 3.5) facilitating the integration of signals from corresponding but not perfectly aligned brain regions. When analyzing data using multivoxel pattern analysis (see Sect. 3.6.5), spatial smoothing is usually avoided or used with very small kernels on the order of the voxel size since differential effects in neighboring voxels may contribute to separating patterns from each other, which would be reduced when performing spatial smoothing.

From the description and discussion of standard preprocessing steps it should have become clear that there are no universally correct criteria to choose preprocessing steps and parameters because choices depend to some extent on the goal of data analysis. Some steps depend also on the experimental design of a study. If, for example, a high-pass temporal filter is used with a cut-off point that is too high, interesting task-related signal fluctuations could easily be removed accidentally from the data.

Besides the described core preprocessing steps, additional procedures may be applied. The next sections will describe three additional preprocessing steps.

3.2.2.6 Mean Intensity Adjustment

Besides drifts in *individual* voxel time courses, the mean intensity level averaged across all voxels might exhibit drifts over time. These global drifts can be corrected by scaling the intensity values of a functional volume in such a way that the new mean value is identical to the mean intensity value of a reference volume. Mean intensity adjustment is not strictly necessary since modern scanners keep a rather constant mean signal level over time. Under this condition, mean intensity adjustment may even produce a negative effect by reducing true activation effects. If, for example, large parts of the brain activate during a main condition as compared to a rest condition, the mean signal level is higher during active periods and a mean intensity adjustment step will "correct" this. A plot of the mean signal level over time might be, however, helpful to identify problems of the scanner quality, especially when such a plot shows "spikes," i.e., strong signal decreases (or increases) at isolated time points.

3.2.2.7 Motion Correction Within and Across Runs

A scanning session typically consists of a series of runs. In such a situation, head movements may occur not only within runs but also between runs. A simple approach to align all functional volumes of all runs of a scanning session with each other consists of specifying the same reference volume for all runs. If a session consists, for example, of three runs, all functional volumes could be aligned to the middle volume of the second run. Since functional data is often aligned with a 3D anatomical dataset recorded in the same session, it is recommended to choose a functional volume as a reference, which is recorded just before (or after) the anatomical dataset. Note, however, that across run motion correction works only if the slice positions are specified identically in all runs. If across-run motion correction is not possible, each run can also be individually coregistered to a common 3D anatomical dataset.

3.3   Statistical Analysis of Functional Data

Statistical data analysis aims at identifying those brain regions exhibiting increased or decreased responses in specific experimental conditions as compared to other (e.g., control) conditions. Due to the presence of physiological and physical noise fluctuations, observed differences between conditions might occur simply by chance. Note that measurements provide only a *sample* of data but we are interested in true effects in the under-lying *population*. At the level of individual functional scans, time points are treated as subjects, i.e., sample corresponds to the obtained repeated measurements at every TR and "population" refers to the estimated but unobservable true condition effects within the subject. In multi-subject (group) analyses, sample usually refers to estimated effects obtained in each subject and population refers to all people from which the sample of subjects has been drawn. Statistical data analysis protects from wrongly accepting effects in small sample datasets by explicitly assessing the effect of measurement variability (noise fluctuations) on estimated condition effects: If it is very unlikely that an observed effect is solely the result of noise fluctuations, it is assumed that the observed effect reflects a true difference between conditions in the population. In standard single-subject statistical fMRI analyses, this assessment is usually performed independently for the time course of each voxel (univariate analysis). The obtained statistical values, one for each voxel, form a three-dimensional *statistical map*. In more complex analyses, each voxel contains one or

more statistical values reflecting *contrasts* esti-mating effects that compare multiple conditions. Since independent testing at each voxel increases the chance to find some voxels with significant differences between conditions simply due to noise fluctuations, further adjustments for *multiple comparisons* need to be made.

3.3.1   From Image Subtraction to Statistical Comparison

Figure 14 shows two fMRI time courses obtained from two different brain areas of an experiment with two conditions, a control condition ("rest") and a main condition ("stim"). Each condition has been measured several times.[1] How can we assess whether the response values are higher in the main condition than in the control condition? One approach consists of subtracting the mean value of the "rest" condition, $\bar{X}_1$, from the mean value of the "stim" condition, $\bar{X}_2$: $d = \bar{X}_2 - \bar{X}_1$. Note that in this example one would obtain the same mean values in both conditions and, thus, the same difference in cases (a) and (b). Despite the fact that the means are identical in both cases, the difference in case (b) seems to be more "trust-worthy" than the difference in case (a) because the measured values exhibit less fluctuations; that is, they *vary less* in case (b) than in case (a).

Statistical data analysis goes beyond simple subtraction by taking the amount of variability of the measured data points into account. Statistical analysis essentially asks how likely it is to obtain a certain effect (e.g., difference of condition means) in a data sample if there is no effect at the population level, i.e., how likely it is that an observed sample effect is solely the result of noise fluctuations. This is formalized by the *null hypothesis* stating that there is no effect, e.g., no true difference between conditions in the popula-tion. In the case of comparing the two means μ_1 and μ_2, the null hypothesis can be formulated as $H_0: \mu_1 = \mu_2$. Assuming the null hypothesis, it can

---

[1] Note that in a real experiment, one would not just present once the control and main condition as in Fig. 14, but sev-eral "on-off" cycles; without repetitions, task-related response might not be distinguishable from potential low-frequency drifts (see Sect. 3.2.2).

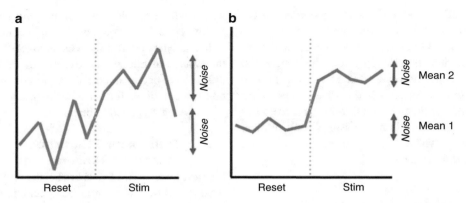

Fig. 14 Principle of statistical data analysis. An experiment with two conditions ("stim" and "rest") has been performed. (**a**) Time course obtained in area 1. (**b**) Time course obtained in area 2. Calculation and subtraction of mean 1 ("rest" condition) from mean 2 ("stim" condition) leads to the same result in (**a, b**). In a statistical analysis, the estimated effect (mean difference) is related to its uncertainty, which is estimated by the variability of the measured values within conditions. Since the variance within the two conditions is smaller in (**b**) than in (**a**), the estimated effect is more likely to correspond to a true difference in (**b**) than in (**a**)

be calculated how likely it is that an observed sample effect would have occurred simply by chance. This requires knowledge about the amount of noise fluctuations (and its distribution), which can be estimated from the data. By incorporating the number of data points and the variability of measurements, statistical data analysis allows to *estimate the uncertainty of effects* (e.g., mean differences) in data samples. If an effect is large enough so that it is very unlikely that it has occurred simply by chance (e.g., the probability is less than $p = 0.05$), one *rejects* the null hypothesis and *accepts* the *alternative hypothesis* stating that there exists a true effect in the population. Note that the decision to accept or reject the null hypothesis is based on a probability value which has been accepted by the scientific community ($p < 0.05$). Since the decision to accept or reject the null hypothesis is based on a probability value, a statistical analysis does not *prove* the existence of an effect; it only suggests to accept in an effect if it is very unlikely that the observed effect is the result of noise fluctuations. Note that a probability of $p = 0.05$ means that if we would repeat the experiment 100 times we would accept the alternative hypothesis in about 5 cases even if there would be no true effect in the population. Since the chosen probability value thus reflects the likelihood of wrongly rejecting

the null hypothesis, it is also called *error probability*. The error probability is also referred to as the *significance level* and denoted with the Greek letter α. If one would know that there is no effect in the population, but one would incorrectly reject the null hypothesis in a particular data sample, a "false-positive" decision would be made (type 1 or α error, "false alarm"). Since a false-positive error depends on the chosen error probability, it is also referred to as alpha error. If one would know that there is a true effect in the population but one would fail to reject the null hypothesis in a sample, a "false-negative" decision would be made, i.e., one would miss a true effect (type 2 or β error).

3.3.2 *T*-Test and Correlation Analysis

The uncertainty of an effect is estimated by calculating the variance of the noise fluctuations from the data. For the case of comparing two mean values, the observed difference of the means is related to the variability of that difference resulting in a *t* statistic:

$$t = \frac{\overline{X}_2 - \overline{X}_1}{\hat{\sigma}_{\overline{X}_2 - \overline{X}_1}}$$

The numerator contains the calculated mean difference while the denominator contains the estimate of the expected variability, the *standard error* of the mean difference. Estimation of the standard error $\hat{\sigma}_{\bar{X}_2 - \bar{X}_1}$ involves pooling of the variances obtained within both conditions. Since we observe a high variability in case (a) of the example data (Fig. 14), we will obtain a small t value. Due to the lower variability of the data points in (b), we will obtain a larger t value in this case (Fig. 14). The higher the t value, the less likely it is that the observed mean difference is just the result of noise fluctuations. It is obvious that measurement of many data points allows a more robust estimation of this probability than the measurement of only a few data points. The error probability p can be calculated exactly from the obtained t value using the incomplete beta function $I_x(a, b)$ and the number of measured data points N:

$$p = I_{\frac{N-2}{N-2+t^2}}\left(\frac{N-2}{2}, \frac{1}{2}\right)$$

If the computed error probability falls below the standard value ($p < 0.05$), the alternative hypothesis is accepted stating that the observed mean difference exists in the population from which the data points have been drawn (i.e., measured). In that case, one also says that the two means differ *significantly*. Assuming in our example that the obtained p value falls below 0.05 in case (b) but not in case (a), we would only infer for brain area 2 that the "stim" condition differs significantly from the "rest" condition.

The described mean comparison method is not the ideal approach to compare responses between different conditions since this approach is unable to capture the gradual rise and fall of fMRI responses, e.g., when a voxel exhibits a strong response to a trial of condition B after having not responded strongly to a preceding trial of condition A. As long as the temporal sampling resolution is low (volume TR >4 s), the mean of different conditions can be calculated easily because transitions of expected responses from different conditions occur within a single time point (Fig. 15). If the temporal resolution is high, the expected fMRI responses change gradually from one condition to the next due to the slug-

gishness of the hemodynamic response (Fig. 15, TR = 1 s). In this case, time points in the "transitional zone" cannot be assigned easily to different conditions. Without special treatment (e.g., dropping transitional data points), the mean response can no longer be easily computed for each condition. As a consequence, the statistical power to detect mean differences may be substantially reduced, especially for short blocks and events.

This problem does not occur when *correlation analysis* is used since this method allows explicitly incorporating the gradual increase and decrease of the expected BOLD signal. The predicted ideal (noise-free) time courses in Fig. 15 can be used as the *reference function* in a correlation analysis. At each voxel, the time course of the reference function is compared with the time course of the measured data from a voxel by calculating the *correlation coefficient r*, indicating the strength of covariation:

$$r = \frac{\sum_{t=1}^{N}(X_t - \bar{X})(Y_t - \bar{Y})}{\sqrt{\sum_{t=1}^{N}(X_t - \bar{X})^2 \sum_{t=1}^{N}(Y_t - \bar{Y})^2}}$$

Index t runs over time points (t for "time") identifying pairs of temporally corresponding values from the reference (X_t) and data (Y_t) time courses. In the numerator the mean of the reference and data time course is subtracted from the respective value of each data pair and the two differences are multiplied. The resulting value is the sum of these cross products, which will be high if the two time courses *covary*, i.e., if the values of a pair are both often above and below their respective mean. The term in the denominator normalizes the covariation term in the numerator so that the correlation coefficient lies in a range of -1 and $+1$. A value of $+1$ indicates that the reference time course and the data time course go up and down in exactly the same way, while a value of -1 indicates that the two time courses run in opposite direction (anticorrelation). A correlation value of 0 indicates that the two time courses do not covary, i.e., the value in one time course cannot be used to predict the corresponding value in the other time course.

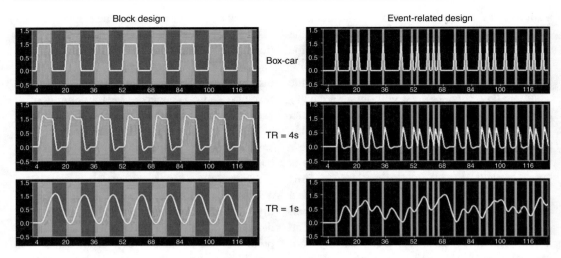

Fig. 15 Calculation of expected fMRI signals for a block and event-related design. The horizontal axis of each plot represents time (data points). The vertical axis represents the amplitude of the modeled fMRI response. The blue vertical segments correspond to intervals of a single main stimulation condition; the grey segments correspond to a control condition. White curves show predicted BOLD responses. The plots in the upper row depict time courses, which do not take into account the delayed hemodynamic response profile ("box-car"). The white curves in the other plots represent the expected time courses after application of a standard hemodynamic response function (two-gamma function) for a temporal resolution (volume TR) of 4 s (middle row) and 1 s (lower row). Correlation analysis is able to capture the gradual increase and decrease of expected time courses for short TRs while it is impossible to unambiguously categorize time points as belonging to stimulation vs. baseline conditions in the context of a *t*-test

While the statistical logic is the same in correlation analysis as described for mean comparisons, the null hypothesis now corresponds to the statement that the population correlation coefficient ρ equals zero ($H0: \rho = 0$). By including the number of data points N, the error probability can be computed assessing how likely it is that an observed correlation coefficient would occur solely due to noise fluctuations in the signal time course. If this probability falls below 0.05, the alternative hypothesis is accepted stating that there is indeed significant covariation between the reference function and the data time course. Since the reference function is the result of a model assuming different response strengths in the two conditions (e.g., "rest" and "stim"), a significant correlation coefficient indicates that the two conditions lead indeed to different mean activation levels in the respective voxel or brain area. The statistical assessment can be performed also by converting an observed r value into a corresponding t value, $t = r\sqrt{N-2} / \sqrt{1-r^2}$.

3.3.3 The General Linear Model

The described *t*-test for assessing the difference of two mean values is a special case of an analysis of a *qualitative (categorical) independent variable*. A qualitative variable is defined by discrete levels, e.g., "stimulus on" vs. "stimulus off" or "male" vs. "female." If a design contains more than two levels, a more general method such as analysis of variance (ANOVA) needs to be used, which can be considered as an extension of the *t*-test to more than two levels and to more than one experimental factor. The described correlation coefficient on the other hand is suited for the analysis of *quantitative independent variables*. A quantitative variable may be defined by any gradual time course. If more than one reference time course has to be considered, *multiple regression analysis* can be used, which can be considered as an extension of the simple linear correlation analysis. The *general linear model*[2] (GLM) is mathematically identical to a multiple regression analysis but stresses its suitability for both multiple qualitative and multiple quantitative variables. The GLM is suited to implement any parametric statistical test with one dependent variable, including any factorial ANOVA design as well as designs with a mixture of qualitative and quantitative variables (covariance analysis, ANCOVA). Because of its flexibility to incorporate multiple quantitative and qualitative independent variables, the GLM has become the core tool for fMRI data analysis after its introduction into the neuroimaging community by Friston et al. (1994, 1995). The following sections briefly describe the mathematical background of the GLM in the context of fMRI data analysis; a comprehensive treatment of the GLM can be found in the standard statistical literature, e.g., Draper and Smith (1998) and Kutner et al. (2005).

From the perspective of multiple regression analysis, the GLM aims to "explain" or "predict" the variation of a dependent variable in terms of a *linear combination* (weighted sum) of several reference functions. The dependent variable corresponds to the observed fMRI time course of a voxel and the reference functions correspond to time courses of expected (noise-free) fMRI responses for different conditions of the experimental paradigm. The reference functions are also called *predictors*, *regressors*, *explanatory variables*, *covariates*, or *basis functions*. A set of specified predictors forms the *design matrix*, also called the *model*. A predictor time course is typically obtained by convolution of a "box-car" (square-wave) time course with a standard hemo-

dynamic response function (Figs. 8 and 15). A box-car time course is usually defined by setting values to 1 at time points at which the modeled condition is defined ("on") and 0 at all other time points.

Each predictor time course X_i is multiplied by an associated coefficient or *beta weight* b_i that quantifies the contribution of a predictor in explaining variance in the voxel time course y. The voxel time course y is modeled as the sum of the defined predictors, each multiplied with the associated beta weight b. Since this linear combination will not perfectly explain the data due to noise fluctuations in the data, an error value e is added to the GLM system of equations with n data points and p predictors:

$$
\begin{aligned}
y_1 &= b_0 + b_1 X_{11} + \cdots + b_p X_{1p} + e_1 \\
y_2 &= b_0 + b_1 X_{21} + \cdots + b_p X_{2p} + e_2 \\
&\vdots \qquad\qquad \ddots \qquad\quad \vdots \\
y_n &= b_0 + b_1 X_{n1} + \cdots + b_p X_{np} + e_n
\end{aligned}
$$

The y variable on the left side corresponds to the data, i.e., the measured time course of a single voxel. Time runs from top to bottom; that is, y_1 is the measured value at time point 1 and y_2 the measured value at time point 2. The voxel time course (left column) is "explained" by the terms on the right side of the equation. The first column on the right side corresponds to the first beta weight b_0. The corresponding predictor time course X_0 has a value of 1 for each time point and is, thus, also called "constant." Since multiplication with 1 does not alter the value of b_0, this predictor time course (X_0) does not explicitly appear in the equation. After estimation (fitting the GLM, see below), the value of b_0 typically represents the signal level of the baseline condition and is also called intercept. While its absolute value is not very informative in the context of fMRI data, it is important to include the constant predictor in a design matrix since it allows the other predictors to model small condition-related fluctuations as increases or decreases relative to the baseline signal level. The other predictors on

---

[2]In the fMRI literature, the term "general linear model" refers to its univariate version where "univariate" refers to the number of dependent variables (one). In its general form, the general linear model has been defined for multiple dependent variables; that is, it encompasses tests as general as multivariate covariance analysis (MANCOVA).

the right side model the expected time courses of different conditions. For multifactorial designs, predictors may be defined coding combinations of condition levels in order to estimate main and interaction effects. The beta weight of a predictor scales the associated predictor time course and reflects (if not correlated strongly with other predictors) the unique contribution of that predictor in explaining part of the variance in the voxel time course. While the exact interpretation of beta values depends on the details of the design matrix, a large positive (negative) beta weight typically indicates that the voxel exhibits strong activation (deactivation) during the modeled experimental condition relative to baseline. All beta values together characterize a voxel's "preference" for one or more experimental conditions. The last column in the system of equations contains error values, also called *residuals*, *prediction errors*, or *noise*. These error values quantify the deviation of the measured voxel time course from the predicted time course.

The GLM system of equations may be expressed elegantly using matrix notation. For this purpose, the voxel time course, the beta values, and the residuals are represented as vectors, and the set of predictors as a matrix:

$$\begin{bmatrix} y_1 \\ \vdots \\ \vdots \\ y_n \end{bmatrix} = \begin{bmatrix} 1 & X_{11} & \cdots & \cdots & X_{1p} \\ \vdots & \vdots & \vdots & \vdots & \vdots \\ \vdots & \vdots & \vdots & \vdots & \vdots \\ 1 & X_{n1} & \cdots & \cdots & X_{np} \end{bmatrix} \begin{bmatrix} b_0 \\ b_1 \\ \vdots \\ b_p \end{bmatrix} + \begin{bmatrix} e_1 \\ e_2 \\ \vdots \\ e_n \end{bmatrix}$$

Representing the indicated vectors and matrix with single letters, we obtain this simple form of the GLM system of equations:

$$\mathbf{y} = \mathbf{Xb} + \mathbf{e}$$

In this notation, the matrix $\mathbf{X}$ represents the design matrix containing the predictor time courses as column vectors. The beta values now appear in a separate vector $\mathbf{b}$. The term $\mathbf{Xb}$ indicates matrix-vector multiplication. Figure 16 shows a graphical representation of the

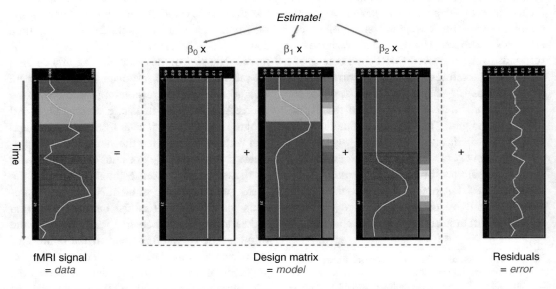

Fig. 16 Graphical display of a general linear model. Time is running from top to bottom. Left side shows observed voxel time course (data). The model (design matrix) consists of three predictors, the constant and two main predictors (middle part). Filled green and red rectangles depict stimulation time while the white curves depict expected BOLD responses. Expected responses are also shown in graphical view using a black-to-white color range (right side of each predictor plot). Beta values have to be estimated (top) to scale the expected responses (predictors) in such a way that their weighted sum predicts the data values as good as possible (in the least squares sense, see text). Unexplained fluctuations (residuals, error) are shown on the right side

GLM. Time courses of the signal, predictors, and residuals have been arranged in column form with time running from top to bottom as in the system of equations.

Given the data $\mathbf{y}$ and the design matrix $\mathbf{X}$, the GLM fitting procedure must find a set of beta values explaining the data as good as possible. The time course values $\hat{\mathbf{y}}$ predicted by the model are obtained by the linear combination of the predictors:

$$\hat{\mathbf{y}} = \mathbf{Xb}$$

A good fit would be achieved with beta values leading to predicted values $\hat{\mathbf{y}}$ that are as close as possible to the measured values $\mathbf{y}$. By rearranging the system of equations, it is evident that a good prediction of the data implies small error values:

$$\mathbf{e} = \mathbf{y} - \mathbf{Xb}$$
$$= \mathbf{y} - \hat{\mathbf{y}}$$

An intuitive idea would be to find those beta values minimizing the sum of error values. Since the error values contain both positive and negative values (and because of additional statistical considerations), the GLM procedure does not estimate beta values minimizing the sum of error values, but finds those beta values *minimizing the sum of squared error values*:

$$\mathbf{e'e} = \left(\mathbf{y} - \mathbf{Xb}\right)' \left(\mathbf{y} - \mathbf{Xb}\right) \rightarrow \min$$

The term $\mathbf{e'e}$ is the vector notation for the sum of squares $\left(\sum_{t=1}^{N} e_t^2\right)$. The apostrophe symbol denotes transposition of a vector (or matrix); that is, a row vector version of $\mathbf{e}$ is multiplied by a column vector version of $\mathbf{e}$ resulting in the sum of squared error values e_t. The optimal beta weights minimizing the squared error values (the "least squares estimates") are obtained non-iteratively by the following equation:

$$\mathbf{b} = \left(\mathbf{X'X}\right)^{-1} \mathbf{X'y}$$

The term in brackets contains a matrix-matrix multiplication of the transposed design matrix $\mathbf{X'}$ and the non-transposed design matrix $\mathbf{X}$. This term results in a square matrix with a number of rows and columns corresponding to the number of predictors. Each cell of the $\mathbf{X'X}$ matrix contains the scalar product of two predictor vectors. The scalar product is obtained by summing all products of corresponding entries of two vectors corresponding to the (non-mean normalized) calculation of covariance. This $\mathbf{X'X}$ matrix, thus, corresponds to the (non-mean normalized) predictor variance-covariance matrix.

The resulting square matrix is inverted as denoted by the "−1" symbol. The resulting matrix $\left(\mathbf{X'X}\right)^{-1}$ plays an essential role not only for the calculation of beta values but also for testing the significance of contrasts (see below). The remaining term on the right side, $\mathbf{X'y}$, evaluates to a vector containing as many elements as predictors. Each element of this vector is the scalar product (non-mean-normalized covariance term) of a predictor time course with the observed voxel time course.

An important property of the least squares estimation method (following from the independence assumption of the errors, see below) is that the variance of the measured time course can be decomposed into the sum of the variance of the predicted values (model-related variance) and the variance of the residuals:

$$\mathrm{Var}\left(\mathbf{y}\right) = \mathrm{Var}\left(\hat{\mathbf{y}}\right) + \mathrm{Var}\left(\mathbf{e}\right).$$

Since the variance of the voxel time course is fixed, minimizing the error variance by least squares corresponds to maximizing the variance of the values explained by the model. The square of the *multiple correlation coefficient R* provides a measure of the proportion of the variance of the data which can be explained by a specified model:

$$R^2 = \frac{\mathrm{Var}\left(\hat{\mathbf{y}}\right)}{\mathrm{Var}\left(\mathbf{y}\right)} = \frac{\mathrm{Var}\left(\hat{\mathbf{y}}\right)}{\mathrm{Var}\left(\hat{\mathbf{y}}\right) + \mathrm{Var}\left(\mathbf{e}\right)}$$

The values of the multiple correlation coefficient vary between 0 (no variance explained) and 1 (all variance explained by the model). A coefficient of $R = 0.7$, for example, corresponds to an explained variance of 49% (0.7). An alternative way to calculate the multiple correlation coefficient consists of computing a standard correlation coefficient between the predicted values and the observed values: $R = r_{\hat{y}y}$. This equation offers another view on the meaning of the multiple correlation coefficient quantifying the interrelationship (correlation) of the *combined* set of optimally weighted predictor variables with the observed time course.

3.3.3.1 GLM Diagnostics

Note that if the design matrix (model) does not contain all relevant predictors, condition-related increases or decreases in the voxel time course will be explained by the error values instead of the model. It is, therefore, important that the design matrix is constructed with all expected effects, which may also include reference functions not related to experimental conditions, for example, estimated motion parameters or drift predictors if not removed during preprocessing (see Sect. 3.2.2). In case that all expected effects are properly modeled, the residuals should reflect only "pure" noise fluctuations. If some effects are not (correctly) modeled, a plot of the residuals may show low-frequency fluctuations instead of a stationary noise time course around zero. A visualization of the residuals (for selected voxels or regions of interest) is, thus, a good diagnostic to assess whether the design matrix has been defined properly.

3.3.3.2 GLM Significance Tests

The multiple correlation coefficient is an important measure of the "goodness of fit" of a GLM. In order to test whether a specified model significantly explains variance in a voxel time course, a F statistic can be calculated for a R value with $p - 1$ degrees of freedom in the numerator and $n - p$ degrees of freedom in the denominator:

$$F_{n-1,n-p} = \frac{R^2(n-p)}{(1-R^2)(p-1)}$$

An error probability value p can then be obtained for the calculated F statistics. A high F value (p value <0.05) indicates that the experimental conditions as a whole have a significant

modulatory effect on the data time course (omnibus effect).

While the overall F statistic answers the question whether the specified model significantly explains a voxel's time course, it does not allow to assess which individual conditions differ significantly from each other. Comparisons between conditions can be formulated as *contrasts*, which are linear combinations of beta values corresponding to null hypotheses. To test, for example, whether activation in a single condition 1 deviates significantly from baseline, the null hypothesis would be that there is no effect in the population, i.e., H_0: $b_1 = 0$. To test whether activation in condition 1 is significantly different from activation in condition 2, the null hypothesis would state that the beta values of the two conditions would be equal, H_0: $b_1 = b_2$ or H_0: $(+1)b_1 + (-1)b_2 = 0$. To test whether the mean of condition 1 and condition 2 differs from the beta value of condition 3, the following contrast could be specified: H_0: $(b_1 + b_2)/2 = b_3$ or H_0: $(+1)b_1 + (+1)b_2 + (-2)b_3 = 0$. The values used to multiply the respective beta values are often written as a *contrast vector* **c**. In the latter example,[3] the contrast vector would be written as **c** = [+1 +1 −2]. Using matrix notation, the linear combination defining a contrast can be written as the scalar product of contrast vector **c** and beta vector **b**. The null hypothesis can then be simply described as $\mathbf{c'b} = 0$. For any number of predictors k, such a contrast can be tested with the following t statistic with $n - p$ degrees of freedom:

$$t = \frac{\mathbf{c'b}}{\sqrt{\mathrm{Var}(\mathbf{e})\mathbf{c'}(\mathbf{X'X})^{-1}\mathbf{c}}}$$

The numerator of this equation contains the described scalar product of the contrast and beta vector. The denominator defines the standard error of $\mathbf{c'b}$, i.e., the variability of the estimate

---

[3] Note that the constant term is treated as a confound and it is not included in contrast vectors; that is, it is implicitly assumed that b_0 is multiplied by 0 in all contrasts. To include the constant explicitly, each contrast vector must be expanded by one entry at the beginning or end.

due to noise fluctuations. The standard error depends on the variance of the residuals Var(**e**) as well as on the design matrix **X**. With the known degrees of freedom, a t value for a specific contrast can be converted in an error probability value p using the equation shown earlier. Note that the null hypotheses above were formulated as $\mathbf{c'b} = 0$ implying a *two-sided* alternative hypothesis, i.e., H_a: $\mathbf{c'b} \neq 0$. For one-sided alternative hypotheses, e.g., H_a: $b_1 > b_2$, the obtained p value from a two-sided test can be simply divided by 2 to get the p value for the one-sided test. If this p value is smaller than 0.05 and if the t value is positive (since b_1 is assumed to be larger than b_2), the null hypothesis may be rejected.

3.3.3.3 Conjunction Analysis

Experimental research questions often lead to specific hypotheses, which can best be tested by the *conjunction* of two or more contrasts. As an example, it might be interesting to test with contrast $\mathbf{c}_1$ whether condition 2 leads to significantly higher activity than condition 1 *and* with contrast $\mathbf{c}_2$ whether condition 3 leads to significantly higher activity than condition 2. This question could be tested with the following conjunction contrast:

$$\mathbf{c}_1 \wedge \mathbf{c}_2 = \begin{bmatrix} -1 & +1 & 0 \end{bmatrix} \wedge \begin{bmatrix} 0 & -1 & +1 \end{bmatrix}.$$

Note that a logical "and" operation is defined for Boolean values (true/false) but that t values associated with individual contrasts can assume any real value. An appropriate way to implement a logical "and" operation for conjunctions of contrasts with continuous statistical values is to use a minimum operation; that is, the significance level of the conjunction contrast is identical to the significance level of the contrast with the smallest t value: $t_{\mathbf{c}_1 \wedge \mathbf{c}_2} = \min\left(t_{\mathbf{c}_1}, t_{\mathbf{c}_2}\right)$. For more details about conjunction testing, see Nichols et al. (2005).

3.3.3.4 Multicollinear Design Matrices

Multicollinearity exists when predictors of the design matrix are highly intercorrelated. To assess multicollinearity, pairwise correlations between predictors are not sufficient. A better way to detect multicollinearity is to regress each predictor variable on all the other predictor variables and examine the resulting R^2 values. Perfect or total multicollinearity occurs when a predictor of the design matrix is a linear function of one or more other predictors, i.e., when predictors are linearly dependent on each other. While in this case solutions for the GLM system of equations still exist, there is no *unique* solution for the beta values. From a mathematical perspective of the GLM, the square matrix $\mathbf{X'X}$ becomes *singular*, i.e., it loses (at least) one dimension, and is no longer invertible in case that **X** exhibits perfect multicollinearity. Matrix inversion is required to calculate the essential term $(\mathbf{X'X})^{-1}$ used for computing beta values and standard error values for contrasts (see above). Fortunately, special methods, including singular value decomposition (SVD), allow obtaining (pseudo-) inverses for singular (rank deficient) matrices. Note, however, that in this case the absolute values of beta weights may be difficult to interpret and statistical hypothesis tests must meet special restrictions.

In fMRI design matrices, multicollinearity occurs if all conditions are modeled as predictors in the design matrix including the baseline (rest, control) condition. Without the baseline condition, multicollinearity is avoided, and beta weights are obtained which are easily interpretable. As an example, consider the case of two main conditions and a rest condition. If we would not include the rest condition (recommended), the design matrix would not be multicollinear and the two beta weights b_1 and b_2 would be interpretable as increase or decrease of activity relative to the baseline signal level modeled by the constant term (Fig. 17, right). Contrasts could be specified to test single beta weights; for example, the contrast $\mathbf{c} = [1\ 0]$ would test whether condition 1 leads to significant (de)activation. Furthermore, the two main conditions could be compared with the contrast $\mathbf{c} = [-1\ 1]$, which would test whether condition 2 leads to significantly more or less

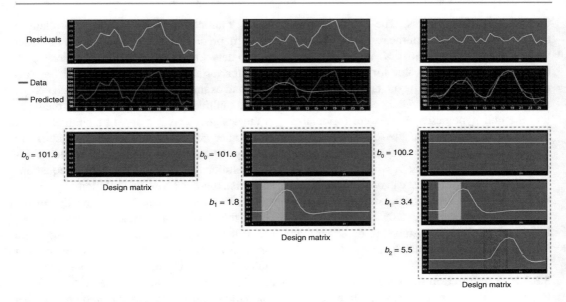

Fig. 17 Three GLMs fitting the same data with different design matrices. Top row shows residuals, and second row predicted (green) and observed (blue) voxel time course. The design matrix on the left contains only one predictor, the constant term. The estimated beta weight (b_0) scales the constant term to the mean signal level. The design matrix in the middle adds a predictor for "green" main condition. The estimated beta weights (b_0, b_1) scale the predictors and the weighted sum explains more variance than the first model, but residual variance is still high. The third model (right) adds a predictor for "red" main condition. The estimated beta weights (b_0, b_1, b_2) scale the predictors and weighted sum now explains all task-related signal fluctuations. The residuals reflect now only noise. The example highlights the importance of modeling all known effects in the design matrix

activation than condition 1. If the design matrix would include a predictor for the rest condition, we would obtain perfect multicollinearity and the matrix $\mathbf{X'X}$ would be singular. Using a pseudo-inverse or singular value decomposition (SVD) approach, we would obtain now three beta values (plus the constant), one for the rest condition, one for main condition 1, and one for main condition 2. While the values of beta weights might not be interpretable, correct inferences of contrasts can be obtained if an additional restriction is met, typically that the sum of the contrast coefficients equals 0. To test whether main condition 1 differs significantly from the rest condition, the contrast $\mathbf{c} = [-1\ +1\ 0]$ would now be used. The contrast $\mathbf{c} = [0\ -1\ +1]$ would be used to test whether condition 2 leads to more or less activation than condition 1.

3.3.3.5 GLM Assumptions

Given a correct model (design matrix), the standard estimation procedure of the GLM—ordinary least squares (OLS)—operates correctly only under the following assumptions. The population error values ε must have an expected value of zero and constant variance at each time point i:

$$E[\varepsilon_i] = 0$$

$$\mathrm{Var}[\varepsilon_i] = \sigma^2$$

Furthermore, the error values are assumed to be uncorrelated:

$$\mathrm{cov}(\varepsilon_i, \varepsilon_j) = 0 \quad \text{for all } i \neq j$$

To justify the use of t and F distributions in hypothesis tests, errors are further assumed to be normally distributed:

$$\varepsilon_i \sim N(0, \sigma^2)$$

In summary, errors are assumed to be normal independent and identically distributed (often abbreviated as "normal i.i.d." or IID). Under these assumptions, the solution obtained by the least squares method is optimal in the sense that it provides the most efficient unbiased estimation of the beta values. While the OLS approach is robust with respect to small violations, assumptions should be checked. In the context of fMRI measurements, the assumption of uncorrelated error values requires special attention.

3.3.3.6 Correction for Serial Correlations

In fMRI data, one typically observes *serial correlations*; that is, high values are followed more likely by high values than low values and vice versa. Assessment of these serial correlations is not performed on the original voxel time course but on the time course of the residuals since serial correlations in the recorded signal are expected to some extent from slow task-related fluctuations. Task-unrelated serial correlations most likely occur because data points are measured in rapid succession; that is, they are also observed when scanning phantoms. Likely sources of temporal correlations are physical and physiological noise components such as hardware-related low-frequency drifts, oscillatory fluctuations related to respiration and cardiac pulsation, and residual head motion artifacts. Serial correlations violate the assumption of uncorrelated errors (see section above). Fortunately, the beta values estimated by the GLM are correct estimates (unbiased) even in the presence of serial correlations. The standard errors of the betas are biased, however, leading to "inflated" test statistics; that is, t or F values are higher than they should be. This can be explained by considering that the presence of serial correlations (serial dependence) reduces the true number of independent observations (effective degrees of freedom) that will, thus, be lower than the nominal number of observations. Without correction, the degrees of freedom are systematically overestimated leading to an underestimation of the error variance resulting in inflated statistical values; that is, t or F values are too high. It is, thus, necessary to correct for serial correlations to obtain valid error probabilities. Serial correlations can be corrected using several approaches. In *pre-whitening*

approaches, autocorrelation is first estimated and removed from the data; the pre-whitened data can then be analyzed with a standard OLS GLM solution. In *pre-coloring* approaches (e.g., Friston et al. 1995), a strong autocorrelation structure is imposed on the data by temporal smoothing and degrees of freedom are adjusted according to the imposed (known) autocorrelation. The pre-coloring (temporal smoothing) operation acts, however, as a low-pass filter, and may weaken experimentally induced signals of interest and is thus not the preferred method. The pre-whitening approach can be expressed in terms of a more powerful estimation procedure than OLS called *generalized least squares* (GLS, Searle et al. 1992). As opposed to the OLS method, GLS works correctly also in case that error values exhibit correlations or when error variances are not homogeneous. Note, however, that this more powerful estimation approach only provides correct results in case that the true (population) variances and covariances of the error values are known. With the known error covariance matrix $\mathbf{V}$, the betas and their (co-)variances can be calculated with GLS as follows:

$$\mathbf{b} = \left(\mathbf{X}'\mathbf{V}^{-1}\mathbf{X} \right)^{-1} \mathbf{X}'\mathbf{V}^{-1}\mathbf{y}$$

$$\mathrm{cov}\left(\mathbf{b} \right) = \left(\mathbf{X}'\mathbf{V}^{-1}\mathbf{X} \right)^{-1}$$

With the obtained b values and their covariances, any contrast can then be assessed statistically as described above for the OLS method. When comparing the GLS solution with the OLS solution it is evident that the inverse of the population error covariance matrix $\mathbf{V}^{-1}$ is needed to properly treat the effect of covariance of the errors on the parameter estimates (betas and their covariances). Note also that when setting $\mathbf{V}$ as a diagonal matrix (entries outside the main diagonal are zero, i.e., no covariation of errors) with equal variance values (all values of the main diagonal are the same, e.g., 1), the GLS equation reduces to the OLS solution; that is, the $\mathbf{V}^{-1}$ term vanishes.

Since the population covariance matrix of the error values $\mathbf{V}$ is usually not known, it needs to be estimated from the data itself. Since there are too many degrees of freedom (number of time points squared: n^2), $\mathbf{V}$ cannot be estimated for the general case of arbitrary covariance matrices. It is, however, often possible to estimate $\mathbf{V}$ for special cases where only some parameters need to be estimated. The two most important special cases in the context of fMRI data analysis are the treatment of serial correlations (see below) and the treatment of unequal variances when integrating data from different subjects in the context of mixed-effects group analyses.

A simple pre-whitening procedure was developed (Cochrane and Orcutt 1949; Bullmore et al. 1996) independently from the GLS approach but can be shown to be identical to a GLS solution. The procedure assumes that the errors follow a first-order autoregressive, or AR(1), process. After calculation of a GLM using OLS, the amount of serial correlation a_1 is estimated using pairs of successive residual values (e_t, e_{t+1}); that is, the residual time course is correlated with itself shifted by one time point (lag = 1). In the second step, the estimated serial correlation is removed from the measured voxel time course by calculating the transformed time course $y_t^n = y_{t+1} - a_1 \cdot y_t$. The superscript "$n$" indicates the values of the new, adjusted time course. The same calculation is also applied to each predictor time course resulting in an adjusted design matrix $\mathbf{X}^n$. In the third step, the GLM is recomputed using the adjusted voxel time course and adjusted design matrix resulting in correct standard errors for beta estimates and, thus, correct significance levels for contrasts (of course under the assumption that the AR(1) model is correct). If autocorrelation is not sufficiently reduced in the new residuals, the procedure can be repeated. If performed using the GLS approach, the first step is identical to the Cochrane-Orcutt method; that is, OLS is used to fit the GLM and the obtained residuals are used to estimate the value of the AR(1) term. The adjustment of the time course y_t and the design matrix described above need, however, not be performed explicitly since these adjustments are handled implicitly in the next step by using a $\mathbf{V}^{-1}$ term in the GLS equations that contains values in the off-

diagonal elements derived from the estimated serial correlation term.

While a AR(1) autocorrelation model substantially reduces serial correlations in fMRI data, better results are obtained when using a AR(2) model; that is, both first-order and second-order autocorrelation terms should be estimated and used to construct the error covariance matrix $\mathbf{V}$ for GLS estimation. Since serial correlations differ across voxels, serial correlation correction should be performed separately for each voxel time course as opposed to the (also used) estimation of serial correlation values from multiple averaged (neighboring) voxel time courses. An AR(2) serial correlation model applied separately for each voxel time course has been shown to be the most accurate approach to treat serial correlations when compared to other models (Lenoski et al. 2008). When using fast sampling with volume TR values below 1 s, higher order autocorrelation terms might be needed to remove serial correlations.

3.3.4   Creation of Statistical Maps

The statistical analysis steps were described for a single voxel's time course since standard statistical methods are performed independently for each voxel (univariate "voxel-wise" analysis). Since a typical fMRI dataset contains several hundred thousand voxels, a statistical analysis is performed independently hundred thousand times. Running a GLM, for example, results in a set of estimated beta values attached to each voxel. A specified contrast $\mathbf{c}'\mathbf{b}_v$ will be performed using the same contrast vector $\mathbf{c}$ for each voxel v, but it will use a voxel's vector of beta values $\mathbf{b}_v$ (and the voxel's error term) to obtain voxel-specific t and p values. Statistical test results for individual voxels are integrated in a 3D dataset called a *statistical map*. To visualize a statistical map, the obtained values, e.g., contrast t values, can be shown at the location of each voxel replacing anatomical intensity values shown as default. As a further useful condition, the statistical values are often only shown for those voxels exceeding a specified *statistical threshold*. This allows visualizing anatomical information in large parts of the brain while statistical information is shown

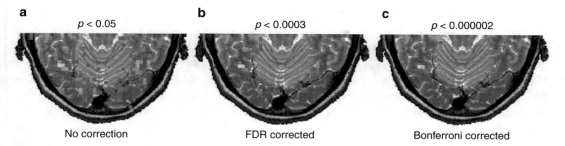

a $p < 0.05$ **b** $p < 0.0003$ **c** $p < 0.000002$

No correction   FDR corrected   Bonferroni corrected

Fig. 18 Comparison of two methods used to solve the multiple comparisons problem. A statistical map has been computed comparing responses to faces and houses. Red/yellow colors depict regions with larger responses to faces than to houses, while blue regions indicate areas with larger responses to houses than to faces. (**a**) No correction for multiple comparisons has been performed. (**b**) Thresholding result when using the false discovery rate approach (FDR). (**c**) Thresholding result when using the Bonferroni method. The p values shown on top of each panel have been used to threshold the map as provided by the respective method. The FDR method shows more voxels as significant because it is less conservative than the Bonferroni method

(overlaid) only in those regions exhibiting suprathreshold (usually statistically significant) signal modulations. While anatomical information is normally visualized using a range of grey values, suprathreshold statistical test values are typically visualized using multiple colors, for example, a red-to-yellow range for positive values and a green-to-blue range for negative values. With these colors, a positive (negative) t value just passing a specified threshold would be colored in red (green), while a very high positive (negative) t value would be colored in yellow (blue) (Fig. 18).

3.3.5 The Multiple Comparison Problem

An important issue in fMRI data analysis is the specification of an appropriate threshold for statistical maps. If there would be only a single voxel's data, a conventional threshold of $p < 0.05$ (or $p < 0.01$) could be used to assess significance of an observed effect quantified by an R, t, or F statistic. Running the statistical analysis separately for each voxel creates, however, a *massive multiple comparison problem*. If a *single test* is performed, the conventional threshold protects from wrongly declaring a voxel as significantly modulated (false positive) with a probability of $p < 0.05$ when there is no effect in the population (α error). Note that in case that the null hypothesis (no effect) holds, an adopted error probability of $p = 0.05$ implies that if the same test would be

repeated 100 times, the alternative hypothesis would be accepted wrongly on average in five cases; that is, we would expect 5% of false positives. If we assume that there is no real effect in any voxel time course, running a statistical test spatially in parallel is statistically identical to repeating the test 100,000 times at a single voxel (each time with new measured data). It is evident that this would lead to about 5000 false positives; that is, about 5000 voxels would be labeled "significant" although these voxels would reach the 0.05 threshold purely due to chance.

Several methods have been suggested to control this massive multiple comparison problem. The *Bonferroni correction* method is a simple multiple comparison correction that controls the α error *across all voxels*, and it is therefore called a *family-wise error* (FWE) correction approach. The method calculates single-voxel threshold values in such a way that an error probability of 0.05 is obtained at the global level. With N independent tests, this is achieved by using a statistical significance level which is N times smaller than usual. The Bonferroni correction can be derived mathematically as follows. Under the assumption of independent tests, the probability that all of N performed tests lead to a subthreshold result is $(1 - p)^N$ and the probability to obtain one or more false-positive results is $1 - (1 - p)^N$. In order to guarantee a family-wise (global) error probability of $p_{FWE} = 1 - (1 - p)^N$, the threshold for a single test, p, has to be adjusted as follows: $p = 1 - (1 - p_{FWE})^{1/N}$. For small p_{FWE} values (e.g., 0.05), this equation can be approximated by $p = p_{FWE}/N$. This means that to obtain a global error probability of $p_{FWE} < 0.05$, the significance level for a single test is obtained by dividing the family-wise error probability by the number of independent tests. Given 100,000 voxels, we would obtain an adjusted single-voxel threshold of $p_v = p_{FWE}/N = 0.05/100,000 = 0.000$ 0005. The Bonferroni correction method ensures that we do not declare even a single voxel wrongly as significantly activated with an error probability of 0.05. For fMRI data, the Bonferroni method would be a valid approach to correct the α error if the data at neighboring voxels would be truly independent from each other. Neighboring voxels, however, show similar response patterns within functionally defined brain regions, such as the fusiform face area (FFA). In the presence of such spatial correlations, the Bonferroni correction method operates too conservative; that is, it corrects the error probability more strongly than necessary. As a result of a too strict control of the α error, the sensitivity (power) to detect truly active voxels is reduced: Many voxels will be labeled as "not significant" although they likely reflect true effects. As described earlier, wrongly accepting (rejecting) a null (alternative) hypothesis is called type II error or β error.

Worsley et al. (1992) suggested a less conservative approach to correct for multiple comparisons taking explicitly the observation into account that neighboring voxels are not activated independently from each other but are more likely to activate together in clusters. In order to incorporate spatial neighborhood relationships in the calculation of global error probabilities, the method describes a statistical map as a *Gaussian random field* (for details, see Worsley et al. 1992). Unfortunately, application of this correction method requires that the fMRI data are spatially smoothed substantially reducing one of its most attractive properties, namely the achievable high spatial resolution. This approach may also lead to inflated alpha errors in certain cases (Eklund et al. 2016).

Another correction method incorporating the observation that neighboring voxels often acti-

vate in clusters is based on Monte Carlo simulations that generate many random images (maps) using the extracted spatial correlation structure of the original map; the generated maps are used to calculate the likelihood to obtain different sizes of functional clusters by chance for specific (less conservative) single-voxel thresholds (Forman et al., 1995). The calculated cluster extent threshold combined with a less strict single-voxel threshold (recommended: $p = 0.001$) is finally applied to the statistical map ensuring that a global error probability of $p < 0.05$ for reported clusters is met. This approach does not require spatial smoothing and appears highly appropriate for fMRI data. A disadvantage is that the method is quite compute intensive and that small functional clusters might not be discovered.

While the described multiple comparison correction methods aim to control the family-wise error rate, the *false discovery rate (FDR) approach* (Benjamini and Hochberg 1995) uses a different statistical logic, and has been proposed for fMRI analysis by Genovese et al. (2002). This approach does not control the overall number of false-positive voxels but the number of false-positive voxels among the subset of voxels labeled as significant. Given a specific threshold, suprathreshold voxels are called "discovered" voxels or "voxels declared as active." With a specified false discovery rate of $q < 0.05$ one would accept that 5% of the discovered (suprathreshold) voxels would be false positives. Given a desired false discovery rate, the FDR algorithm calculates a single-voxel threshold, which ensures that the voxels above that threshold contain on average not more than the specified proportion of false positives. With a q value of 0.05 this also means that one can "trust" 95% of the suprathreshold (i.e., color-coded) voxels since the null hypothesis has been rejected correctly. Since the FDR logic relates the number of false positives to the amount of truly active voxels, the FDR method adapts to the amount of activity in the data: The method is very strict if there is not much evoked activity in the data, but assumes less conservative thresholds if a larger number of voxels show task-related effects. In the extreme case that not a single voxel is truly active, the

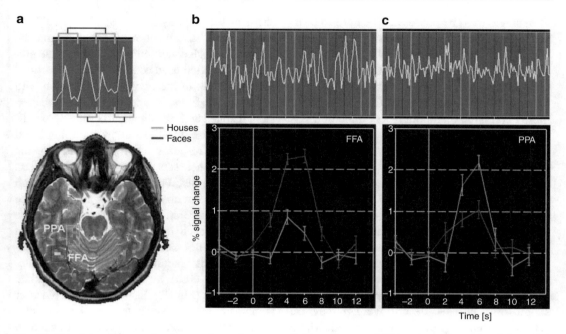

Fig. 19 Principle of event-related averaging and event-related averaging plots from a slow event-related design. (a) The thresholded statistical map shows in red/yellow color brain regions responding more to faces than to houses and in blue color brain regions responding more to houses than to faces. The areas demarcated with red and green rectangles in the lower panel correspond well to *fusiform face area* (FFA) and *parahippocampal place area* (PPA), respectively (O'Craven and Kanwisher 2000). (b) Time course from FFA (upper panel) and event-related averaging plot (lower panel) obtained by selectively averaging all responses belonging to the same condition. (c) Time course (upper panel) and event-related averaging plot (lower panel) from PPA

calculated single-voxel threshold is identical to the one computed with the Bonferroni method. The FDR method appears ideal for fMRI data because it does not require spatial smoothing and it detects voxels with a high sensitivity (low β error) if there are true effects in the data.

Another simple approach to the multiple comparisons problem is to reduce the number of tests by using anatomical masking. Most correction methods, including Bonferroni and FDR, can be combined with this approach since a smaller number of tests leads to a less strict control of the α error and thus a smaller β error is made as compared to inclusion of all voxels. In a simple version of an anatomical mask, an intensity threshold for the basic signal level can be used to remove voxels outside the head. The number of voxels can be further reduced by masking the brain, e.g., after performing a brain extraction step. These simple steps typically reduce the number of voxels by more than 50%. In a more advanced ver-

sion, statistical data analysis may be restricted to grey matter voxels (Goebel and Singer 1999), which may be identified by standard cortex segmentation procedures (e.g., Kriegeskorte and Goebel 2001). This approach not only removes voxels outside the brain but also excludes voxels in white matter and ventricles. Note that anatomically informed correction methods do not require spatial smoothing of the data and reduce not only the multiple comparisons problem but also the computation time since fewer tests (e.g., GLM calculations) have to be performed (Fig. 19).

3.3.6 Event-Related Averaging

Event-related designs can be used to not only *detect* activation effects but also *estimate* the time course of task-related responses. Visualization of mean response profiles can be achieved by averaging all responses of the same condition across corresponding time points with respect to stimulus onset (Fig. 19). Averaged (or even single trial) responses can be used to characterize the temporal dynamics of brain activity within and across brain areas by comparing estimated features such as response latency, duration, and amplitude (e.g., Kruggel and von Cramon 1999; Formisano and Goebel 2003). In more complex, temporally extended tasks, responses to sub-processes may be identified. In working memory paradigms, for example, encoding, delay, and response phases of a trial may be separated. Note that event-related selective averaging works well only for slow event-related designs. In rapid event-related designs, responses from different conditions lead to substantial overlap and event-related averages are often meaningless. In this case, deconvolution analysis is recommended (see below).

To avoid circularity, event-related averages should only be used descriptively if they are selected from significant clusters identified from a whole-brain statistical analysis of the same data. Even a merely descriptive analysis visualizing averaged condition responses is, however, helpful in order to ensure that significant effects are caused by "BOLD-like" response shapes and not by, e.g., signal drifts or measurement artifacts. If ROIs are determined using independent (localizer) data, event-related averages extracted from these regions in a subsequent (main) experiment can be statistically analyzed. For a more general discussion of ROI vs. whole-brain analyses, see Friston and Henson (2006), Friston et al. (2006), Saxe et al. (2006), and Frost and Goebel (2013).

3.3.7 Deconvolution Analysis

While standard design matrix construction (convolution of box-car time course with two-gamma function) can be used to estimate condition amplitudes (beta values) in rapid event-related designs, results critically depend on the appropriateness of the assumed standard BOLD response shape: Due to variability in different brain areas within and across subjects, a *static* model of the response shape might lead to nonoptimal fits. Furthermore, the isolated responses to different conditions cannot be visualized due to overlap of condition responses over time. To model the

shape of the hemodynamic response more flexibly, multiple basis functions (predictors) may be defined for each condition instead of a single predictor. Two often used additional basis functions are derivatives of the two-gamma function with respect to two of its parameters, delay and dispersion. If added to the design matrix for each condition, these basis functions allow capturing small variations in response latency and width of the response. Other sets of basis functions (i.e., gamma basis set, Fourier basis set) are much more flexible but obtained results are often more difficult to interpret. *Deconvolution analysis* is a general approach to estimate condition-related response profiles using a flexible and interpretable set of basis functions. It can be easily implemented as a GLM by defining an appropriate design matrix (Fig. 20) that models each bin after stimulus onset by a separate condition predictor (delta or "stick" functions). This is also called a finite impulse response (FIR) model because it allows estimating any response shape evoked by a short stimulus (impulse). To capture the BOLD response for short events, about 20 s is typically modeled after stimulus onset. This would require, for each condition, 20 predictors in case of a TR of 1 s, or 10 predictors in case of a TR of 2 s (Fig. 20). Despite overlapping responses, fitting such a GLM "recovers" the underlying condition-specific response profiles in a series of beta values, which appear in plots as if event-related averages have been computed in a slow event-related design (Fig. 20). Since each condition is modeled by a series of temporally shifted stick predictors, hypothesis tests can be performed that compare response amplitudes *at different moments in time* within and between conditions. Note, however, that the deconvolution analysis assumes a linear time invariant system (see Sect. 3.1). In order to uniquely estimate the large number of beta values from overlapping responses, variable ITIs must be used in the experimental design (see Sect. 3.1). The deconvolution model is very flexible allowing to capture any response shape. This implies that also non-BOLD-like time courses will be detected easily since the trial responses are not "filtered" by the ideal BOLD response shape as in conventional analysis.

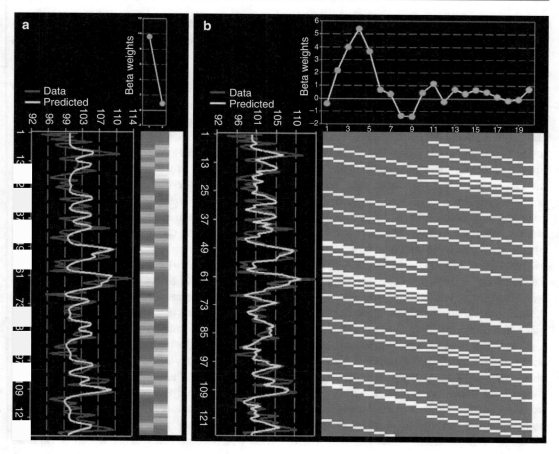

Fig. 20 Deconvolution analysis of a rapid event-related design. Time runs from top to bottom, design matrix depicted in graphical view. Beta values are plotted horizontally at positions corresponding to the respective predictor. (**a**) Standard analysis with two main predictors obtained by convolution of stimulus times with standard hemodynamic response model (two-gamma function). Beta values can be compared with a standard contrast. (**b**) Deconvolution analysis fitting the same data. Each condition is modeled with 10 "stick" predictors allowing to estimate the time course of condition-related responses as if stimuli were presented in a slow event-related design. Beta values may be compared within and across conditions

3.4   Integration of Anatomical and Functional Data

The localization of the neural correlates of sensory, motor, and cognitive functions requires a precise relationship between voxels in calculated statistical maps with voxels in high-resolution anatomical datasets. This is especially important in single-subject analyses and, thus, for presurgical mapping. While it is recommended to also view statistical maps overlaid on a volume of the functional data itself, EPI datasets often do not contain sufficient anatomical detail to specify the precise location of an active cluster in a subject's brain. 3D renderings of high-resolution anatomical datasets may greatly aid in visualizing activated brain regions. Advanced visualization requires that a high-resolution 3D dataset is recorded for a subject and that the functional data is *coregistered* to the 3D dataset as precisely as possible. Anatomical datasets are also important for most brain normalization methods, which is a prerequisite of the analysis of whole-brain group studies. High-resolution anatomical datasets are typically recorded with T_1-weighted MRI sequences. A typical structural scan covering the whole brain with a resolution of 1 mm in all three dimensions (e.g., 180 sagittal slices) lasts between 5 and 20 min on current 1.5 and 3.0 T scanners.

3.4.1 Visualizing Statistical Maps on Anatomical Images

Having identified a statistically significant region in the functional dataset does not easily allow a precise statement about its location in the brain of the subject since the functional data itself does not often contain enough anatomical details.[4] If anatomical, coplanar images are available, it is already helpful to overlay the functional results (thresholded statistical maps) on these "in-plane" images. Figure 19a shows, for example, a statistical map on a high-resolution, coplanar, T_2-weighted image. While high-resolution, coplanar images improve localization within the recording plane, the direction along slices is sampled with low resolution due to typical distances between slices of 2–4 mm (slice distance = slice thickness + slice gap). Identification of the anatomical substrate of an activated cluster greatly benefits from visualizing functional data over isotropic high-resolution (1 mm) 3D datasets. Overlaying or fusing images from functional data (MRI, PET, SPECT) with high-resolution anatomical MRI datasets is a common visualization method in functional imaging. To correctly fuse functional and anatomical datasets, appropriate coregistration transformations have to be performed.

3.4.2 Coregistration of Functional and Anatomical Datasets

If functional images are superimposed on coplanar images, spatial transformations (translations and rotations) to align the two datasets are not necessary (except maybe the correction of small

head movements and small geometric distortions), since the respective slices are measured at the same 3D positions. Since the coplanar anatomical images are usually recorded with a higher resolution (typically with a 256 × 256 matrix) than the functional images (typically 64 × 64 or 128 × 128 matrices), only a scaling factor has to be applied. To allow high-quality visualization of the functional data in arbitrary resliced anatomical planes, the functional data must be coregistered with high-resolution 3D datasets.

These high-resolution 3D datasets are usually recorded with different voxel size, slice orientation, and position than the functional data and the coregistration step and, thus, require an affine spatial transformation including translation, rotation, and scaling to coregister the two datasets. These three elementary spatial transformations can be integrated in a single transformation step expressed in a standard 4x4 spatial transformation matrix. If the high-resolution 3D dataset has been recorded in the same scanning session as the functional data, the coregistration matrix can be constructed simply by using the scanning parameters (slice positions, voxel size) from both recordings. The alignment based on this information would be perfect if there would be no head movement between the anatomical and functional images. To further improve coregistration results, an additional intensity- or gradient-driven alignment step is usually performed after the initial (mathematical) alignment correcting for head displacements (and eventually geometric distortions) between the functional and anatomical recordings. While this step operates similar to that described for motion correction, it is likely not possible to align the two datasets perfectly well in all regions of the brain due to signal dropouts and distortions in the functional EPI images. For neurosurgical purposes, it is important to ensure that at least the most relevant regions of the brain do not suffer from EPI distortions and that they are perfectly coregistered with the anatomical data. EPI distortions and signal dropouts can be corrected to some extent with special MRI sequence modifications as well as with image processing software (see Sect. 3.2.2.1). Using appropriate visualization tools, it is also possible

---

[4]While functional sequences are T_2^* weighted, the first functional volume of a run contains the richest anatomical detail because it is T_1 weighted. Unfortunately, this dataset is often thrown away either by the scanner directly (during "prep scans") or by transfer of the data to the researcher. We recommend keeping the first functional volume and to use it for visualization and coregistration because of its relative richness in anatomical details.

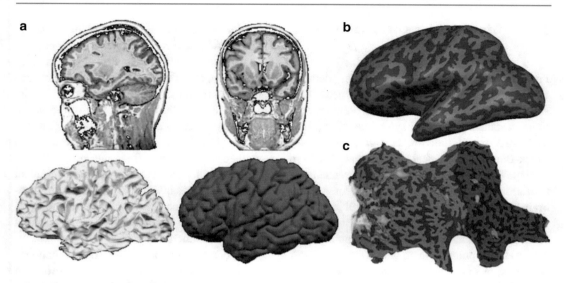

Fig. 21 Cortex representations used for advanced visualization. (**a**) Segmentation and surface reconstruction of the inner (white/grey matter, yellow) and outer (grey matter/CSF, magenta) boundary of grey matter. (**b**) Inflated "cortex representation of the left hemisphere obtained by iterative morphing process." (**c**) "Flat map" of the right cortical hemisphere with superimposed functional data

to manually align a functional volume with an anatomical 3D dataset. The precision of manual alignment depends, however, strongly on acquired expertise.

3.4.3 Visualizing Statistical Maps on Reconstructed Cortex Representations

High-resolution anatomical datasets can be used to create 3D volume or surface renderings of the brain, which allow additional helpful visualizations of functional data on a subject's brain (Fig. 21c). These visualizations require segmentation of the brain, which can be performed automatically with most available software packages. For more advanced visualizations, segmentation of cortical voxels allows to construct topologically correct mesh representations of the cortical sheet, one for the left and one for the right cortical hemisphere (e.g., Fischl et al. 1999; Kriegeskorte and Goebel 2001). The obtained meshes (Fig. 21a) may be further transformed into inflated (Fig. 21b) and flattened (Fig. 21c) cortex representations. Functional data can then be superimposed on folded, inflated, and flattened representations

(Fig. 21c), which is particularly useful for topologically organized functional information, for example, in the context of retinotopic, tonotopic, and somatotopic mapping experiments. To help in orientation, inflated and flattened cortex representations indicate gyral and sulcal regions by color-coding local curvature; concave regions, indicating sulci, may be depicted, e.g., with a dark grey color while convex regions, indicating gyri, may be depicted, e.g., with a light grey color (Fig. 21). A general advantage of visualizing functional data on flat maps is that all cortical activation foci from different experiments can be visualized at once at their correct anatomical location in a canonical view. In contrast, visualizing several activated regions using a multi-slice representation depends on the chosen slice orientation and number of slices. Note that anatomical data is not only important to visualize functional data. Anatomical information may also be used to constrain statistical data analysis as has been described in Sect. 3.3.5. Furthermore, the explicit segmentation of cortical voxels is also the prerequisite for advanced anatomical analyses, including cortical thickness analysis.

3.5   Group Analysis of Functional Datasets

Presurgical neuroimaging requires detailed single-subject analyses, which can be performed with the methods described in the previous sections. A standardized routine for analyzing (clinical) fMRI data in individuals is given in chapter "Task-Based Presurgical Functional MRI in Patients with Brain Tumors." If, however, characterization and statistical assessment of general brain patterns are desired, multiple subjects have to be integrated in groups. Such *group studies* allow generalizing findings from a sample of subjects to the population from which the patients or healthy subjects have been drawn. Group analysis of functional datasets is of clinical relevance when the effects of various brain pathologies or different therapies (e.g., pharmacological effects) on brain function are subject to study.

The integration of fMRI data from multiple subjects is challenging because of the *spatial correspondence problem* between different brains. This problem manifests itself already at a purely anatomical level but presents a fundamental problem of neuroscience when considered as a question of the consistency of structure-function relationships across individual brains. At the anatomical level, the correspondence problem refers to the differences in brain shape, and more specifically to differences in the gyral and sulcal pattern varying substantially across subjects. At this macroanatomical level, the correspondence problem would be solved, if brains could be matched in such a way that for each macroanatomical structure in one brain, the corresponding region in the other brain would be known. In neuroimaging, the matching of brains is usually performed by a process called *brain normalization*, which involves warping each brain into a common space allowing averaging over (more or less) corresponding regions in different subjects. After brain normalization, a point in the common space identified by its x, y, and z coordinates is assumed to refer to a similar region in any other normalized brain. The most commonly used target space for normalization is the *Talairach space* (see below) and the closely related *MNI* (*Montreal*

Neurological Institute) *space*. Unfortunately, warping brains in a common space does not solve the anatomical correspondence problem very well; that is, macroanatomical structures such as banks of prominent sulci are often still misaligned with deviations in the order of 0.5–1 cm. To increase the chance that corresponding regions overlap, functional data is therefore often smoothed with a large Gaussian kernel with a width of about 1 cm. More advanced anatomical matching schemes attempt to directly align macroanatomical structures such as gyri and sulci (see below) and require less (or no) spatial smoothing of functional data.

The deeper version of the correspondence problem addresses the fundamental question of the existence of an identical relationship between certain brain functions and neuroanatomical structures across brains such as cytoarchitectonic brain regions. While neuroimaging has successfully demonstrated that there are common structure-function relationships across brains, a high level of variability has also been observed, especially for higher cognitive functions. A more satisfying answer to this fundamental question might only emerge after much more careful investigations, e.g., by letting the same subjects perform a large battery of tasks (Frost and Goebel 2012). An interesting approach to the functional correspondence problem has been proposed that aims to only align those brain regions of interest (ROIs), which are activated in a given task in all (or at least most) subjects.

3.5.1   Talairach Transformation

The most often used standard space for brain normalization is the MNI space, which is closely related to *Talairach space* (Talairach and Tournoux 1988). MNI and Talairach transformation is performed by a data-driven alignment of a subject's brain to a target (average) brain (typically the MNI template brain) that has been previously transformed in (near-)Talairach space. Talairach transformation can also be performed by the original explicit specification of prominent landmarks (Talairach and Tournoux 1988). In this approach, the midpoint of the anterior commissure (AC) is located first, serving as the origin of

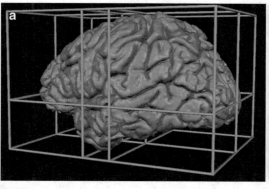 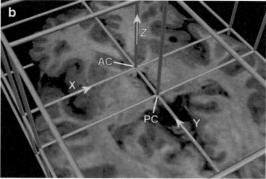

Fig. 22 Definition of Talairach space. (**a**) View from left. (**b**) View from top. Talairach space is defined by three orthogonal axes pointing from left to right (*x*-axis), posterior to anterior (*y*-axis), and inferior to superior (*z*-axis). The origin of the coordinate system is defined by the anterior commissure (AC). Coordinates are in millimeters. The posterior commissure (PC) is located on the *y*-axis

($y = -23$ mm). The borders of the Talairach grid (**a**) correspond to the borders of the cerebrum. The most right point of the brain corresponds to $x = 68$ mm, the most left one to $x = -68$ mm, the most anterior one to $y = 70$, the most posterior one to $y = -102$, the most upper one to $z = 74$, and the most lower one to $z = -42$

Talairach space. The brain is then rotated around the new origin (AC) so that the posterior commissure (PC) appears in the same axial plane as the anterior commissure (Fig. 22). The connection of AC and PC in the middle of the brain forms the *y*-axis of the Talairach coordinate system. The *x*-axis runs from the left to the right hemisphere through AC orthogonal to the *y*-axis. The *z*-axis runs from the inferior part of the brain to the superior part through AC orthogonal to both other axes. In order to further constrain the *x*- and *z*-axes, a *y*–*z* plane is rotated around the *y* (AC-PC) axis until it separates the left and right hemisphere (midsagittal plane). The obtained AC-PC space is attractive for individual clinical applications, especially presurgical mapping and neuronavigation since it keeps the original size of the subject's brain intact while providing a common orientation for each brain anchored at important landmarks. For a full Talairach transformation, a cuboid is defined running parallel to the three axes enclosing precisely the cortex. This cuboid or bounding box requires specification of additional landmarks specifying the borders of the cerebrum. The bounding box is subdivided by several sub-planes. The midsagittal *y*–*z* plane separates two sub-cuboids containing the left and right hemisphere, respectively. An axial (*x*–*y*)

plane through the origin separates two sub-cuboids containing the space below and above the AC-PC plane. Two coronal (*x*–*z*) planes, one running through AC and the other running through PC, separate three sub-cuboids; the first contains the anterior portion of the brain anterior to the AC, the second contains the space between AC and PC, and the third contains the space posterior to PC. These planes separate 12 sub-cuboids. In a final Talairach transformation step, each of the 12 sub-cuboids is expanded or shrunken linearly to match the size of the corresponding sub-cuboid of the standard Talairach brain. To reference any point in the brain, *x*, *y*, and *z* coordinates are specified in millimeters of Talairach space. Talairach and Tournoux (1988) also defined the "proportional grid," to reference points within the defined cuboids.

In summary, Talairach normalization ensures that the anterior and posterior commissures obtain the same coordinates in each brain and that the sub-cuboids defined by the AC and PC points and the borders of the cortex will have the same size. Note that the specific distances between landmarks in the original postmortem brain are not important for establishing the described spatial relationship between brains. The important aspect of Talairach transformation is that correspondence is established across brains by linearly interpolating the space between important landmarks.

While Talairach transformation provides a recipe to normalize brains, regions at the same coordinates in different individuals do not necessarily point to corresponding brain areas. This holds especially true for cortical regions (e.g., Frost and Goebel 2012). For subcortical structures around the AC and PC landmarks, however, the established correspondence is remarkably good even when analyzing high-resolution fMRI data (e.g., De Martino et al. 2013).

As an alternative to specify crucial landmarks, a direct approach of stereotactic normalization has been proposed (e.g., Evans et al., 1993; Ashburner and Friston 1999) that automatically aligns each individual brain as good as possible to an average target brain, called *template brain*. The most often used template brain is provided by the Montreal Neurological Institute (MNI) and has been created by averaging many (>100) single brains after manual Talairach transformation. Although automatic alignment to a template brain has the potential to result in a better correspondence between brain regions, comparisons have shown that the achieved results are not substantially improved as compared to the explicit landmark specification approach, even when using nonlinear spatial transformation techniques. This can be explained by noting that the template brain has lost anatomical details due to extensive averaging. In order to bring functional data of a subject into Talairach space, the obtained spatial transformation for the anatomical data may be applied to the functional data if it has been coregistered with the unnormalized anatomical dataset. Using the intensity-driven matching approach, functional datasets may also be directly normalized (without the help of anatomical datasets) because versions of the MNI template brain for functional (EPI) scans are also available. If possible, it is, however, recommended to apply the transformation obtained for the anatomical data also to the functional data because this approach guarantees that the precision of functional-anatomical alignment achieved during coregistration is not changed during the normalization step.

More advanced volume-based normalization schemes have been proposed that replace the presented simple intensity-driven approaches (e.g., DARTEL, Ashburner 2007).

3.5.2 Cortex-Based Normalization

In recent years, more advanced brain normalization techniques have been proposed going beyond simple volume space alignment approaches. A particular interesting method attempts to explicitly align the cortical folding pattern (macroanatomy) across subjects (Fischl et al. 1999; Goebel et al. 2004, 2006; Frost and Goebel 2012) starting with topologically correct cortex mesh representations (see Sect. 3.4.3). The folded cortex meshes are first morphed to spherical representations since the restricted space of a sphere allows alignment using only two dimensions (longitude and latitude) instead of three dimensions as needed in volume space. Since the inflation of cortex hemispheres to spheres removes ("flattens") information of the gyral/sulcal folds, the respective information is retained by calculating curvature maps prior to inflation that are projected on the spherical representations. Cortex meshes from different subjects are then aligned on the sphere by *increasing the overlap of curvature information*. Since the curvature of the cortex reflects the gyral/sulcal folding pattern of the brain, this brain matching approach essentially aligns corresponding gyri and sulci across brains. It has been shown that cortex-based alignment substantially increases the statistical power and spatial specificity of group analyses by increasing not only the overlap of macroanatomical regions but also the overlap of corresponding functionally defined specialized brain areas (Frost and Goebel 2012).

3.5.3 Correspondence Based on Functional Localizer Experiments

An interesting approach to establish correspondence between brains is to use functional information directly. Using standardized stimuli, a specific region of interest (ROI) may be functionally identified in each subject. The ROIs identified in such *functional localizer experiments* are then used to extract time courses in subsequent main experiments avoiding double dipping. The extracted time courses of individual subjects are then integrated in group analyses (see below). An extension of this functionally driven approach is hyperalignment (Haxby et al. 2011). If the assumption is correct that functional localizer experiments reveal corresponding brain regions in different subjects, the approach provides an optimal solution to the correspondence problem and will allow detection of subtle differences in fMRI responses at the group level with high statistical power. Statistical sensitivity is further enhanced by avoiding the massive multiple comparison correction problem. Instead of hundreds of thousand voxel-wise tests, only a few tests must be performed—one for each considered ROI. The approach is statistically sound (no circularity) because the considered regions have been determined *independently* from the main data using special localizer runs. It may also be acceptable to use the same functional data for both localizer and main analysis as long as the contrast to localize ROIs is orthogonal to any contrast used to statistically test more subtle differences. The localizer approach has been applied successfully in many experiments, most notably in studies of the ventral visual cortex (e.g., O'Craven and Kanwisher 2000).

Unfortunately, it is often difficult to define experiments localizing the same pattern of activated brain areas in all subjects, especially in studies of higher cognitive functions, such as attention, mental imagery, working memory, and planning. If at all possible, the selection of corresponding functional brain areas in these experiments is very difficult and depends on the investigator's choice of thresholding statistical maps and often on additional decisions such as grouping sub-clusters to obtain the same number of major clusters for each subject. Note that the increased variability of activated regions in more complex experiments could be explained by at least two factors. On the one hand the location of functionally corresponding brain regions may vary substantially across subjects with respect to aligned macroanatomical structures. On the other hand, subjects may engage in different cognitive

strategies to solve the same task leading to a (partially) different set of activated brain areas. Most likely, the observed variability is caused by a mixture of both sources of variability. Another problem of the localizer approach is the tendency to focus only on a few brain areas, namely those which can be mapped consistently in different subjects. This tendency bears the danger to overlook other important brain regions. This can be avoided by functionally informed cortex-based alignment (Frost and Goebel 2013) that integrates ROI-based and whole-cortex analysis using a modified version of cortex-based alignment that uses corresponding pre-mapped ROIs as alignment targets in addition to anatomical curvature information.

3.5.4 Statistical Analysis of Group Data

After brain normalization, the whole-brain data from multiple subjects can be statistically analyzed simply by concatenating time courses at corresponding locations. The corresponding locations can be voxel coordinates in MNI space, vertex coordinates in cortex space, or identified ROIs in the localizer approach. Note that the power of statistical analysis depends on the quality of brain normalization. If the achieved alignment of corresponding functional brain areas is poor, suboptimal group results may be obtained since active voxels of some subjects will be averaged with non-active voxels (or active voxels from a non-corresponding brain area) from other subjects. In order to increase the overlap of activated brain areas across subjects in volume space, the functional data of each subject is often smoothed, typically using rather large Gaussian kernels with a full width at half maximum (FWHM) of 8–12 mm. While such an extensive spatial smoothing ("blurring") increases the overlap of active regions, it reduces selectivity of neighboring specialized brain areas. Furthermore, functional clusters smaller than the smoothing kernel will be suppressed reducing detection sensitivity of truly active but small functional clusters. Extensive spatial smoothing may not be necessary when using advanced volumetric normalization schemes (e.g., Ashburner 2007), cortex-based alignment (e.g., Frost and Goebel 2012, 2013), hyperalignment (Haxby et al. 2011), or functional localizers.

After concatenating the data, the statistical analysis described for single-subject data (see Sect. 3.3) can be applied to the integrated time courses. In the context of the GLM, the multi-subject voxel time courses as well as the multi-subject predictors may be obtained by concatenation. After estimating the beta values, contrasts can be tested in the same way as described for single-subject data. While the described concatenation approach leads to a high statistical power due to the large number of blocks or events, the obtained results cannot be generalized to the population level since the data is analyzed as if it stems from a single subject. Significant findings only indicate that the results are replicable for the same "subject" (group of subjects). In order to test whether the obtained results are valid at the population level, the statistical procedure must assess the variability of observed effects across subjects (*random effects analysis*) as opposed to the variability across individual measurement time points as performed in the concatenation approach (*fixed effects analysis*). There are many statistical methods to assess the variability across subjects for the purpose of proper population inferences. A simple and elegant method is provided by *multilevel summary statistics approach* (e.g., Kirby 1993; Holmes and Friston 1998; Worsley et al. 2002; Beckmann et al. 2003; Friston et al. 2005). In the first analysis stage, parameters (*summary statistics*) are estimated for each subject independently (level 1, fixed effects). Instead of the full-time courses, only the resulting first-level parameter estimates (betas) from each subject are carried forward to the second analysis stage where they serve as the *dependent variables*. The second-level analysis assesses the consistency of effects within or between groups based on the variability of the first-level estimates across subjects (level 2, random effects). This hierarchical analysis approach reduces the data for the second-stage analysis enormously since the time course data of each subject has been "collapsed" to only one or a few condition-related parameter estimates per sub-

ject. Since the summarized data at the second level reflects the variability of the estimated parameters across subjects, obtained significant results can be generalized to the population from which the subjects were drawn as a random sample.

To summarize the data at the first level, a standard GLM may be used to estimate effects—beta values—separately for each subject. Instead of one set of beta values in fixed effects analysis, this step will provide a *separate set of beta values for each subject*. The obtained beta values or calculated contrast values can be analyzed at the second level using again a GLM or a standard ANOVA with one or more within-subjects factors for factorial designs. If the data represent multiple groups of subjects, one or more between-subjects factors for group comparisons can be added.

These short explanations indicate that the statistical analysis at the second level does not differ from the usual statistical approach in medical studies. The only major difference to standard statistics at the second level is that the analysis is performed separately for each voxel (or vertex) requiring correction for a massive multiple comparison problem as has been described above. Note that in addition to the estimated subject-specific effects of the fMRI design (beta values or contrast values of first-level analysis), additional external variables (e.g., an IQ value for each subject) may be incorporated as covariates at the second level.

3.6 Selected Advanced Data Analysis Methods

The analysis steps described in previous sections for single subjects and for group comparisons represent essential components of a standard fMRI analysis, which are performed in a similar way for most fMRI studies. Such a standard analysis involves proper preprocessing that includes drift removal and 3D motion correction, coregistration of functional and anatomical data, brain normalization, and a thorough statistical analysis usually based on the general linear model. The standard procedure produces statistical maps that localize regions showing differential responses with respect to specified experimental hypotheses. Random effects group analyses allow generalization of observed findings from a sample of subjects to the population level. Event-related averages of active brain regions or pre-specified ROIs can be used to compare estimated condition time courses within and across brain areas, often revealing additional interesting insights. The following sections shortly describe a selected list of further analysis methods aiming at improving or extending the standard analysis procedure.

3.6.1 Nonparametric Statistical Approaches

As stated in Sect. 3.3.3.5, GLM hypothesis testing requires normally distributed residuals with equal variance. Fortunately, the GLM is robust with respect to minor violations of the normality assumption. To avoid, however, wrong inferences due to non-normal distributions, nonparametric methods may be used, especially when analyzing small data samples. Extensive analyses of many datasets have shown that permutation-based nonparametric approaches do indeed not suffer from inflated false-positive rates as observed with parametric methods (Eklund et al. 2016).

3.6.2 Bayesian Statistics

It has been proposed to use Bayesian statistics because it provides an elegant framework for multilevel analyses (Friston et al. 2002). In the Bayesian approach, the data of a single experiment (or the data of a single subject) is not considered in isolation, but in light of available a priori knowledge. This a priori knowledge is formalized with prior probabilities $p(H_i)$ for relevant initial hypotheses H_i. Obtained new data D modifies the a priori knowledge resulting in posterior conditional probabilities $p(H_i|D)$, which are updated probabilities of the initial hypotheses given the new data. To calculate these probabilities, the inverse conditional probabilities $p(D|H_i)$ must be known describing the probability to obtain certain observations given that the hypotheses H_i are true. In the context of the *empirical Bayes approach*, these conditional probabilities

can be estimated from the data. The empirical Bayes approach is appropriate for the analysis of fMRI data, since it allows an elegant formulation of hierarchical random effects analyses. It is, for example, possible to enter estimated parameters at a lower level as prior probabilities at the next higher level. Furthermore, the approach allows integrating correction for multiple comparisons resulting in thresholding values similar to the ones obtained with the false discovery rate approach.

3.6.3 Brain Normalization

As described earlier, brain normalization methods have an important influence on the quality of group analyses, since optimization of the standard analysis does not lead to substantial improvements if voxel time courses are concatenated from nonmatching brain regions. The described cortex-based normalization technique may substantially improve the alignment of corresponding brain regions across subjects. For more complex tasks, different, nonmatching activity patterns might reflect different cognitive strategies used by subjects. To cope with this situation, it would be desirable to use methods allowing automatic estimation of the similarity of activity patterns across subjects. Such methods could suggest splitting a group into subgroups with different statistical maps corresponding to the neural correlate of (automatically detected) different cognitive strategies. Such a clustering approach has been recently implemented in the context of group-level ICA analyses (Esposito et al. 2005).

3.6.4 Data-Driven Analysis Methods

When considering the richness of fMRI data, it may be useful to apply *data-driven analysis methods*, which aim at discovering interesting spatiotemporal relationships in the data, which would be eventually overlooked with a purely hypothesis-driven approach. Data-driven methods, such as *independent component analysis* (ICA, e.g., McKeown et al. 1998a, 1998b; Formisano et al. 2002), do not require a specification of expected, stimulus-related responses since they are able to extract interesting information automatically ("blindly") from the data. It is, thus, not necessary to specify an explicit statistical model (design matrix). This is particularly interesting with respect to paradigms for which the exact specification of event onsets is difficult or impossible. Spatial ICA of fMRI data has been successfully applied in many tasks including the automatic detection of active networks during perceptual switches of ambiguous stimuli (Castelo-Branco et al. 2002) and the automatic detection of spontaneous hallucinatory episodes in schizophrenic patients (van de Ven et al. 2005). Data-driven methods are exploratory in nature, and should not be viewed as replacements, but as complementary tools for hypothesis-driven methods: If interesting, unexpected events have been discovered with a data-driven method, one should test these observations in succeeding studies with a hypothesis-driven standard statistical analysis. More generally, ICA has become an important method to reveal functionally connected networks, especially in the context of resting-state fMRI (see below). Furthermore ICA is often used to denoise fMRI data by removing artifacts (e.g., Murphy et al. 2013).

3.6.5 Multivariate Analysis of Distributed Activity Patterns

Multi-voxel pattern analysis (MVPA) has been established in the neuroimaging community as an important analysis tool because it allows to detect differences between conditions with higher sensitivity than conventional univariate analysis by focusing on the analysis and comparison of distributed patterns of activity (Haxby et al. 2001). In such a multivariate approach, data from individual voxels within a region are jointly analyzed. Furthermore, MVPA is often presented in the context of "brain reading" applications reporting that specific mental states or representational content can be decoded from fMRI activity patterns after performing a "training" or "learning" phase. In this context, MVPA tools are often referred to as classifiers or, more generally, learning machines. The latter names stress that many MVPA tools originate from a field called machine learning, a branch of artificial intelligence. In fMRI research, the support vector machine (SVM, Vapnik 1995) has become a particular popular machine learning classifier, which is used both for analyzing patterns in ROIs and for discriminating patterns that are potentially spread out across the whole brain.

Another popular MVPA approach is the "searchlight" method (Kriegeskorte et al. 2006). In this approach, each voxel is visited, as in a standard univariate analysis, but instead of using only data of the visited voxel for analysis, several voxels in the neighborhood are included forming a set of features for joined multivariate analysis. The neighborhood is usually defined roughly as a sphere; that is, voxels within a certain (Euclidean) distance from the visited voxel are included. The result of the multivariate analysis is then stored at the visited voxel (e.g., a t value resulting from a *multivariate* statistical comparison or an accuracy value from a support vector machine classifier). By visiting all voxels and analyzing their respective (partially overlapping) neighborhoods, one obtains a whole-brain map in the same way as when running univariate statistics.

Representational similarity analysis (RSA) is another important multivariate pattern analysis approach used to analyze the pattern similarity between fMRI responses evoked by trials from different experimental conditions (Kriegeskorte et al. 2008). For the responses from a region of interest a representational distance (or dissimilarity) matrix (RDM) is computed containing distance measures (usually "1—correlation") between pairs of distributed activity patterns. The calculated dissimilarity matrix can itself be compared to RDMs from other regions producing second-level RDMs that characterize the specific representational structure of a brain region by revealing what distinctions between conditions are emphasized and what distinctions are de-emphasized in a specific ROI. In a visual study, for example, the similarity structure in V1 will be based on the topographic overlap of presented stimuli while in higher level visual cortex the similarity structure will represent more categorical and semantic information (Khaligh-Razavi and Kriegeskorte 2014). Since the comparison of first-level RDMs does not require correspondence at the level of measurement channels (voxels, electrode recordings, units in computational models), RSA circumvents the correspondence problem enabling comparison of data across subjects, measurement modalities, as well as representations in brains and models.

3.6.6 Real-Time Analysis of fMRI Data

The described steps and techniques to analyze functional MRI data are very computation intensive and are, thus, performed in most cases hours or days after data acquisition has been completed. There are many scenarios that would benefit greatly from a *real-time analysis of fMRI data*, especially when studying single subjects as in presurgical mapping. Using appropriately modified analysis tools and state-of-the-art computer hardware, it is nowadays possible to perform real-time fMRI analysis during an ongoing experiment, including 3D motion correction and incremental GLM statistics of whole-brain recordings (Goebel 2012; Weiskopf 2012). It is even possible to run multivariate data-driven tools in real time, including ICA (Esposito et al. 2003) and multi-voxel pattern analyses (LaConte et al. 2007; Sorger et al. 2010). One obvious benefit of real-time fMRI analysis is *quality assurance*. If, for example, one observes during an ongoing measurement that a patient moves too much, or that the (absence of) activity patterns indicates that the task was not correctly understood, the running measurement may be stopped and repeated after giving the subject further instructions. If the ongoing statistical analysis on the other hand indicates that expected effects have reached a desired significance level earlier than expected, one could save scanning time by stopping the measurement ahead of schedule. Real-time fMRI also offers the possibility to plan optimal slice positioning for subsequent runs based on the results obtained of an initial run. Based on the results of a first run, it would be, for example, possible to position a small slab of slices at an identified functional region for subsequent high-resolution spatial and/or temporal scanning. More advanced applications of real-time fMRI include neurofeedback (Weiskopf et al. 2003; Goebel 2021) and communication BCIs (Sorger et al. 2012). In fMRI neurofeedback studies, subjects learn to voluntarily control the level of activity in circumscribed brain areas by engaging in mental tasks such as inner speech, visual or auditory imagery, spatial navigation, mental calculation, or recalling (emotional) memories. In recent years, fMRI neurofeedback has been successfully employed as a therapeutic tool for various psychiatric and neurological diseases (e.g., Linden et al. 2012; Subramanian et al. 2011; Mehler et al. 2018).

4 Functional Connectivity and Resting-State Networks

The last two sections of this chapter provide a brief overview of the basic aspects of the important topic of connectivity. Generally, three types of brain connectivity are distinguished in brain research (Sporns 2010). *Structural connectivity* (or anatomical connectivity) refers to the physical presence of an axonal projection from one brain area to another. This type of connectivity and how diffusion MRI and computational tractography can be used to identify large axon bundles in the human brain are described in Sect. 5. *Functional connectivity* refers to the correlation structure in the data that can be used to reveal functional coupling between specific brain regions and to reveal functional networks. Finally, *effective connectivity* refers to models that go beyond correlation (or more generally statistical dependency) to more advanced measures of directed influence and causality within networks (Friston, 1994).

4.1 Functional and Effective Connectivity

Functional and effective connectivity methods aim to reveal the *functional integration* of brain areas, whereas the classical voxel-wise statistical approach (Sect. 3) is suited to reveal the *functional segregation* (functional specialization) of brain regions. Besides data-driven methods such as independent component analysis (ICA), many approaches have been used to model the interaction between spatially remote brain regions more explicitly. In the simplest case, the time courses from two regions are correlated resulting in a measure (e.g., linear correlation coefficient) of functional connectivity. Functional connectivity can be calculated separately for different experimental conditions, which allows to assess whether two brain areas change their *functional coupling* in different cognitive contexts (Büchel et al. 1999). In conditions of attention, for example, two remote areas might work more closely with each other than in conditions of no attention.

Models of effective connectivity go beyond simple pair-wise correlation analysis and assess the validity of models containing directed interactions between brain areas. These directed effective connections are often symbolized by arrows connecting boxes each representing a different brain area. Structural equation models (SEM, e.g., McIntosh and Gonzalez-Lima 1994) and the more elaborate dynamic causal modeling (DCM, e.g., Penny et al. 2004) can be used to test effective connectivity models. An interesting *data-driven* approach to effective connectivity modeling is provided by methods based on the concept of *Granger causality*. This approach does not require specification of connectivity models but enables to automatically detect effective connections from the data by mapping Granger causality for any selected reference voxel or region of interest (Goebel et al. 2003; Roebroeck et al. 2005; Roebroeck et al. 2011).

4.2   Resting-State Networks

Functional connectivity studies have gained increased interest where the subject is in a relaxed resting state, i.e., in the absence of experimental tasks and behavioral responses. These *resting-state fMRI* (RS-fMRI) studies allow measuring the amount of spontaneous BOLD signal synchronization within and between multiple regions across the entire brain (Biswal et al. 1995). The measured RS-fMRI activity is characterized by low-frequency (0.01–0.1 Hz) BOLD signal fluctuations, which are topologically organized as

multiple spatially distributed functional connectivity networks called *resting-state networks* (RSNs) (e.g., van de Ven et al. 2004; De Luca et al. 2006). Spatial ICA (see Sect. 3.6.4) at the individual and group level is commonly applied in resting-state fMRI. ICA provides a set of spatial maps and corresponding time courses. The selection of components corresponding to RSNs is not trivial and is usually performed by visual inspection or correlation with a predefined RSN template. This procedure reveals RSNs that are consistently found in individuals including the default-mode network (often separated in an anterior and posterior sub-network), a visual and a auditory network, a sensorimotor network, and two (lateralized) dorsolateral frontoparietal networks (Fig. 23; for further details, see, e.g., Allen et al. 2011). The extracted independent components are usually scaled to spatial z-scores (i.e., the number of standard deviations of their whole-brain spatial distribution). These values express the relative amount a given voxel is modulated by the activation of the component (McKeown et al. 1998b) and hence reflect the amplitude of the correlated fluctuations within the corresponding functional connectivity network.

An alternative (less objective, historically first) approach to retrieve RSNs is to calculate whole-brain correlations from seed regions that correspond to core locations of RSNs. In this approach the DMN, for example, can be retrieved by selecting a region in the posterior cingulate cortex as the seed region and then correlating each brain voxel's time course with the reference time course from the seed region; the RSN is then determined as the subset of voxels with highest correlation values with the seed region, eventually inside a provided RSN-specific mask. For both the seed-based correlation and ICA approach it is recommended to identify and possibly remove BOLD artifacts due to residual motion, cardiac pulsation, and respiratory cycle using ICA denoising (Birn et al. 2008; Murphy et al. 2013) as well as explicit physiological noise correction methods such as RETROICOR (Glover et al. 2000).

In contrast to early resting-state fMRI analysis approaches that are based on the assumption of

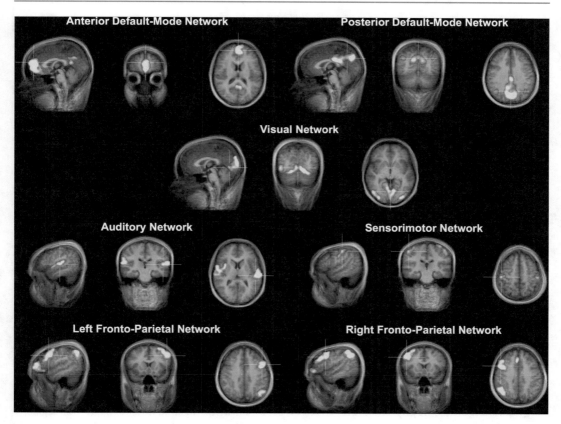

Fig. 23 A subset of major resting-state networks (RSNs) obtained by ICA analysis of the resting-state fMRI data of a group of healthy individuals ($n = 8$); the default mode network (DMN) is split into an anterior and posterior part (upper row)

stationarity, dynamic functional connectivity (dFC) addresses the temporal component of spontaneous BOLD signals. The technique can be implemented using, for example, a sliding window correlations approach (Hindriks et al. 2016). Dynamic FC analysis has the potential to clarify the changes in patterns of neural activity over time and may be a more appropriate choice for the analysis of RS-fMRI studies. For further details about the analysis and application of resting-state networks, see chapter "Presurgical Resting-State fMRI."

The obtained functional networks during rest conditions demonstrate that the brain is never "at rest" and the description of RSNs is, thus, a useful approach to explore the brain's functional organization in healthy individuals as well as to examine if it is altered in neurological or psychi-

atric diseases. Furthermore, it has been possible to relate RSNs to externally modifiable factors, such as different pharmacological treatments or psychological experiences (Khalili-Mahani et al. 2012; Esposito et al. 2014). The default mode network (DMN) has gained particular attention; the term "default mode" has been introduced by Raichle et al. (2001) to describe resting-state brain function. The DMN is a network of brain regions that include part of the medial temporal lobe (presumed memory functions), part of the medial prefrontal cortex (presumed theory of mind functions), posterior cingulate cortex along with the adjacent ventral precuneus, and medial, lateral, and inferior parietal cortex. The DMN is active when the individual is not focused on the outside world and the brain is at wakeful rest corresponding likely to task-independent introspection, mind-wandering, and self-referential thought. During goal-oriented activity, the DMN is deactivated and other regions are active that are sometimes described as the task-positive network (TPN). The DMN has been hypothesized to be relevant to disorders including Alzheimer's disease, autism, and schizophrenia (Buckner et al. 2008).

5   Diffusion-Weighted MRI and Tractography

In recent years, MRI has not only revolutionized functional brain imaging targeting grey matter neuronal activity but also enabled insights into human white matter structure using diffusion-weighted magnetic resonance imaging (DW-MRI, dMRI, or DWI). Pulse sequences for dMRI measure the diffusion of water molecules in each voxel providing information about the fibers in that voxel that can be used to assess the "intactness" of white matter structure. Furthermore, diffusion measurements may serve as the basis for *computational tractography* since the diffusion process is hindered by the boundaries of the fibers forcing the majority of water molecules to diffuse along these fibers.

A diffusion-weighted MR measurement consists of several volumes each measuring the reduction of the signal resulting from diffusion along a specific axis in space that is selected by setting the x, y, and z gradients of the scanner accordingly using a pulsed gradient spin echo sequence (PGSE) developed by Stejskal and Tanner (1965).

5.1   Diffusion Tensor Imaging

It has been proposed to model the diffusion measured in a voxel as a 3D Gaussian probability function from which a *diffusion tensor* (3 × 3 matrix) can be calculated (Basser et al. 1994), which has led to the name *diffusion tensor imaging* (DTI) for the most widely used diffusion-weighted MRI acquisition and modeling approach. While there are more advanced bio-

physical multi-compartment models to analyze diffusion-weighted data (e.g., Panagiotaki et al. 2012; Jelescu and Budde 2017), this section focuses on the DTI model. To construct the diffusion tensor a minimum of six diffusion-weighted volumes and a non-diffusion-weighted image need to be measured. From the diffusion tensor, the principal diffusion directions (three eigenvectors of the tensor) and associated diffusion coefficients (three eigenvalues λ_1, λ_2, λ_3) can be derived. Note that although eigenvectors mathematically represent directions, DTI cannot distinguish opposing directions from each other; that is, the resulting values estimate diffusion along opposing directions, i.e., along principal axes of diffusion. The eigenvectors and eigenvalues can be visualized as an ellipsoid. If water molecules diffuse without restrictions in all directions, the resulting "ellipsoid" will have the shape of a sphere; that is, all three axes (eigenvectors) have the same length ($\lambda_1 = \lambda_2 = \lambda_3$) and there is no preferred axis of diffusion. This situation is described as *isotropic diffusion*. In case that water molecules diffuse with low restrictions along one axis but diffusion is hindered in other directions, a strongly elongated (cigar shaped) ellipsoid will be obtained ($\lambda_1 \gg \lambda_2 \approx \lambda_3$). This case of restricted diffusion occurs within and around white matter fibers and is described as *anisotropic diffusion*. In this case, the main (longest) axis of the resulting ellipsoid will likely coincide with the main orientation of fiber bundles running through the measured voxel. This is the principal assumption of DTI. Note, however, that the tensors estimated in each voxel do not provide fibers but only local discrete measurements; that is, putative fibers need to be reconstructed using *computational tractography*; that is, orientation of estimated tensors needs to be "concatenated" across neighboring voxels. Since results of specific tractography procedures are dependent on many factors (see below), visualized fibers need to be interpreted with care.

Several interesting quantities can be derived from the diffusion tensor in each voxel. The *mean diffusivity* quantifies the overall movement of water molecules in a voxel, which depends on tissue type (e.g., CSF vs. white matter) and presence

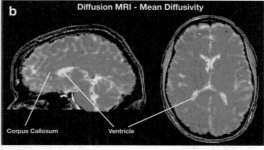

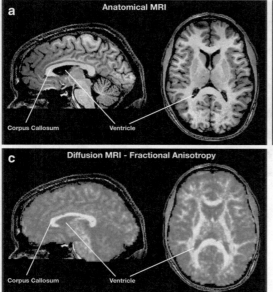

Fig. 24 Important voxel-wise measures that can be extracted from diffusion-weighted MRI scans. (**a**) Anatomical scan shown as reference. (**b**) Mean diffusivity map coregistered with anatomy shown in (**a**); note that diffusivity is high in CSF (ventricles, yellow color) but low in grey matter and white matter fiber bundles such as the corpus callosum (orange color). (**c**) Fractional anisotropy (FA) map coregistered with anatomy shown in (**a**); note that FA is low (orange color) in the presence of low diffusion restrictions (ventricles) but high in white matter fiber bundles such as the corpus callosum containing coherently oriented fibers within voxels

of diffusion restrictions (e.g., axons). Figure 24b shows that the mean diffusivity is high in the ventricles (yellow color) while it is low in white and grey matter (orange color). The most commonly derived scalar quantity is *fractional anisotropy* (FA) that characterizes the overall shape of the diffusion; that is, it quantifies the fraction of the diffusion tensor that can be ascribed to anisotropic diffusion:

$$FA = \frac{\sqrt{\left(\lambda_1 - \lambda_2\right)^2 + \left(\lambda_2 - \lambda_3\right)^2 + \left(\lambda_1 - \lambda_3\right)^2}}{\sqrt{2\left(\lambda_1^2 + \lambda_2^2 + \lambda_3^2\right)}}$$

The FA value varies between 0 (isotropic diffusion, shape of a sphere) and 1 (maximal anisotropy, shape of a line). Figure 24c shows that fractional anisotropy is high (yellow color) in white matter (e.g., in the corpus callosum) but low (orange color) in grey matter and ventricles. The FA value disregards the specific diffusion axis. A value of 0 indicates no preferred diffusion

axis (sphere) while a value of 1 indicates diffusion precisely along a single axis. Since white matter contains parallel fibers within larger tracts, it contains usually high FA values (>0.3) whereas FA values are low (0.0–0.2) in grey matter. The FA quantity has gained increasing interest in recent years since it has been shown that FA values in specific tracts can be related to specific diseases; furthermore, FA values correlate with cognitive performance measures such as reading capability (see Sect. 5.3).

5.1.1 Tractography: From Tensors to Fiber Bundles

Based on the preferred orientation of the tensors in neighboring voxels, computational tractography or *fiber tracking* procedures aim to reconstruct the trajectory of fibers in white matter by "concatenating" neighboring tensors. Fiber tracking is usually launched (seeded) in all voxels (even in sub-voxel coordinate grids) except those with low FA values since they do not reflect

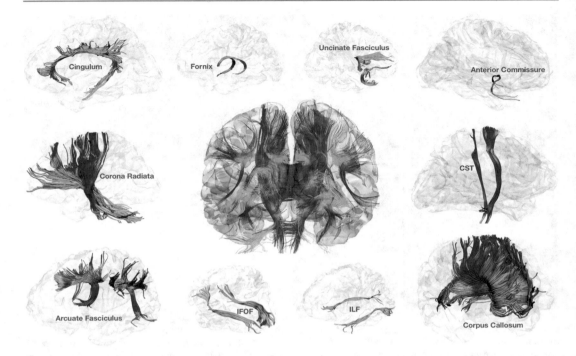

Fig. 25 A subset of major fiber tracts revealed by computational tractography from the diffusion-weighted MRI data of a healthy individual. *CST* corticospinal tract, *IFOF* inferior fronto-occipital fasciculus, *ILF* inferior longitudinal fasciculus

strong directionality. The tracking process then generates a large amount of short and long reconstructed ("software") fibers. Specific fiber tracts are extracted from the dense fiber field by using regional constraints (e.g., Catani and Thiebaut de Schotten 2008); that is, fibers belonging to a specific tract are included if they pass through one or more specified volumes of interest (VOIs). Since the main axis of the tensor indicates an oriented axis and not a direction, fiber tracking is performed in two opposing directions. After both "half-fibers" have been reconstructed, they are finally integrated into a single fiber. In order to reconstruct a (half-) fiber, a small (sub-voxel) step is performed in one of the two directions provided by the main (longest) axis of the ellipsoid at a seed position. At the reached position, the direction for the next small step will be calculated using the tensor orientation and the direction of the previous step. Since the reached position usually does not correspond to integral coordinates (i.e., it falls between voxels), the cal-culation of the next direction is based on the tensors surrounding the current 3D position; in this interpolation process, tensors influence the calculation with respect to the distance of the corresponding voxels to the current position. After updating the direction, the next step is performed. Again a new direction is calculated at the new position for the next step and so on producing a connected trajectory of short line segments. This process continues until certain stop criteria are reached such as when an FA value is encountered that falls below a specified threshold or in case that the reconstructed fiber leaves white matter. In order to create smooth reconstructed fibers (Fig. 25), the chosen step size needs to be smaller than the distance of the voxels.

5.2 Validation and Improvements

While tractography usually creates interesting results, it is important to realize that visualized fibers are reconstructed from diffusion estimates that are measured at discrete 3D positions (voxels) and, thus, may not necessarily reflect true fiber tracts in the brain. A central concern in current tractography research concerns the question how much one can trust the beautiful pictures generated by fiber tracking procedures. The answer depends on many factors including the quality of the diffusion-weighted measurement which is influenced by scanner parameters (e.g., signal-to-noise ratio) as well as by parameters of the participant such as head motion and physiological noise. The most important limiting factor is related to the voxel size used for in vivo studies that is a few orders of magnitudes larger than the small scale at which the diffusion of water molecules happens. With a typical spatial resolution of about 2 mm only the average diffusion of water molecules in a large cube (voxel) is captured, which does not allow to resolve fine-grained white matter fiber bundles or fiber bundles in grey matter. The resolution issue relates also to the "kissing or crossing" problem; that is, it often cannot be decided in a large voxel whether two (or more) incoming fiber bundles cross in that voxel or whether they merely touch each other and part by changing direction.

Despite its usefulness in many applications, the diffusion tensor model has the drawback of being a unidirectional model. Its orientation estimation works very well in areas characterized by prominent fiber pathways following one direction, giving rise to a unimodal water diffusivity profile. When, however, several different diffusion directions are present in one voxel, the estimated diffusion tensor contains directionality information which has high uncertainty at best (low precision) or is even biased to a wrong average orientation. In order to obtain more valid results from diffusion-weighted measurements, several advanced measurement schemes and analysis methods have been proposed. The most complete approach to estimate the full fiber orientation density function is diffusion spectrum imaging (DSI) that requires, however, very long measurement times (Wedeen et al. 2005). Somewhat less time-consuming advanced approaches are q-ball imaging (Tuch 2004) and

spherical deconvolution (Tournier et al. 2004). These modeling approaches go beyond the simple tensor model and fit more complex models to the measured diffusion data that do no longer assume a single major diffusion axis but explicitly allow multiple (crossing) fibers in a voxel. In order to provide sufficient constraints for these more complex models, many more diffusion directions (e.g., 100) need to be measured as for conventional DTI scans that require only 6 diffusion directions. Because of the high number of direction measurements, these approaches are also called "HARDI" (high-angular-resolution diffusion imaging) methods. Since HARDI measurements (Tuch 2002) need much longer scanning time than DTI measurements, they are not common in clinical MRI measurements. Even with more advanced measurement and analysis approaches, reconstructed fiber tracts may vary substantially depending on the used tractography algorithm (Bastiani et al. 2012). To validate fiber tracking algorithms, it is important to have ground-truth data, i.e., knowledge about the true trajectory of fiber bundles. One way to perform ground-truth validation is to use "DTI phantoms" that contain known, artificially created, fibers, including challenging cases with crossing and kissing fibers (Pullens et al. 2010). Another important validation approach uses postmortem brain tissue that is analyzed both with dMRI and with tracers that are released in specific brain areas. Since these tracers traverse backwards along axons through other regions, they reveal true region-to-region connectivity that can be used as ground-truth data for DWI-based connectivity analyses of the same tissue (e.g., Seehaus et al. 2013).

5.3   Applications

In recent years, diffusion MRI has led to several interesting applications. Especially the fractional anisotropy measure has become an important biomarker of white matter integrity serving as a local index to diagnose neurological or psychiatric diseases or to predict (lack of) cognitive performance. It has been, for example, shown that

FA values extracted from dMRI measurements from good and poor readers differ, and the size of the difference is largest within a region within the left hemisphere temporoparietal white matter (Klingberg et al. 2000; Deutsch et al. 2005). FA values could also be related to the level of creativity in several brain areas including prefrontal cortex, basal ganglia, and at the border of the temporal and parietal lobe (Takeuchi et al. 2010). Note, however, that FA values are not fixed ("hardwired") properties of white matter but can change depending on the usage of the underlying fibers. It has been, for example, shown that FA values in white matter in regions of the posterior parietal cortex (containing fibers that presumably mediate visuospatial transformation) significantly increase when subjects train on an intensive visual motor coordination task such as learning to juggle (Scholz et al. 2009). It has also been discovered that FA values reflect the development of cognitive abilities including systematic increases in the corpus callosum and prefrontal cortex during childhood (Barnea-Goraly et al. 2005); the changes observed in prefrontal cortical areas are discussed as related to the development of working memory, attention, and behavioral control. FA measures are also increasingly used for early diagnosis of stroke since reduced diffusion in affected brain regions is often detected already minutes after the stroke. It is important to note that FA measurements are quantitative values (as opposed to fMRI measurements) that can be compared across people, labs, and scanners.

While computational tractography produces less objective results than FA estimates, reconstructed white matter fiber tracts are especially important to guide neurosurgical procedures potentially reducing the risk of lesioning important fiber tracts, e.g., related to language functions. For this and similar purposes, several tools (e.g., Yeatman et al. 2012) are now available that allow extracting major long-range fiber tracts from dMRI data, including *commissural tracts* (e.g., corpus callosum) connecting both cortical hemispheres, *association tracts* (e.g., arcuate fasciculus) connecting regions within the same hemisphere, and *projection tracts* (e.g., cortico-

spinal tract) connecting cortical regions to subcortical areas, the cerebellum and spinal cord. Figure 25 shows selected major fiber tracts that have been reconstructed from the dMRI data of a healthy individual; further details about the depicted (as well as other) fiber tracts are described, e.g., by Catani and Thiebaut de Schotten (2008) and Yeatman et al. (2012). For more details about the analysis and application of diffusion-weighted MRI see chapter "Diffusion Imaging with MR Tractography for Brain Tumor Surgery."

5.3.1   The Human Connectome

An important aim of recent brain research is to understand how brain areas communicate with each other. This aim is pursued by investigating anatomical connectivity with dMRI to reconstruct in vivo the macroscale human connectome (Sporns et al. 2005), which is the map of all the structural connections in the human brain. This is complemented by functional and effective connectivity studies using fMRI (see Sect. 4.1) and other modalities such as EEG and MEG. In integrative multimodal modeling approaches, the anatomical connectome may serve as an important structural constraint for functional connectivity models since only brain areas that are connected via fiber bundles may communicate directly with each other. Diffusion MRI may even help to estimate the strength of connectivity between brain areas. The *Human Connectome Project* (HCP, see http://www.neuroscienceblueprint.nih.gov/connectome/) has made substantial progress in deriving a complete map of all major macroscale connections between brain areas by measuring dMRI as well as functional connectivity and genetic data in more than 1000 individuals (twin pairs and their siblings from 300 families). Besides deriving a connectivity map—the human connectome—the measured data of structural and functional connectivity has been shared to stimulate research in the field of *human connectomics*. Furthermore, the HCP provided the basis for a number of large-scale follow-up projects using its paradigm to study the brain in health and disease. The *HCP Lifespan Projects*, for example, focus on the healthy brain across the human life span. Very early stages of development are being covered by the *Lifespan Baby Connectome* project and by the Developing Human Connectome Project that studies prenatal and neonatal brain development. The HCP also stimulated more than ten projects focusing on brain disorders operating under the general umbrella of the *Connectomes Related to Human Disease* effort. These connectome projects will unravel new insights into disease-related brain connectivity abnormalities contributing to a better understanding, diagnosis, and ultimately treatment of psychiatric, neurological, and neurodegenerative disorders.

References

Allen EA, Erhardt EB, Damaraju E, Gruner W, Segall JM et al (2011) A baseline for the multivariate comparison of resting-state networks. Front Syst Neurosci 5:2

Andersson JLR, Skare S, Ashburner J (2003) How to correct susceptibility distortions in spin-echo echo-planar images: application to diffusion tensor imaging. NeuroImage 20(2):870–888

Ashburner J (2007) A fast diffeomorphic image registration algorithm. NeuroImage 38:95–113

Ashburner J, Friston KJ (1999) Nonlinear spatial normalization using basis functions. Hum Brain Mapp 7:254–266

Bandettini PA, Cox RW (2000) Event-related fMRI contrast when using constant interstimulus interval: theory and experiment. Magn Reson Med 43:540–548

Bandettini PA, Birn RM, Donahue KM (2000) Functional MRI: background, methodology, limits, and implementation. In: Cacioppo JT, Tassinary LG, Berntson GG (eds) Handbook of psychophysiology. Cambridge University Press, New York, pp 978–1014

Barnea-Goraly N, Menon V, Eckert M, Tamm L, Bammer R, Karchemskiy A, Dant CC, Reiss AL (2005) White matter development during childhood and adolescence: a cross-sectional diffusion tensor imaging study. Cereb Cortex 15:1848–1854

Basser PJ, Mattiello J, LeBihan D (1994) Estimation of the effective self-diffusion tensor from the NMR spin echo. J Magn Reson B 103:247–254

Bastiani M, Shah NJ, Goebel R, Roebroeck A (2012) Human cortical connectome reconstruction from diffusion weighted MRI: the effect of tractography algorithm. NeuroImage 62:1732–1749

Beckmann CF, Jenkinson M, Smith SM (2003) General multilevel linear modeling for group analysis in FMRI. NeuroImage 20:1052–1063

Benjamini Y, Hochberg Y (1995) Controlling the false discovery rate: a practical and powerful approach to multiple testing. J R Stat Soc Ser B 57:289–300

Birn RM, Murphy K, Bandettini PA (2008) The effect of respiration variations on independent component analysis results of resting state functional connectivity. Hum Brain Mapp 29:740–750

Biswal B, Yetkin FZ, Haughton VM, Hyde JS (1995) Functional connectivity in the motor cortex of resting human brain using echo-planar MRI. Magn Reson Med 34:537–541

Blamire AM, Ogawa S, Ugurbil K et al (1992) Dynamic mapping of the human visual cortex by high-speed magnetic resonance imaging. Proc Natl Acad Sci U S A 89:11096–11073

Bledowski C, Cohen Kadosh K, Wibral M, Rahm B, Bittner RA, Hoechstetter K, Scherg M, Maurer K, Goebel R, Linden DE (2006) Mental chronometry of working memory retrieval: a combined functional magnetic resonance imaging and event-related potentials approach. J Neurosci 26:821–829

Boynton GM, Engel SA, Glover GH, Heeger DJ (1996) Linear systems analysis of functional magnetic resonance imaging in human V1. J Neurosci 16:4207–4221

Breman H, Mulders J, Fritz L, Peters J, Pyles J, Eck J, Bastiani M, Roebroeck A, Ashburner J, Goebel R (2020) An image registration-based method for EPI distortion correction based on opposite phase encoding (COPE). In: Špiclin Ž, McClelland J, Kybic J, Goksel O (eds) Biomedical image registration. WBIR 2020, Lecture notes in computer science, vol 12120. Springer, Cham

Brown MA, Semelka RC (1999) MRI—basic principles and applications. Wiley-Liss, New York

Büchel C, Coull JT, Friston KJ (1999) The predictive value of changes in effective connectivity for human learning. Science 283:1538–1541

Buckner RL, Bandettini PA, O'Craven KM, Savoy RL, Petersen SE, Raichle ME, Rosen BR (1996) Detection of cortical activation during averaged single trials of a cognitive task using functional magnetic resonance imaging. Proc Natl Acad Sci U S A 93:14878–14883

Buckner RL, Andrews-Hanna JR, Schacter DL (2008) The brain's default network: anatomy, function, and relevance to disease. Ann N Y Acad Sci 1124:1–38

Bullmore E, Brammer M, Williams SC et al (1996) Statistical methods of estimation and inference for functional MR image analysis. Magn Reson Med 35:261–277

Buxton RB, Wong EC, Frank LR (1998) Dynamics of blood flow and oxygen metabolism during brain activation: the balloon model. Magn Reson Med 39:855–864

Buxton RB, Uludağ K, Dubowitz DJ, Liu TT (2004) Modeling the hemodynamic response to brain activation. NeuroImage 23:S220–S233

Castelo-Branco M, Formisano E, Backes W, Zanella F, Neuenschwander S, Singer W, Goebel R (2002) Activity patterns in human motion-sensitive areas depend on the interpretation of global motion. Proc Natl Acad Sci U S A 99:13914–13919

Catani M, Thiebaut de Schotten M (2008) A diffusion tensor imaging tractography atlas for virtual in vivo dissections. Cortex 44:1105–1132

Cheng K, Waggoner AK, Tanaka K (2001) Human ocular dominance columns as revealed by high-field functional magnetic resonance imaging. Neuron 32:359–374

Cochrane D, Orcutt GH (1949) Application of least squares regression to relationships containing autocorrelated error terms. J Am Stat Assoc 44:32–61

Dale AM, Buckner RL (1997) Selective averaging of rapidly presented individual trials using fMRI. Hum Brain Mapp 5:329–340

Dale AM, Halgren E (2001) Spatiotemporal mapping of brain activity by integration of multiple imaging modalities. Curr Opin Neurobiol 11:202–208

De Luca M, Beckmann CF, De Stefano N, Matthews PM, Smith SM (2006) fMRI resting state networks define distinct modes of long-distance interactions in the human brain. NeuroImage 29:1359–1367

De Martino F, Moerel M, van de Moortele PF, Ugurbil K, Goebel R, Yacoub E, Formisano E (2013) Spatial organization of frequency preference and selectivity in the human inferior colliculus. Nat Commun 4:1386

De Martino F, Moerel M, Ugurbil K, Goebel R, Yacoub E, Formisano E (2015) Frequency preference and attention effects across cortical depths in the human primary auditory cortex. Proc Natl Acad Sci U S A 112(52):16036–16041

Deutsch GK, Dougherty RF, Bammer R, Siok WT, Gabrieli JD, Wandell B (2005) Children's reading performance is correlated with white matter structure measured by diffusion tensor imaging. Cortex 41:354–363

Draper NR, Smith H (1998) Applied regression analysis, 3rd edn. John Wiley & Sons, New York

Duvernoy HM, Delon S, Vannson JL (1981) Cortical blood vessels of the human brain. Brain Res Bull 7:519–579

Eklund A, Nichols TE, Knutsson H (2016) Cluster failure: why fMRI inferences for spatial extent have inflated false-positive rates. Proc Natl Acad Sci 113:7900–7905

Esposito F, Seifritz E, Formisano E, Morrone R, Scarabino T, Tedeschi G, Cirillo S, Goebel R, Di Salle F (2003) Real-time independent component analysis of fMRI time-series. NeuroImage 20:2209–2224

Esposito F, Scarabino T, Hyvarinen A, Himberg J, Formisano E, Comani S, Tedeschi G, Goebel R, Seifritz E, Di Salle F (2005) Independent component analysis of fMRI group studies by self-organizing clustering. NeuroImage 25:193–205

Esposito F, Otto T, Zijlstra FRH, Goebel R (2014) Spatially distributed effects of mental exhaustion on resting-state FMRI networks. PLoS One 9:e94222

Evans AC, Collins DL, MIlls SR, Brown ED, Kelly RL, Peters TM (1993) 3D statistical neuroanatomical models from 305 MRI volumes. In: Proceedings of IEEE-Nuclear Science Symposium and Medical Imaging Conference. pp 1813–1817.

Fischl B, Sereno MI, Tootell RBH, Dale AM (1999) High-resolution inter-subject averaging and a coordinate system for the cortical surface. Hum Brain Mapp 8:272–284

Forman SD, Cohen JD, Fitzgerald M, Eddy WF, Mintun MA, Noll DC (1995) Improved assessment of significant activation in functional magnetic resonance imaging (fMRI): use of a cluster size threshold. Magn Reson Med 3(5):636–647

Formisano E, Goebel R (2003) Tracking cognitive processes with functional MRI mental chronometry. Curr Opin Neurobiol 13:174–181

Formisano E, Esposito F, Kriegeskorte N, Tedeschi G, Di Salle F, Goebel R (2002) Spatial independent component analysis of functional magnetic resonance imaging time-series: characterization of the cortical components. Neurocomputing 49:241–254

Fox PT, Raichle ME, Mintun MA, Dence C (1988) Nonoxidative glucose consumption during focal physiological neural activity. Science 241:462–464

Friston KJ, Henson RN (2006) Commentary on: divide and conquer; a defense of functional localisers. NeuroImage 30:1097–1099

Friston KJ, Jezzard P, Turner R (1994) The analysis of functional MRI time-series. Hum Brain Mapp 1:153–171

Friston KJ, Holmes AP, Worsley KJ, Poline JP, Frith CD, Frackowiak RSJ (1995) Statistical parametric maps in functional imaging: a general linear approach. Hum Brain Mapp 2:189–210

Friston KJ, Fletcher P, Josephs O, Holmes A, Rugg MD, Turner R (1998) Event-related fMRI: characterizing differential responses. NeuroImage 7:30–40

Friston KJ, Penny W, Phillips C, Kiebel S, Hinton G, Ashburner J (2002) Classical and Bayesian inference in neuroimaging: theory. NeuroImage 16:465–483

Friston KJ, Stephan KE, Lund TE, Morcom A, Kiebel S (2005) Mixed-effects and fMRI studies. NeuroImage 24:244–252

Friston KJ, Rotshtein P, Geng JJ, Sterzer P, Henson RN (2006) A critique of functional localisers. NeuroImage 30:1077–1087

Frost M, Goebel R (2012) Measuring structural-functional correspondence: spatial variability of specialised brain regions after macro-anatomical alignment. NeuroImage 59:1369–1381

Frost M, Goebel R (2013) Functionally informed cortex based alignment: an integrated approach for whole-cortex macro-anatomical and ROI-based functional alignment. NeuroImage 83:1002–1010

Fujita I, Tanaka K, Ito M, Cheng K (1992) Columns for visual features of objects in monkey inferotemporal cortex. Nature 360:343–346

Genovese CR, Lazar NA, Nichols T (2002) Thresholding of statistical maps in functional neuroimaging using the false discovery rate. NeuroImage 15:870–878

Gentile F, van Atteveldt N, De Martino F, Goebel R (2017) Approaching the ground truth: revealing the functional organization of human multisensory STC using ultra-high field fMRI. J Neurosci 37(42):10104–10113

Glover GH, Li TQ, Ress D (2000) Image-based method for retrospective correction of physiological motion effects in fMRI: RETROICOR. Magn Reson Med 44:162–167

Goebel R (2012) BrainVoyager—past, present, future. NeuroImage 62:748–756

Goebel R (2021) Analysis methods for real-time fMRI neurofeedback. In: Hampson M (ed) fMRI neurofeedback. Elsevier, Amsterdam

Goebel R, Singer W (1999) Cortical surface-based statistical analysis of functional magnetic resonance imaging data. NeuroImage 9(6):S64

Goebel R, Roebroeck A, Kim DS, Formisano E (2003) Investigating directed cortical interactions in time-resolved fMRI data using vector autoregressive modeling and Granger causality mapping. Magn Reson Imaging 21:1251–1261

Goebel R, Hasson U, Lefi I, Malach R (2004) Statistical analyses across aligned cortical hemispheres reveal high-resolution population maps of human visual cortex. NeuroImage 22(Supplement 2)

Goebel R, Esposito F, Formisano E (2006) Analysis of functional image analysis contest (FIAC) data with BrainVoyager QX: from single-subject to cortically aligned group general linear model analysis and self-organizing group independent component analysis. Hum Brain Mapp 27:392–401

Goebel R, Zilverstand A, Sorger B (2010) Real-time fMRI-based brain–computer interfacing for neurofeedback therapy and compensation of lost motor functions. Imag Med 2:407–414

Handwerker DA, Ollinger JM, D'Esposito M (2004) Variation of BOLD hemodynamic responses across subjects and brain regions and their effects on statistical analyses. NeuroImage 21(4):1639–1651

Haxby JV, Gobbini MI, Furey ML, Ishai A, Schouten JL, Pietrini P (2001) Distributed and overlapping representations of faces and objects in ventral temporal cortex. Science 293:2425–2430

Haxby JV, Guntupalli JS, Connolly AC, Halchenko YO, Conroy BR, Gobbini MI, Hanke M, Ramadge PJ (2011) A common, high-dimensional model of the representational space in human ventral temporal cortex. Neuron 72(2):404–416

Hindriks R, Adhikari MH, Murayama Y, Ganzetti M, Mantini D, Logothetis NK et al (2016) Can sliding-window correlations reveal dynamic functional connectivity in resting-state fMRI? NeuroImage 127:242–256

Holmes AP, Friston KJ (1998) Generalisability, random effects & population inference. In: Fourth int. conf. on functional mapping of the human brain. NeuroImage 7:S754

Huettel SA, Song AW, McCarthy G (2004) Functional magnetic resonance imaging. Sinauer Associates, Sunderland, MA

Jelescu IO, Budde MD (2017) Design and validation of diffusion MRI models of white matter. Front Phys 5:61

Jezzard P, Balaban B (1995) Correction for geometric distortion in echo planar images from B0 field variations. Magn Reson Med 34(1):65–73

Khaligh-Razavi SM, Kriegeskorte N (2014) Deep supervised, but not unsupervised, models may explain IT cortical representation. PLoS Comput Biol 10(11):e1003915

Khalili-Mahani N, Zoethout RM, Beckmann CF, Baerends E, de Kam ML et al (2012) Effects of morphine and alcohol on functional brain connectivity during "resting state": a placebo-controlled cross-over study in healthy young men. Hum Brain Mapp 33:1003–1018

Kim DS, Duong TQ, Kim SG (2000) High-resolution mapping of iso-orientation columns by fMRI. Nat Neurosci 3:164–169

Kirby KN (1993) Advanced data analysis with SYSTAT. Van Nostrand Reinhold, New York

Klingberg T, Hedehus M, Temple E, Salz T, Gabrieli JD, Moseley ME, Poldrack RA (2000) Microstructure of temporo-parietal white matter as a basis for reading ability: evidence from diffusion tensor magnetic resonance imaging. Neuron 25:493–500

Krause F, Benjamins C, Eck J, Lührs M, van Hoof R, Goebel R (2019) Active head motion reduction in magnetic resonance imaging using tactile feedback. Hum Brain Mapp 40(14):4026–4037

Kriegeskorte N, Goebel R (2001) An efficient algorithm for topologically correct segmentation of the cortical sheet in anatomical MR volumes. NeuroImage 14:329–346

Kriegeskorte N, Goebel R, Bandettini P (2006) Information-based functional brain mapping. Proc Natl Acad Sci U S A 103:3863–3868

Kriegeskorte N, Mur M, Bandettini P (2008) Representational similarity analysis—connecting the branches of systems neuroscience. Front Syst Neurosci 2:1–28

Kruggel F, von Cramon DY (1999) Temporal properties of the hemodynamic response in functional MRI. Hum Brain Mapp 8:259–271

Kutner MH, Nachtsheim CJ, Neter J, Li W (2005) Applied linear statistical models, 5th edn. McGraw-Hill, Boston

LaConte SM, Peltier SJ, Hu XP (2007) Real-time fMRI using brain-state classification. Hum Brain Mapp 28:1033–1044

Lenoski B, Baxter LC, Karam LJ, Maisog J, Debbins J (2008) On the performance of autocorrelation estimation algorithms for fMRI analysis. IEEE J Sel Top Signal Proc 2:828–838

Linden DEJ, Habes I, Johnston SJ, Linden S, Tatineni R, Subramanian L, Sorger B, Healy D, Goebel R (2012) Real-time self-regulation of emotion networks in patients with depression. PLoS One 7:e38115

Logothetis NK, Wandell B (2004) Interpreting the BOLD signal. Annu Rev Physiol 66:735–769

Logothetis NK, Pauls J, Augath M, Trinath T, Oeltermann A (2001) Neurophysiological investigation of the basis of the fMRI signal. Nature 412:150–157

Magistretti PJ, Pellerin L, Rothman DL, Shulman RG (1999) Energy on demand. Science 283:496–497

Mathiesen C, Caesar K, Lauritzen M (2000) Temporal coupling between neuronal activity and blood flow in rat cerebellar cortex as indicated by field potential analysis. J Physiol 523:235–246

Maus B, van Breukelen GJ, Goebel R, Berger MP (2010a) Optimization of blocked designs in fMRI studies. Psychom Theory 75:373–390

Maus B, van Breukelen GJ, Goebel R, Berger MP (2010b) Robustness of optimal design of fMRI experiments with application of a genetic algorithm. NeuroImage 49:2433–2443

McIntosh AR, Gonzalez-Lima F (1994) Structural equation modeling and its application to network analysis in functional brain imaging. Hum Brain Mapp 2:2–22

McKeown MJ, Makeig S, Brown GG, Jung TP, Kindermann SS, Bell AJ, Iragui V, Sejnowski TJ (1998a) Blind separation of functional magnetic resonance imaging (fMRI) data. Hum Brain Mapp 6:368–372

McKeown MJ, Makeig S, Brown GG, Jung TP, Kindermann SS, Bell AJ, Sejnowski TJ (1998b) Analysis of fMRI data by blind separation into independent spatial components. Hum Brain Mapp 6:160–188

Mehler DMA, Sokunbi MO, Habes I, Barawi K, Subramanian L, Range M, Evans J, Hood K, Lührs M, Keedwell P, Goebel R, Linden DEJ (2018) Targeting the affective brain-a randomized controlled trial of real-time fMRI neurofeedback in patients with depression. Neuropsychopharmacology 43(13):2578–2585

Menon RS, Kim SG (1999) Spatial and temporal limits in cognitive neuroimaging with fMRI. Trends Cogn Sci 3:207–216

Moeller S, Yacoub E, Auerbach E, Strupp JP, Harel N, Ugurbil K (2010) Multi-band multi-slice GE-EPI at 7 Tesla, with 16 fold acceleration using partial parallel imaging with application to high spatial and temporal whole brain fMRI. Magn Reson Med 63: 1144–1143

Mulert C, Jager L, Schmitt R, Bussfeld P, Pogarell O, Moller HJ, Juckel G, Hegerl U (2004) Integration of fMRI and simultaneous EEG: towards a comprehensive understanding of localization and time-course of brain activity in target detection. NeuroImage 22:83–94

Murphy K, Birn RM, Bandettini PA (2013) Resting-state fMRI confounds and cleanup. NeuroImage 80:349–359

NessAiver M (1997) All you really need to know about MRI physics. Simply Physics, Baltimore

Nichols TE, Brett M, Andersson J, Wager T, Poline JB (2005) Valid conjunction inference with the minimum statistic. NeuroImage 25:653–660

Nowogrodzki A (2018) The world's strongest MRI machines are pushing human imaging to new limits. Nature 563:24–26

O'Craven KM, Kanwisher N (2000) Mental imagery of faces and places activates corresponding stimulus-specific brain regions. J Cogn Neurosci 12:1013–1023

Ogawa S, Lee TM, Kay AR, Tank DW (1990) Brain magnetic resonance imaging with contrast dependent on blood oxygenation. Proc Natl Acad Sci U S A 87:9868–9872

Panagiotaki E, Schneider T, Siow B, Hal MG, Lythgoe MF, Alexander DC (2012) Compartment models of the diffusion MR signal in brain white matter: a taxonomy and comparison. NeuroImage 59(3):2241–2254

Penny WD, Stephan KE, Mechelli A, Friston KJ (2004) Comparing dynamic causal models. NeuroImage 22:1157–1172

Pruessmann KP, Weiger M, Scheidegger MB, Boesiger P (1999) SENSE: sensitivity encoding for fast MRI. Magn Reson Med 42:952–962

Pullens P, Roebroeck A, Goebel R (2010) Ground truth hardware phantoms for validation of diffusion-weighted MRI applications. J Magn Reson Imaging 32:482–488

Raichle ME, MacLeod AM, Snyder AZ, Powers WJ, Gusnard DA, Shulman GL (2001) A default mode of brain function. Proc Natl Acad Sci U S A 98:676–682

Robson MD, Dorosz JL, Gore JC (1998) Measurements of the temporal fMRI response of the human auditory cortex to trains of tones. NeuroImage 7:185–198

Roebroeck A, Formisano E, Goebel R (2005) Mapping directed influence over the brain using Granger causality and fMRI. NeuroImage 25:230–242

Roebroeck A, Formisano E, Goebel R (2011) The identification of interacting networks in the brain using fMRI: model selection, causality and deconvolution. NeuroImage 58:296–302

Saxe R, Brett M, Kanwisher N (2006) Divide and conquer: a defense of functional localizers. NeuroImage 30:1088–1096; discussion 1097–1089

Scherg M, Linden DEJ, Muckli L, Roth R, Drüen K, Ille N, Zanella FE, Singer W, Goebel R (1999) Combining MEG with fMRI in studies of the human visual system. In: Yoshimoto T, Kotani M, Karibe H, Nakasato N (eds) Recent advances in biomagnetism. Tohoku University Press, Sendai

Schild HH (1990) MRI made easy. Schering AG, Berlin

Schneider M, Kemper VG, Emmerling TC, De Martino F, Goebel R (2019) Columnar clusters in the human motion complex reflect consciously perceived motion axis. Proc Natl Acad Sci U S A 116(11): 5096–5101

Scholz J, Klein MC, Behrens TEJ, Johansen-Berg H (2009) Training induces changes in white-matter architecture. Nat Neurosci 12:1370–1371

Searle SR, Casella G, McCulloch CE, (1992) Variance Components. Wiley, New York.

Seehaus AK, Roebroeck A, Chiry O, Kim DS, Ronen I, Bratzke H, Goebel R, Galuske RAW (2013)

Histological validation of DW-MRI tractography in human postmortem tissue. Cereb Cortex 23:442–450

Setsompop K, Gagoski BA, Polimeni JR, Witzel T, Wedeen VJ, Wald LL (2012) Blipped-controlled aliasing in parallel imaging for simultaneous multislice echo planer imaging with reduced g-factor penalty. Magn Reson Med 67:1210–1224

Sorger B, Peters J, van den Boomen C, Zilverstand A, Reithler J, Goebel R (2010) Real-time decoding of the locus of visuospatial attention using multi-voxel pattern classification. In: Human brain mapping, 16th edn., Barcelona, Spain

Sorger B, Reithler J, Dahmen B, Goebel R (2012) A real-time fMRI-based spelling device immediately enabling robust motor-independent communication. Curr Biol 22:1333–1338

Sporns O (2010) Connectome. Scholarpedia 5:5584

Sporns O, Tononi G, Kotter R (2005) The human connectome: a structural description of the human brain. PLoS Comput Biol 1:e42

Stejskal EO, Tanner JE (1965) Spin diffusion measurements: spin echoes in the presence of a time-dependent field gradient. J Chem Phys 42:288–292

Subramanian L, Hindle JV, Johnston S, Roberts MV, Husain M, Goebel R, Linden D (2011) Real-time functional magnetic resonance imaging neurofeedback for treatment of Parkinson's disease. J Neurosci 31:16309–16317

Takeuchi H, Taki Y, Sassa Y, Hashizume H, Sekiguchi A, Fukushima A, Kawashima R (2010) White matter structures associated with creativity: evidence from diffusion tensor imaging. NeuroImage 51:11–18

Talairach G, Tournoux P (1988) Co-planar stereotaxic atlas of the human brain. Thieme, New York

Thesen S, Heid O, Mueller E, Schad LR (2000) Prospective acquisition correction for head motion with image-based tracking for real-time fMRI. Magn Reson Med 44(3):457–465

Todd N, Josephs O, Zeidman P, Flandin G, Moeller S, Weiskopf N (2017) Functional sensitivity of 2D simultaneous multi-slice echo-planar imaging: effects of acceleration on g-factor and physiological noise. Front Neurosci 11:158

Tournier JD, Calamante F, Gadian DG, Connelly A (2004) Direct estimation of the fiber orientation density function from diffusion-weighted MRI data using spherical deconvolution. NeuroImage 23:1176–1185

Tuch DS (2002) High angular resolution diffusion imaging reveals intravoxel white matter fiber heterogeneity. Magn Reson Med 48:577–582

Tuch DS (2004) Q-ball imaging. Magn Reson Med 52:1358–1372

Uludağ K, Uğurbil K, Berliner L (2015) MRI: from nuclear spins to brain functions. Springer, New York

van de Ven VG, Formisano E, Prvulovic D, Roeder CH, Linden DE (2004) Functional connectivity as revealed by spatial independent component analysis of fMRI measurements during rest. Hum Brain Mapp 22:165–178

van de Ven VG, Formisano E, Roder CH, Prvulovic D, Bittner RA, Dietz MG, Hubl D, Dierks T, Federspiel A, Esposito F, Di Salle F, Jansma B, Goebel R, Linden DE (2005) The spatiotemporal pattern of auditory cortical responses during verbal hallucinations. NeuroImage 27:644–655

Vapnik V (1995) The nature of statistical learning theory. Springer Verlag, New York

Wager TD, Nichols TE (2003) Optimization of experimental design in fMRI: a general framework using a genetic algorithm. NeuroImage 18:293–309

Wedeen VJ, Hagmann P, Tseng WY, Reese TG, Weisskoff RM (2005) Mapping complex tissue architecture with diffusion spectrum magnetic resonance imaging. Magn Reson Med 54:1377–1386

Weiskopf (2012) Real-time fMRI and its application to neurofeedback. NeuroImage 62:682–692

Weiskopf N, Veit R, Erb M, Mathiak K, Grodd W, Goebel R, Birbaumer N (2003) Physiological self-regulation of regional brain activity using real-time functional magnetic resonance imaging (fMRI): methodology and exemplary data. NeuroImage 19:577–586

Weiskopf N, Hutton C, Josephs O, Deichmann R (2006) Optimal EPI parameters for reduction of susceptibility-induced BOLD sensitivity losses: a whole-brain analysis at 3 T and 1.5 T. NeuroImage 33:493–504

Worsley KJ, Marrett S, Neelin P, Evans AC (1992) A three-dimensional statistical analysis for CBF activation studies in human brain. J Cereb Blood Flow Metab 12:900–918

Worsley KJ, Liao CH, Aston J, Petre V, Duncan GH, Morales F, Evans AC (2002) A general statistical analysis for fMRI data. NeuroImage 15:1–15

Yacoub E, Harel N, Ugurbil K (2008) High-field fMRI unveils orientation columns in humans. PNAS USA 105:10607–10612

Yeatman JD, Dougherty RF, Myall NJ, Wandell BA, Feldman HM (2012) Tract profiles of white matter properties: automating fiber-tract quantification. PLoS One 7:e49790

Zaitsev M, Dold C, Sakas G, Hennig J, Speck O (2006) Magnetic resonance imaging of freely moving objects: prospective real-time motion correction using an external optical motion tracking system. NeuroImage 31(3):1038–1050

Zimmermann J, Goebel R, De Martino F, van de Moortele PF, Feinberg D, Adriany G, Chaimov D, Shmuel A, Uğurbil K, Yacoub E (2011) Mapping the organization of axis of motion selective features in human area MT using high-field fMRI. PLoS One 6:e28716

Functional Neuroanatomy

Thomas P. Naidich and Tarek A. Yousry

Contents

T. P. Naidich
Mount Sinai School of Medicine,
New York, NY, USA

Department of Neuroradiology and Neurosurgery,
Irving and Dorothy Regenstreif Research,
New York, NY, USA

T. A. Yousry (✉)
Lysholm Department of Neuroradiology, The
National Hospital for Neurology and Neurosurgery,
Institute of Neurology, London, UK
e-mail: t.yousry@ucl.ac.uk

Abstract

We present the surface anatomy of the brain describing in detail the typical configuration of the sulci and gyri and their most frequent variations. After describing the borders of the lobes, we give guidance on the methods of localizing functionally important atomic structures such as the pericentral cortex, Heschl's gyrus, and calcarine sulcus.

© The Author(s), under exclusive license to Springer Nature Switzerland AG 2022
C. Stippich (ed.), *Clinical Functional MRI*, Medical Radiology Diagnostic Imaging,
https://doi.org/10.1007/978-3-030-83343-5_3

On the basis of the surface anatomy and the cytoarchitectonic subdivision of the cortex, we describe the function of selected areas related to the motor system and to speech.

1   Introduction

Modern neurophysiology and fMRI have refined our concepts of cerebral organization. This section presents the surface anatomy of the brain and begins to address the functional interrelationships among the cortical areas.

2   Surface Anatomy

2.1   Convexity Surface

2.1.1   Sylvian Fissure

The convexity face of the sylvian fissure displays five major arms (rami) that help to define the surface anatomy of the convexity (Fig. 1). The long nearly horizontal portion of the sylvian fissure is the posterior horizontal ramus. At its anterior end, the anterior horizontal ramus and the anterior ascending ramus arise together in a "V" or "Y" configuration. At its posterior end, the prominent posterior ascending ramus and the small posterior descending ramus branch outward in a "T" or "fishtail" configuration. The anterior subcentral sulcus and the posterior subcentral sulcus form two minor arms that extend superiorly into the frontoparietal operculum to delimit the subcentral gyrus. One or multiple transverse temporal sulci extend inferiorly into the temporal lobe in relation to the transverse temporal gyrus of Heschl.

2.1.2   Frontal Lobe

The convexity surface of the frontal lobe is formed by four gyri and three sulci (Fig. 2). The superior frontal gyrus (SFG) is a horizontally oriented, roughly rectangular bar of tissue that

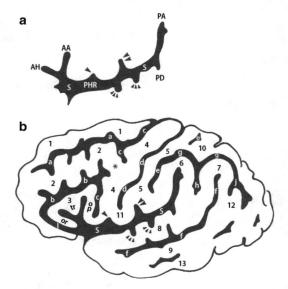

Fig. 1 (**a**, **b**) Surface anatomy of the convexity. (**a**) Sylvian fissure (*dark area*). The margins of the frontal, parietal, and temporal opercula are defined by the configuration of the sylvian fissure (*S*), its five major rami (the anterior horizontal ramus (*AH*), anterior ascending ramus (*AA*), posterior horizontal ramus (*PHR*), posterior ascending ramus (*PA*), and posterior descending ramus (*PD*)), and its minor arms, the anterior subcentral sulcus (*single arrowhead*), posterior subcentral sulcus (*double arrowheads*), and transverse temporal sulci (*triple arrowheads*). (**b**) Cerebral convexity. The configuration of the sylvian fissure then permits identification of the adjoining gyri and sulci. GYRI: *1* superior frontal gyrus (*SFG*), *2* middle frontal gyrus (*MFG*), *3* inferior frontal gyrus (or, pars orbitalis; tr, pars triangularis; op, pars opercularis), *4* precentral gyrus (*pre-CG*), *5* postcentral gyrus (*post-CG*), *6* supramarginal gyrus (*SMG*), *7* angular gyrus (*AG*), *8* superior temporal gyrus (*STG*), *9* middle temporal gyrus (*MTG*), *10* superior parietal lobule (*SPL*), *11* subcentral gyrus, *12* temporo-occipital arcus, *13* inferior temporal gyrus: * union of the MFG (*2*) with the pre-CG (*4*). SULCI; *a* superior frontal sulcus (*SFS*), *b* inferior frontal sulcus (*IFS*), *c* precentral sulcus (*pre-CS*), *d* central sulcus (*CS*), *e* postcentral sulcus (*post-CS*), *f* superior temporal sulcus (*STS*), *g* intraparietal sulcus (*IPS*), *h* primary intermediate sulcus, *j* secondary intermediate sulcus, *k* accessory intermediate sulcus (not shown in this image), *S* sylvian fissure, *single black arrowhead* anterior subcentral sulcus, *double black arrowheads* posterior subcentral sulcus, *triple black arrowheads* transverse temporal sulci. Note specifically how the anterior horizontal and anterior ascending rami of the sylvian fissure divide the inferior frontal gyrus into the three parts orbitalis (*or*), triangularis (*tr*), and opercularis (*op*). The lateral orbital sulcus (*l*) separates the pars orbitalis from the lateral orbital gyrus. (From Naidich et al. (1995); with permission)

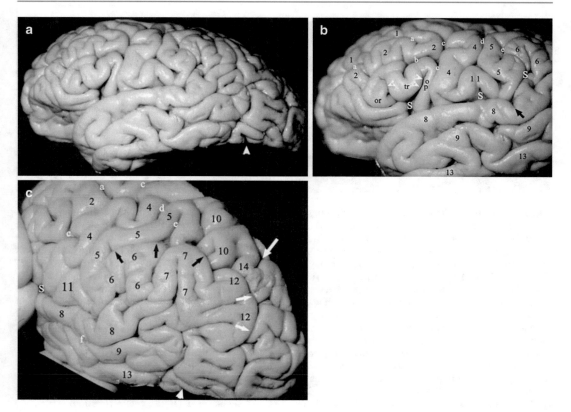

Fig. 2 (**a–c**) Normal cerebral convexity. (**a**) Anatomic specimen full surface. (**b**) Magnified view of the low-middle convexity. (**c**) Magnified oblique view of the parietal lobe. The surface vessels and the pia-arachnoid have been removed to expose the gyri and sulci more clearly (labels as in Fig. 1). In (**a**), the *single large white arrowhead* = preoccipital notch. In (**b**), the portions of the sylvian fissure (*S*) are indicated: *first white S* = vallecula leading to the anterior horizontal ramus (*single white arrow*) and the anterior ascending ramus (*double white arrow*); *second white S* = posterior horizontal ramus; *third white S* = posterior ascending ramus; *short black arrow* = posterior descending ramus of the sylvian fissure. In (**c**), the anterior border of the occipital lobe extends from the lateral end of the parieto-occipital sulcus (*large white arrow*) above to the preoccipital notch (*large white arrowhead*) below. The intraparietal sulcus (*multiple large black arrows*) crosses the theoretical lobar border to become the intraoccipital sulcus (*multiple large white arrows*). The inferior parietal lobule is composed of the SMG (*6*), the AG (*7*), and the temporo-occipital arcus (second *pli de passage* of Gratiolet) (*12*). The superior parietal lobule merges into the superior occipital gyrus across the parieto-occipital border through the parieto-occipital arcus (first *pli de passage* of Gratiolet) (*14*). ((**a**, **b**) From Naidich et al. (1997); (**c**) from Naidich and Brightbill (1995); with permission)

forms the uppermost margin of the frontal lobe. The middle frontal gyrus (MFG) is a horizontally oriented, undulant length of tissue that zigzags posteriorly to merge with the anterior face of the precentral gyrus. The inferior frontal gyrus (IFG) is a triangular gyrus that nestles inferiorly against the anteriormost portion of the sylvian fissure. The precentral gyrus (pre-CG) is a nearly vertical gyrus that forms the posterior border of the fron-

tal lobe, behind the SFG, MFG, and IFG. The superior frontal sulcus (SFS) separates the SFG from the MFG. At its posterior end, the SFS bifurcates to form the superior precentral sulcus. The inferior frontal sulcus (IFS) separates the MFG from the IFG. At its posterior end, the IFS bifurcates to form the inferior precentral sulcus. Together, the superior and inferior portions of the pre-CS delimit the anterior face of the precentral

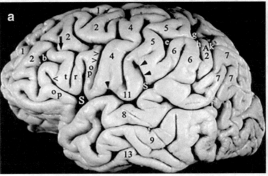
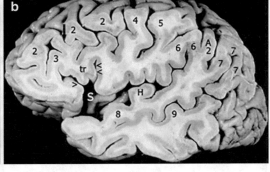

Fig. 3 (**a**, **b**) Normal variations in convexity anatomy. (**a**) Convexity surface of a prepared left hemisphere. (**b**) Sagittal section of a prepared left hemisphere. A vertically oriented connecting gyrus (*short black arrow*) crosses the inferior frontal sulcus (IFS) (*b*) to unite the pars triangularis (*tr*) with the middle frontal gyrus (MFG) (*2*). A sulcus triangularis (between the *t* and the *r*) deeply notches the superior surface of the pars triangularis making it appear bifid. The precentral gyrus (*4*) and the postcentral gyrus (*5*) unite beneath the central sulcus to form the subcentral gyrus (*11*), which is delimited by a shallow anterior subcentral sulcus (*single black arrowhead*) and a deep posterior subcentral sulcus (*double black arrowheads*). The inferior portion of the postcentral sulcus (*e*) forms the initial upswing of the arcuate intraparietal sulcus (IPS) (*g*). The posterior ascending ramus of the sylvian fissure

(*S*) indents the inferior parietal lobule (IPL) to form the supramarginal gyrus (SMG) (*6*). The superior temporal sulcus (STS) (*f*) indents the posterior portion of the IPL to form the angular gyrus (AG) (*7*). The entire STS parallels the sylvian fissure, hence its synonym: parallel sulcus. The distal end of the STS within the AG may be designated the angular sulcus. In this specimen, an intercalated accessory preangular gyrus (*A2*) separates the SMG from the AG. Note the relationships of the IPS (*g*), the SMG (*6*), the AG (*7*), and the accessory preangular gyrus (*A2*) with the primary intermediate sulcus (*h*), the secondary intermediate sulcus (*j*), and the accessory intermediate sulcus (*k*). In (**b**), the sagittal section exposes the characteristic appearance of the transverse temporal gyrus of Heschl (*H*) on the superior surface of the temporal lobe. (From Naidich et al. (1995); with permission)

gyrus, except where the MFG merges with the pre-CG between the superior and inferior precentral sulci.

The frontal gyri display characteristic configurations (Fig. 1) and variations (Albanese et al. 1989; Naidich et al. 1995, 1997). The IFG has an overall triangular configuration (hence, its synonym: triangular gyrus). The IFS courses above the IFG, bifurcates into the inferior pre-CS, and thereby separates the triangular IFG from the MFG above and from the pre-CG behind. The anterior horizontal and anterior ascending rami of the sylvian fissure extend upward into the triangular IFG, partially subdividing it into three portions: the *pars orbitalis*, which abuts the orbital gyri of the frontal lobe; the *pars triangularis* in the center; and the *pars opercularis*, which forms the anteriormost portion of the frontal operculum. Together, the three parts of the IFG resemble an oblique letter "M" (Figs. 1, 2, 3, and 4). Because the anterior ascending ramus of

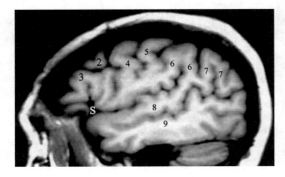

Fig. 4 Sagittal T1-weighted MR imaging of the language-related areas of the normal cerebral convexity. T1-weighted image of a 78-year-old man. Labels as in Figs. 1 and 2. (From Naidich et al. (1997); with permission)

the sylvian fissure cuts through the full thickness of the IFG to reach the insula, the cortex of the *pars opercularis* presents both a superficial cortex visible on the surface and a deep cortex within the depths of the fissure (Naidich et al. 2001a).

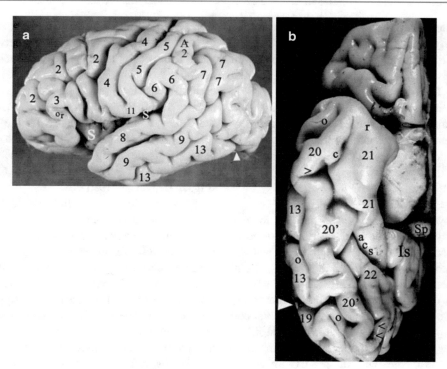

Fig. 5 (**a, b**) The temporal lobe. Prepared anatomic specimen of the right hemisphere from a 1-day-old girl. (**a**) Convexity (reversed to match the other lateral views). The simplified gyral and sulcal pattern reflects the young age. The inferior temporal gyrus (*13*) extends posteriorly to the preoccipital notch (*large white arrowhead*). An accessory preangular gyrus (*A2*) is situated superior to the SMG (*6*) and anterior to the AG (*7*). Labels as in Figs. 1 and 2. (**b**) Inferior surface. The brain stem and the inferior thalamus have been removed to reveal the medial surface more clearly. The inferior temporal gyrus (*13*) and the inferior occipital gyrus (*19*) form the inferior margin of the hemisphere, separated by the preoccipital notch (*large white arrowhead*). The lateral occipitotemporal sulcus (*o*) delineates their medial border and separates them from the lateral occipitotemporal gyrus (LOTG) (*20*) further medially. The medial occipitotemporal sulcus (synonym: collateral sulcus) (*c*) delimits the medial border of the LOTG over its full length. Anteriorly, the collateral sulcus approximates the rhinal sulcus (*r*), and may run into it, or may parallel it. The parahippocampal gyrus (PHG) (*21*) forms the medial surface of the temporal lobe over its full length and extends posteriorly to become the isthmus (*Is*) of the cingulate gyrus inferior to the splenium (*Sp*). In the anterior half of the temporal lobe, the collateral sulcus (*c*) separates the LOTG (*20*) from the PHG (*21*). In the posterior half, the medial occipitotemporal gyrus (MOTG) (lingual gyrus) (*22*) intercalates itself between the LOTG and the PHG. The collateral sulcus stays with the medial border of the LOTG, so the collateral sulcus (*c*) separates the LOTG (*20*) from the MOTG (*22*), while the anterior calcarine sulcus (*acs*) separates the MOTG (*22*) from the PHG (*21*). The anterior and posterior transverse collateral sulci (*single and double black arrowheads*) delimit a midportion of the LOTG (*20'*) that has been designated by Duvernoy (1991) as the fusiform gyrus. (From Daniels et al. (1987); with permission)

2.1.3 Temporal Lobe

The convexity surface of the temporal lobe is formed by three horizontal gyri: the superior temporal gyrus (STG), the middle temporal gyrus (MTG), and the inferior temporal gyrus (ITG), separated by the superior temporal sulcus (STS) and the inferior temporal sulcus (ITS) (Fig. 5). The superior and middle temporal gyri extend posteriorly and then swing upward to join with the parietal lobe. The inferior temporal gyrus forms the inferior edge of the convexity surface of temporal lobe and curves onto the inferior surface of the temporal lobe. It is delimited posteriorly by a small notch, the preoccipital notch (synonyms: temporo-occipital notch or incisura), which separates the inferior temporal gyrus anteriorly from the inferior occipital gyrus posteriorly. The STS courses parallel to the posterior horizontal and the posterior ascending rami of the sylvian fissure (hence its synonym, parallel sulcus). The posterior portion of the STS is directed superiorly and is sometimes designated the angular sulcus. The ITS courses approximately parallel to the inferior margin of the convexity and may become continuous posteriorly with the inferior occipital sulcus.

2.1.4   Parietal Lobe

The convexity surface of the parietal lobe is formed by three portions: the vertically oriented postcentral gyrus (post-CG) anteriorly, and the two superior parietal (SPL) and inferior parietal (IPL) lobules posteriorly (Figs. 1, 2, 3, and 4). The post-CG courses vertically just posterior and parallel to the pre-CG. The post-CG is separated from the pre-CG by the intervening central sulcus (CS) over most of its length. However, inferiorly, the post-CG merges with the pre-CG inferior to the CS along the subcentral gyrus (sub-CG) just above the sylvian fissure. Superiorly, the post-CG merges with the pre-CG superior to the CS along the paracentral lobule (para-CL) on the medial surface of the hemisphere. Thus, the precentral and postcentral gyri actually form a continuous band of tissue that circles around the central sulcus from the precentral gyrus through the subcentral gyrus, into the postcentral gyrus and the paracentral lobule, returning into the precentral gyrus.

The posterior border of the post-CG is delimited by the superior and inferior postcentral sulci. The superior post-CS separates the upper post-CG from the superior parietal lobule. The inferior post-CS separates the post-CG from the inferior parietal lobule. The inferior post-CS may be considered the upswing of a long, deep, arcuate intraparietal sulcus (IPS) that ascends behind the lower post-CG and then slashes posteriorly across the convexity surface of the parietal lobe, dividing it into the SPL situated superomedial to the IPS and the IPL situated inferolateral to the

IPS. The posterior downswing of the arcuate IPS then crosses the theoretical border between the parietal and occipital lobes and continues into the occipital lobe, where it is designated the intraoccipital sulcus (IOS) (synonym: superior occipital sulcus, SOS) (Figs. 1, 2, 3, and 4). Posteriorly, the SPL becomes continuous with the superior occipital gyrus (SOG) behind it through a narrow band of tissue designated the arcus parieto-occipitalis (first *pli de passage* of Gratiolet) (Fig. 2) (Duvernoy 1991).

Within the inferior parietal lobule, the posterior ascending ramus of the sylvian fissure swings upward into the anterior portion of the IPL and is capped by a horseshoe-shaped gyrus designated the supramarginal gyrus (SMG). In parallel fashion, the distal STS swings upward into the posterior portion of the IPL where it is capped by a second horseshoe-shaped gyrus designated the angular gyrus (AG). The AG usually lies just posterior to the SMG, but may be displaced from that position by variant accessory gyri (Figs. 1, 2, 3, and 4) (Naidich et al. 1995, 1997). Together the SMG and the AG constitute most of the IPL. An additional small horseshoe of tissue, designated the second parieto-occipital arcus (second *pli de passage* of Gratiolet), connects the AG with the middle OG posterior to it, completing the IPL (Fig. 2) (Duvernoy 1991). A small primary intermediate sulcus descends from the IPS to separate the SMG from the AG. A small secondary intermediate sulcus descends from the IPS to define the posterior border of the AG, separating the AG from the rest of the IPL posterior to it (Naidich et al. 2001a).

2.1.5   Occipital Lobe

The convexity surface of the occipital lobe has also been divided into three horizontal gyri: the superior occipital gyrus (SOG), the middle occipital gyrus (MOG), and the inferior occipital gyrus (IOG). These are separated by the superior and inferior occipital sulci (SOS and inferior OS). The SOS (synonym: intraoccipital sulcus) is the direct continuation of the IPS (Figs. 1, 2, 3, and

4). The inferior OS is usually coextensive with the inferior temporal sulcus. Therefore, the MOG lies just posterior to the confluence of the temporal and parietal lobes at the SMG, the AG, the STG, and the MTG. The MOG is the largest portion of the occipital lobe on the convexity. It is usually subdivided into a superior and an inferior portion by a horizontally oriented middle OS (synonym: lateral OS).

2.1.6   Insula

Separating the superior and inferior covers (opercula) of the sylvian fissure discloses the Island of Reil (insula). The insula is delimited circumferentially by the peri-insular sulcus (synonym: circular sulcus), composed of the anterior, superior, and inferior perisylvian sulci (Ture et al. 1999). The central sulcus of the convexity extends over the insula as the central sulcus of the insula, dividing the insula into a larger anterior and a smaller posterior lobule (Fig. 6) (Naidich et al. 2004; Nieuwenhuys et al. 1988; Ture et al. 1999). The anterior lobule typically has three vertically oriented short insular gyri designated the anterior short, middle short, and posterior short insular gyri. These three converge anteroinferolaterally to form the apex of the insula. The posterior lobule of the insula typically displays two oblique gyri: the anterior and posterior long insular gyri. The anterior insula is connected exclusively to the frontal lobe, whereas the posterior insula is connected to both the temporal and the parietal lobes (Naidich et al. 2004; Ture et al. 1999).

2.2   Inferior Surface

2.2.1   The Frontal Lobe

The inferior (orbital) surface of the frontal lobe is formed by the gyrus rectus medially and four orbital gyri laterally, separated by the olfactory and orbital sulci. The gyrus rectus forms the medial margin of the orbital surface of frontal lobe for the full length of the frontal lobe. The lateral border of the gyrus rectus is delimited by the olfactory sulcus (Fig. 7). The orbital gyri are arranged around an "H-shaped" orbital sulcus as the medial orbital, lateral orbital, anterior orbital, and posterior orbital gyri.

2.2.2   The Temporo-Occipital Lobes

The inferior surface of the temporo-occipital lobe is formed by the inferior temporal gyrus, the lateral occipitotemporal gyrus (LOTG), the medial occipitotemporal gyrus (MOTG) (synonym: lingual gyrus), and the parahippocampal gyrus (PHG), separated by the lateral occipitotemporal sulcus, the collateral sulcus, and the anterior calcarine sulcus (Fig. 5). Medially, the parahippocampal gyrus forms the medial border of the temporal lobe for the full length of the temporal lobe, from just posterior to the temporal pole to the level of the splenium. Posterior to the splenium, the medial occipitotemporal gyrus forms the medial border of the occipital lobe. Laterally, along the full length of the temporo-occipital lobes, the inferior temporal gyrus and the inferior occipital gyrus curve medially form the inferior cerebral margin, and pass onto the inferior surface, where they constitute the lateral-most portion of the inferior surface of the temporo-occipital lobes. Only the small preoccipital notch delimits the inferior temporal gyrus from the inferior occipital gyrus. Centrally, the LOTG runs the full length of the temporo-occipital lobes from the temporal pole to the occipital pole. Throughout its length, the LOTG remains just medial to the ITG and the IOG and is separated from them by the lateral occipitotemporal sulcus. Medially, the medial occipitotemporal sulcus (synonym: collateral sulcus) runs the full length of the LOTG (Fig. 5b). In the anterior half of the temporal lobe, the lateral occipitotemporal sulcus separates the LOTG from the parahippocampal gyrus. In the posterior half of the temporal lobe, the medial occipitotemporal gyrus intercalates itself between the LOTG and the parahippocampal gyrus. Therefore, in the posterior half of the temporal lobe, the lateral occipitotemporal sulcus separates the LOTG from the MOTG, while the

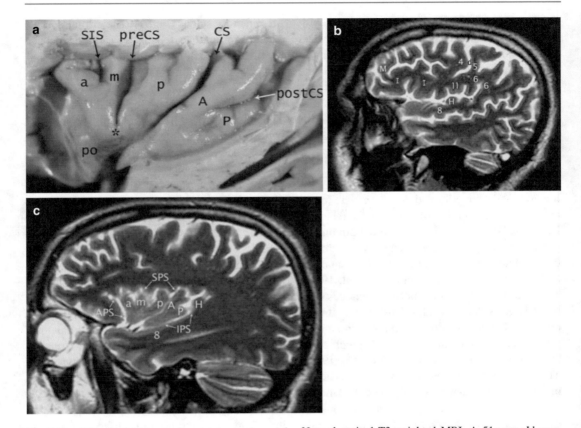

Fig. 6 (**a–c**) Insula. (**a**) Prepared anatomic specimen of the convexity surface of the insula, after removal of the overhanging opercula. A 71-year-old man. The central sulcus (*CS*) extends across the triangular insula like a "hockey stick," dividing it into a larger anterior lobule and a smaller posterior lobule. The anterior lobule typically displays three gyri, the anterior short (*a*), middle short (*m*), and posterior short (*p*) insular gyri, separated by the short insular sulcus (*SIS*) and the precentral sulcus (*pre-CS*). These three characteristically converge inferiorly to form the apex of the insula. The posterior insular lobule typically displays two gyri, the anterior long (*A*) and the posterior long (*P*) insular gyri, separated by the postcentral sulcus (*post-CS*). These too often merge together, anteriorly, just behind the central sulcus. Just inferomedial to the apex, the pole of the insula (*po*) forms the most anteroinferomedial portion of the insula. The central sulcus courses under the apex and the pole and then abruptly swings medially toward the suprasellar cistern. (**b, c**)

Normal sagittal T2-weighted MRI. A 51-year-old man. Laterally (**b**), the convexity gyri form two opercula that cover the insula. Superiorly, the inferior frontal gyrus (*I*), the inferior ends of the precentral (*4*) and postcentral (*5*) gyri, the subcentral gyrus (*11*), and the supramarginal gyrus (*6*) form the frontoparietal operculum. The superior temporal gyrus (*8*) and Heschl's gyrus (*H*) form the temporal operculum. *M* middle frontal gyrus. Medially (**c**), the insula is delimited by the peri-insular sulcus, composed of three segments: the anterior (*APS*), superior (*SPS*), and inferior (*IPS*) peri-insular sulci. The anterior (*a*), middle (*m*), and posterior (*p*) short insular gyri constitute the larger anterior lobule, while the anterior (*A*) and posterior (*P*) long insular gyri form the smaller posterior lobule. The central sulcus courses between the two lobules. Heschl's gyrus (*H*) snugs up against the posteromedial portion of the posterior long insular gyrus. *8* = superior temporal gyrus. (From Naidich et al. (2004); with permission)

anterior calcarine sulcus separates the MOTG from the PHG.

Two synonyms are commonly used for temporo-occipital gyri. The term *lingual gyrus* usually refers to the MOTG (Duvernoy 1991; Ono et al. 1990). The term *fusiform gyrus* is most

often used to designate either the LOTG (Ono et al. 1990) or a large middle portion of the LOTG that crosses the arbitrary border of the temporal and the occipital lobes between the anterior and the posterior transverse collateral sulci (Duvernoy 1991). However, in another usage, Williams et al.

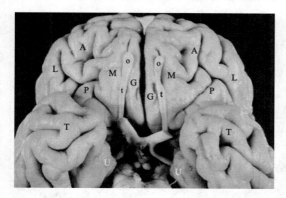

Fig. 7 Inferior surface of frontal lobe. Prepared anatomic specimen of the inferior surfaces of the anterior brain. The inferior surface of the frontal lobes is divided into two portions. The paired paramedian linear gyri recti (*G*) flank the interhemispheric fissure and are delimited laterally by the olfactory sulci, largely obscured here by the olfactory bulbs (*o*) and tracts (*t*). Lateral to the olfactory sulci, the orbital gyri of the frontal lobe are arranged around approximately H-shaped orbital sulci as the paired medial (*M*), lateral (*L*), anterior (*A*), and posterior (*P*) orbital gyri. In true base view, the anterior temporal lobes (*T*) overlap the posterior orbital gyri. Note the paired unci (*U*)

(1989) group the MOTG and the LOTG together as the fusiform gyrus. In most brains, the fusiform gyrus is larger on the left (Kopp et al. 1977; Naidich et al. 2001a).

2.3 Superior Surface of the Temporal Lobe

Opening the margins of the sylvian fissure, or resecting the overlying superior operculum, displays the superior surface of the temporal lobe, designated the superior temporal plane. The prominent features of this plane are one or more transverse temporal gyri (of Heschl) (Fig. 8). Heschl's gyrus or gyri (HG) arise just posteromedial to the insula and course obliquely across the superior temporal surface from posteromedial to anterolateral and may be visible at the external surface of the sylvian fissure. The presence of an HG is constant. The number of HG on each side and their symmetry are highly variable. Heschl's gyri may be single (66–75%), double (25–33%), or triple (1%), both unilaterally and bilaterally (Yoshiura et al. 2000; Yousry et al. 1997a).

Heschl's gyrus is often larger and longer on the left side than the right, but there is no constant relationship between HG and the side of handedness or cerebral dominance (Carpenter and Sutin 1983; Yousry et al. 1997a). A shallow longitudinal sulcus (of Beck) may groove the superior surface of HG, especially laterally, giving it a partially bifid appearance. A deep transverse temporal sulcus (Heschl's sulcus [HS]) typically defines the posterior border of HG.

The oblique Heschl's gyrus divides the superior surface of the temporal lobe into three parts. (1) The flat superior surface of the temporal lobe anterior to HG is designated the planum polare. (2) From HS at the posterior border of HG to the posterior end of the sylvian fissure, the flat superior surface of the temporal lobe is designated the planum temporale. (3) The posterosuperior extension of the planum temporale along the posterior bank of the posterior ascending ramus of the sylvian fissure may be designated the planum parietale. The planum temporale is triangular. It is typically asymmetric on the two sides and most often is larger on the left in humans, chimpanzees, and other great apes (Fig. 8) (Gannon et al. 1998). The size of the planum temporale seems to correlate with the side of language dominance (and perhaps with right- or left-handedness, gender, or both) (Galaburda and Sanides 1980; Galaburda et al. 1998; Geschwind 1965a, b, 1970; Geschwind and Levitsky 1968; Pieniadz and Naeser 1984; Steinmetz and Seitz 1991; Steinmetz et al. 1989b, 1990a, b, 1991). Most of the variation in the sizes of the planum temporale may be ascribed to differing sizes of a cytoarchitectonic zone designated area Tpt (Galaburda and Sanides 1980). Area Tpt has a homologue in nonhuman primates that shows significant asymmetry (left > right) at the cellular level (Gannon et al. 1998).

2.4 Medial Surface

The medial surface of the cerebrum is arranged as a radial array of gyri and sulci that are oriented either co-curvilinear with the corpus callosum or perpendicular to it (Fig. 9). The major gyri of the

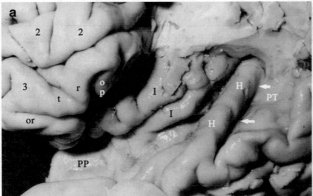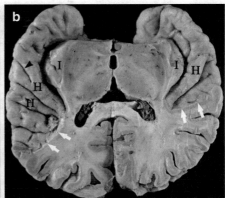

Fig. 8 (**a**, **b**) The superior surface of the temporal lobe from prepared anatomic specimens. (**a**) Anatomy of Heschl's gyrus in relation to the insula. Resection of the frontal and parietal opercula exposes the middle frontal gyrus (*2*); the pars orbitalis (*or*), triangularis (*tr*), and the residual portion of the opercularis (*op*) of the inferior frontal gyrus (*3*); the oblique long gyri (*black I*) of the posterior insula; the length of a single Heschl's gyrus (*H*) which courses obliquely across the superior surface of the temporal lobe from just posterior to the insula (postero-medially) toward the convexity surface of the superior temporal gyrus (anterolaterally); Heschl's sulcus (*white arrows*) immediately posterior to Heschl's gyrus; the planum polare (*PP*) anterior to the HG; and the planum temporale (*PT*) posterior to HG (from Naidich and Matthews

(2000) with permission). (**b**) Exposure of the superior surfaces of both temporal lobes by resection of the overlying frontal and parietal opercula. Right is to the reader's right. The single right and the dual left Heschl's gyri (*H*) course obliquely across the upper surface of the temporal lobe from just posterior to the insulae (*I*) (posteromedially) to the convexity surface (anterolaterally). A shallow Beck's sulcus (*small black arrowhead*) grooves the left HG laterally. Heschl's sulcus delimits the posterior border of HG. The planum polare extends from the temporal pole to the anterior aspect of HG. The planum temporale extends between Heschl's sulcus and the posterior limit of the sylvian fissure (*white arrows*) and is substantially larger on the left

medial surface are the cingulate gyrus (cing-G), the superior frontal gyrus (SFG) (whose medial surface may also be designated the medial frontal gyrus), the paracentral lobule (para-CL), the pre-cuneus (pre-Cu), the cuneus (Cu), and the medial occipitotemporal gyrus (MOTG) (synonym: lingual gyrus). The major sulci are the callosal sulcus (cal-S), the cingulate sulcus (cing-S), the paracentral sulcus (para-CS), the subparietal sulcus (sub-PS), the parieto-occipital sulcus (POS), the calcarine sulcus (CaS), and the anterior calcarine sulcus (ant-CaS). The cingulate gyrus encircles the corpus callosum. It is delimited from the corpus callosum centrally by the callosal sulcus and from the superior frontal gyrus and paracentral lobule superficially by the cingulate sulcus.

The gyri that form the medial surface of the brain peripheral to the cingulate gyrus and sulcus are nothing more than the medial aspects of the gyri that constitute the high convexity of the brain. The superior frontal gyrus of the convexity

curves over the cerebral margin onto the medial surface to form a broad arc of tissue designated the SFG or medial frontal gyrus. The precentral gyrus and the postcentral gyrus curve over the cerebral margin from the convexity onto the medial surface and join together to form the paracentral lobule. The superior parietal lobule curves over the cerebral margin onto the medial surface to form the precuneus. The superior occipital gyrus curves over the cerebral margin onto the medial surface to form the cuneus. The SFG is separated from the paracentral lobule posterior to it by the paracentral sulcus. The posterior end of the cingulate sulcus sweeps upward to reach the cerebral margin. This radially oriented distal portion of the cingulate sulcus is the pars marginalis (pM). The pars marginalis separates the paracentral lobule anteriorly from the precuneus posteriorly. The upper end of the central sulcus typically curves over the margin onto the medial surface of the hemisphere just anterior to the pars marginalis. This medial portion of the CS courses posteriorly nearly perpendicular to the pars marginalis. The "H"-shaped subparietal sulcus lies posterior to the pars marginalis and separates the inferior end of the precuneus from the cingulate gyrus

deep to it. The parieto-occipital sulcus courses parallel to the pars marginalis, joins with the anterior end of the calcarine sulcus, and continues anteriorly as the anterior calcarine sulcus. The POS separates the precuneus anteriorly from

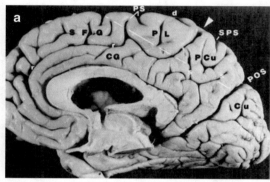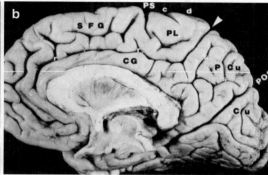

Fig. 9 (**a–c**) Medial and superior surfaces of both hemispheres. Prepared anatomic specimens. (**a, b**) Medial surfaces. The major sulci subdivide the medial surface of each cerebral hemisphere into the cingulate gyrus (*CG*), medial surface of the superior frontal gyrus (*SFG*), paracentral lobule (*PL*), precuneus (*PCu*), and cuneus (*Cu*). The posterior end of the cingulate sulcus sweeps sharply upward toward the superior cerebral margin as the marginal portion of the cingulate sulcus (pars marginalis, *white arrowhead*), which separates the paracentral lobule anteriorly from the precuneus posteriorly. Anterior to the pars marginalis, the paracentral sulcus (*PS*) arises from the cingulate sulcus and/or from the cerebral margin to separate the superior frontal gyrus from the paracentral lobule. The vertical and horizontal arms of the "H-shaped" subparietal sulcus (*s*) groove the medial surface of the precuneus and delimit it from the cingulate gyrus inferior to it. The superior ends of the vertical arms of the subparietal sulcus may reach to and notch the superior margin. The superior medial end of the central sulcus (*d*) usually crosses over the cerebral margin onto the medial surface and then recurves sharply posteriorly to course nearly perpendicular to the pars marginalis, just millimeters in front of the pars marginalis. As a consequence, the most superior medial portion of the precentral gyrus (*4*) merges with the most superior medial portion of the postcentral gyrus (*5*) around the uppermost end of the central sulcus to form the paracentral lobule anterior to the pars marginalis. A posterior portion of the postcentral gyrus passes posterior to the pars marginalis to merge with the precuneus. The prominent parieto-occipital sulcus (*POS*) courses approximately parallel to the pars marginalis, but posterior to the splenium, and delimits the parietal lobe plus cingulate gyrus anterosuperiorly from the occipital plus temporal lobes postero-inferiorly. (**c**) Superior surface of the two

hemispheres. The two cerebral hemispheres border the interhemispheric fissure (*IHF*). Multiple sulci oriented at right angles to the IHF form a series of transverse grooves or "crossbars" across the IHF. The paired pars marginalis (*white arrowheads*) is often the most prominent of these grooves and extends laterally into the hemispheres for a substantial distance. At the vertex, the lateral edges of the two pars marginalis often curve anteriorly to form a bracket, open anteriorly. The paired central sulci (*d*) undulate across the cerebral convexity between the precentral gyri (*4*) and the postcentral gyri (*5*). They typically hook sharply posteriorly as they circumscribe the hand motor region of the precentral gyrus, and then reverse curvature, become concave posteriorly, and converge toward the IHF just anterior to the pars marginalis. The two central sulci (*d*) characteristically (but not invariably) pass anterior to and medial to the lateral edges of the pars marginalis ("enter the bracket") and reach to or cross the superior margins of the hemispheres. The postcentral gyri course superiorly, behind the precentral gyri, toward or to the cerebral margins. The medial ends of the postcentral sulci (*e*) usually bifurcate around the pars marginalis to form a prominent "parenthesis" configuration (*e, e* in the right hemisphere). The interlocking curves of the precentral gyri (*d*), postcentral gyri (*e*), and pars marginalis (*white arrowheads*) form a characteristic set of interlocking curves that usually identifies these sulci and the adjacent gyri. Other labels: (*1*) superior frontal gyrus, (*2*) middle frontal gyrus, (*4*) precentral gyrus, (*5*) postcentral gyrus, (*16*) precuneus, (*a*) superior frontal sulcus, (*c*) precentral sulcus, (*d*) central sulcus, (*e*) postcentral sulcus, (*g*) intraparietal sulcus, (*r*) cingulate sulcus, (*s*) subparietal sulcus, (*t*) superior parietal sulcus, and (*w*) parieto-occipital sulcus. (From Naidich and Brightbill (1996b); with permission)

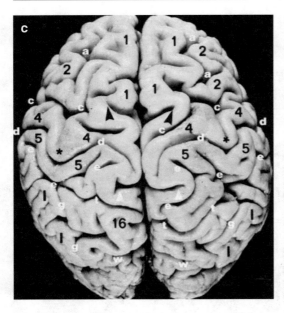

Fig. 9 (continued)

the cuneus posteriorly. The calcarine sulcus separates the cuneus superiorly from the MOTG (lingual gyrus) inferiorly. The anterior calcarine sulcus separates the cingulate gyrus anteriorly from the MOTG posteriorly. The calcarine sulcus may remain entirely on the medial surface of the hemisphere, extend posteriorly to reach the occipital pole, or extend beyond medial surface onto either the convexity or the inferior surfaces of the occipital lobe.

3   Lobar Borders

The precise borders of the temporal, parietal, and occipital lobes on the convexity are highly arbitrary. Published diagrams from different authors indicate substantially different criteria for partitioning the TPO lobes along the convexity (Yousry 1998). The very definitions of these borders and their lobes have evolved substantially over the years (Yousry 1998). In one common system of nomenclature, one identifies the lobes by first finding the lateral end of the deep parieto-occipital sulcus near the superior margin of the

hemisphere. Then one identifies the inconstant preoccipital notch (Gusmão et al. 2002) in the inferior margin of the hemisphere (Fig. 10). The arbitrary anterior border of the occipital lobe is then defined by drawing the "lateral parietotemporal line" along the convexity from the lateral end of the parieto-occipital sulcus above to the preoccipital notch inferiorly.

Next one demarcates the borders of the temporal and parietal lobes that abut onto the occipital lobe. To do this, one draws the "temporo-occipital line," defined variably as (1) an arc from the distal end of the posterior descending ramus of the sylvian fissure to the midpoint of the anterior border of the occipital lobe (Ono et al. 1990); (2) an arc from the posterior descending ramus of the sylvian fissure to the anterior border of the occipital lobe, taking care to make sure that the arc is co-curvilinear with the IPS above (Duvernoy 1991; Schwalbe 1881; Yousry 1998); (3) an arc from the posterior descending ramus of the sylvian fissure to the anterior border of the occipital lobe at the preoccipital notch (Jensen 1871; Yousry 1998); or (4) a straight linear extension from the distal end of the posterior horizontal ramus of the sylvian fissure to the anterior border of the occipital lobe (Dejerine 1895; Talairach and Tournoux 1988; Yousry 1998).

On the medial surface, the deep parieto-occipital sulcus clearly divides the parietal lobe from the occipital lobe and is the landmark used to define the anterior border of the medial occipital lobe in all systems of nomenclature. On the inferior surface, the demarcation of the lobes again becomes arbitrary. On the infero-medial surface, one may delineate the temporal lobe from the occipital lobe by drawing a basal parietotemporal line from the preoccipital notch to, variably, (1) the inferior end of the parieto-occipital sulcus where it joins the calcarine sulcus (Fig. 10) (Ono et al. 1990), (2) the anterior calcarine sulcus beneath the splenium (Fig. 11) (Duvernoy 1991), or (3) the anterior end of the anterior calcarine sulcus (Jensen 1871; Yousry 1998).

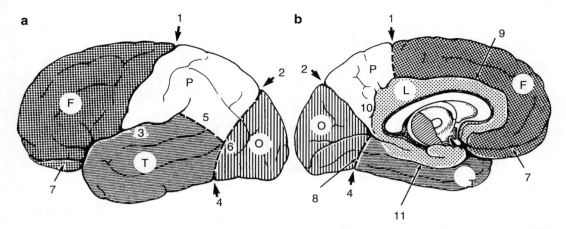

Fig. 10 (**a**, **b**) Lobar borders according to Ono, Kubik, and Abernathy. (**a**) Convexity. (**b**) Medial surface. The anterior border of the occipital lobe is delimited by the lateral parietotemporal line (*6*) drawn between the parieto-occipital sulcus and the preoccipital notch. On the convexity, the temporal lobe is separated from the parietal lobe by the temporo-occipital line (*5*) drawn from the sylvian fissure to the middle of the anterior border of the occipital lobe. On the basal surface, the temporal lobe is separated from the occipital lobe by the basal parietotemporal line (*8*) drawn from the preoccipital notch to the union of the parieto-occipital sulcus with the calcarine sulcus (unlabeled). *F* frontal lobe, *O* occipital lobe, *P* parietal lobe, *T* temporal lobe, *1* central sulcus, *2* parieto-occipital sulcus, *3* sylvian fissure, *4* preoccipital notch, *5* temporo-occipital line, *6* lateral parietotemporal line, *7* orbital surface, *8* basal parietotemporal line, *9* cingulate sulcus, *10* subparietal sulcus, *11* collateral sulcus. (From Ono et al. (1990), p. 9; with permission)

Because the patterns of sulcal branching, the gyral configurations, and the very definitions of the lobes used for anatomic description are so highly variable in this region, it may ultimately prove more accurate to designate the entire region as the TPO confluence. One could then choose to divide the convexity surface of the TPO confluence along the line of the multimodal association cortex from the lateral end of the parieto-occipital sulcus downward to, and then along, the superior temporal sulcus to define three functional compartments, a temporoparietal lobe rostral to the multimodal area (for somatosensory and auditory processing), a temporo-occipital lobe caudal to the multimodal area (for visual processing), and a TPO multimodal association lobe (for integrating the diverse modalities). On the medial surface, one could similarly use the multimodal association cortex that extends along the parieto-occipital sulcus and the anterior calcarine sulcus to divide the medial surface of the hemisphere into a medial parietal region rostral to the multimodal cortex (for somatosensory processing), a caudal temporo-occipital lobe (for visual processing), and the interposed multimodal lobe (for integration) (Naidich et al. 2001a).

The term limbic lobe signifies a broad band of tissue on the medial surfaces of the two hemispheres that, considered together, encircle the brain stem, creating a limbus about the stem. Specifically, the limbic lobe includes the subcallosal area, the cingulate gyrus, the isthmus of the cingulate gyrus, the parahippocampal gyrus, and the piriform lobe, which according to Duvernoy corresponds to the anterior parahippocampal gyrus (Duvernoy 1991).

Recently, Yasargil emphasized the arbitrary and uncertain borders between the lobes and proposed a new lobar classification in which the continuous circle of tissue formed by the precentral gyrus, subcentral gyrus, postcentral gyrus, and paracentral gyrus was considered to be a separate, distinct *central* lobe. Thus, the Yasargil classification would include seven lobes, the frontal, central, parietal, occipital, temporal, insular, and limbic lobes (Yasargil 1994).

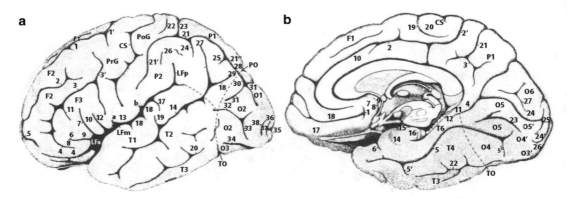

Fig. 11 (**a**, **b**) Lobar borders according to Duvernoy. (**a**) Convexity. (**b**) Inferomedial surface. The anterior border of the occipital lobe is delimited by the same lateral parietotemporal line drawn between the parieto-occipital sulcus and the preoccipital notch. On the convexity, the temporal lobe is separated from the parietal lobe by a temporo-occipital line drawn co-curvilinear with the intraparietal sulcus from the posterior descending ramus of the sylvian fissure to the anterior border of the occipital lobe. On the basal surface, the temporal lobe is separated from the occipital lobe by a basal parietotemporal line drawn from the preoccipital notch to the anterior calcarine sulcus inferior to the splenium. The posterior end of the superior temporal sulcus bifurcates as it extends into the inferior parietal lobule, making a large angular gyrus (a common variation). The fusiform gyrus is formed from portions of the temporal lobe (*T4*) and the occipital lobe (*O4*) that occupy the midportion of the lateral occipitotemporal gyrus between the anterior (*5′*) and posterior (*5″*) transverse collateral sulci. Convexity surface (**a**) *LFa*, *LFm*, and *LFp* = lateral fissure (anterior, middle, and pos-

terior segments); *CS* central sulcus; *PO* parieto-occipital fissure; *TO* temporo-occipital incisure; *F1*, *F2*, and *F3* = superior, middle, and inferior frontal gyri; *PrG* precentral gyrus; *T1*, *T2*, and *T3* = superior, middle, and inferior temporal gyri; *P1* = superior parietal gyrus (lobule); *P2* = inferior parietal gyrus (lobule); *PoG* postcentral gyrus; *O1*, *O2*, and *O3* = superior, middle (synonym: lateral), and inferior occipital gyri; *21*, *21′*, and *21″* = intraparietal sulcus; *33* = sulcus lunatus. Inferomedial surface (**b**) *P1* precuneus, *T3* inferior temporal gyrus, *T4* temporal portion of the fusiform gyrus, *T5* parahippocampal gyrus, *TO* temporo-occipital incisure, *O3* inferior occipital gyrus, *O4* occipital portion of the fusiform gyrus, *O5* lingual gyrus, *O6* cuneus, *2* cingulate sulcus, *2′* marginal segment of the cingulate sulcus (pars marginalis), *3* subparietal sulcus, *4* anterior calcarine sulcus, *22* lateral occipitotemporal sulcus, *24* calcarine sulcus. The caudal portions of *O3*, *O4*, and *O5* merge together at the inferior aspect of the occipital lobe. (From Duvernoy (1991), pp. 5–9; with permission)

4   Localizing Anatomic Sites Independent of Lobar Anatomy

Several attempts have been made to identify functionally relevant anatomic sites, *independent of* the variable lobar and sulcal borders. These systems depend on first establishing reference planes that are based upon a very limited number of deep anatomic structures, then designating all locations in space in terms of coordinates based upon those limited reference planes, and finally identifying all other anatomic features in terms of these coordinates. These attempts may be extended to "correct for" differences in overall head and brain shape by "morphing" the anatomy of any individual brain to superimpose its gross

contours on those of a single standard anatomic reference brain. Applied to groups of patients, such systems may detect commonalities otherwise obscured by individual variation, but at the costs of (1) information specific to each individual and (2) understanding of the range of normal variation.

4.1   Talairach-Tournoux Coordinate System and "Talairach Space"

Talairach and Tournoux took a horizontal plane that extended through the brain along a line drawn from the top of the anterior commissure (AC) to the bottom of the posterior commissure

(PC). The line is the AC-PC line. The horizontal plane through the anterior and posterior commissures is the Talairach-Tournoux baseline. From this baseline, a vertical plane is raised perpendicular to the baseline at the top of the anterior commissure. This is the VAC (vertical at the anterior commissure). A second similar vertical plane is raised perpendicular to the baseline at the bottom of the posterior commissure. This is the VPC (vertical at the posterior commissure). These planes define the coronal position. The third orthogonal plane is taken as the midline vertical plane through the AC-PC line. All anatomic positions are then defined by their coordinates in the vertical direction (designated from superior to inferior as 1–12), anteroposterior direction (A to I), and transverse direction (designated from the midline to lateral as a–d). Thus, the central sulcus is found in "a, 1–2, F" of the left or right hemisphere. These coordinates are considered to exist in "Talairach space" independent of any sulcal or lobar borders.

5 Identification of Specific Anatomic Structures

5.1 The Pericentral Cortex

The pericentral region consists of two parallel gyri, the precentral and postcentral gyri, separated by the CS. Superiorly, the CS nearly always reaches the cerebral margin and may extend onto the medial interhemispheric surface of the brain. In this location, the precentral and postcentral gyri fuse to each other to form the paracentral lobule around the upper end of the CS. Inferiorly, the CS rarely reaches the sylvian fissure. Instead, the pre-CG and post-CG fuse together to form the subcentral gyrus between the inferior end of the CS and the sylvian fissure. This is partially delimited anteriorly and posteriorly by the anterior and posterior subcentral sulci (Fig. 9). Functional and anatomical MRI have both been used to define significant regions along the pre-CG (primary motor cortex) and the post-CG (primary sensory cortex).

5.1.1 Functional Methods

Functional MRI (fMRI) shows that the motor hand area is located at the middle genu of the CS in a portion of the pre-CG that displays a characteristic omega or epsilon-shaped "knob" or "knuckle" (Naidich and Brightbill 1996b; Yousry et al. 1997b). Using MEG (magnetoencephalography), it is possible to identify the post-CG reliably (Sobel et al. 1993). Using positron-emission tomography (PET), it can be shown that the cortical representation of the sensory hand area is located along the anterior bank of the post-CG at a characteristic curve of the CS immediately posterior to the motor hand area (Rumeau et al. 1994). On fMRI, detection of an "activated" vein can assist in the identification of the CS, especially in patients with tumors distorting the cortical anatomy (Yousry et al. 1996). Currently fMRI is increasingly used to define the central region preoperatively.

5.1.2 Anatomical Methods

CT has shown that the marked normal variability of the cortical anatomy can limit the use of standard systems for localizing anatomy, such as the Talairach space (Steinmetz et al. 1989a). Therefore, specific signs have been developed to help to identify the individual portions of the pericentral region more directly (Iwasaki et al. 1991; Naidich and Brightbill 1995, 1996a, b; Naidich et al. 1995; Yousry et al. 1995, 1997b). The sensitivity and specificity of these signs have been evaluated and the multiple signs combined into a system for localizing the CS and related gyri (Naidich and Brightbill 1996b). Three axial and three sagittal signs are most important. These signs should always be used together, systematically, so that the failure of any one sign is corrected by the concordance of localization given by the other signs (Naidich and Brightbill 1996b).

- Axial plane images
  The precentral knob: a focal, posteriorly directed protrusion of the posterior surface of the pre-CG, designated the precentral knob, has been shown by fMRI to be the site of the hand motor area. This focal

motor region is seen on axial CT and MRI images as an inverted omega (90%) or as a horizontal epsilon (10%) in all cases (Fig. 12). This sign has a high inter-rater reproducibility (Yousry et al. 1997b) as well as high "applicability" (Naidich and Brightbill 1996b).

The pars bracket sign: in axial plane CT and MRI, the pars marginalis of the cingulate sulcus of the left and the right cerebral hemispheres appears together as a horizontal bracket. The medial end of the CS enters the pars bracket immediately anterior to the pars marginalis in 94–96% of cases (Fig. 12), whereas the postcentral sulcus enters the pars bracket in only 3%. Thus, the relationship of a sulcus to the pars bracket permits accurate identification of the CS (the "bracket sign"). This sign is also characterized by a high applicability (Naidich and Brightbill 1996a, b).

Thickness of the pre- and postcentral gyri: the full sagittal dimension of the pre-CG is thicker than that of the post-CG (Fig. 12) (Naidich and Brightbill 1996b; Naidich et al. 1995). Further, the posterior *cortex* of the pre-CG is also thicker than the anterior cortex of the post-CG at the corresponding site on the other side of the central sulcus (Meyer et al. 1996). Using T1-weighted turbo inversion recovery sequences, the mean cortical thicknesses of the anterior (pre-CG) and posterior (post-CG) banks of the CS were found to be 2.70 and 1.76 mm for both hemispheres with a mean cortical thickness ratio of 1.54 (Fig. 12) (Meyer et al. 1996). The difference in cortical thickness is based on and explained by cytoarchitectonic studies (Brodmann 1909; Naidich and Brightbill 1996b; von Economo and Koskinas 1925). These three signs are the most important and most reliable for attempting to localize the CS in the axial plane (Naidich and Brightbill 1996b).

• Sagittal plane images

Lateral sagittal plane. The "M" shape of the inferior frontal gyrus. The anterior horizontal and anterior ascending rami of the

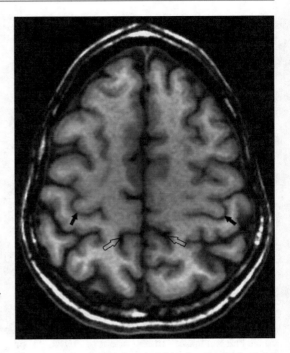

Fig. 12 Pericentral region. Axial landmarks. In the axial plane (T1-weighted MPRAGE sequence), the Ω-shaped knob of the precentral gyrus is easily identified (*arrows*). The pars marginalis of the cingulate sulcus of both hemispheres appears as a horizontal bracket (*open arrows*). The medial end of the central sulcus enters the pars bracket immediately anterior to the pars. The full sagittal dimension of the precentral gyrus is thicker than that of the postcentral gyrus. The cortex of the precentral gyrus is thicker than the cortex of the postcentral gyrus

sylvian fissure extend upward into the IFG, giving it the shape of a letter "M." The first vertical line of the "M" represents the pars orbitalis. The middle "v" of the "M" represents the pars triangularis. The posterior vertical line of the "M" represents the pars opercularis of the IFG. Identification of the "M" provides the starting point for subsequent, sequential identification of the pre-CS, pre-CG, CS, and post-CG (Fig. 13) (Naidich et al. 1995, 1997; Steinmetz et al. 1990a).

Middle sagittal plane: the precentral knob. The posteriorly directed expansion of the pre-CG at the hand motor area may be identified at the level of the insula as a posteriorly directed hook, which fits neatly into the concavity of the hand sensory region of the postcentral gyrus. This configuration defines the position of the pre-CG, the CS, and the post-CG in 92% of cases (Fig. 13) (Yousry et al. 1997b).

Medial sagittal plane: the pars marginalis. The posterior portion of the cingulate sulcus, which sweeps upward to reach the cerebral margin, is the pars marginalis. The CS lies millimeters anterior to the pars marginalis. Characteristically the portion of the CS that lies on the medial surface of the brain curves posteriorly to course nearly perpendicular to the pars marginalis (Fig. 13) (Naidich and Brightbill 1996b).

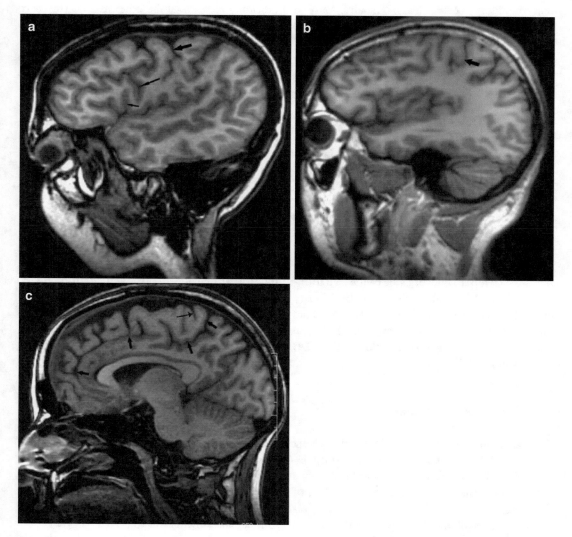

Fig. 13 (a–c) Pericentral region. Sagittal landmarks (T1-weighted MPRAGE sequence). (**a**) In the sagittal plane, the anterior horizontal ramus (unlabeled anteriorly) and anterior ascending ramus (*short thin arrow more posteriorly*) of the sylvian fissure are first identified on the lateral sections and used to identify the M shape of the inferior frontal gyrus. Posterior to this gyrus, in order, lie the precentral gyrus (*long thin arrow*), the subcallosal gurus, the central sulcus (*short thick arrow*), and the postcentral gyrus. (**b**) At the level of the insula, the posteriorly directed hook (*arrow*) of the motor hand area defines the precentral gyrus. (**c**) The cingulate sulcus and its ramus marginalis (*arrows*) are first identified. The central sulcus (*thin arrow*) lies immediately anterior to the pars marginalis and is oriented such that it curves posteriorly, to course nearly perpendicular to the ramus marginalis

5.2   The Superior Temporal Plane

The transverse temporal gyrus of Heschl courses anterolaterally over the superior surface of the temporal lobe from the posterior border of the insula medially to the convexity surface of the temporal lobe laterally. HG corresponds to Brodmann's area 41 (Brodmann 1909), the primary auditory cortex (A1). Usually, only a restricted posteromedial portion of HG can be considered the true site of A1 (Liegeois-Chauvel et al. 1991). A second HG may be present posterior and parallel to the first and may occasionally be functionally included in A1 (Liegeois-Chauvel et al. 1995).

Using MRI, HG may be identified accurately in the axial, sagittal, and coronal planes. In the *sagittal plane*, HG has a characteristic shape easily identified on the supratemporal surface just lateral to the insula. Depending on the number of HG present, HG may assume the form of a single "omega," a "mushroom," a "heart," or a double Ω (Fig. 14) (Yousry et al. 1997a). In the *coronal plane* perpendicular to the Talairach-Tournoux baseline, HG is found best in the section that displays the (tentlike) convergence of the two fornices and the eighth cranial nerves (Fig. 14) (Yousry et al. 1997a). In the *axial plane*, HG is found most easily in the section which displays the massa intermedia of the thalamus (Fig. 14) (Yousry et al. 1997a).

5.3   The Occipital Lobe

The occipital lobe is important for the visual areas (V1–V3, Brodmann's areas 17–19) it contains. The primary visual area (V1, Brodmann's area 17) is located in the striate cortex. Most of the striate cortex extends along the calcarine sulcus (Korogi et al. 1996). However, the precise site of the striate cortex is variable. The striate cortex may be exposed on the medial surface of the occipital lobe, lie hidden within the depths of the calcarine sulcus, extend into the parieto-occipital or anterior calcarine sulci, and/or lie on the tentorial surface of the occipital lobe (Korogi et al. 1996). The precise configuration of the cal-

carine sulcus also varies (Fig. 15). Korogi et al. found that the sulcus could be a single continuous sulcus without major branches (50%), could give off major branches (26%), and could even show significant disruptions (24%) (Korogi et al. 1996). In the coronal plane, the calcarine sulci and parieto-occipital sulci were symmetric in only 60% of cases. One calcarine sulcus was significantly lower than the other in 24% (by more than 10 mm in 12% of cases) (Korogi et al. 1996). The calcarine and the parieto-occipital sulci formed a "V" in 16% (Korogi et al. 1996). The exact positions and (a) symmetries of the calcarine and parieto-occipital sulci are also influenced by the magnitude of any occipital petalia. These variations complicate the identification of the calcarine sulcus (Yousry et al. 2001).

6   Cortical Architecture

6.1   Cytoarchitectonics

The neocortex exhibits six cell layers characterized by differing proportions of cell types, cell densities, and myelination of fibers. From superficial to deep, the six neocortical layers are designated by Roman numerals: (I) molecular layer, (II) external granule cell layer, (III) external pyramidal cell layer, (IV) internal granule cell layer, (V) internal pyramidal cell layer, and (VI) multiform layer. Further variations within each layer may lead to subdivisions such as layers IVA and IVB. In general, afferent fibers to the cortex synapse in layers I–IV. Afferents from specific thalamic nuclei end predominantly in layer IV. Efferents from the cortex arise in layers V and VI. Those efferents directed to the brain stem and spinal cord arise mainly in layer V (Carpenter and Sutin 1983; Gilman and Newman 1996).

Granule cells are small polymorphic (stellate, tufted, or bipolar) cells that form the major component of the external and internal granule cell layers (II and IV). These are mainly γ-aminobutyric acid-(GABA)-ergic inhibitory neurons. Pyramidal cells are pyramid-shaped cells with their apical dendrites directed superfi-

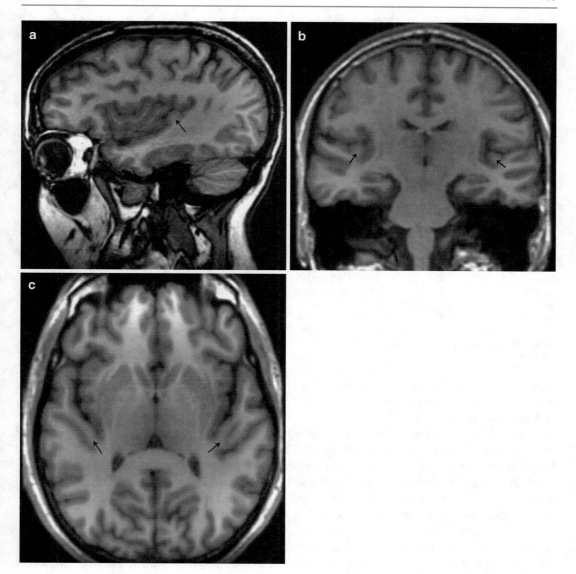

Fig. 14 (**a–c**) Heschl's gyrus. Landmarks in three planes (T1-weighted MPRAGE sequence). (**a**) In the sagittal plane just lateral to the insula, the shape of HG (*arrow*) is so characteristic that it can easily be identified directly on the supratemporal surface without the need for additional landmarks. Depending on the presence and extent of any intermediate sulcus, HG may appear Ω-shaped, on medial sections of the temporal lobe and insula. (**b**) In a coronal plane perpendicular to the bicommissural plane, the sec- tion on which HG (*arrows*) is identified best is character- ized by (*1*) a tentlike shape formed as the two fornices converge to join with each other and (*2*) the presence of the eighth cranial nerves. (**c**) In the axial plane, HG (*arrows*) is identified by its temporal location and its char- acteristic anterolateral course on the section in which the interthalamic adhesion (massa intermedia) can be identified

cially to layer I. The basal dendrites span outward laterally. The major axon arises from the base of each pyramidal cell to pass to its target. Small pyramidal cells found in layers II, III, and IV project to intracortical regions (Gilman and Newman 1996). Large pyramidal cells in layer V project to the brain stem and the spinal cord (Gilman and Newman 1996). Giant pyramidal cells with direct corticomotoneuronal connec- tions to the (alpha) motoneurons of the brain

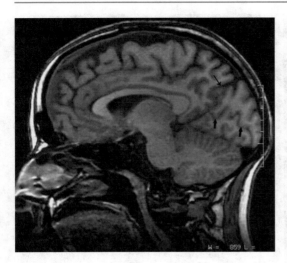

Fig. 15 Occipital lobe (T1-weighted MPRAGE sequence). The calcarine sulcus (*arrows*) runs obliquely in an anterosuperior direction from the occipital pole to its junction with the parieto-occipital sulcus (*thin arrow*) to form the anterior calcarine sulcus. The calcarine sulci show a gradual posterior declination

stem and the spinal cord are designated Betz cells. In humans, Betz cells are found exclusively in the primary motor cortex (M1).

Throughout the cortex, the cell layers differ in their total thickness, the thickness of each layer, the concentrations of cells within each layer, the conspicuity of each layer, the degree of myelination of the fibers within the layer, and the presence or absence of special cells, like the Betz cells. These variations give each region a specific cytoarchitecture that subserves the function of that region. The cytoarchitectonic variations in the cortex lead to classifications of cortical regions by their cytoarchitecture. If the six-layered neocortical organization is readily discernable, the cortex is designated homotypical. If focal specialization of the cytoarchitecture partly obscures these layers, the cortex is designated heterotypical (von Economo and Koskinas 1925). von Economo and Koskinas (1925) grouped the cortical regions into five types (Fig. 16). Three types were considered homotypical: frontal cortex, parietal cortex, and polar cortex. Two were considered heterotypical cortices: the agranular cortex (specialized for motor function) and the

koniocortex (specialized for sensory function). Brodmann (1909) recognized additional variations in cortical architecture, subdivided the cortex into approximately 40 distinct cytoarchitectonic areas, and tried to relate the cortical architecture to function. These regions are now designated the Brodmann's areas (BA) (Fig. 17).

In humans, the motor cortex is formed of three major cortical types:

- The heterotypical agranular isocortex is characterized by increased overall thickness, significantly reduced to absent granule cells in layer IV, and thick well-developed layers of large pyramidal cells in layers III and V (Zilles et al. 1996). In this agranular cortex, even the small cells in layers II (and the region of IV) are predominantly pyramidal in shape. Type (a) corresponds predominantly to BA 4, 6, 8, 24, 44, and 45 and is found in the posterior half of the precentral gyrus, the anterior half of the cingulate gyrus, and the anterior portion of the insula, and in a narrow strip which extends from the retrosplenial portion of the cingulate gyrus into the parahippocampal gyrus (Figs. 16 and 17). Within these areas, the primary motor cortex, designated M1 (Brodmann's area 4), is characterized by the presence of giant Betz cells in lower layer V (Zilles et al. 1996). The motor speech areas, BA 44 and BA 45, are found in the inferior frontal gyrus.
- The homotypical frontal cortex is characterized by narrow granule cell layers composed of loosely arrayed small granule cells and by prominent small- and medium-sized pyramidal cells in layers III and V (Carpenter and Sutin 1983). Giant Betz cells are absent. This frontal cortex corresponds to BA 9, 10, 11, 46, and 47 and is found along the convexity and the anteriormost medial surfaces of the superior and middle frontal gyri.
- The homotypical polar cortex is characterized by overall cortical thinness, well-developed granule cell layers, and a comparative wealth of cells (Carpenter and Sutin 1983; Naidich et al. 2001b). It corresponds to BA 10.

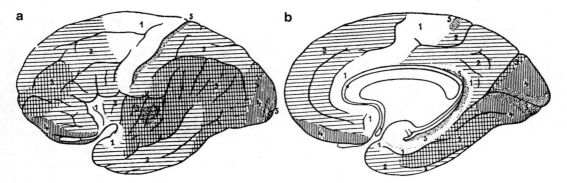

Fig. 16 (**a**, **b**) The five types of cerebral isocortex are distributed over the convexity (**a**) and medial surface (**b**) of the cerebral hemisphere. Cortex type *1* agranular (motor) heterotypical, *2* frontal homotypical, *3* parietal homotypical, *4* polar homotypical, *5* granulous (sensory) hetero- typical (koniocortex). Note that the words frontal and parietal used in this way signify types of isocortex and not anatomic locations or lobes. (From von Economo and Koskinas (1925); with permission)

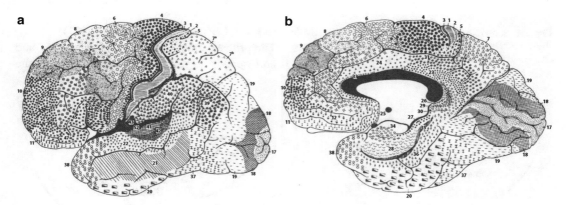

Fig. 17 (**a**, **b**) Cytoarchitecture of the human cortex. Convexity (**a**) and medial (**b**) surface views of Brodmann's areas. Symbols indicate Brodmann's parcellation of the cortex into the cytoarchitectonic areas that are designated by the Brodmann's area (BA) numbers assigned. Compare with Fig. 1. (Parts **a**, **b** from Carpenter and Sutin (1983); with permission)

6.2 Somatotopy

The term somatotopy refers to the topographic organization of function along the cortex. It is a map of the sites at which smaller or larger regions of cortex form functional units that correspond to body parts or to motions across a joint. In specific regions like the primary auditory cortex, the somatotopy may be described by a more specific word such as tonotopy. For white matter, the preferred term is myelotopy. The presence of somatotopy signifies that the functional activity of the cortex is organized topographically along the cortex. Absence of somatotopy signifies that medi- cine has failed, thus far, to appreciate any topographic organization of that cortex. Somatotopy may be fine, as in the primary motor cortex (BA 4), where relatively restricted zones of cortex correspond to defined manipulation units (Fig. 18). It may be very fine, as in the hand motor area along the precentral gyrus, where there may be representation for the motion of each individual digit. Alternatively, somatotopy may be very crude, as in the SMA, the pre-SMA, and the cingulate motor cortex (CMC), where cortical zones seem to correspond to broad regions, such as head, trunk, and upper and lower extremities, rather than to individual motion units (Fig. 19).

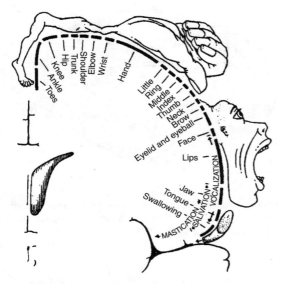

Fig. 18 Somatotopy of the primary motor cortex (M1): the motor homunculus, as described by Penfield and Jasper. (From Williams et al. (1989); with permission)

Using PET to measure regional cerebral blood flow (rCBF), Grafton et al. (1993) have shown within-arm somatotopy of the primary motor cortex, the SMA, and the CMA. Kleinschmidt et al. (1997) used fMRI to show somatotopy for digits in the human hand motor area and concluded that "… somatotopy within the hand area of the primary motor cortex does not present as qualitative functional segregation but as quantitative predominance of certain movement or digit representation embedded in an overall joint hand area" (Naidich et al. 2001b).

6.3 Selected Areas Involved in Motor and Speech Function

6.3.1 Primary Motor Cortex (M1)

The primary motor cortex is designated M1 and corresponds to BA 4. M1 extends from the

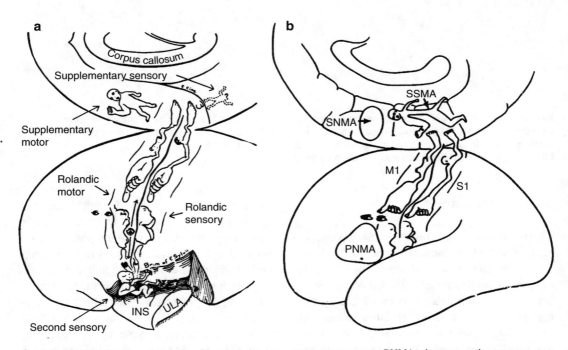

Fig. 19 (a) Somatotopy of the supplementary motor areas (*SMA*) as represented by Penfield and Jasper. (b) Somatotopy of the pre-SMA (the supplementary negative motor area [*SNMA*]) and the relation of the pre-SMA to the SMA, simplified from Penfield and Jasper. *M1* primary motor cortex, *PNMA* primary negative motor cortex, *S1* primary sensory cortex, *SSMA* supplementary somatosensory cortex. ((a) From Luders (1996); (b) from Freund (1996b); with permission)

anterior part of the paracentral lobule on the medial surface, over the cerebral margin, and down the convexity along the crown and posterior face of the precentral gyrus (Figs. 3 and 17). Its anteroposterior extent is broader superiorly and on the medial surface. From there, BA 4 tapers progressively downward toward the sylvian fissure. Just above the sylvian fissure and behind the inferior frontal gyrus, BA 4 becomes restricted to a narrow strip along the posterior face of the precentral gyrus, within the central sulcus (Fig. 17).

M1 is heterotypical agranular isocortex characterized by significant overall cortical thickness, reduced to absent granule cells in layer IV, prominent pyramidal cells in layers III and V, and prominent giant Betz cells in lower layer V (Zilles et al. 1996). The individual Betz cells are largest in size superomedially at the paracentral lobule and smallest inferolaterally at the operculum (Carpenter and Sutin 1983). Classically, the somatotopy of M1 is given by the motor homunculus (Fig. 18). Each functional zone was considered to be responsible for directing the action of a group of muscles that effects motion across a joint. Individual neurons within this group innervate different muscles, so that individual muscles are innervated repeatedly in different combinations by multiple different cell clusters to effect action across different joints. In the classic concept, therefore, the motor map represents motion of the joint, rather than any single body part. More recently, Graziano et al. (2002) have shown that the motor homunculus may better be considered a map of final body postures.

M1 activates anterior horn cells within the spinal cord to generate specific patterns of movement (Marsden et al. 1996). It serves to execute voluntary activity of the limbs, head, face, and larynx, both contralaterally and ipsilaterally. Contralaterally, M1 excites all muscle groups of the extremity. Ipsilaterally, M1 excites the proximal musculature most strongly, especially the shoulder. By direct stimulation of neurons in monkeys, Tanji et al. (1987, 1988) found that 77.2% of movement-related M1 neurons are contralateral motor neurons, affecting the action of the contralateral side; 8.2% are ipsilateral motor neurons, responsible for the action on the ipsilateral side; and 4.5% are bilateral motor neurons. Stimulation of M1 produces simple motions, such as flexion and extension at one or more joints, and not skilled movements. Regions of M1 exhibit different thresholds for inciting action. These thresholds are lowest for the thumb and highest for the face.

Activation studies confirm activation of the ipsilateral hemisphere by sensorimotor tasks (Li et al. 1996). The ipsilateral activation is greater for motor than for sensory tasks and is greater for the nondominant hand than for the dominant hand (Li et al. 1996). The left and the right primary motor cortices show reciprocal actions. Transcranial magnetic stimulation of the motor cortex may inhibit the contralateral cortex (Allison et al. 2000). Direct focal stimulation of M1 causes excitation of a homologous area in the contralateral M1, surrounded by a zone of inhibition (Allison et al. 2000; Asanuma and Okuda 1962). In fMRI studies, unilateral finger movements activate M1 ipsilaterally. The same movements may also deactivate portions of M1 ipsilaterally (Allison et al. 2000).

6.3.2 Supplementary Motor Area (SMA)

The SMA (Figs. 18 and 19) (Penfield and Welch 1951) is also known by a large number of synonyms, including the SMA proper, caudal SMA, posterior SMA, supplementary sensorimotor area M2, and BA 6a α (medial) (Olivier 1996; Rizzolatti et al. 1996; Seitz et al. 1996). In this chapter, the term SMA refers to the SMA proper, distinct from the more anteriorly situated pre-SMA. Anatomically, the SMA proper corresponds to BA 6a α (medial) situated along the medial cerebral cortex in the paracentral lobule and posterior portion of the superior (medial) frontal gyrus. Its specific site varies among individuals, but it is typically found in relation to the medial precentral sulcus (Zilles et al. 1996). Zilles et al. (1996) report that the SMA is located between the VAC and the VPC (Fig. 20).

The SMA is bordered anteriorly by the pre-SMA, posteriorly by the primary motor cortex,

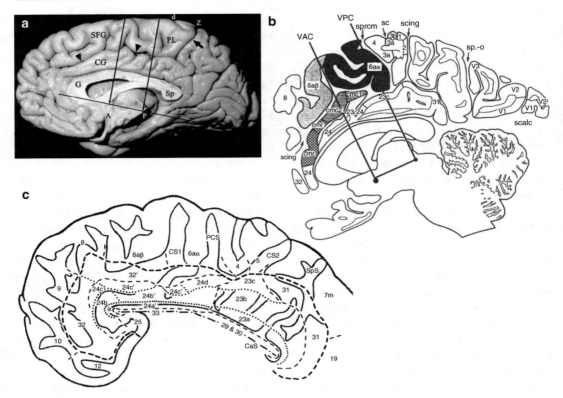

Fig. 20 (**a–c**) Mesial motor areas: SMA, pre-SMA, and CMA. (**a**) Gross anatomy of the medial surface of the hemisphere. Prepared specimen, oriented anterior to the reader's left. This hemisphere displays the co-curvilinearity of the fornix (*F*), genu (*G*), and splenium (*Sp*) of the corpus callosum; the callosal sulcus (not labeled), the cingulate gyrus (*CG*); the single cingulate sulcus (*arrowheads*); the superior frontal gyrus (*SFG*); and the paracentral lobule (*PL*). The pars marginalis (*arrow, z*) of the cingulate sulcus sweeps upward to the cerebral margin to define the posterior aspect of the paracentral lobule. The central sulcus (*d*) cuts the cerebral margin just anterior to the pars marginalis and then courses a short (and variable) distance down the medial face of the paracentral lobule, almost perpendicular to the pars marginalis. To illustrate the anatomic relationships, the AC-PC line has been drawn from the superior surface of the anterior commissure (AC, here labeled *A*) to the inferior surface of the posterior commissure (PC, here labeled *P*) and the perpendiculars are erected to this line at the AC and the PC. The AC-PC line is the baseline for the Talairach-Tournoux coordinate system (Talairach and Tournoux 1988). (**b**) The medial parasagittal plane, oriented anterior to the readers' left. *CC* corpus callosum, *AC*

anterior commissure, *PC* posterior commissure. The VAC and VPC are the vertical lines erected perpendicular to the AC-PC line at AC (*VAC*) and PC (*VPC*). The cytoarchitectonic areas are numbered after Brodmann and Vogt. *Black areas* show the position of the SMA on the medial surface of the hemisphere. *Solid gray* shows the position of the pre-SMA. *Cross hatching* indicates the rostral portion of the cingulate motor area (*cmr*), whereas the *horizontal lines* show the caudal portion of the cingulate motor area (*cmc*), itself divided into parts one and two. *Scing* cingulate sulcus, *sc* central sulcus. *V1–V3* are the visual cortical areas. (**c**) Flat map of the cytoarchitectonic areas of the human cingulate cortex and the locations of adjacent areas. The cingulate sulcus is shown with two separate segments (*CS1, CS2*). *Thick lines* outline the cingulate areas, *thin lines* divide each major cingulate area, *stippling* borders of each sulcus, *dotted lines* show the subdivisions of each area, *dot-dash line* shows the fundus of the callosal sulcus; the fundi of the other sulci are not marked for simplicity. *PCS* paracentral sulcus. ((**a**) From Naidich et al. (2001b); (**b**) from Zilles et al. (1996) and Vogt et al. (1997); (**c**) adapted from Vogt et al. (1995); with permission)

laterally by the premotor cortex on the convexity, and ventrally (inferiorly) by the posterior CMA (Fried 1996; Zilles et al. 1996).

The SMA is a heterotypical agranular isocortex characterized by reduced to absent granule cell layers and by absence of Betz cells in pyramidal cell layer V. The SMA (BA 6a α on the medial surface) can be distinguished from the laterally adjacent premotor area (BA 6a α on the convexity), because the SMA has increased cell density in the lower part of layer III and in layer Va (Zilles et al. 1996). The SMA can be distinguished from the pre-SMA, because the SMA shows poorer delineation of the laminae and poorer distinction of layer III from layer V (Zilles et al. 1996).

The SMA exhibits crude somatotopy. From anterior to posterior, one finds representations of the head, trunk, and upper and lower extremities (Fried et al. 1991). In humans, one stimulation study with subdural electrode grids placed along the mesial cortex elicited a finer somatotopy (Fried et al. 1991). In order from anterior to posterior, these authors found the face, neck, distal upper extremity, proximal upper extremity, proximal lower extremity, and distal lower extremity. The SMA clearly shows greater representation of the contralateral side than the ipsilateral side. The dominant SMA exerts more control than the non-dominant SMA, both contralaterally and ipsilaterally. The supplementary eye fields lie in relation to the head portion of the SMA but are distinct from the SMA (Lim et al. 1996; Tanji 1994).

The SMA appears to act in several different ways:

- *Connections to the cervical motor neurons.* The SMA has tight, probably monosynaptic, connections to the cervical motoneurons (94% contralateral, 6% ipsilateral). SMA activity in one hemisphere is associated with movement of either arm, especially whole-arm prehension involving the shoulder and trunk muscles. Stimulation of the SMA causes a characteristic posture with raising of the opposite arm (abduction and external rotation at the shoulder with flexion at the elbow) and turning of the head and eyes to gaze at the elevated hand (Carpenter and Sutin 1983; Chauvel et al. 1996; Freund 1996a, b). The trunk and lower extremities show bilateral synergic contractions (Carpenter and Sutin 1983). Distal hand muscles are weakly represented in the SMA. Isolated finger movements, easily elic-

ited by stimulation of MI, are rarely elicited by stimulating SMA. The SMA appears less involved with distal grasping.

- *Posture.* The SMA plays a role in posture, especially in anticipating and correcting posture during motor tasks, so that the final position or task is performed successfully. In normal subjects, when a heavy object is lifted from one hand by the other, there is anticipatory adjustment of the posture of the forearm flexors, so position is maintained despite the unloading (Brust 1996; Viallet et al. 1992).

- *Action.* Stimulation of the SMA leads to an urge to act and an anticipation of action (Fried et al. 1991). In monkeys, Tanji et al. (1987, 1988) used intracellular recording to demonstrate that 38% of SMA cells fire before any action is performed. At least some SMA neurons fire before M1 neurons.

- *Laterality.* The SMA is involved with selecting the laterality of the task. In monkeys, 27% of motor-related SMA neurons only fire before deciding on which side to perform an action (Tanji et al. 1987, 1988). Considering SMA neurons and premotor neurons together as one group of non-M1 neurons, Tanji et al. (1987, 1988) showed that when choosing the upper extremity to use for a job, 16% of non-M1 cells fire before deciding right, not both; 20% fire before deciding left, not both; 20% fire before deciding either, not both; and 40% fire before deciding both, not either.

- *Coordination and cooperation.* The SMA serves to assist bimanual coordination and cooperation between the paired upper and the paired lower extremities, especially for self-initiated action. The SMA appears to be required for independent control of the contralateral hand.

- *Sequences of action.* The SMA is heavily involved in learning and generating sequences of actions and with executing multiple actions involving both sides of the body (Gilman and Newman 1996; Passingham 1996; Shibasaki et al. 1993). It may serve in selecting a specific action from among a group of remembered tasks. In monkeys, Tanji and Shima (1994) found one group of SMA cells that were preferentially activated in relation to a particular order of forthcoming movements, guided by memory. A second group of SMA cells became active after the performance of one particular movement and then remained active during the waiting period before performing a second specific movement. These cells were not active if the preceding or subsequent movement was different. Thus, these cells seem to signal a temporal linkage combining two specific movements (Tanji and Shima 1994). Single unit discharges were also observed in the SMA before the performance of the remembered sequence of movements (preparatory sequencing of neurons) and in the midst of the sequence of movements (tonic sequencing of neurons) (Tanji 1994; Tanji et al. 1987, 1988; Tanji and Shima 1994). Similarly, rCBF in the SMA increases with ideation about sequential motor tasks (e.g., when subjects plan but do not execute fast, isolated finger movements) (Roland 1999). When these tasks are actually executed, increased rCBF can be seen contralaterally in M1 and bilaterally in the SMA. From these data, the SMA seems to be crucial for learned, internally generated (i.e., self-initiated) voluntary motor behavior (Burton et al. 1996; Freund 1996a, b; Freund and Hummelsheim 1985; Rao et al. 1993), especially in the preparation and initiation of such voluntary motor behavior (Freund 1996b; Luders 1996). The SMA seems to be less related to performance of the movements themselves. Simple repetition of fast finger motion does not stimulate SMA (Freund 1996b).

Stimulation studies also show a relation between the complexity of a task and the speed with which the action itself is performed. Simple tasks, like flexion of one joint, are commonly performed rapidly. More complex tasks involving multiple joints, multiple body regions, or both evolve more slowly. In some stimulations, the responses elicited were repeated several times until stimulation stopped (Fried 1996).

- *Attention-intention network.* The SMA may form part of an attention-intention network. Fried (1996) found that most ipsilateral and

bilateral sequences can be elicited from the right, nondominant SMA. The right hemisphere has an attention mechanism that spans both hemispheres, whereas the left hemisphere seems to mediate only contralateral attention (Fried et al. 1991). Therefore, the lateralization of attention to the right hemisphere and the lateralization of motor intention to the right SMA may signify a right cerebral dominance for attention and motor intention directed at the external milieu in which the motor action takes place (Fried 1996; Fried et al. 1991; Naidich et al. 2001b).

6.3.3 Pre-supplementary Motor Area (Pre-SMA)

The term pre-SMA signifies a motor area that has also been called rostral SMA, anterior SMA, BA 6a β (medial), and supplementary negative motor area (Figs. 19 and 20). It corresponds to BA 6a β (medial) (Seitz et al. 1996). The pre-SMA lies along the medial face of the superior (medial) frontal gyrus just anterior to the SMA. It shows individual variability. According to Zilles et al. (1996), the pre-SMA lies predominantly anterior to VAC (Fig. 20). It borders posteriorly on the SMA, laterally on the anterior portion of the premotor cortex on the convexity, and ventrally (inferiorly) on the anterior cingulate motor area (Zilles et al. 1996).

The pre-SMA is a heterotypical agranular isocortex with no Betz cells. It can be distinguished from the SMA posterior to it because the pre-SMA has more pronounced lamination and clearer demarcation of layer III from layer V (Zilles et al. 1996). The pre-SMA exhibits a somatotopy similar in form to the SMA, but even cruder in detail. From anterior to posterior, there are areas for the head and upper and lower extremities.

The pre-SMA seems to serve in sequencing and preparing complex tasks, especially internally generated, visually guided tasks. Stimulation of the pre-SMA may elicit negative motor activity for diverse tasks. Fried (1996) found that pre-SMA stimulation causes slowing or arrest of the entire spectrum of motor activity tested, including speech. When a patient executes a repetitive task, such as rapid alternating movements of the hand, stimulation of the pre-SMA causes the movements to gradually slow down and come to a halt. Activation studies suggest that the pre-SMA is involved in the decision whether to act, whereas the SMA proper plays a similar role in directing motor action once the decision to act is made (Humberstone et al. 1997; Naidich et al. 2001b).

6.3.4 Cingulate Motor Area (CMA)

The CMA is composed of two portions (Fig. 20), which appear to correspond to the functionally defined anterior cingulate motor area (CMA rostral; cmr) and a posterior cingulate motor area (CMA caudal; cmc). The CMA corresponds to BA 24c and BA 24d (and perhaps the posterior portion of BA 32, BA 32′ of Vogt) (Vogt and Vogt 1919, 1926). It lies in the superior (dorsal) and inferior (ventral) banks of the cingulate sulcus and, in macaques, does not extend onto the medial surface of the cingulate gyrus (Shima et al. 1991). From the callosal sulcus (inferiorly) to the superior frontal gyrus (superiorly), the cerebral cortex undergoes transition from true allocortex (BA 33), through intermediate stages (lower and upper BA 24), to true isocortex (BA 32) (Zilles et al. 1996). Intermediate area BA 24, therefore, is subdivided into three bands coextensive with the cingulate gyrus and sulcus. These three bands are designated BA 24a (ventral band), 24b (intermediate band), and 24c and 24d (dorsal bands). BA 32 lies superior to BA 24c and BA 24d. Dorsal bands BA 24c and 24d are then subdivided further into a rostral zone (cmr), conforming approximately to BA 24c, and a caudal zone (cmc) conforming approximately to BA 24d (Vogt et al. 1995, 1997; Zilles et al. 1996). The cmr lies entirely rostral to VAC. The cmc flanks VAC but lies entirely anterior to the VPC (Fig. 20).

BA 24c and 24d (cmr and cmc) are heterotypical agranular motor cortices (Zilles et al. 1996). In fine detail, both cmr and cmc appear heterogeneous, leading to further subdivisions of their cytoarchitecture and nomenclature (Zilles et al. 1996). Compared with BA 24c, BA 24d shows a thinner overall width of layer V, clearer borders between layers III and V, larger cells in layers III and VI, and larger cells in layer V.

The CMA exhibits crude somatotopy with multiple representations of the body (Freund 1996b). BA 24c includes representations of the head and the forelimbs (Freund 1996b). Posterior to BA 24c, BA 24d has representations for the forelimbs and the hindlimbs, but with the forelimbs situated caudal to the hindlimbs (Luppino et al. 1991). Thus, the CMA (cmr and cmc) exhibits mixed somatotopy that is partially reversed from that seen in the SMA and in the pre-SMA (Freund 1996b; Luppino et al. 1991; Zilles et al. 1996).

The CMA projects directly to M1 with somatotopic organization (Shima et al. 1991). CMA fibers also project directly to the spinal cord (Shima et al. 1991). Stimulation of the CMA causes contralateral or bilateral movements of the lower and the upper extremities (Freund 1996b). Single-cell studies in macaques show that more than 60% of CMA motoneurons fire before movement-related activity (Shima et al. 1991). Most are involved in simple movements of the distal forelimb. These cells may show either a short lead time or a long lead time between firing and action. Long lead time cells (500 ms to 2 s) are more common in the anterior than the posterior cingulate area and show this long lead time in response to self-paced tasks, not stimulus-triggered tasks. Few CMA cells respond to visual, auditory, or tactile stimuli. Overall, the anterior CMA appears to be significant for self-paced internally guided tasks. According to Paus et al. (1993), the anterior CMA participates in motor control by facilitating the execution of appropriate responses or by suppressing the execution of inappropriate responses.

The zone designated rostral CMA (cmr) is involved with autonomic function. Cells project to the hypothalamus and periaqueductal gray matter. Stimulation of cmr causes nonvolitional vocalization and fear reactions involving the heart, gut, bladder, and genitalia (Jurgens 1983; Nimchinsky et al. 1995, 1997; Naidich et al. 2001b; Vogt et al. 1995, 1997).

6.3.5 Premotor Area

The premotor area (pre-MA) may be designated M2. It extends along the frontal convexity to occupy contiguous portions of the superior frontal gyrus, the middle frontal gyrus, and the pre-central gyrus (Figs. 19 and 20). The dorsal pre-MA lies within the posterior portions of the superior and middle frontal gyri. The ventral pre-MA occupies the anterior face and part of the crown of the precentral gyrus anterior to the primary motor area (M1). Like M1, the ventral portion of pre-MA progressively tapers inferiorly. An additional small area, BA 6b, lies further inferiorly, superior to the sylvian fissure and anterior to the motor face area. The pre-MA corresponds to BA 6a α (convexity), BA 6a β (convexity), and BA 6b (Carpenter and Sutin 1983).

The pre-MA is a heterotypical agranular isocortex with large, well-formed pyramidal cells in layers III and V. Betz cells are absent. Large pyramidal cells that resemble Betz cells are present in the border zone abutting onto BA 4 posteriorly, but these cannot be designated Betz cells, by definition. Granule cell layer IV is thin and difficult to discern. The pre-MA exhibits somatotopy that is similar to, but cruder than, the motor homunculus of the primary motor cortex (M1; BA 4).

Stimulation of BA 6a α (convexity) causes responses similar to those elicited by stimulation of the primary motor cortex M1 (BA 4) but requires higher current to elicit the response. Stimulation of BA 6a β (convexity) elicits more general movement patterns, characterized by abduction and elevation of the arm (frequently associated with rotation of the head, eyes, and trunk to the opposite side). Stimulation of the leg region causes synergic patterns of flexion and extension of the contralateral extremity (Carpenter and Sutin 1983; Freund 1996a). These movements resemble the effect of stimulating the SMA (Freund 1996a). Stimulation of BA 6b produces rhythmic, coordinated, complex movements of the face, masticatory, and laryngeal and pharyngeal musculature (Carpenter and Sutin 1983). Like the pre-SMA, the pre-MA contains cells that fire before a motion is initiated and that appear to determine the usage of the extremities: right, left, or both (Tanji et al. 1987, 1988). Intracellular recordings in monkeys indicate that 48% of motor-related pre-MA neurons fire before all types of motion. Of motor-related pre-MA neurons, 18% fire exclusively before decisions as to the laterality of subsequent activity, not in rela-tion to the performance of the movement (Tanji et al. 1987, 1988). The pre-MA responds more to visual signals and is active in visually guided sequential movements. The pre-MA appears active (1) during mental preparation for a motor task directed by verbal instructions; (2) when voluntary movements are performed under somatosensory, auditory, or visual guidance; and (3) when sensory input is necessary to execute the task. The pre-MA appears especially active when a new motor program is established or an old motor program is modified on the basis of new sensory input (Roland et al. 1980a, b). In monkeys, some of the neurons seem to be stimulated both in performing a task and in observing a similar task being performed by the experimenter (especially when the monkey uses manual or oral "observation"). These neurons are designated mirror neurons (Gallese et al. 1996; Naidich et al. 2001b).

6.3.6 Prefrontal Cortex (Pre-FC)

The term prefrontal cortex designates the cortex that is situated anterior to the pre-MA, corresponding to BA 9, BA 10, and BA 46. It lies along the frontal convexity in the superior and middle frontal gyri and extends onto the medial surface of the frontal lobe along the superior (medial) frontal gyrus (Figs. 3, 16, and 17). The pre-FC is a homolateral frontal type of isocortex characterized by a more or less clearly recognizable granule cell layer IV and an absence of Betz cells (Zilles et al. 1996). No somatotopy is known.

The pre-FC is involved with executive functions, behavior, and memory. Brodmann's area 46 on the dorsolateral pre-FC appears to be involved with the selection of items, whether selecting different items from an internal memory of possible tasks or selecting freely between movements needed to perform a voluntary action (Rowe et al. 2000). Right dorsolateral pre-FC (BA 9 and BA 46) is involved in decisions of what to do and when to do it (Marsden et al. 1996; Passingham 1996). Neurons of the pre-FC are involved with inhibitory responses to stimuli that require a delay in the motor responses (Gilman and Newman 1996). They are thought to integrate motivational elements with complex sensorimotor stimuli (Gilman and Newman 1996). Hasegawa et al. (2000) have detected pre-FC neurons that appear to track long periods of time (as long as 30 s). Activity of these cells correlates with success of past or future performance of complex tasks, not the immediate activity. These cells may set the tone for general behavior, in a fashion similar to that accomplished by stimulants, enthusiasm, arousal, or fatigue (Hasegawa et al. 2000). Using PET measurement of rCBF during a simple motor task of sequential opposition of the thumb to each finger, Kawashima et al. (1993) showed activation of the contralateral pre-FC for both right- and left-handed tasks. Tasks performed with the nondominant hand, however, additionally activated the ipsilateral primary motor area and ipsilateral pre-FC. Thus, the pre-FC exhibits asymmetric activity with dominant or nondominant simple motor tasks (Naidich et al. 2001b).

6.3.7 Broca's Area

Broca's area is the motor speech area. It conforms to BA 44 and to the posterior portion of BA 45. Broca's area occupies the inferior frontal gyrus (*pars opercularis* and a small posterior portion of *pars triangularis*) in the dominant hemisphere. Some data indicate that many women, but not men, have motor speech areas in the inferior frontal gyri bilaterally (Pugh et al. 1996; Shaywitz et al. 1995). The motor speech area traditionally assigned to the inferior frontal gyrus has recently been suggested to lie instead in the anterior insula (Price 2000). Broca's area is a heterotypical agranular isocortex, characterized by reduced thickness of the granule cell layer IV and by the presence of large pyramidal cells in layers III and V. Betz cells are absent. No somatotopy is known.

Broca's area is believed to generate the signals for the musculature to produce meaningful sound. It may also be involved in the initiation of speech (Alexander et al. 1989; Demonet et al. 1992), the organization of articulatory sequences (Demonet et al. 1992), and the covert formation of speech (inner speech). Lesions of Broca's area are associated with a form of aphasia termed, variably, motor aphasia, anterior aphasia, non-fluent aphasia, executive aphasia, and Broca's aphasia.

Patients who have this form of aphasia exhibit difficulty with the production of speech and, therefore, produce little speech. The speech produced is emitted slowly, with great effort and with poor articulation (Geschwind 1970). There are phonemic deficits. Small grammatical words and word endings are omitted (Geschwind 1970). There is a characteristic, comparable disorder in their written output. Surprisingly, these patients may retain musical ability and, despite severe motor aphasia, may sing melodies correctly and even elegantly (Geschwind 1970). Patients who have Broca's aphasia maintain good comprehension of the spoken and written language. Patients who have lesions restricted to the traditional Broca's area in the inferior frontal gyrus do not exhibit persisting speech apraxia (Dronkers 1996). Recovery after Broca's aphasia appears to involve a transient shift of function to the right hemisphere, followed by a return to normal laterality (Neville and Bavelier 1998). A new capability for speech production has been observed to arise within the right hemisphere of an adult several years after corpus callosotomy (Neville and Bavelier 1998).

Broca's area and its right hemispheric homologue are also involved with auditory hallucinations (Cleghorn et al. 1990; Lennox et al. 2000; Mcguire et al. 1993). Schizophrenics experiencing auditory hallucinations show increased metabolism and activation in Broca's area, left anterior cingulate region, and left and right superior temporal regions, among other sites (Cleghorn et al. 1990; Lennox et al. 2000; Mcguire et al. 1993).

6.3.8 Dronkers' Area

Dronkers' area (Dronkers 1996) has no other specific designation. Brodmann did neither parcellate nor number the insular cortex in his final work. Dronkers' area occupies the precentral gyrus of the anterior lobule of the insula. The cortex is a heterotypical agranular isocortex, characterized by a poorly defined layer IV and medium-sized pyramids in layers III and V. No somatotopy has yet been established.

Electrocortical stimulation of the insula during epilepsy surgery has been reported to cause word-finding difficulties, but the specific site on the insula was not specified (Ojemann and Whitaker 1978). The anterior insula has been suggested to be the true site of the function that Broca ascribed to the inferior frontal gyrus (Price 2000). Lesions of the precentral gyrus of the insula are associated with speech apraxia (Fig. 21). This is a disorder of the motor planning of speech, i.e., a disorder in programming the speech musculature to produce correct sounds in the correct order with the correct timing (Dronkers 1996). Such patients exhibit inconsistent articulatory errors that approximate the target word. They grope toward the desired word with disruption of prosody and rate (Dronkers 1996). These patients maintain good perception of language and can perceive and recognize speech sounds, including their own articulatory errors.

An alternate conception of speech apraxia is that it represents a disorder in temporal coordination that disrupts the timing or the integration of movements between two independent articulators. Speech apraxia is distinct from oral apraxia. Oral apraxia is a defect in planning and performing voluntary oral movements with the muscles of the larynx, pharynx, lips, and cheeks, although automatic movements of the same muscles are preserved (Tognola and Vignolo 1980). Oral apraxia often coexists with speech apraxia and has been related to lesions in the left frontal and central opercula, in the anterior insula, and in a small area of the STG (Dronkers 1996; Tognola and Vignolo 1980). The insula has also been reported to be involved in conductive aphasia and Broca's aphasia, where articulatory errors are prominent (Dronkers 1996).

6.3.9 Sensory Appreciation of Speech

The sensory speech area may be designated Wernicke's area (WA). The site(s) of Wernicke's area are very poorly defined (Roland 1999). Most of WA appears to lie along the most caudal part of BA 22 in the STG and the planum temporale (area Tpt of Galaburda and Sanides 1980) or TA 1 of Von Economo and Koskinas (1925). Wernicke's area also includes part of the multimodal belt in the STS (Nieuwenhuys 1994; Nieuwenhuys et al. 1988). Thus, one may also include in WA BA 40, BA 39, BA 22, and BA

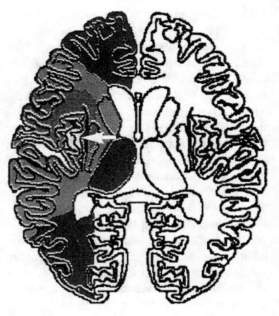

Fig. 21 Speech apraxia. Complete double dissociation in Dronkers' area. Pooled data from 25 patients with speech apraxia show that the only region of involvement common to all cases is the precentral gyrus (*white arrow*) of the insula. Pooled data from 19 other patients with similar infarctions but no speech apraxia showed no involvement in this same area. (From Dronkers (1996); with permission)

37. Anatomically, WA is the least well-defined area, largely due to the significant variation in gyral and sulcal anatomy of this region of the brain (von Economo and Koskinas 1925). In most individuals, WA involves parts of the dominant hemisphere around the posterior sylvian fissure, i.e., the SMG, the angular gyrus, the bases of the STG and the MTG, and the planum temporale. Price reports that the role ascribed by Wernicke to WA is actually found along the posterior superior TS (Price 2000). Cytoarchitectonically, Wernicke's area is a homotypical granular cortex.

Wernicke's area serves to recognize speech relayed to it from the left HG. Direct cortical stimulation of WA intraoperatively causes impairment of language (Ojemann 1983; Ojemann and Whitaker 1978; Ojemann et al. 1989). Patients who have lesions in WA exhibit a form of aphasia designated, variably, sensory aphasia, fluent aphasia, posterior aphasia, and Wernicke's aphasia. These patients produce

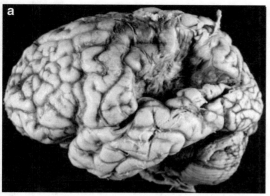

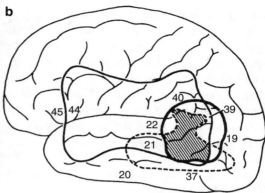

Fig. 22 (**a, b**) Lesions of the posterior language area. (**a**) Large depressed area representing an old infarction of the temporoparietal language area in the dominant left hemisphere. (**b**) Site of pure semantic deficit for single-word comprehension. Area of *broken line* indicates the cortical projection of an extensive subcortical hematoma cavity. (From Hart and Gordon (1990); with permission)

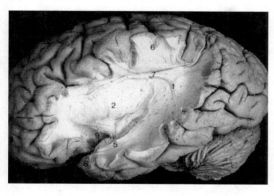

Fig. 23 The arcuate fasciculus interconnects the language areas. Immediately deep to the gyri and sulci of the language areas lie interconnecting fiber tracts, specifically the arcuate fasciculus (*1*), extreme capsule (*2*), inferior longitudinal fasciculus (*5*), short association fibers (*6*), superior longitudinal fasciculus (*7*), and uncinate fasciculus (*9*); (*8*) = temporal pole. (From England and Wakely (1991), p. 95, with permission)

speech fluently, effortlessly, and rapidly, often too rapidly. The output has the rhythm and melody of normal speech but is remarkably empty of content. These patients show poor comprehension of language and poor ability to repeat language. They use poor grammar and exhibit many errors in word usage (termed *paraphasias*), including well-articulated replacements of simple sounds, such as spoot for spoon (Geschwind 1970). Patients who have Wernicke's aphasia show the same errors in written output. Recovery of function after Wernicke's aphasia appears to involve a long-lasting shift of function to the right hemisphere (Naidich et al. 2001a).

6.3.10 Interconnection of Speech Areas: Arcuate Fasciculus

The term *arcuate fasciculus* signifies a broad bundle of fibers that interconnect WA with Broca's area. The arcuate fasciculus may also be designated the anterior limb of the superior longitudinal fasciculus (Nieuwenhuys et al. 1988). It extends between BA 22 and BA 44. The arcuate fasciculus courses from the posterior temporal lobe around the posterior edge of the sylvian fissure to the inferior parietal lobule deep to the SMG and then forward deep to the insula to reach the inferior frontal gyrus. More rostral parts of the STG are also connected with successively more rostral parts of the prefrontal cortex (Nieuwenhuys et al. 1988). The temporal pole is connected with the medial frontal and orbitofrontal cortices through the uncinate fasciculus (Nieuwenhuys et al. 1988). The auditory association areas, particularly the rostral areas, establish connections with the paralimbic cortex of the cingulate gyrus and the PHG (Nieuwenhuys et al. 1988). No myelotopy has yet been determined.

Lesions of the arcuate fasciculus disconnect Wernicke's area from Broca's area, causing a conduction aphasia (Figs. 22 and 23). Patients who have conduction aphasia exhibit good comprehension of the spoken language (WA intact) and fluency of speech (Broca's area intact) but have phonetic errors and poor ability to repeat language. The patient has fluent paraphasic speech and writing with good comprehension of spoken and written language (Geschwind 1970). The inability to repeat speech indicates disruption of the arcuate fasciculus. The disorder in repetition is greatest for the small grammatical words (the, if, is). Repetition of numbers is relatively preserved (Naidich et al. 2001a).

7   Conclusion

Understanding of the structure and function of the brain depends, in part, on an understanding of the basic anatomic structure of the parts, the cytoarchitecture of the cortex, the functional somatotopy, and the interconnections and dominances among the diverse regions. This chapter has tried to present some of the relevant data and to provide a guide to our current, necessarily limited, understanding of brain function. It is hoped that it may serve as one foundation for advances in understanding the brain.

References

Albanese E, Merlo A, Albanese A, Gomez E (1989) Anterior speech region. Asymmetry and weight-surface correlation. Arch Neurol 46:307–310

Alexander MP, Hiltbrunner B, Fischer RS (1989) Distributed anatomy of transcortical sensory aphasia. Arch Neurol 46:885–892

Allison JD, Meador KJ, Loring DW, Figueroa RE, Wright JC (2000) Functional MRI cerebral activation and deactivation during finger movement. Neurology 54:135–142

Asanuma H, Okuda O (1962) Effects of transcallosal volleys on pyramidal tract cell activity of cat. J Neurophysiol 25:198–208

Brodmann K (1909) Vergleichende Lokalisationlehre der Grosshirnrinde. Verlag von Johann Ambrosius Barth, Leipzig

Brust JC (1996) Lesions of the supplementary motor area. Adv Neurol 70:237–248

Burton DB, Chelune GJ, Naugle RI, Bleasel A (1996) Neurocognitive studies in patients with supplementary sensorimotor area lesions. Adv Neurol 70:249–261

Carpenter MB, Sutin J (1983) Human neuroanatomy. In the cerebral cortex. Williams and Wilkins, Baltimore, pp 643–705

Chauvel PY, Rey M, Buser P, Bancaud J (1996) What stimulation of the supplementary motor area in humans tells about its functional organization. Adv Neurol 70:199–209

Cleghorn JM, Garnett ES, Nahmias C, Brown GM, Kaplan RD, Szechtman H et al (1990) Regional brain metabolism during auditory hallucinations in chronic schizophrenia. Br J Psychiatry 157:562–570

Daniels OL, Haughton VM, Naidich TP (1987) Cranial and spinal magnetic resonance imaging. An atlas and guide. Raven Press, New York

Dejerine J (1895) Anatomie des centres nerveux. Rueff et Cie, Paris

Demonet JF, Chollet F, Ramsay S, Cardebat D, Nespoulous JL, Wise R et al (1992) The anatomy of phonological and semantic processing in normal subjects. Brain 115:1753–1768

Dronkers NF (1996) A new brain region for coordinating speech articulation. Nature 384:159–161

Duvernoy H (1991) The human brain: surface. Three-dimensional sectional anatomy and MRI. Springer, Berlin

England MA, Wakely J (1991) Color atlas of the brain and spinal cord. Mosby Year Book, St Louis

Freund HJ (1996a) Functional organization of the human supplementary motor area and dorsolateral premotor cortex. Adv Neurol 70:263–269

Freund HJ (1996b) Historical overview. Adv Neurol 70:17–27

Freund HJ, Hummelsheim H (1985) Lesions of premotor cortex in man. Brain 108:697–733

Fried I (1996) Electrical stimulation of the supplementary sensorimotor area. Adv Neurol 70:177–185

Fried I, Katz A, McCarthy G, Sass KJ, Williamson P, Spencer SS et al (1991) Functional organization of human supplementary motor cortex studied by electrical stimulation. J Neurosci 11:3656–3666

Galaburda A, Sanides F (1980) Cytoarchitectonic organization of the human auditory cortex. J Comp Neurol 190:597–610

Galaburda AM, LeMay M, Kemper TL (1998) Right-left asymmetries in the brain. Structural differences between the hemispheres may underlie cerebral dominance. Science 199:852–856

Gallese V, Fadiga L, Fogassi L, Rizzolatti G (1996) Action recognition in the premotor cortex. Brain 119:593–609

Gannon PJ, Holloway RL, Broadfield DC, Braun AR (1998) Asymmetry of chimpanzee planum temporale: humanlike pattern of Wernicke's brain language area homolog. Science 279:220–222

Geschwind N (1965a) Disconnection syndromes in animals and man. I. Brain 88:237–294

Geschwind N (1965b) Disconnection syndromes in animals and man. II. Brain 88:585–644

Geschwind N (1970) The organization of language and the brain. Language disorders after brain damage help in elucidating the neural basis of verbal behavior. Science 170:940–944

Geschwind N, Levitsky W (1968) Human brain: left-right asymmetries in temporal speech region. Science 161:186–187

Gilman S, Newman SW (1996) Manter and Gatz's essentials of clinical neuroanatomy and neurophysiology. In the cerebral cortex. FA Davis, Philadelphia

Grafton ST, Woods RP, Mazziotta JC (1993) Within-arm somatotopy in human motor areas determined by positron emission tomography imaging of cerebral blood flow. Exp Brain Res 95:172–176

Graziano M, Taylor CS, Moore T (2002) Complex movements evoked by microstimulation of precentral cortex. Neuron 34:841–851

Gusmão S, Reis C, Tazinaffo U, Mendonça C, Silveira RL (2002) Definition of the anterolateral occipital lobe limit in anatomical specimens and image examination. Arq Neuropsiquiatr 60(1):41–46. (in Portuguese)

Hart J Jr, Gordon B (1990) Delineation of single-word semantic comprehension deficits in aphasia, with anatomical correlation. Ann Neurol 27:226–231

Hasegawa RP, Blitz AM, Geller NL, Goldberg ME (2000) Neurons in monkey prefrontal cortex that track past or predict future performance. Science 290:1786–1789

Humberstone M, Sawle GV, Clare S, Hykin J, Coxon R, Bowtell R et al (1997) Functional magnetic resonance imaging of single motor events reveals human presupplementary motor area. Ann Neurol 42:632–637

Iwasaki S, Nakagawa H, Fukusumi A, Kichikawa K, Kitamura K, Otsuji H et al (1991) Identification of pre- and postcentral gyri on CT and MR images on the basis of the medullary pattern of cerebral white matter. Radiology 179:207–213

Jensen J (1871) Die Furchen und Windungen der menschlichen Großhirnhemisphären. Allgemeine Zeitschrift fur Psychiatrie und psychisch-gerichtliche Medizin 27:465–473

Jurgens U (1983) Afferent fibers to the cingular vocalization region in the squirrel monkey. Exp Neurol 80:395–409

Kawashima R, Yamada K, Kinomura S, Yamaguchi T, Matsui H, Yoshioka S et al (1993) Regional cerebral blood flow changes of cortical motor areas and prefrontal areas in humans related to ipsilateral and contralateral hand movement. Brain Res 623:33–40

Kleinschmidt A, Nitschke MF, Frahm J (1997) Somatotopy in the human motor cortex hand area. A high-resolution functional MRI study. Eur J Neurosci 9:2178–2186

Kopp N, Michel F, Carrier H (1977) Etude de certaines asymetries hemispheriques du cerveau humain. J Neurol Sci 34:349–363

Korogi Y, Takahashi M, Okuda T, Ikeda S, Kitajima M, Yoshizumi K et al (1996) MR topography of the striate cortex: correlation with anatomic sections. Int J Neuroradiol 2:534–540

Lennox BR, Park SB, Medley I, Morris PG, Jones PB (2000) The functional anatomy of auditory hallucinations in schizophrenia. Psychiatry Res 100:13–20

Li A, Yetkin FZ, Cox R, Haughton VM (1996) Ipsilateral hemisphere activation during motor and sensory tasks. AJNR Am J Neuroradiol 17:651–655

Liegeois-Chauvel C, Musolino A, Chauvel P (1991) Localization of the primary auditory area in man. Brain 114:139–151

Liegeois-Chauvel C, Laguitton V, Badier JM, Schwartz D, Chauvel P (1995) Cortical mechanisms of auditive perception in man: contribution of cerebral potentials and evoked magnetic fields by auditive stimulations. Rev Neurol (Paris) 151:495–504

Lim SH, Dinner DS, Luders HO (1996) Cortical stimulation of the supplementary sensorimotor area. Adv Neurol 70:187–197

Luders HO (1996) The supplementary sensorimotor area. An overview. Adv Neurol 70:1–16

Luppino G, Matelli M, Camarda RM, Gallese V, Rizzolatti G (1991) Multiple representations of body movements in mesial area 6 and the adjacent cingulate cortex: an intracortical microstimulation study in the macaque monkey. J Comp Neurol 311:463–482

Marsden CD, Deecke L, Freund HJ, Hallett M, Passingham RE, Shibasaki H et al (1996) The functions of the supplementary motor area. Summary of a workshop. Adv Neurol 70:477–487

McGuire PK, Shah GM, Murray RM (1993) Increased blood flow in Broca's area during auditory hallucinations in schizophrenia. Lancet 342:703–706

Meyer JR, Roychowdhury S, Russell EJ, Callahan C, Gitelman D, Mesulam MM (1996) Location of the central sulcus via cortical thickness of the precentral and postcentral gyri on MR. AJNR Am J Neuroradiol 17:1699–1706

Naidich TP, Brightbill TC (1995) The intraparietal sulcus. A landmark for localization of pathology on axial CT-scans. Int J Neuroradiol 1:3–16

Naidich TP, Brightbill TC (1996a) The pars marginalis: part 1. A "bracket" sign for the central sulcus in axial plane CT and MRI. Int J Neuroradiol 2:3–19

Naidich TP, Brightbill TC (1996b) Systems for localizing fronto-parietal gyri and sulci on axial CT and MRI. Int J Neuroradiol 2:313–338

Naidich TP, Matthews VP (2000) Integrating neuroanatomy and functional MR imaging: language lateralisation. ASNR Am Soc Neuroradiol 75–83

Naidich TP, Valavanis AG, Kubik S (1995) Anatomic relationships along the low-middle convexity: part I—normal specimens and magnetic resonance imaging. Neurosurgery 36:517–532

Naidich TP, Valavanis AG, Kubik S (1997) Anatomic relationships along the low-middle convexity: part II—lesion localization. Int J Neuroradiol 3:393–409

Naidich TP, Hof PR, Gannon PJ, Yousry TA, Yousry I (2001a) Anatomic substrates of language. Neuroimaging Clin N Am 11:305–341

Naidich TP, Hof PR, Yousry TA, Yousry I (2001b) The motor cortex: anatomic substrates of function. Neuroimaging Clin N Am 11:171–193

Naidich TP, Kang E, Fatterpekar GM, Delman BN, Gultekin SH, Wolfe D et al (2004) The insula: anatomic study and MR imaging display at 1.5 T. AJNR Am J Neuroradiol 25:222–232

Neville HJ, Bavelier D (1998) Neural organization and plasticity of language. Curr Opin Neurobiol 8:254–258

Nieuwenhuys R (1994) The human brain: an introductory survey. Med Mundi 39:64–79

Nieuwenhuys R, Voogd J, van Huijzen C (1988) The human central nervous system. A synopsis and atlas. Springer, Berlin, pp 247–292

Nimchinsky EA, Vogt BA, Morrison JH, Hof PR (1995) Spindle neurons of the human anterior cingulate cortex. J Comp Neurol 355:27–37

Nimchinsky EA, Vogt BA, Morrison JH, Hof PR (1997) Neurofilament and calcium-binding proteins in the human cingulate cortex. J Comp Neurol 384:597–620

Ojemann GA (1983) Brain organization for language from the perspective of electrical stimulation mapping. Behav Brain Sci 6:189–230

Ojemann GA, Whitaker HA (1978) Language localization and variability. Brain Lang 6:239–260

Ojemann G, Ojemann J, Lettich E, Berger M (1989) Cortical language localization in left, dominant hemisphere. An electrical stimulation mapping investigation in 117 patients. J Neurosurg 71:316–326

Olivier A (1996) Surgical strategies for patients with supplementary sensorimotor area epilepsy. The Montreal experience. Adv Neurol 70:429–443

Ono O, Kubik S, Abernathy CD (1990) Atlas of the cerebral sulci. Thieme, New York

Passingham RE (1996) Functional specialization of the supplementary motor area in monkeys and humans. Adv Neurol 70:105–116

Paus T, Petrides M, Evans AC, Meyer E (1993) Role of the human anterior cingulate cortex in the control of oculomotor, manual, and speech responses: a positron emission tomography study. J Neurophysiol 70:453–469

Penfield W, Welch K (1951) The supplementary motor area of the cerebral cortex; a clinical and experimental study. AMA Arch Neurol Psychiatry 66:289–317

Pieniadz JM, Naeser MA (1984) Computed tomographic scan cerebral asymmetries and morphologic brain asymmetries. Correlation in the same cases postmortem. Arch Neurol 41:403–409

Price CJ (2000) The anatomy of language: contributions from functional neuroimaging. J Anat 197:335–359

Pugh KR, Shaywitz BA, Shaywitz SE, Constable RT, Skudlarski P, Fulbright RK et al (1996) Cerebral organization of component processes in reading. Brain 119:1221–1238

Rao SM, Binder JR, Bandettini PA, Hammeke TA, Yetkin FZ, Jesmanowicz A et al (1993) Functional magnetic resonance imaging of complex human movements. Neurology 43:2311–2318

Rizzolatti G, Luppino G, Matelli M (1996) The classic supplementary motor area is formed by two independent areas. Adv Neurol 70:45–56

Roland PE (1999) Brain activation. In: Motor functions. Language. Wiley, New York, pp 269–290

Roland PE, Larsen B, Lassen NA, Skinhoj E (1980a) Supplementary motor area and other cortical areas in organization of voluntary movements in man. J Neurophysiol 43:118–136

Roland PE, Skinhoj E, Lassen NA, Larsen B (1980b) Different cortical areas in man in organization of voluntary movements in extrapersonal space. J Neurophysiol 43:137–150

Rowe JB, Toni I, Josephs O, Frackowiak RS, Passingham RE (2000) The prefrontal cortex: response selection or maintenance within working memory? Science 288:1656–1660

Rumeau C, Tzourio N, Murayama N, Peretti-Viton P, Levrier O, Joliot M et al (1994) Location of hand function in the sensorimotor cortex: MR and functional correlation. AJNR Am J Neuroradiol 15:567–572

Schwalbe G (1881) Lehrbuch der neurologie. Verlag von Eduard Besold, Erlangen

Seitz RJ, Schlaug G, Knorr U, Steinmetz H, Tellmann L, Herzog H (1996) Neurophysiology of the human supplementary motor area. Positron emission tomography. Adv Neurol 70:167–175

Shaywitz BA, Shaywitz SE, Pugh KR, Constable RT, Skudlarski P, Fulbright RK et al (1995) Sex differences in the functional organization of the brain for language. Nature 373:607–609

Shibasaki H, Sadato N, Lyshkow H, Yonekura Y, Honda M, Nagamine T et al (1993) Both primary motor cortex and supplementary motor area play an important role in complex finger movement. Brain 116:1387–1398

Shima K, Aya K, Mushiake H, Inase M, Aizawa H, Tanji J (1991) Two movement-related foci in the primate cingulate cortex observed in signal-triggered and self-paced forelimb movements. J Neurophysiol 65:188–202

Sobel DF, Gallen CC, Schwartz BJ, Waltz TA, Copeland B, Yamada S et al (1993) Locating the central sulcus: comparison of MR anatomic and magnetoencephalographic functional methods. AJNR Am J Neuroradiol 14:915–925

Steinmetz H, Seitz RJ (1991) Functional anatomy of language processing: neuroimaging and the problem of individual variability. Neuropsychologia 29:1149–1161

Steinmetz H, Furst G, Freund HJ (1989a) Cerebral cortical localization: application and validation of the proportional grid system in MR imaging. J Comput Assist Tomogr 13:10–19

Steinmetz H, Rademacher J, Huang YX, Hefter H, Zilles K, Thron A et al (1989b) Cerebral asymmetry: MR planimetry of the human planum temporale. J Comput Assist Tomogr 13:996–1005

Steinmetz H, Ebeling U, Huang YX, Kahn T (1990a) Sulcus topography of the parietal opercular region: an anatomic and MR study. Brain Lang 38:515–533

Steinmetz H, Rademacher J, Jancke L, Huang YX, Thron A, Zilles K (1990b) Total surface of temporoparietal intrasylvian cortex: diverging left-right asymmetries. Brain Lang 39:357–372

Steinmetz H, Volkmann J, Jancke L, Freund HJ (1991) Anatomical left-right asymmetry of language-related temporal cortex is different in left- and right-handers. Ann Neurol 29:315–319

Talairach J, Tournoux P (1988) Co-planar stereotaxic atlas of the human brain. 3-Dimensional proportional system. An approach to cerebral imaging. Thieme, New York

Tanji J (1994) The supplementary motor area in the cerebral cortex. Neurosci Res 19:251–268

Tanji J, Shima K (1994) Role for supplementary motor area cells in planning several movements ahead. Nature 371:413–416

Tanji J, Okano K, Sato KC (1987) Relation of neurons in the nonprimary motor cortex to bilateral hand movement. Nature 327:618–620

Tanji J, Okano K, Sato KC (1988) Neuronal activity in cortical motor areas related to ipsilateral, contralateral, and bilateral digit movements of the monkey. J Neurophysiol 60:325–343

Tognola G, Vignolo LA (1980) Brain lesions associated with oral apraxia in stroke patients: a clinico-neuroradiological investigation with the CT scan. Neuropsychologia 18:257–272

Ture U, Yasargil DC, Al-Mefty O, Yasargil MG (1999) Topographic anatomy of the insular region. J Neurosurg 90:720–733

Viallet F, Massion J, Massarino R, Khalil R (1992) Coordination between posture and movement in a bimanual load lifting task: putative role of a medial frontal region including the supplementary motor area. Exp Brain Res 88:674–684

Vogt C, Vogt O (1919) Allgemeinere ergebnisse unserer hirnforschung. J Psychol Neurol 25:279–461

Vogt O, Vogt C (1926) Die vergleichend-architektonische und vergleichend-reizphysiologische felderung der grobhirnrinde unter besonderer berücksichtigung der menschilchen. Naturwissenchaften 14:1190–1194

Vogt BA, Nimchinsky EA, Vogt LJ, Hof PR (1995) Human cingulate cortex: surface features, flat maps, and cytoarchitecture. J Comp Neurol 359:490–506

Vogt BA, Vogt LJ, Nimchinsky EA (1997) Primate cingular cortex chemoarchitecture and its disruption in Alzheimer's disease. In: Bloom FE, Bjorklund A, Hokfelt T (eds) Handbook of chemical neuroanatomy, vol 13. Elsevier Science, Amsterdam, pp 455–528

von Economo C, Koskinas GN (1925) Die Cytoarchitektonik der Hirnrinde des erwachsenen Menschen. Springer, Berlin

Williams PL, Warwick R, Dyson M (1989) Gray's Anatomy, 37th edn. Churchill Livingstone, Edinburgh/New York, pp 1047–1063

Yasargil MG (1994) Microneurosurgery. Thieme, Stuttgart

Yoshiura T, Higano S, Rubio A, Shrier DA, Kwok WE, Iwanaga S et al (2000) Heschl and superior temporal gyri: low signal intensity of the cortex on T2-weighted MR images of the normal brain. Radiology 214:217–221

Yousry TA (1998) Historical perspective: the cerebral lobes and their boundaries. Int J Neuroradiol 4:342–348

Yousry TA, Schmid UD, Jassoy AG, Schmidt D, Eisner WE, Reulen HJ et al (1995) Topography of the cortical motor hand area: prospective study with functional MR imaging and direct motor mapping at surgery. Radiology 195:23–29

Yousry TA, Schmid UD, Schmidt D, Hagen T, Jassoy A, Reiser MF (1996) The central sulcal vein: a landmark for identification of the central sulcus using functional magnetic resonance imaging. J Neurosurg 85:608–617

Yousry TA, Fesl G, Buttner A (1997a) Heschl's gyrus: anatomic description and methods of identification on magnetic resonance imaging. Int J Neuroradiol 3:2–12

Yousry TA, Schmid UD, Alkadhi H, Schmidt D, Peraud A, Buettner A et al (1997b) Localization of the motor hand area to a knob on the precentral gyrus. A new landmark. Brain 120:141–157

Yousry TA, Yousry I, Naidich TP (2001) Progress in neuroanatomy. In: Demaerel P (ed) Recent advances in diagnostic neuroradiology. Springer, Berlin

Zilles K, Schlaug G, Geyer S, Luppino G, Matelli M, Qu M et al (1996) Anatomy and transmitter receptors of the supplementary motor areas in the human and non-human primate brain. Adv Neurol 70:29–43

Task-Based Presurgical Functional MRI in Patients with Brain Tumors

Christoph Stippich, Maria Blatow,
and Meritxell Garcia Alzamora

Contents

C. Stippich (✉)
Department of Neuroradiology and Radiology,
Schmieder Clinic, Allensbach, Germany

M. Blatow
Department of Neuroradiology, University Hospital
Zürich, Zürich, Switzerland
e-mail: maria.blatow@usz.ch

M. G. Alzamora
European Telemedicine Clinic (TMC)—A Unilabs
Company, Barcelona, Spain

© The Author(s), under exclusive license to Springer Nature Switzerland AG 2022
C. Stippich (ed.), *Clinical Functional MRI*, Medical Radiology Diagnostic Imaging,
https://doi.org/10.1007/978-3-030-83343-5_4

Abstract

Neurosurgery in functionally important brain areas carries a high risk for postoperative neurological deficits. In patients with brain tumors, functional magnetic resonance imaging (fMRI) facilitates presurgical planning and evaluation of surgical outcome for the estimation of an as good as possible balance between maximal tumor resection and minimal loss of function. To this end fMRI is also applied intraoperatively for functional neuronavigation preferably in combination with DTI-tractography. However, fMRI has not reached the status of a standard diagnostic neuroimaging procedure, yet. Preoperative task-based fMRI represents the best established and validated clinical application of fMRI, is increasingly performed in larger medical neurocenters, and in this context can only be performed exclusively in individual patients. Therefore, it differs fundamentally from research application in neuroscience.

This chapter provides a review of the current literature and presents optimized task-based presurgical fMRI protocols for motor, somatosensory, and language function, along with a standardized data evaluation protocol using a dynamic statistical threshold. Examples of physiological brain activation are given, criteria for the selection of candidates for presurgical fMRI are provided, and illustrative cases with typical and atypical presurgical fMRI findings are presented. Complementary applications with diffusion tensor imaging (DTI) and DTI-tractography (DTT) are highlighted. Finally, important diagnostic capabilities and limitations of presurgical fMRI are discussed. In this context some novel options are indicated by using resting-state fMRI.

In conclusion, fMRI is feasible for advanced multimodal MR neuroimaging in the clinical setting and provides important diagnostic information noninvasively, which is otherwise unavailable. Task-based preoperative fMRI is valid, reasonably sensitive, and accurate to localize the different representa-

tions of the human body in the primary motor and somatosensory cortex prior to brain tumor surgery, which in general also applies to language localization and lateralization. Although there is a substantial body of studies on presurgical language fMRI available, the results are still heterogeneous. Here, fMRI has at least the potential to help to reduce the number of invasive diagnostic measures needed and to guide their targeted application. It may substitute Wada testing in many patients. If, and to what extent, intraoperative electrocorticography (ECoG) can be replaced is still not decided, yet. The integration of fMRI with DTI and DTT is complementary and increasingly used, providing important pretherapeutic and intraoperative information on essential cortical and subcortical functional structures in relation to the surgical target. For the in-depth information on presurgical resting-state fMRI we refer the reader to chapter "Presurgical Resting-State fMRI."

1　Brain Tumors and Brain Tumor Surgery

The age-adjusted incidence of brain tumors (benign and malignant) has been estimated at approximately 19 per 100,000 person years (Parkin and Muir 1992; Ohgaki 2009; Ostrom and Barnholtz-Sloan 2011). Mortality rates from all tumors of the CNS range between 4 and 7 per 100,000 persons/year in men and between 3 and 5 per 100,000 persons/year in women (McKinney 2004; Ohgaki 2009). With the exception of pilocytic astrocytoma, the survival rate of brain neoplasms is poor (Landis et al. 1999) and correlates with the grade of malignancy. Most gliomas are infiltrative and have ill-defined margins making complete surgical removal often impossible. Patients with low-grade gliomas have a median survival of 6–10 years, but these tumors tend to have a malignant transformation. For instance, the mean 5-year survival rate for anaplastic astrocytoma is 11% and for glioblastoma 1.2%

(Ohgaki 2009), comparable to primary CNS lymphoma or metastatic disease where prolonged survival is rather exceptional.

Histologically, brain tumors can be classified as "primary," that is, arising from the brain or its linings, or as "secondary" or "metastatic" affecting the CNS predominantly from lung, breast, kidney, gastrointestinal, and skin cancer. In adults, primary and secondary brain tumors can be approximated equiprevalent, whereas in children metastatic disease is rare (Stefanowicz et al. 2011).

Extra-axial tumors are typically noninvasive and affect the brain by displacement or compression. Clinical symptoms may also be related to occlusive hydrocephalus caused by impaired circulation of cerebrospinal fluid (CSF) due to compression of the ventricles or connecting foramina. The primary goal of treatment is complete removal. Intra-axial tumors grow inside the brain parenchyma. The spectrum of appearance is wide ranging from focal and well-defined masses to diffusely infiltrating processes. Clinical signs and symptoms depend mainly on the location and mass effect. According to protocols of the World Health Organization (WHO), brain tumors are classified in four grades based on a malignancy scale, that is, on pleomorphism, mitotic activity, endothelial proliferation, and necrosis. Based on cell origin, 12 groups have been defined (Louis et al. 2007).

Of note, the WHO 2016 revision on brain tumor classification marks an important update and change. The revised 2016 WHO classification accounts for various molecular and genetic patterns of brain malignancies in addition to the abovementioned "classical" microscopic histology. This has led to some important corrections such as addition of newly recognized tumor entities, variants, and patterns; eliminations of others; or reclassifications, e.g., in former astrocytoma, oligoastrocytoma, and oligodendroglioma by using IDH mutations and 1p/19q codeletion, but also of numerous other CNS neoplasms (Louis et al. 2016). This impacts not only treatment (Banan and Hartmann 2017), but also brain tumor imaging (Johnson et al. 2017). Meanwhile, there are numerous publications available on imaging and molecular genetic findings in brain tumors (Delfanti et al. 2017; Lewis et al. 2019; Iv

and Bisdas 2021). The field is very dynamic and molecular diagnostic criteria are considered highly relevant for brain tumor diagnosis and treatment.

The treatment of brain tumors and metastases is traditionally based on surgery, radiation, or chemotherapy or a combination of these treatments, tailored to the target location and pathology (Kaye and Laws 2011; DeMonte et al. 2007; Jovčevska et al. 2013). Also here, cellular and molecular biology has opened up new diagnostic and novel targeted therapeutic options. Advanced neuroimaging—based on morphological, metabolic, and functional assessment—provides very detailed diagnostic information on intracranial pathologies, has helped to guide and refine treatment strategies in individual patients and to estimate procedural risks and prognosis (Jacobs et al. 2005). Reduction of morbidity associated with treatment is of utmost importance, which especially applies to patients in whom complete removal of the pathology is impossible and complete cure cannot be achieved. Here, the goal of neurosurgery is to eliminate as much of the tumor as safely as possible while preserving the eloquent areas of the brain. To achieve this, cutting-edge technology is applied for image-guided neurosurgery and functional neuronavigation (Nimsky et al. 2006; Nimsky 2011; Archip et al. 2007; Kuhnt et al. 2012; Kumar et al. 2014; Sang et al. 2018). Recent research indicates that presurgical functional neuroimaging helps to achieve benefit regarding postoperative morbidity, better functional outcome, and longer term survival (Kundu et al. 2013; Bailey et al. 2015; Vysotski et al. 2018; Liouta et al. 2019).

2   Presurgical Functional Neuroimaging: Rationale and Diagnostic Aims

Neurosurgical procedures in or next to functionally relevant brain tissue invariably carry the risk of surgery-induced postoperative neurological deficits. Although all brain areas are to a certain extent of functional importance, in clinical practice the term "functionally relevant" or "eloquent" is limited to those brain structures where damage can result in severe neurological compromise and consequently in a significant reduction of the patient's quality of life. Resection of the so-called Rolandic or synonymously "central" brain tumors, for example, can lead to injury of the primary motor and somatosensory cortices and therefore cause permanent movement and sensibility impairment. Patients with frontal or temporal lesions of the left hemisphere are particularly prone to suffer from postoperative motor or sensory language deficits, while mesiotemporal interventions can affect memory function. Therefore, the indication for neurosurgery in such patients has to be set rigorously, and other, less invasive, therapeutic options like radiotherapy or neuroradiological interventions—as in the case of vascular malformations—should be considered. This applies especially to patients where curative treatment is not possible. Here, preservation of brain function and reduction of treatment-associated morbidity are crucial. Prudent preoperative consideration of the optimal surgical access and resection borders for each patient can be of utmost importance to avoid damage to functionally relevant brain structures (Duffau 2006; Voss et al. 2013; Kundu et al. 2013; Håberg et al. 2004; Kumar et al. 2014; Jia et al. 2013). Similar to brain tumor surgery, epilepsy surgery aims at complete removal of the epileptogenic zone with minimal damage to eloquent brain areas. To this end latest technologies are employed (Dorfer et al. 2020) (see chapter "Presurgical EEG-fMRI in Epilepsy"). Thus, depending on the location of the pathology, the determination of the hemispheric dominance and the precise spatial relationship between the brain tumor or epileptogenic zone and the functionally relevant brain area can be mandatory for the selection of the appropriate therapeutic option and its approach. Ideally, this information should be available before initiation of any therapy in order to minimize postoperative neurosurgical morbidity and duration of postoperative hospitalization. In this view, functional neuroimaging not only offers a variety of novel options for clinical diagnostics and research but also opens up a new

diagnostic field of neuroradiology, with a shift from a strictly morphological imaging to the measurement and visualization of brain function (Stippich et al. 2002a).

The standard and probably most accurate procedure for the mapping of human brain function is intraoperative electrocorticography (ECoG) (Penfield 1937, 1950; Woolsey et al. 1979; Ojemann et al. 1989; Ojemann 1991; Cedzich et al. 1996; Duffau et al. 1999; Cordella and Acerbi 2013; Robertson et al. 2019; Roessler et al. 2019), consisting of electrophysiological recordings from the cerebral cortex with surface electrodes, which is a demanding technique offered only by highly specialized medical centers. Application of ECoG considerably increases surgery duration and involves distressing awake craniotomy, since mapping of language and memory-related brain structures requires active collaboration of the patient. A particular disadvantage of ECoG is the fact that it is applied during surgery so that the obtained results cannot be incorporated in the preoperative process of treatment selection and planning. Presurgical determination of hemispheric dominance is traditionally achieved by the invasive Wada test (Wada and Rasmussen 1960; Rausch et al. 1993; Sharan et al. 2011; Cunningham et al. 2008; Wagner et al. 2012; Kundu et al. 2019), where language and memory functions are assessed neuropsychologically during intra-arterial injection of barbiturates (amobarbital). This method bears all the risks of cerebral angiography with complication rates in up to 11% of cases (Sharan et al. 2011), is discomforting for the patient, and requires several days of hospitalization (see also Handbook of Neuro-Oncology Neuroimaging, 2nd edition, 2016). Correspondence to fMRI lateralization is not always congruent (Janecek et al. 2013). Other methods for the identification of functionally important brain structures are positron-emission tomography (PET) (Csaba 2003; La Fougère et al. 2009) and single-photon emission computed tomography (SPECT) (La Fougère et al. 2009), which detect changes of cerebral blood flow and glucose metabolism. These techniques, however, are also invasive, utilize ionizing radiation, and thus carry a certain risk of morbidity. In addition, their temporal resolution is low (Müller et al. 1998), and discordance of the results for presurgical diagnostics is recognized. Today, the use of PET or SPECT for presurgical localization of eloquent brain areas has decreased inversely to the application of fMRI and represents an alternative functional imaging modality when less invasive measures cannot be employed. However, nuclear medicine plays a very important role in the characterization of brain tumors, posttreatment effects, and recurrence (Fink et al. 2015; Humbert et al. 2019; Drake et al. 2020; Sharma and Kumar 2020) as well as in epilepsy (Sidhu et al. 2018). Besides fMRI, other frequently used noninvasive techniques for the assessment of human brain function are electrophysiological methods which measure neuronal activity directly via the detection of electromagnetic fields with an excellent temporal resolution (ms range)—these include electroencephalography (EEG) (Berger 1929; Gevins 1995; Gevins et al. 1995) and magnetoencephalography (MEG) (Hari and Ilmoniemi 1986; Findley et al. 2012; Choudhri et al. 2013; Zimmermann et al. 2019, 2020). Spatial resolution, however, is lower than that obtained from fMRI, and localization of electromagnetic sources requires complicated mathematical modeling and calculations (based on single- or multidipole models and various spherical head models) and is therefore limited in precision and accuracy (Hämäläinen et al. 1993; Schmid et al. 2018; Ellis et al. 2020; Liu et al. 2021).

The diagnostic potential of presurgical morphological imaging in the clinical routine with magnetic resonance imaging (MRI) is limited regarding the localization of functionally relevant brain structures (Villanueva-Meyer et al. 2017). For instance, structural MRI provides detailed information of the brain parenchyma and intracranial pathologies (Osborn et al. 2010), but cannot assess brain function. Anatomically identifiable landmarks for specific functions could be described solely for the central region (see chapter "Functional Neuroanatomy"), where reliability reaches a maximum of approximately 95% in healthy volunteers (Fig. 1). In the presence of anatomical variants, malformations of the brain, or patients with large or vastly infiltrating tumors, these morphological landmarks are not consistently identifiable. Pathological signal changes involving the pre- or postcentral gyrus further challenge presurgical morphological imaging diagnostics. A trustworthy attribution of a functional representation to a defined anatomical landmark is—even with an intact Rolandic anatomy—only feasible for the hand motor area, identified as a characteristically dorsally oriented convexity in the precentral gyrus, the so-called hand knob (Yousry et al. 1997). However, motor activity can also be detected outside of typical landmarks and the pattern of motor cortex activation is modulated by different physiological factors (Yousry et al. 2001). Other representations of the human body in the pre- or postcentral gyrus lack any reliable morphological correlate (Fesl et al. 2003). Their localization can be merely estimated knowing the somatotopic organization of the Rolandic cortex in the motor and somatosensory homunculi (Penfield 1937, 1950). Moreover, the localization and extent of activated brain sites can vary under pathological conditions as well as the pattern of brain activation. Besides local mass effects and hemodynamic alterations, brain tumors and arteriovenous malformations (AVMs) may also induce neuroplastic changes, that is, an altered pattern of activation as compared to the normal brain, known as lesion-induced reorganization or plasticity (Baciu et al. 2003; Bogomolny et al. 2004; Deng et al. (2016); Peck and Holodny 2007; Holodny et al. 2002, 2011; Tuntiyatorn et al. 2011; Briganti et al. 2012; Rösler et al. 2014; Kong et al. 2020) which is also observed in patients with epilepsy (Wunderlich et al. 1998; Fandino et al. 1999; Holodny et al. 1999, 2000; Alkadhi et al. 2000; Bittar et al. 2000; Duffau et al. 2000; Lehericy et al. 2002; Roux et al. 2000; Carpentier et al. 2001b; Duffau 2001; Krings et al. 2002a; Rutten et al. 2002b; Baciu et al. 2003; Bogomolny et al. 2004; Peck and Holodny 2007; Wellmer et al. 2009; Kasprian and Seidel 2010; Niu et al. 2014), which is moreover a consequence of surgical intervention (Shinoura et al. 2006, 2009). This also applies to language-associated brain structures (Duffau et al. 2001; Lazar et al. 1997; Springer et al.

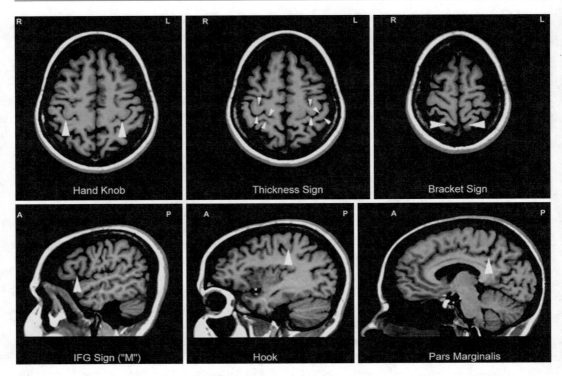

Fig. 1 Anatomical landmarks on morphological MRI according to Naidich and Yousry in transverse (*upper row*) and sagittal (*lower row*) views. *White arrows* indicate the relevant anatomical structures. The "hand knob" and "hook" are synonyms for the "precentral knob" (see chapter "Functional Neuroanatomy"). (Modified from Stippich et al. 2003a, with permission)

1999; Spreer et al. 2001; Duffau et al. 2002a, b; Hertz-Pannier et al. 2002; Lehericy et al. 2002; Petrovich et al. 2004; Stippich et al. 2007a, b; Partovi et al. 2012a; Briganti et al. 2012; Rösler et al. 2014; Balter et al. 2019; Cirillo et al. 2019; Deverdun et al. 2020; Zimmermann et al. 2020) which, other than motor cortex representations, display a marked anatomical variability even in healthy subjects (Bogen 1976; Price 2000; Naidich et al. 2001). Additionally, many cognitive brain functions are under the influence of individual factors, such as multilinguality (Bello et al. 2006; Hasegawa et al. 2002; Hernandez et al. 2001; Illes et al. 1999; Kim et al. 1997; Klein et al. 1995; Roux and Tremoulet 2002; Andrews et al. 2013; Centeno et al. 2014; Leung et al. 2020), handedness (Szaflarski et al. 2002; Wiberg et al. 2019), age (Gaillard et al. 2000a, b, 2001a, b; Schlaggar et al. 2002), or gender (Shaywitz et al. 1995; Frost et al. 1999; Nenert

et al. 2017), as published with partly incongruent or conflicting results (Allendorfer et al. 2016). This variability suggests the need for the assessment of functional localization in each patient individually.

The use of functional neuroimaging methods is especially valuable prior to neurosurgery (Stopa et al. 2020) in Rolandic (Jack et al. 1994; Baumann et al. 1995; Yousry et al. 1995, 1996; Atlas et al. 1996; Mueller et al. 1996; Pujol et al. 1996, 1998; Krings et al. 1997, 1998; Roux et al. 1997, 1999a, b; Schlosser et al. 1997; Stapleton et al. 1997; Yetkin et al. 1997; Dymarkowski et al. 1998; Lee et al. 1998b, 1999; Nitschke et al. 1998; Schulder et al. 1998; Achten et al. 1999; Hirsch et al. 2000; Lehericy et al. 2000b; Kober et al. 2001; Krings et al. 2001; Ozdoba et al. 2002; Liu et al. 2003; Schiffbauer et al. 2003; Stippich et al. 2003a; Towle et al. 2003; Krishnan et al. 2004; Parmar et al. 2004; Reinges et al.

2004; Majos et al. 2005; Roessler et al. 2005; Van Westen et al. 2005; Nimsky et al. 2006; Holodny et al. 2011; Fisicaro et al. 2015), frontal or temporoparietal (Desmond et al. 1995; Binder et al. 1996; Bahn et al. 1997; FitzGerald et al. 1997; Herholz et al. 1997; Hertz-Pannier et al. 1997; Worthington et al. 1997; van der Kallen et al. 1998; Yetkin et al. 1998; Benson et al. 1999; Bittar et al. 1999a, b; Killgore et al. 1999; Ruge et al. 1999; Rutten et al. 1999; Springer et al. 1999; Bazin et al. 2000; Grabowski 2000; Hirsch et al. 2000; Lehericy et al. 2000a; Lurito et al. 2000; Gaillard et al. 2002; Pouratian et al. 2002; Rutten et al. 2002c; Roux et al. 2003; Stippich et al. 2003b, 2010; Van Westen et al. 2005; Grummich et al. 2006; Voss et al. 2013; Benjamin et al. 2017), and mesiotemporal (Deblaere et al. 2002; Avila et al. 2006; Stippich 2010; Spritzer et al. 2012; Fakhri et al. 2013; Voss et al. 2013) brain areas for the individual functional localization of motor, somatosensory, and language- and memory-related brain activation, as well as for the determination of the hemispheric dominance and epileptogenic zone (Tyndall et al. 2017). At present, functional magnetic resonance imaging (fMRI) is the most widely used method for functional neuroimaging. This modern imaging technique measures brain function indirectly (Kwong et al. 1992) with a higher spatial accuracy, but lower temporal resolution than other noninvasive techniques such as EEG (Gevins et al. 1995) or MEG (Hämäläinen et al. 1993; Tarapore and Matthew 2012). Advantages of fMRI over PET (Fox et al. 1986) (Mazziotta et al. 1982; Raichle 1983), SPECT (Holman and Devous 1992), ECoG, and the Wada test are its noninvasiveness, lack of need for radiation, and broad availability of MR scanners.

FMRI assesses brain activity indirectly via detection of local hemodynamic changes in capillaries (Menon et al. 1995) and draining veins (Frahm et al. 1994) of functional areas. The blood oxygen level-dependent (BOLD) technique makes use of blood as an intrinsic contrast agent (Ogawa et al. 1990a, b, 1992). BOLD signals have been shown to reflect actual neuronal activity with high spatial accuracy (Logothetis et al. 2001; Logothetis 2002, 2003; Logothetis and Pfeuffer 2004; Logothetis and Wandell 2004). For details, please refer to chapter "Revealing Brain Activity and White Matter Structure Using Functional and Diffusion-Weighted Magnetic Resonance Imaging" giving information about the physiological basics and methodological-technical aspects of fMRI also in the context of clinical applications. Although fMRI has been quickly established in the research field of basic neuroscience—and high-performance gradient systems with higher field scanners and development of ultrafast MR sequences have allowed examination of the entire brain in clinically feasible scanning times—this technique is still rarely used for clinical diagnostics and research mostly due to its higher technical and methodological requirements as compared to clinical morphological MRI. Again, it should be kept in mind that presurgical fMRI has to be performed in individual patients with the goal of a neuroradiological "functional" diagnosis and therefore fundamentally differs from research experiments in basic neuroscience, where the general understanding of brain function in groups of healthy subjects or patients is in the center of interest.

The vast majority of clinical task-based fMRI measurements are performed at 1.5 T systems due to their more widespread distribution, but increasingly at 3 T, which is ideal for clinical fMRI studies (Scarabino et al. 2007; Tyndall et al. 2017). During the last years the first ultrahigh-field clinical MR imagers with a main magnetic field strength of 7 T have been installed in leading neurocenters around the globe for basic and clinical research (Beisteiner et al. 2011; Batson et al. 2015; Springer et al. 2016; Lima Cardoso et al. 2017; Trattnig et al. 2018; Beckett et al. 2020). Human 9.4 T units are used in experimental setup (Huber et al. 2018). fMRI profits from higher main magnetic fields mainly through higher signal-to-noise ratio (SNR), higher BOLD signal, and better spatial resolution (Garin et al. 2021). This is further supported by high-performance gradients and the multichannel head coil technique. An increased sensitivity (determined as the increase in percentage of voxels activated) for motor and somatosensory stimulation and more specific localization in the gray matter have been shown for 3 T fMRI compared to 1.5 T fMRI (Krasnow et al. 2003; García-Eulate et al. 2011). A further study has demonstrated an earlier onset of the hemodynamic response at 7 T in comparison to 1.5 T, hereby reducing the undesired venous contribution to the BOLD response (Van der Zwaag et al. 2009).

Real-time fMRI with immediate data analysis was developed and pushed forward for fMRI neurofeedback and brain-computer interfacing (Esposito et al. 2003; Weiskopf et al. 2003, 2004, 2007; Lührs et al. 2017; Sorger and Goebel 2020) and requires ultrafast computing capabilities. Online processing also facilitates the use under clinical conditions (Fernandez et al. 2001; Moller et al. 2005; Schwindack et al. 2005; Feigl et al. 2008; Vakamudi et al. 2020) (see Sect. 4.1). Hence, most new-generation MR imagers come along with software packages that have some functionality for processing fMRI data already at the scanner console. These products are designed to be user friendly and are easy to apply. However, the options to monitor the different steps of the underlying data processing are limited as well as the options to analyze and control the fMRI results in detail. This lacking in fundamental functionality may be problematic in cases of unclear, ambiguous, or unexpected fMRI results; during determination of artifacts; or when imaging quality is reduced.

Presurgical diagnostic assessment in patients with brain tumors and epilepsy is to date the most commonly established clinical application of fMRI. Historically, due to its good spatial resolution and direct correlation with surface anatomy, BOLD fMRI was used shortly after its first description (Bandettini et al. 1992; Kwong et al. 1992; Ogawa et al. 1992) for presurgical localization of the primary sensorimotor cortex in patients with Rolandic brain tumors (Jack et al. 1994) (see Sect. 4) and shortly after for the determination of the language-dominant hemisphere and localization of the Broca's and Wernicke's language areas (FitzGerald et al. 1997) in patients with left frontal or temporoparietal tumors (Desmond et al. 1995) (see Sect. 5). There is substantial evidence from validation studies with established reference procedures (see chapter "Presurgical Functional Localization Possibilities, Limitations and Validity") and from multimodal investigations comparing fMRI with other functional neuroimaging methods (see chapter "Multimodality in Functional Neuroimaging"), suggesting a good reliability of fMRI data for the (presurgical) localization of functional areas and—not unisono however—for the determination of the language-dominant hemisphere, considering the indications and limitations of this technique. Of note, neurovascular uncoupling induced by the brain pathology may interfere with and alter the fMRI BOLD response (Agarwal et al. 2021).

Basically, the predominant diagnostic aims of presurgical functional neuroimaging are the following:

- Localization of eloquent brain areas with respect to the envisaged site of surgery
- Determination of the dominant hemisphere for specific brain functions
- Localization of the epileptic zone and lateralization of epileptic activity
- Delineation of neuroplastic changes in brain activity

Presurgical fMRI is now commonly used in combination with diffusion tensor imaging (DTI) to additionally delineate functionally important fiber bundles such as the pyramidal tract or the arcuate fascicle (see chapter "Diffusion Imaging with MR Tractography for Brain Tumor Surgery"). The diagnostic information of both modalities is complementary and can be integrated and used for functional neuronavigation (see chapter "Functional Neuronavigation"). Resting-state fMRI (rsfMRI) has been extensively used in the last years in the field of neuroscience imaging to study different functional networks of the human brain without the need to actively stimulate the brain. Meanwhile rsfMRI has found its way into the clinical arena and was employed as a new modality for presurgical functional neuroimaging (see chapter "Presurgical Resting-State fMRI").

Standardization of the imaging procedures, data processing, and neuroradiological interpretation of the results is an ongoing issue (Beisteiner 2017; Black et al. 2017; Agarwal et al. 2019a, b; Gene et al. 2021). Therefore, a relevant amount of clinical fMRI studies should still be performed in the framework of research trials. Initial, but very general instructions for clinical fMRI have been published in the "current protocols in magnetic resonance imaging" (Thulborn 2006). By now, attempts of the responsible medical associations have been made to release instructions for established clinical applications of fMRI (https://www.asfnr.org/clinical-standards/) based on continuous evaluation, optimization, and implementation of novel technical solutions. This is an important step for clinical fMRI towards becoming a routine diagnostic neuroimaging procedure (for details see Sect. 3.1).

3 Presurgical Task-Based fMRI: Practical, Technical, and Methodological Considerations

3.1 Practical Issues

In contrast to experimental applications of fMRI, in research laboratories where permanent test setups can be installed, generally healthy subjects are examined, and measured results do not necessarily need to be immediately available, the clinical application of fMRI in a hospital setting faces particular challenges. Technically and methodologically custom-tailored developments including hardware, software, imaging protocols, and data evaluation processes (see Sects. 3.3 and 3.4) are required to allow a successful examination of patients with existing deficits, uncooperative or sedated patients, and children (Hajnal et al. 1994; Baudendistel et al. 1996; Buckner et al. 1996; Cox 1996; Friston 1996; Lee et al. 1996, 1998a, b, c; Gold et al. 1998; Stippich et al. 1999, 2000, 2002a; Thulborn and Shen 1999; Bookheimer 2000; Hammeke et al. 2000; Hirsch et al. 2000; Gaillard et al. 2001a, b; Hsu et al. 2001; Roux et al. 2001; Hoeller et al. 2002; Rutten et al. 2002c, d; Roberts 2003; Steger and Jackson 2004; Hulvershorn et al. 2005a, b; Weiskopf et al.

2005; Liu and Ogawa 2006; Priest et al. 2006; Wienbruch et al. 2006; Stopa et al. 2020; Manan et al. 2020; Gene et al. 2021). Instructions for dealing with sources of error and solving specific problems arising in clinical fMRI are given in chapter "Clinical BOLD fMRI and DTI: Artifacts, Tips and Tricks."

The principal element of any task-based fMRI measurement consists of a "paradigm," defined by a functional measurement including a stimulation adjusted to the respective brain area to be investigated. Altogether, a complete fMRI protocol comprises one or several different paradigms in addition to at least one morphological 3D data set for image overlay procedures. Clinical fMRI protocols need to be optimized for clinically acceptable examination times, low susceptibility to artifacts, good signal yield, and a reliable localization of functional brain areas. In this context, block-designed paradigms, with cyclically alternating "stimulation" and "baseline" or synonymously "control" conditions, are usually more feasible than the methodologically more demanding event-related paradigms (Fig. 2) (Tie et al. 2009). Ideally, it should be possible to use clinical fMRI protocols even in patients with existing neurological and cognitive deficits. Thus, particularly when creating complex protocols, such as for language or other cognitive brain functions, a close cooperation with neuropsychological experts is strongly advisable. Prior to any clinical fMRI examination, an accurate documentation of relevant neurological and neuropsychological deficits has to be available in order to avoid erroneous data interpretation. Individual training and stimulation adjustment according to the patient's abilities are also indispensable. The time required for the pre-measurement training generally exceeds the actual measurement time and can vary in own experience between 20 min and 3 h dependent on the patient's abilities (Stippich et al. 2002a). By using optimized and standardized protocols, fMRI examinations can be integrated in the clinical MR imaging routine without major problems. To investigate motor function, self-triggered movements are most commonly used (see Sect. 4.3), and non-standardized tactile

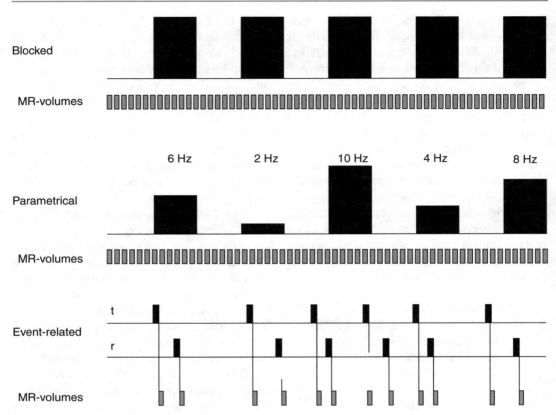

Fig. 2 Schematic illustration of different paradigm designs used for fMRI studies. Conventional "blocked design" consists of different stimulation periods that repeatedly alternate over time, while images are acquired continuously (MR volumes). Usually a series of identical stimuli (or tasks) is applied during each period. "Parametrical design" is a modification of blocked design with a systematic variation of the applied stimulation between periods (e.g., trigger frequency). "Event-related" design requires triggering and enables to measure BOLD responses to single events (e.g., a single finger movement) with improved temporal resolution. Images can be acquired continuously or discontinuously (shown). To achieve a higher SNR averaging of a larger number of events is required (for details see chapter "Revealing Brain Activity and White Matter Structure Using Functional and Diffusion-Weighted Magnetic Resonance Imaging"). (Modified from Stippich et al. 2002a, with permission)

stimuli (e.g., manual touching of the hand by the examiner) are applied to measure somatosensory function (Hammeke et al. 1994). Language functions are examined using various paradigms involving acoustic or visual stimulation (see Sect. 5.3). In the published studies on preoperative fMRI, the required measurement times per paradigm show a high variability between 1 min (Stippich et al. 2004) and above 20 min (Rutten et al. 2002c); technical and methodological differences are also considerable. To make "getting started" in preoperative fMRI easier, sample established protocols are presented in Sects. 4.4,

4.5, and 5.4. In our experience, these protocols ensure a robust functional localization at 1.5 T and sufficient BOLD signal (measured parameters: r = correlation of the measured BOLD signals to the applied hemodynamic reference function, $\Delta S\%$ = relative BOLD signal change). It seems possible to use the proposed protocols also on EPI-capable MR imagers with a lower main magnetic field strength up from 1.0 T, but this has not been tested systematically. Scan times per paradigm are 66 or 105 s (fully automatic somatosensory stimulation) (Stippich et al. 2004, 2005), 140 s (motor) (Stippich et al.

2002b), and 234 s (language) (Stippich et al. 2003b). Reproducibility of functional localization and BOLD signal during one MR session as well as on different examination days is high. However, due to the persisting lack of consensus on the performance of clinical fMRI examinations, it is not yet possible to make definitive recommendations on how these should be carried out—thus, we also allude the reader to the large body of data available on this field (see Sects. 4.1 and 5.1, https://www.asfnr.org/paradigms/).

Examination times in the clinical neuroimaging routine are in general limited and rarely exceed 1 h. Within this time, the entire stimulation equip-

ment needs to be set up at the scanner and subsequently dismantled (Fig. 3). Positioning of the pre-trained patient for MRI is more time consuming than preparation for routine morphological MR imaging. Head fixation should be optimized to reduce motion artifacts and all stimulation devices have to be installed and calibrated (Figs. 4 and 5). Once all is set up, a final performance test prior to the beginning of the fMRI examination is strongly recommended—that is, each patient should shortly repeat the task inside the scanner under the supervision of the investigator. In general, all clinical fMRI measurements should be closely monitored by the investigator to document

Fig. 3 Scheme of a typical fMRI setup. Electrical equipment placed inside the scanner room requires sufficient shielding. Test measurements should be performed to exclude imaging artifacts. For all electrical stimulation devices and critical metal implants, safety measurements on phantoms are recommended (Georgi et al. 2004; Akbar et al. 2005)

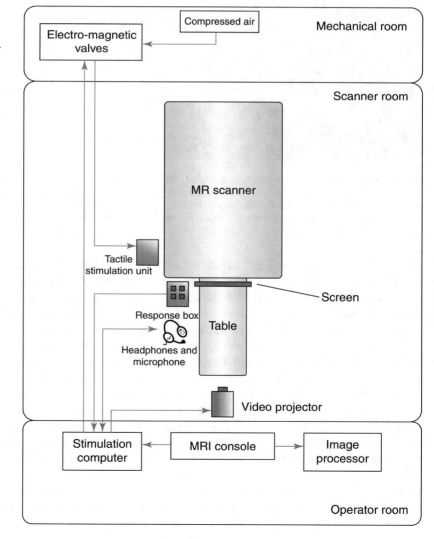

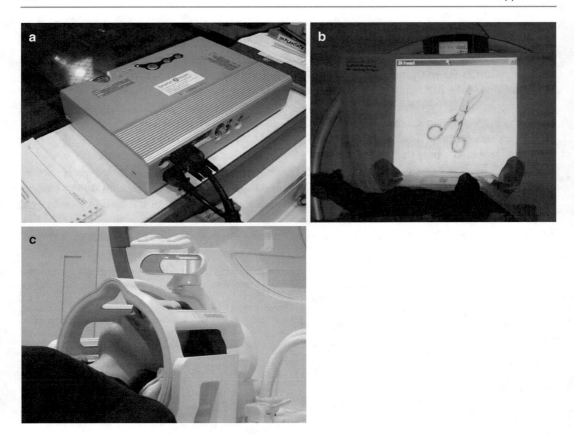

Fig. 4 Typical equipment for visual stimulation. (**a**) High-resolution video beamer. As for all electronic devices, placement of the device outside the scanner room should be preferred to avoid imaging artifacts. (**b**) Semitransparent projection screen mounted to the scanner bore. (**c**) Commercial mirror system for back projection mounted on the head coil. (Reprinted from Stippich 2005, 2010, with permission)

errors arising while the paradigms are carried out. For this reason, our investigators remain in the scan room or observe the patient from outside while the motor paradigms are carried out by the patients. For language fMRI, the patient is asked immediately after each measurement for correct task performance before initiation of the next task. This is also recommended for clinical fMRI of other cognitive functions, such as memory. These brief post-scan interviews are also important to document incorrect task performance accounting for the sometimes unavoidable and time-consuming manual post-processing of erroneous data from patients who are difficult to examine. However, erroneous measurements should be immediately repeated, whenever possible. Some commercially available clinical fMRI devices come with functionalities for patient monitoring. However, such apparatus cannot substitute proper supervision of the patient's performance by the investigator. It is highly recommended to follow the abovementioned procedure to ensure reliable clinical fMRI scanning.

The results of clinical fMRI measurements usually need to be already available on the examination day in order to ensure that fMRI data can be considered in the early therapeutic decision-making process. Traditionally, fMRI data are processed right after the fMRI examination (off-line) using freely available or commercial software (Cox 1996; Friston 1996; Gold et al. 1998; Roberts 2003; Bowring et al. 2019; see also: www.mriquestions.com/best-fmri-software.html). Today, most MR scanners come with

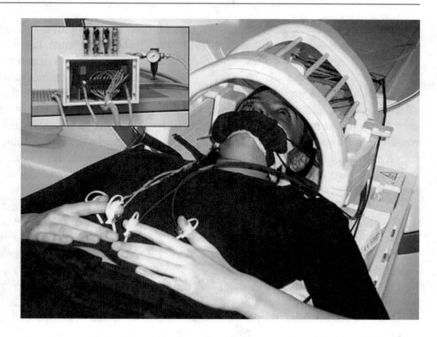

Fig. 5 Fully automated pneumatically driven tactile stimulation. Flexible membranes (4D neuroimaging, Aachen, Germany) connected to pressure-resistant pneumatic tubes transmit the stimuli to the lips, fingers, or toes (not shown). *Upper left*: The 24-channel high-precision electromagnetic valve system was designed to investigate somatosensory somatotopy. (Reprinted from Stippich 2005, 2010, with permission)

optional software packages for an immediate "online" processing of fMRI data (Fernandez et al. 2001; Moller et al. 2005; Schwindack et al. 2005) (see Sect. 4.1). The functionality of such online processing software tools is variable. The choice of the appropriate programs is usually made on the basis of individual criteria. However, any data processing software for fMRI should at least include image alignment, motion correction, temporal and spatial data smoothing, and multiple statistical tests to assess functional activation (see chapter "Revealing Brain Activity and White Matter Structure Using Functional and Diffusion-Weighted Magnetic Resonance Imaging"). It is also important to note that tools for superimposition of the functional images on morphological images and for data export (e.g., neuronavigation) are essential in presurgical fMRI, whereas the capabilities for spatial normalization can be considered as optional. Of note is that the use of software not certified for medical applications may be critical when it comes to direct intraoperative applications, for example, for neuronavigation or radiation therapy. On the other hand, research software tools and processing pipelines often provide better access to the different underlying data processing steps, which may be relevant for the meaningful interpretation of clinical fMRI data,

as well as for the detection of imaging artifacts and for fMRI quality assurance. As a consequence it may be necessary to perform the data analysis in parallel using different software, dedicated to medical application and dedicated to research.

Since the availability of accepted guidelines or recommendations for the evaluation and interpretation of clinical fMRI is very limited, appropriate imaging protocols and criteria for the diagnostic interpretation often need to be defined by the individual institutions. As an important step towards a more standardized diagnostic application of fMRI, the American Society for Functional Neuroradiology (ASFNR) provides instructions and recommendations for clinical fMRI including BOLD-fMRI paradigms, educational videos, and fMRI CPT codes (for further information please visit the ASFNR homepage, https://www.asfnr.org). The proposed paradigms cover motor, somatosensory, language, and memory function as well as vision. They are of special value for clinical neurocenters which intend to start with presurgical fMRI, wish to adopt their existing imaging protocols, or aim to participate in multicenter trials.

However, most larger medical centers offering clinical fMRI studies still use their own internal routines, which are typically the result of a long-standing own "evolutionary" process and thus of specific in-house expertise (Tyndall et al. 2017). An intrinsic advantage of this situation is the thorough understanding of the whole process associated with presurgical fMRI between the different medical partner disciplines involved in each respective neuro- and imaging center (neuroradiology, neurosurgery, neurology, radio-oncology, etc.). This highly interdisciplinary process of using presurgical fMRI includes the following:

1. FMRI indication, data acquisition, analysis, and diagnostic interpretation
2. Clinical decision-making also considering fMRI (and DTI) results
3. Planning of an optimal treatment tailored to the specific findings in each individual patient
4. Detailed information of patients about the desired treatment, its side effects, other possible consequences, and therapeutical alternatives
5. Application of the optimized treatment based on profound knowledge of its methodological and medical limitations
6. Assessment of the post-therapeutic outcome with respect to the pretherapeutic findings

On the other hand, such methodological variability considerably affects the comparability of fMRI studies between different investigators, especially when it is about imaging cognitive brain function (e.g., language or memory). As a consequence the following sections provide recent and in-depth information on legal, methodological, technical, and medical aspects to implement and employ state-of-the-art presurgical task-based fMRI.

3.2 Legal Aspects

Today, there exists a substantial body of evidence that task-based BOLD fMRI is robust, valid, and reasonably precise to localize different cortical representations of the human body within the primary motor and somatosensory cortices, to local-ize essential motor and receptive language areas, and to determine language dominance prior to brain surgery. More and more stimulation devices and software solutions have become commercially available that facilitate the clinical application of fMRI and that have been certified for medical use. However, fMRI can still not be considered as a standard routine application in clinical diagnostic neuroimaging, since in most countries worldwide (except for the USA), no recommendations or guidelines have been issued by the responsible domestic medical associations. Until then, individual routine procedures and standards need to be established for measuring techniques and examination protocols, data processing, and evaluation, as well as for medical evaluation and documentation of clinical fMRI findings (Pernet and Poline 2015; Pernet et al. 2016; Beisteiner 2017). Validation of preoperative fMRI using established reference procedures (e.g., ECoG, Wada test) (Spritzer et al. 2012; Janecek et al. 2013; Ojemann et al. 2013; Siero et al. 2014; Massot-Tarrús et al. 2020) by the operator is indispensable, even if the examination protocols suggested in this book are used. As a prerequisite clinical fMRI examinations should be performed, evaluated, and interpreted by trained and experienced investigators with particular expertise in this area, since careless use of this very promising technique could endanger patients.

3.3 Evaluation of Presurgical fMRI Data

Presurgical fMRI examinations are always carried out in individual patients with the primary goal of an individual "functional" diagnosis. To achieve this, the surgically relevant functional brain areas need to be reliably localized and their spatial relationship to the brain tumor or epileptogenic zone needs to be accurately identified. Precise localization of the anatomical correlate of the center of gravity of a functional area (focus of activation) and correct naming of the corresponding anatomical structure (gyrus) are of utmost importance, as far as the pathology allows. When determining the language-dominant hemisphere, limitations of the method need to be considered (see Sect. 6).

The use of dynamic statistical thresholds in the data processing helps to reliably localize functional brain areas and to provide defined BOLD signal readings (see Sect. 3.4). Regardless of the software used and of the level of automation achieved, the superposition of the intrinsically distorted echo planar MR images (EPI) onto anatomical 3D data sets and the definition of the appropriate display parameters for intraoperative representation of the functional data remain manual procedures or require at least control and refinement. Just like the medical evaluation and documentation of clinical fMRI findings, they require a certain level of experience of the investigator. These investigator-related factors in particular underline the need for the establishment of standardized fMRI protocols, data processing strategies, and evaluation procedures to achieve a consistent quality among the clinical fMRI examinations.

In general, it is important to note that the *spatial extent* of a functional brain area cannot be reliably and accurately determined with BOLD fMRI, since the extent of the local signal display varies according to the statistical threshold chosen for data evaluation (of note, the same applies to DTI-tractography regarding the size and extent of important white matter tracts). Therefore, defining resection margins on the basis of BOLD activations alone is not safe enough and should not be permitted until sufficient data from prospective clinical trials on this topic are available. In addition, the spatial coordinates of the focus of activation change with the statistical threshold as well as with the cluster size and BOLD signal (Fig. 6). When evaluating clinical fMRI data, the use of one or more predetermined (fixed) statistical thresholds—a common approach in research fMRI—does not solve the problem, since BOLD signal intensities and cluster sizes differ significantly between single patients and different paradigms (e.g., foot movement, hand movement), respectively, even if the examinations are carried out in a standardized way. This holds also true for different fMRI mea-

surements performed in the same patient, regardless of whether they are acquired on different days or within the same scanning session. More importantly, inaccuracies in localizing functional cortical representations may mislead the neurosurgeon with respect to presurgical assurance, a security which in reality is unfounded and could consequently put the patient at risk. This problem can be overcome by the adoption of the individual fMRI analyses on the basis of clearly defined criteria using dynamic statistical thresholding (Fig. 7) (see Sect. 3.4).

Determination of the dominant hemisphere with fMRI is at least equally challenging. Typically, activated voxels in defined target regions in both hemispheres (e.g., Broca's and Wernicke's areas and their anatomically homologous areas in the contralateral hemisphere) are counted at a particular statistical threshold; upon them lateralization indices (LI) are calculated from interhemispheric quotients (Stippich et al. 2003b). This procedure has intrinsic problems for several reasons: (1) The BOLD activation measured depends on the paradigm used, but the application of several different paradigms for the identification of language-related brain areas has proven to be more reliable to localize and lateralize language as compared to the application of one single paradigm alone (Ramsey et al. 2001; Rutten et al. 2002c; Zacà et al. 2013; Black et al. 2017). In addition, some linguistically different paradigms do better account for the complexity of language assessment in presurgical fMRI. The single results of the various paradigms are rarely identical, but often congruent. There are, however, no scientific data indicating how conflicting results should be medically interpreted. (2) BOLD activation varies independently between hemispheres if the frequency of stimuli is varied, even when the same paradigm is used (Konrad et al. 2005). This means that the lateralization measured depends on both the statistical threshold chosen and the "cerebral workload" associated with the respective task. (3) In contrast to imaging modalities based on ionizing radiation (e.g., CT), MRI yields "relative" rather than "absolute" measurements, so that the results of

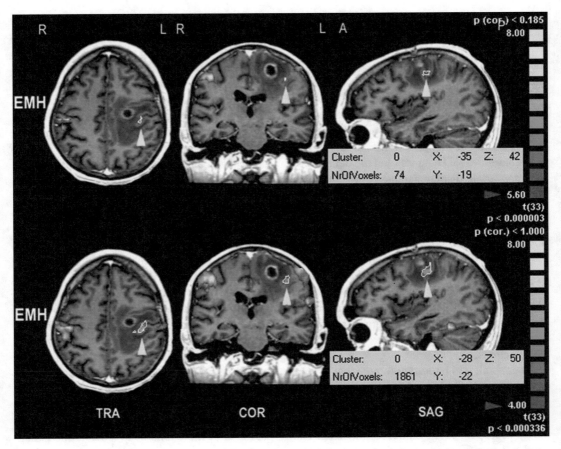

Fig. 6 Influence of the statistical threshold on spatial extent and localization of the center of gravity of BOLD fMRI activation. With decreasing statistical threshold, BOLD clusters increase in size and show a marked shift of spatial coordinates (please compare *upper and lower rows*). The *yellow arrowheads* indicate primary senso- rimotor activation obtained from contralateral finger opposition in a hemiparetic patient; *red arrowheads* indi- cate the statistical threshold used to display functional activation. *Gray boxes*: spatial coordinates (*x, y, z*) of the center of gravity of BOLD clusters (cluster size in mm³, 1 voxel = 1 mm³)

BOLD fMRI have to be interpreted semiquantita- tively. (4) Brain tumors induce neuroplastic changes which may affect motor (Tozakidou et al. 2013) and language lateralization (Partovi et al. 2012a) or may even cause neurovascular uncoupling leading to pseudo-reorganization (Ulmer et al. 2003, 2004a, b). A right-sided lan- guage dominance, for example, as calculated based on preoperative fMRI data in patients with brain tumors affecting the language system, does not mean that the (relatively) reduced language activation in the left hemisphere is no longer essential to maintain language function. The same holds true for the reduced primary motor activation in Rolandic lesions. In contrast, the functional reorganization in these patients reflects the brain's attempts to functionally cope with the brain tumor. Consequently, tumor-induced altered functional lateralization, which is repro- ducible in different paradigms, should therefore be considered as an indicator for very "watchful" resections. In such situations, additional intraop- erative measures (ECoG) and/or awake cranioto- mies may be considered.

In spite of the limitations mentioned, fMRI yields—in the vast majority of patients—impor- tant diagnostic information noninvasively which is otherwise unavailable. Functional landmarks

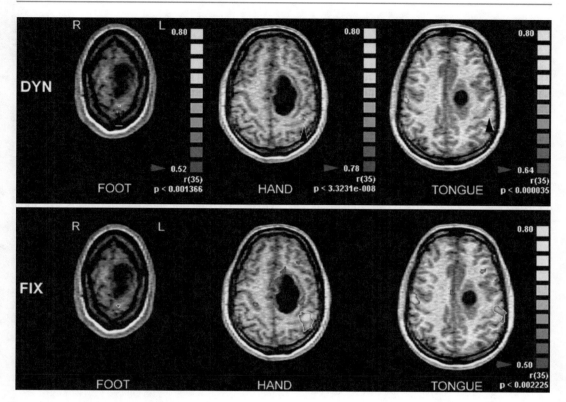

Fig. 7 Comparison of dynamic thresholding (DYN, *upper row*) and fixed thresholding (FIX, *lower row*) in somatotopic mapping of the left primary sensorimotor cortex. Dynamic thresholding enables to adapt the data evaluation to different fMRI measurements in a standardized way. Using the empirically proven cluster size of 36 mm³ as a standard for data evaluation allows to achieve well-outlined fMRI activations (*black arrowheads*) and enables to precisely assess their anatomical correlates and spatial coordinates as well as to measure BOLD signals under defined conditions (r = correlation of the measured BOLD signals to the hemodynamic reference function (hrf), ΔS = relative BOLD signal change [%]). Fixed thresholding (here adapted to the "weakest" activation (foot)) results in BOLD clusters of variable size and spatial coordinates precluding a reliable assessment of their anatomical correlates as well as of BOLD signal characteristics. In this patient, at low statistical threshold, artificial activations occurred around the tumor, obscuring diagnostic information and potentially confusing the neurosurgeon (please compare hand, *upper and lower rows*)

facilitate pretherapeutic assessment of the most function-sparing therapy upon a careful consideration of the benefits and risks, as well as the planning and execution of function-preserving interventions. At the same time, preoperative fMRI has the potential to better prove the indication and reduce the number of invasive diagnostic procedures, such as the Wada test or ECoG, either before or during neurosurgery. There is substantial evidence available from studies comparing preoperative fMRI with Wada test, indicating that invasive catheter testing can be replaced in many instances, when fMRI yields robust and reliable language or memory lateralization (Dym et al. 2011; Bohm et al. 2020; Massot-Tarrús et al. 2020). However, preoperative functional neuroimaging has relevant limitations (Metwali et al. 2019; Azad and Duffau 2020) and—in case of conflicting results—many surgeons rely on invasive procedures (Stopa et al. 2020). Consequently, fMRI cannot fully replace the abovementioned invasive measures and should therefore be considered as a supportive diagnostic modality playing a major role in the pretherapeutic assessment of brain tumors and epilepsies.

3.4 Analyzing fMRI Data in Individual Patients

Defining standard analysis processes is a significant prerequisite for the medical interpretation of clinical fMRI data, alongside standardized clinical examination protocols, defined reference values, and automated data processing. These are the minimum requirements if clinically diagnostic information is to be gleaned from fMRI. Diagnostic and pretherapeutic evaluation of non-standardized fMRI examinations in "interesting" patients is highly inadvisable and may put the patients at risk.

A number of freely available and commercial programs are available for fMRI data processing and evaluation (Cox 1996; Friston 1996; Gold et al. 1998; Roberts 2003, Bowring et al. 2019; see also: www.mriquestions.com/best-fmri-software.html). Due to the diversity of these programs and the varying requirements and preferences of the individual user, no program can be recommended in particular. The following three-step procedure using dynamic thresholding has been developed for BrainVoyager (BV) but is transferable to other programs.

Preprocessing (step 1, for details see chapter "Revealing Brain Activity and White Matter Structure Using Functional and Diffusion-Weighted Magnetic Resonance Imaging"): Any interpretation of clinical fMRI data should begin with processing of the raw data, including at minimum image alignment, correction of motion artifacts, and temporal-spatial smoothing. Generally, functional activation maps are then calculated on the basis of a number of successive images (2D fMRI maps), for which various statistical processes can be alternatively used [e.g., t-test, cross correlations, general linear model (GLM)]. As a basic principle, a reference function corrected for the delayed hemodynamic response should be used. A volume map of activations (3D fMRI maps) can be calculated following (manual) superposition of the EPI image layers onto anatomical 3D data sets (Fig. 8). The minimal number of voxels within a cluster to be

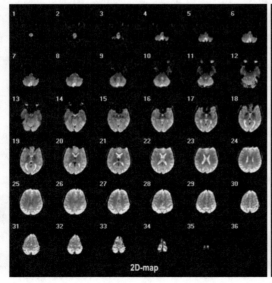
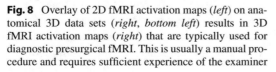
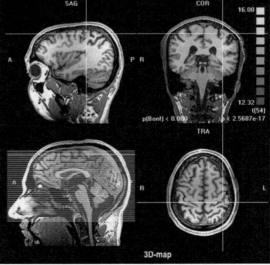

Fig. 8 Overlay of 2D fMRI activation maps (*left*) on anatomical 3D data sets (*right, bottom left*) results in 3D fMRI activation maps (*right*) that are typically used for diagnostic presurgical fMRI. This is usually a manual procedure and requires sufficient experience of the examiner to cope with the distortions of the functional EPI images and other imaging artifacts (movement artifacts, BOLD signal of venous origin, etc.). The fit should be optimized to the different anatomical structures of interest in patients with Rolandic, frontal, or temporoparietal brain tumors

shown can be freely predetermined, but should be standardized. On the basis of empirical experience, we consider a cluster size of 36 mm³ appropriate and define this as a standard parameter for all 3D analyses. On the one hand, randomly scattered activations are barely shown at this cluster size; on the other hand, clusters are not so large that small anatomic details are obscured. When defining own standards, it should be borne in mind that the representation of the clusters also depends on spatial smoothing.

Dynamic thresholding (step 2): This evaluation process for individual fMRI data typically begins at the maximal statistical threshold, so that no activation is displayed (empty map). The statistical threshold is then progressively lowered, until an activation is detected, which best correlates with the hemodynamic reference function (HRF). Much like the tip of an iceberg, this activation is small and well outlined, in such a way that the anatomic correlate of the activation focus and the spatial coordinates can be accurately determined. The associated correlation of the measured BOLD signal to the HRF (r), the relative BOLD signal changes ($\Delta S\%$), and the cluster size can be measured under defined conditions. By further reducing the statistical threshold, activations in other functional areas appear, to which the measurements mentioned can be applied (Stippich et al. 2000, 2003a, b, 2007a, b; Stippich 2010). Thus, for each fMRI data set there is an individual hierarchy of the various functional activations associated with the applied paradigm. Simultaneously, the size of clusters already shown on a higher statistical level increases with decreasing threshold. This can be used to determine the dominant hemisphere by calculating the lateralization index according to the established formula LI = (LH − RH): (LH + RH), where "LH" is the number of voxels in the left and "RH" the number of voxels in the right hemisphere (Stippich et al. 2003b; Partovi et al. 2012a, b). Due to the well-outlined clusters separate LIs can be calculated, for example, for the Broca's and Wernicke's speech areas, enabling a highly detailed analysis of atypical language activation as, for example, influenced by the presence of a brain tumor (Fig. 9). In order

to reliably distinguish the measured BOLD signals from noise, $r > 0.5$ for motor and language function and $r > 0.4$ for somatosensory brain activation have empirically been proven as appropriate lower threshold limits, each with $p < 0.05$. Alternatively, or additionally, an error rate can be determined which should not be exceeded in order to evaluate a BOLD activation as "real," for example, a false discovery rate (FDR) <0.001 (0.1%).

Checking BOLD signal characteristics (step 3, for details see chapters "Revealing Brain Activity and White Matter Structure Using Functional and Diffusion-Weighted Magnetic Resonance Imaging" and "Clinical BOLD fMRI and DTI: Artifacts, Tips and Tricks"): Measuring BOLD signals under defined conditions can help to separate real activations from artifacts. Both the correlation with HRF (r) and the signal intensity ($\Delta S\%$) should remain within normal range (Fig. 10). Unphysiologically high signal intensity can arise from activation of "venous" origin—an assumption supported by a sulcal localization of the cluster focus—or by motion artifacts. In the latter case, the strongest usually ring-shaped activations tend to occur in the frontal circumference of the brain opposite the supporting point of the head (occipital). Depending on the dominant motion components, other localizations may also account for erroneous signal. Here, the onset of the measured signal time course corresponds better to the box-car function of the block design than to the HRF (for details see chapter "Clinical BOLD fMRI and DTI: Artifacts, Tips and Tricks"). A reduction or loss of BOLD signal can occur in functional areas compressed or infiltrated by a tumor by limiting the capability of the affected brain tissue to hemodynamically respond to the applied stimulation. Also, the opposite effect has been observed in highly vascularized pathologies, such as arteriovenous malformations that may induce a "steal phenomenon" in the respective functional areas. For more detailed information on relevant hemodynamical and pathophysiological mechanisms underlying BOLD fMRI failure we refer the reader also to publications on cerebrovascular reactivity mapping and a phenomenon called "neurovascular

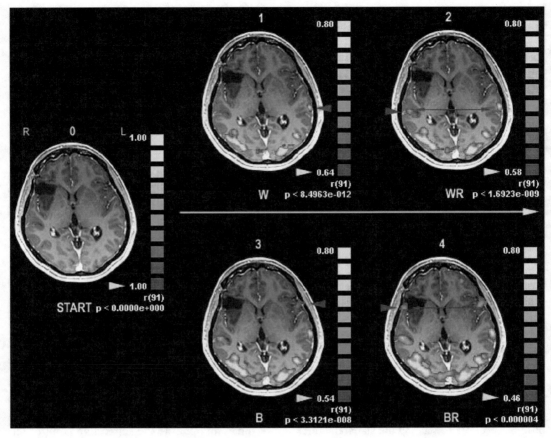

Fig. 9 Dynamic thresholding: evaluation routine for individual clinical fMRI data. Continuous reduction of the statistical threshold (*yellow arrowheads*) results in a hierarchy of different functional activations (*red arrowheads*) associated with a given task (e.g., word generation). The starting point (0) is at the maximum statistical threshold (*r* = 1.0) where no activation is displayed. Wernicke's activation (*W*) correlates best with the HRF (*1, r* = 0.64) followed by WR (*2, r* = 0.58), *B* (*3, r* = 0.54), and BR (*4, r* = 0.46). Regional lateralization indexes (LI) are calculated from BOLD cluster sizes in corresponding functional brain areas in the left and right hemispheres (*red double-headed arrows*). Empirically proven default parameters: cluster size >35 mm³, correlation to the HRF: *r* > 0.4 with *p* < 0.05. Note the strong occipital activation related to the visual trigger presentation

uncoupling" (Zaca et al. 2011, 2013, 2014; Pillai and Zaca 2012; Pillai and Mikulis 2015; Agarwal et al. 2016, 2019a, b, 2021; Pak et al. 2017).

4 Presurgical fMRI of Motor and Somatosensory Function

Surgery on Rolandic brain tumors entails a high risk of motor and sensory deficits. Task-based fMRI of motor function is the most frequently used presurgical application due to the compara-tively low equipment requirements for this examination (no stimulation devices are necessary), the relative ease with which it is performed, and the generally stable functional activation. The diagnostic aim is to localize the primary motor cortex in relation to Rolandic tumors. On the basis of morphological MR imaging and clinical findings (motor and/or sensory deficits), the indication for presurgical fMRI should be assessed (see Sect. 4.2) and the appropriate examination protocol individually adjusted (see Sects. 4.4–4.6). Even patients with tumor-associated pareses can be examined using special paradigms (see

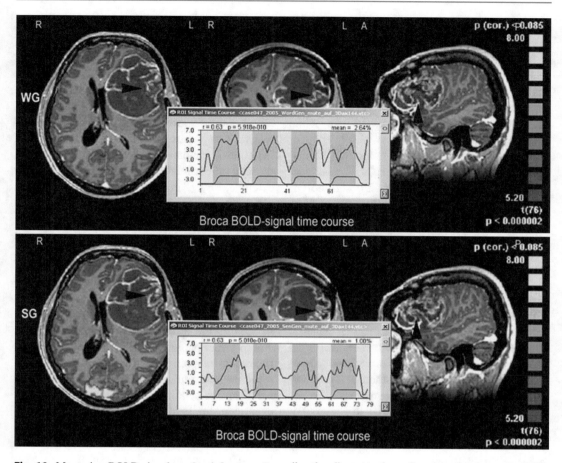

Fig. 10 Measuring BOLD signals under defined conditions helps to distinguish between "true" activation and "artifacts." In this left-handed patient with a giant left frontal high-grade glioma (WHO grade IV), presurgical fMRI was performed to assess language dominance. FMRI indicated left dominance and functional tissue directly adjacent to the malignancy. Good reproducibility of the functional localization of Broca's area using two different paradigms (*WG* word generation, *SG* sentence generation) and "physiological" BOLD signal parameters (WG: $r = 0.63$, $\Delta S = 2.64\%$, SG: $r = 0.63$, $\Delta S = 1.00\%$) made artifacts unlikely

Sects. 4.5 and 4.6). According to the site and extent of the tumor, a single fMRI reading can suffice. However, it is often necessary to examine the entire motor and, where appropriate, somatosensory somatotopy. Today, presurgical localization of various body representations in the pre- and postcentral gyrus by fMRI can be considered reliable (see chapter "Presurgical Functional Localization Possibilities, Limitations and Validity"). Even neuroplastic changes (Baciu et al. 2003; Bogomolny et al. 2004; Peck and Holodny 2007; Kasprian and Seidel 2010; Holodny et al. 2011; Tuntiyatorn et al. 2011; Tozakidou et al. 2013; Cirillo et al. 2019; Kong et al. 2020) can be examined, although in the presence of brain tumors, shifts in different body representations can be observed as well as changes in functional hemispheric lateralization and in activation of secondary cortical areas (see chapter "Brain Plasticity in fMRI and DTI").

4.1 Review of Literature

Shortly after the first reports on BOLD fMRI in healthy subjects (Belliveau et al. 1991; Bandettini et al. 1992; Kwong et al. 1992; Ogawa et al. 1993), the potential usefulness of functional imaging techniques in the clinical context and particularly in the presurgical identification of motor and somatosensory cortices was postulated. The literature concerning functional imaging in patients with tumoral lesions in and adjacent to the "central" or synonymously "Rolandic" region will be reviewed here, while specific literature on patients with epilepsy or lesions near language-related areas will be discussed in Sect. 5.1 and in chapter "Presurgical EEG-fMRI in Epilepsy." The first description of presurgical fMRI as a clinically useful application dates from 1994, when Jack et al. provided proof of concept in two patients with brain tumors in the sensorimotor cortex, validating their preliminary results with established electrophysiological techniques (Jack et al. 1994). Soon after, several case studies (Baumann et al. 1995) (Cosgrove et al. 1996) and reports on small patient populations (Puce et al. 1995; Mueller et al. 1996; Krings et al. 1998) harboring glial tumors or arteriovenous malformations (AVM) confirmed the technical and practical feasibility of fMRI using motor and sensory tasks in the clinical context and stressed the high potential of this new upcoming technique for preoperative risk assessment, therapeutic decision-making, and surgical planning.

During the following years investigations on larger numbers of tumor patients (up to 50) were carried out, whose results had been claimed to represent an important factor for surgical decision-making (Schlosser et al. 1997; Pujol et al. 1998). Comparisons of presurgical fMRI data with the established reference procedure, intracortical stimulation (ICS), are numerous, and only those specifically dealing with brain tumor patients will be mentioned here, since a detailed description of validation studies referring to this is offered in chapter "Presurgical Functional Localization Possibilities, Limitations and Validity." Virtually all studies report highly concordant results between presurgical fMRI and ICS data in patients with lesions around the central sulcus (Dymarkowski et al. 1998; Achten et al. 1999; Roux et al. 1999a, b) with an accor-

dance ranging from 83% in 33 patients (Majos et al. 2005) to 92% in 60 patients (Lehericy et al. 2000b). Task sensitivity for the identification of the sensorimotor region estimated in large groups of tumor patients was 85% in 103 patients (Krings et al. 2001) and 97% in 125 patients (Hirsch et al. 2000). Furthermore, it should be briefly noted that various groups focused on the correlation of fMRI results in patients with central lesions with those of other functional imaging procedures, for example, PET (Bittar et al. 1999a, b); for details please refer to chapter "Multimodality in Functional Neuroimaging."

One of the first attempts to evaluate the impact of fMRI on neurosurgical planning was published by Lee et al. The authors applied preoperative fMRI sensorimotor mapping in 32 tumor patients and reported that the results were used to determine the feasibility of surgical resection in 55%, to aid in the surgical planning in 22%, and to select patients for invasive intraoperative functional mapping in 78%. Overall, the fMRI results were useful in one or more of these surgical decision-making categories in 89% of all examined tumor patients (Lee et al. 1999). Similar numbers were described by Ternovoi et al. who found that presurgical fMRI results had an influence on therapeutic strategies in 69% of 16 tumor patients (Ternovoi et al. 2004). Other investigators tried to establish a functional risk prediction (or estimation) for postoperative clinical outcome: Haberg et al. examined 25 patients with primary brain tumors in the near of sensorimotor regions. In 80% of the patients, successful fMRI measurements were obtained, out of which 75% were used for preoperative planning. The risk of postoperative loss of function was significantly lower when the distance between the tumor margin and the BOLD activation was 10 mm or more (Håberg et al. 2004). Similar observations have been described by Berntsen et al. (2010). Krishnan et al. who evaluated BOLD activation in 54 patients found that a lesion-to-activation distance of less than 5 mm and incomplete resection were predictors for new postoperative neurological deficits and recommended cortical stimulation within a 10 mm range, given that for a lesion-to-activation distance of >10 mm a complete resection can be safely achieved (Krishnan et al. 2004). In patients with medial frontal lesions, preoperative fMRI was used to establish the area at risk for the resection of specific parts of the supplementary motor area associated with transient postoperative motor deficits and speech disorders (Krainik et al. 2001, 2003, 2004). In a further study, Hall et al. used fMRI-guided resection in 16 patients with low-grade gliomas. Since these tumors are generally not contrast enhancing, resection borders are particularly difficult to define based on morphological imaging alone. Using fMRI for the determination of resection borders, no permanent neurological deficits and no radiological tumor progression within a median follow-up of 25 months were observed (Hall et al. 2005). However, the data available to calculate a safe resection distance between functional activation and lesion borders for prevention of surgically induced neurological deficits are still very limited and do not justify any general conclusion or recommendation (Gil-Robles and Duffau 2010).

Overall, although the abovementioned studies clearly demonstrate the feasibility of presurgical fMRI in the clinical environment and militate for the preoperative contribution of the additional clinical information obtained from fMRI to pre-therapeutic decision-making, an effect on the decrease in the post-therapeutic morbidity has not been corroborated at this time. Although most investigators agree on the necessity of a standardized procedure in the clinical routine and several methodological studies presenting optimized protocols for the clinical use have been published (Hirsch et al. 2000; Ramsey et al. 2001; Rutten et al. 2002a, b, c, d; Springer et al. 1999; Stippich et al. 2000, 2002b, 2004, 2005), no large-scale clinical trials addressing the actual benefit for the patient in terms of decrease in morbidity were available. In order to achieve this, a number of controlled clinical trials using site-specific but optimized and standardized fMRI protocols were

conducted during the last decade. Meanwhile, there is some evidence for improved postoperative morbidity, extent of resection, and longer term survival when fMRI is employed (Kundu et al. 2013; Bailey et al. 2015; Vysotski et al. 2018; Liouta et al. 2019).

Although sensorimotor areas are identified with high success rates using fMRI in patients with central lesions by most investigators, a frequently encountered phenomenon is neuroplasticity (Tuntiyatorn et al. 2011; Tozakidou et al. 2013) which is also found in the language network (Stippich et al. 2007b; Partovi et al. 2012a; Briganti et al. 2012; Rösler et al. 2014). In an early study in seven patients with intracerebral gliomas of the primary sensorimotor cortex, activation was found to be displaced or reduced (Atlas et al. 1996). Roux et al. correlated the type of activation with histologic tumor characteristics in 17 patients. In infiltrating tumors, intratumoral activation was detected, which was displaced and scattered, and correlated with the degree of infiltration, whereas in noninfiltrating tumors activation showed extra-tumoral shift. In tumors at some distance from the motor cortex, no intratumoral activation was measured (Roux et al. 1997). Likewise, a PET study on 51 patients described that central lesions were more frequently associated with altered patterns of activation than lesions in noncentral locations (Bittar et al. 2000). Other studies found significant BOLD signal decrease in areas adjacent to tumor tissue in motor and sensory cortices as compared to the contralateral side. This effect was present in glial tumors, most pronounced in glioblastoma, and presumably related to tumor-induced changes in local cerebral hemodynamics (Holodny et al. 1999, 2000; Schreiber et al. 2000; Krings et al. 2002a; Ludemann et al. 2006; Jiang and Krainik 2010; Tozakidou et al. 2013), while in non-glial tumors (metastasis, cavernoma, abscess, AVM), no BOLD signal decrease was found (Schreiber et al. 2000). A report on 33 patients with different intra- and extra-axial tumors established the influence of tumor type and distance from the eloquent cortex on activation volumes in fMRI (Liu et al. 2005). In addition to a displacement or a reduction of activation in the primary sensorimotor cortex harboring the tumor, other patterns of lesion-induced reorganization encompass the activation of solely the contralesional cortex (Tozakidou et al. 2013) or an enhanced activation of non-primary sensorimotor areas with increasing degree of paresis (Alkadhi et al. 2000; Carpentier et al. 2001b; Krings et al. 2002b; Reinges et al. 2005). Also in patients with prior surgery (Kim et al. 2005) or newly developed central paresis after tumor resection (Reinges et al. 2005), a significant decrease in BOLD activation was observed. One possible explanation for this tumor-induced BOLD signal loss has been proposed by an fMRI study where tumor blood volume and perfusion were measured. The authors concluded that the BOLD amplitude correlated with total intratumoral blood volume and thus reduced peritumoral perfusion due to a sucking effect by the tumor core (i.e., blood is siphoned off by the tumor similar to the steal phenomenon known from AVMs) was responsible for the reduced BOLD activation (Ludemann et al. 2006; Jiang and Krainik 2010). Of note is, however, that resection of gliomas whose preoperatively acquired images show perilesional hyperintensity on T2w images, likely reflecting edema, may cause a transient increase in BOLD activation ipsilateral to the tumor, presumably by a decrease of perfusion pressure on the brain tissue adjacent to the resection (Kokkonen et al. 2005). Lesion-induced functional reorganization may reflect the recruitment of plastic neuronal networks to compensate for sensory or motor impairment. On the level of a functional diagnosis in presurgical fMRI, these reorganization phenomena are of major clinical significance for the presurgical planning of resections, since they can potentially cause false-negative results. For further information, please refer to chapter "Brain Plasticity in fMRI and DTI" on brain plasticity.

In the last decade, the use of combined presurgical fMRI and diffusion tensor imaging (DTI) (see Sect. 6) for tractography has been suggested to provide a better estimation of the proximity of the tumor borders to the eloquent cortex than

fMRI measurements alone. In particular for space-occupying lesions affecting the central region, visualization of the origin, direction, and functionality of large white matter tracts allowing imaging of functional connectivity was promoted to improve surgical outcome and to aim for a decrease in patient morbidity (Parmar et al. 2004; Ulmer et al. 2004a, b; Shinoura et al. 2005; Stippich et al. 2003a, 2010; Holodny et al. 2001; Wengenroth et al. 2011; Jia et al. 2013; Kumar et al. 2014; Leclercq et al. 2011; Potgieser et al. 2014; Bailey et al. 2015; Conti Nibali et al. 2019; Mancini et al. 2019; Hazzaa et al. (2019); Henderson et al. 2020).

Another practically relevant innovation was the introduction of real-time fMRI in the clinical environment (Moller et al. 2005; Feigl et al. 2008; Vakamudi et al. 2020). Real-time fMRI enables for a quick online analysis of fMRI data, which is particularly useful in presurgical diagnostics, considering that fMRI data acquisition and off-line processing are very time consuming. Moller et al. first demonstrated the technical feasibility of presurgical real-time fMRI in ten patients with tumors in the central area immediately prior to surgery (Moller et al. 2005). In another study, motor and language tasks were used for real-time fMRI in 11 tumor patients. The authors reported satisfactory activation for hand motor tasks, weaker activation for foot motor tasks, and no useful activation for language tasks at the chosen threshold, concluding that real-time fMRI needed to be optimized, but was generally practicable in the clinical routine (Schwindack et al. 2005). Furthermore, Gasser et al. could obtain the recording of intraoperative fMRI in four anesthetized patients with lesions in the vicinity of the central region. Using a passive stimulation paradigm and analyzing the data during acquisition by online statistical evaluation, they could identify eloquent brain areas taking into account intraoperatively occurring brain shift (Gasser et al. 2005). For further details on intraoperative imaging techniques and specific problems caused by intraoperative brain shift (Kuhnt et al. 2012; Shahar et al. 2014; Gerard et al. 2017; Fan et al. 2018), see chapter "Functional Neuronavigation." Since those early studies real-time fMRI has been used more widely for preoperative application and has demonstrated usefulness, but did not replace the established and validated processing routines in most neuro- and imaging centers performing routine clinical fMRI studies.

Finally, with the introduction of higher magnetic field scanners for clinical diagnostics, practicability of presurgical fMRI at 3 T has been established in patients with brain tumors (Roessler et al. 2005; Van Westen et al. 2005; Scarabino et al. 2007). Today, it is recommended to perform clinical fMRI studies at 3 T where available. For a general review on the role of imaging in disease management and the development of improved image-guided therapies in neuro-oncology see Jacobs et al. (2005), Brindle et al. (2017), and Villanueva-Meyer et al. (2017).

4.2 Selection of Candidates for Presurgical Motor and Somatosensory fMRI

In patients with Rolandic brain tumors, presurgical fMRI is usually performed when neurological symptoms indicate involvement of the sensorimotor cortex and when insufficient information is obtained from morphological imaging. Four different scenarios can be distinguished:

- Due to tumor growth, MR morphologic Rolandic landmarks cannot be identified (see Fig. 15). In these patients, it is possible neither to localize the pre- or postcentral gyrus on the basis of anatomic criteria alone nor to reliably estimate putative surgery-related sensorimotor deficits. Here, fMRI offers somatotopic motor and somatosensory mapping of up to six functional landmarks in the pre- and postcentral cortical representations of the lower and upper extremities, as well as of the facial area. As patients with tumors invading the pre- or postcentral gyrus often present with contralateral motor and/or sensory deficits, the application of appropriate paradigms for the respective deficit may be required.
- Although the Rolandic region is morphologically localizable, the "hand knob" and/or

precentral hook is no longer clearly identifiable because of a displacement or compression by the tumor. In this case, the MR morphologic reference of the motor hand area as an orientation point for the somatotopic mapping of the precentral gyrus is absent: Surgery-related neurological deficits cannot be reliably estimated, and the planning and performance of low-risk interventions are problematic. Any presurgical fMRI should at least image the motor hand area while somatotopic mapping can, with relatively little additional effort, increase the diagnostic value of the examination.

- The tumor lies directly above or below the identifiable motor hand area (see Figs. 16, 17, and 18). In this case, somatotopic mapping is indicated in order to assess the local relationship between the tumor and functional areas and hence better estimate surgery-related neurological deficits in the lower extremities or facial area, as well as to provide the operator with additional functional landmarks.
- Presurgical fMRI can also be helpful in cases with a discrepancy between the morphological findings and the clinical status of the patient, for example, when there are little or no neurological deficits despite verifiable tumor growth into the central region. This and similar constellations should prompt a search for atypical brain activation as a result of tumor-associated cerebral plasticity and reorganization. The same applies to patients with recurrent malignancies, where the functional system has already been affected by former treatment (see Fig. 19). A study assessing surgical outcome in patients with primary or metastatic brain tumors based on the lesion-to-activation distance (LAD) showed that the LAD to the primary sensorimotor cortex does affect the incidence of motor deficits, while the LAD to the supplementary motor area (SMA) does not (Voss et al. 2013). Nevertheless more studies are needed to draw more robust conclusion on whether damage to secondary areas during surgery in such patients actually leads to additional and permanent neurological deficits.

Despite all these resources helping in the localization of relevant eloquent areas fMRI is still not able to answer the following question: What is the risk of functional deficits after resection of the contrast-enhancing tumor areas in the pre- or postcentral gyrus? The reason is simply that the definition of the resection margins using fMRI has still to be considered non-reliable—as outlined earlier only very limited data are available on that topic (Håberg et al. 2004; Krishnan et al. 2004; Hall et al. 2005; Berntsen et al. 2010; González-Darder and González-López 2010; Zimmermann et al. 2019) that do not justify general conclusions on how to determine the "safe" borders for function-preserving resection based on presurgical fMRI (Gil-Robles and Duffau 2010; Azad and Duffau 2020) (see Sect. 4.1). Such interventions are hazardous, for jeopardizing not only the eloquent cortex but also the deep white matter tracts (Rasmussen et al. 2007; Berntsen et al. 2010; Oda et al. 2018; Beckett et al. 2020).

Note The selection criteria mentioned here are meant as suggestions arising from typical morphological and clinical findings in patients with Rolandic brain tumors. It is currently not possible to define a medical indication in the strict sense for fMRI. This is due to the still limited number of controlled prospective studies demonstrating the clinical benefit of presurgical fMRI in terms of reduced postoperative morbidity or mortality.

4.3   Motor and Somatosensory Paradigms for Presurgical fMRI

A complex neuronal network of functional areas in both hemispheres of the human brain is recruited for the planning and execution of arbitrary movements, whereby somatosensory impulses are processed and consequently motor functions carried out (see chapter "Functional Neuroanatomy"). Knowledge of an identification of the reliable localization of the various body representations in the primary motor and somatosensory cortices is essential in presurgical fMRI diagnostics, since permanent paralysis or sensory deficits can result from surgery-related injury to the respective functional areas. Neurological deficits resulting from damage to the secondary areas can also occur; however, those are typically transient and not as severe as compared to damage to the primary sensorimotor cortices (Voss et al. 2013), but may cause motor neglect (Shinoura et al. 2010) or induce motor dysfunction (Wilkins et al. 2020). Nevertheless, the functional localization of premotor activations may be of clinical relevance as an additional functional landmark of the precentral gyrus in hemiplegic patients (Stippich et al. 2000) (see Sect. 4.6).

Most investigators use self-triggered movements to assess motor activation and sensorimotor somatotopy, for example, various movements of the tongue or lips, the hand or fingers, and the foot or toes (see Sect. 4.4). Some groups use mechanical devices to better assess movements or to measure various physical parameters (force, acceleration) (Baudendistel et al. 1996; Schaechter et al. 2006; Diciotti et al. 2007; Newton et al. 2008; Farrens et al. 2018). To ensure a successful examination in the clinical setting, it is essential that the paradigms are feasible, motion artifacts are kept to a minimum, and examination time is kept short. Under these conditions, BOLD activations in the primary motor cortex are generally very robust and reliable.

When defining motor paradigms in a block design, it is essential to decide whether only the primary motor cortex or also the secondary areas should be analyzed. In the case where only the primary motor cortex is the target, paradigms may include movements of both sides of the body (e.g., right hand vs. left hand). Since unilateral movements lead to activation of secondary areas in both hemispheres (Stippich et al. 2000, 2007a; Blatow et al. 2007; Tozakidou et al. 2013), secondary areas are active during both alternating movements of the right and left sides of the body (right vs. left contrast) throughout the entire measurement. This results in a continuous activation of the secondary cortical areas that are involved in bilateral movements and is therefore not depicted in the statistical evaluation of fMRI data acquired using conventional block designs due to the lack of "contrast" between the various stimulation blocks. Therefore, if information needs to be obtained regarding secondary motor activation, paradigms with strictly unilateral movements of a single part of the body (e.g., right hand only) need to be applied with true "resting" as the control condition. Alternatively, three different stimulation conditions could be integrated in the paradigm, that is, right movement–rest–left movement. However, in this case the number of blocks per paradigm is increased as compared to unilateral movements only and consequently also examination time and susceptibility to motion artifacts. In addition, it should be borne in mind that—sensu stricto—information on brain activation in the tumor-unaffected hemisphere is largely insignificant for the resec-

tion itself, except for the assessment of tumor-induced neuroplastic changes. More importantly, paradigms enabling the examination of several different cortical body representations within one single fMRI measurement are problematic in brain tumor patients (e.g., foot–hand–face: complete somatotopy). Although with this paradigm the total scan time for the functional mapping of the body's somatotopy could be reduced compared to three individual measurements, the time needed would substantially exceed the scanning time required for a short paradigm that is focused on a single cortical body representation. Short scanning times are particularly important in the case of agitated patients or patients with paresis, as the probability of motion artifacts increases with the scan time needed, subsequently affecting accurate identification of functional localizations. In conclusion, short paradigms that provide robust activation and focus on the examination of a single cortical body representation are considered the most clinically feasible (Fig. 11). The

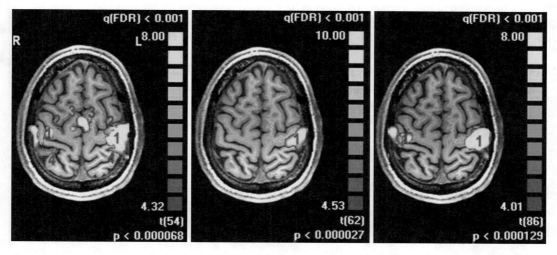

Fig. 11 Variation of paradigms to localize the motor hand area results in different activation patterns. *Left*: Complex finger opposition of the right hand vs. rest; strong activation of the cortical motor network in both hemispheres. The large contralateral cluster (*left*) covers the primary sensorimotor cortex (1), premotor cortex (2), and parietal cortex (4). Bilateral supplementary motor activation (3, 3) is displayed in the midline, as well as ipsilateral (*right*) premotor activation (2), primary sensorimo-tor coactivation (1), and parietal activation (4). *Middle*: Complex finger opposition of the right vs. left hand; strong contralateral (*left*) primary sensorimotor activation (1), but no activation of secondary areas. *Right*: Complex finger opposition of the right hand vs. right toe movements and tongue movements; strong contralateral (*left*) primary sensorimotor activation (1) and ipsilateral primary sensorimotor coactivation (1), but no activation of secondary areas

investigator needs to decide whether only the primary motor representations should be mapped functionally (in this case the paradigm should consist of alternating blocks with identical movements on both sides of the body, e.g., right vs. left hand) or whether additional information on functional reorganization in secondary cortical areas is of interest (in this case unilateral movements need to be performed vs. "resting"). This decision depends on the individual medical questions to be answered with preoperative fMRI.

Clinical feasibility tests performed on neurosurgical patients with and without tumor-related pareses or sensory disturbances showed that self-triggered movement tasks are better suited to presurgical fMRI than externally controlled paradigms, since only in this way each patient can perform the respective task within his or her range of ability. To keep the likelihood of motion artifacts to a minimum (Hoeller et al. 2002; Krings et al. 2001; Seto et al. 2001; Todd et al. 2015), the following movement tasks were chosen: repetitive tongue movements with the mouth closed, opposition of finger digits D2–D5 against the thumb (D1) with free choice of the opposition order, and repetitive flexion and extension of all five toes without moving the ankle. Relaxed positioning of the large joints (knees, elbows) using foam cushions is recommended. The prerequisite for this examination is again "resting" as a control condition (Stippich et al. 2002b) (Fig. 12). Alternatively, in the case of a mild paresis of the upper extremity, fist clenching/releasing can be tested. Face, arm, and leg movements, or movement of the feet, can often lead to a poor diagnostic evaluation of the data due to strong motion artifacts and should therefore be avoided. A paradigm with a block duration of 20 s and three repeating cycles resulting to an examination time of 140 s is a suitable compromise between a robust functional localization of the primary motor cortex, high BOLD signal, and an acceptable scan time (Fig. 13). Of note, the widely used "traditional" block design consists of five repetitive stimulation–rest cycles plus one baseline condition (rest) at the end of the fMRI measurement with a block duration of 30 s each. This sums up to a scanning time of 330 s per paradigm, does not provide more robust functional motor cortex localization nor higher BOLD signals, increases the chance for movement artifacts, and is therefore less well suited to map the full somatotopy when compared to the abovementioned time-optimized paradigm.

Determination of motor function with task-based presurgical fMRI is limited in patients with high-grade paresis (Pujol et al. 1998; Krings et al. 2002b). In this case, a reliable preoperative fMRI diagnosis is not guaranteed, if the fMRI protocol is based solely on self-triggered

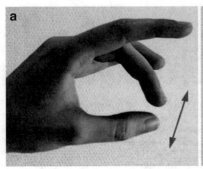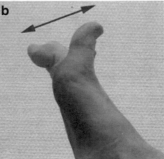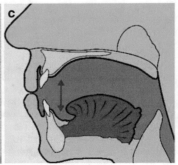

Fig. 12 Recommended self-paced movements to investigate sensorimotor somatotopy in clinical fMRI. (**a**) Complex finger opposition of digits 2–5 against the thumb in a random order. Movement frequency ~3 Hz. (**b**) Toe up and down movements, frequency >1 Hz. (**c**) Tongue up and down movements with the mouth closed. Movement frequency ~3 Hz. (Reprinted from Stippich et al. 2005, with permission)

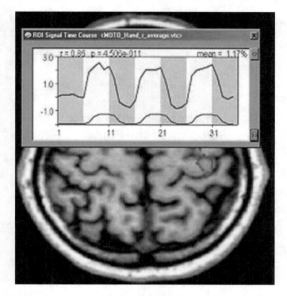

Fig. 13 Clinical standard protocol for motor paradigms. The block-designed paradigm consists of four rest periods (*light gray*) alternating with three stimulation periods (*white*), each of 20-s duration. The BOLD signal time course of the motor hand area activation (*red line*) shows a task-related increase in regional hemodynamics. The *black line* indicates the hemodynamic reference function (HRF)

movements contralateral to the tumor. Typically, paresis results from insufficient residual function of the primary motor cortex, which is in turn reflected by a reduced BOLD activation. Nevertheless, many patients with tumor-related paresis can be successfully examined by activating the primary somatosensory lip, finger, and toe representations of the postcentral gyrus (Stippich et al. 1999). The somatosensory stimulation does not require patient cooperation; can also be applied in children and poorly cooperative or sedated patients; and activates both contralateral primary (Stippich et al. 2004) and bilateral secondary (Stippich et al. 2005) somatosensory areas. Even at 1.5 T fMRI sensitivity is sufficient to localize the cortical somatosensory representations in most patients. It is possible to distinguish various body representations in the postcentral gyrus (Stippich et al. 1999) (see Sect. 5.5) and even individual finger representations (Kurth et al. 1998). While most published studies used non-standardized stimuli, such as manual hand touching, automatic stimuli guarantee reproducible stimulation conditions. Electric (Kurth et al. 1998; Kampe et al. 2000; Golaszewski et al. 2004), tactile (Stippich et al. 1999; Wienbruch et al. 2006), or vibrotactile (Golaszewski et al. 2002, 2006) stimulators are the most commonly used.

Passive movements of the fingers or toes may also elicit BOLD responses in the contralateral primary sensorimotor cortex and could potentially help when self-paced movements or somatosensory stimulation fails (Shriver et al. 2013). Unfortunately mechanical devices that generate controlled and reproducible passive movements are hardly available commercially or difficult to apply during routine clinical fMRI. In practice such passive movements usually need to be generated by the investigator through direct manipulation on the patient during the actual fMRI measurement.

As a further adjunct in preoperative motor fMRI in patients with paresis, complex finger opposition of the non-paretic hand (ipsilateral to the brain tumor) can be used to elicit robust premotor activation as an additional functional landmark for the precentral gyrus on the tumor's side (Stippich et al. 2000). Using this paradigm not only supplementary motor and premotor activation may be achieved but also additional ipsilateral primary motor coactivation (Blatow et al. 2007) that helps to directly localize the primary motor cortex on the tumor's side. If combined with somatosensory stimulation, a total of three functional landmarks for the cortical hand representations on the tumor's side are available for the localization of the precentral sulcus via premotor activation, the precentral gyrus via ipsilateral primary motor coactivation, and the postcentral gyrus using primary somatosensory activation, respectively (see Sect. 4.6, Fig. 22).

Of note, resting-state fMRI represents a valuable adjunct in paretic patients and can be applied successfully as active cooperation and execution of movements are not required (Lee et al. 2013, 2016; Sparacia et al. 2019, 2020; Vakamudi et al. 2020).

4.4 Presurgical Somatotopic Mapping of the Primary Motor Cortex

Somatotopic motor cortex mapping is the most frequently used presurgical fMRI protocol in patients with Rolandic brain tumors (Stippich et al. 2002b). This standard protocol contains three different fMRI measurements. Paradigms should include tongue movements as well as finger and toe movements contralateral to the tumor to localize the primary motor homunculus in relation to the brain tumor (Fig. 14). Even in the case of a completely obscured Rolandic anatomy fMRI can provide diagnostic information which may be relevant for the confirmation of the surgical indication as well as for the planning and implementation of function-preserving surgery (Fig. 15). In patients with small tumors that are—by anatomical consideration—not critical for any body representation, it seems appropriate to shorten the protocol by leaving the least relevant body representations unexamined (Figs. 16, 17, and 18). However, the examination of a single body representation alone, for example, the motor hand representation, is often not sufficient to provide the required diagnostic information. Somatotopic mapping also enables

assessment of neuroplastic changes of cortical motor activation, for example, in patients with recurrent malignancies prior to repeated surgery (Fig. 19).

4.5 Presurgical Somatotopic Mapping of the Primary Somatosensory Cortex

This fMRI protocol was designed to localize the different primary somatosensory body representations of the postcentral gyrus (Stippich et al. 1999) (Fig. 20). In presurgical fMRI, somatotopic somatosensory mapping is mostly used as a diagnostic adjunct, when motor paradigms are difficult to apply—for example, in uncooperative, sedated, or hemiparetic patients or in children, but there is also potential for standardized follow-up measurements on neuroplastic changes of the somatosensory system. The fully automated pneumatically driven 24-channel tactile stimulation used in our institution is artifact free and produces reproducible stimuli and consistent examination conditions for comparative and outcome studies. The whole unit can be set up and dismantled within 5 min. Scan time per measurement is 66 s for the localization of the primary

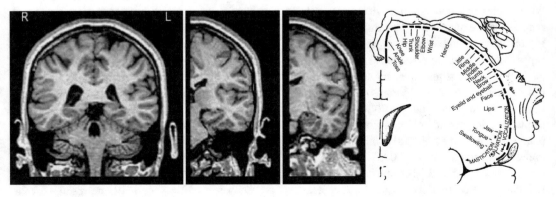

Fig. 14 FMRI motor cortex somatotopy. From *left to right*: foot, hand, and tongue representations, drawing of the motor homunculus

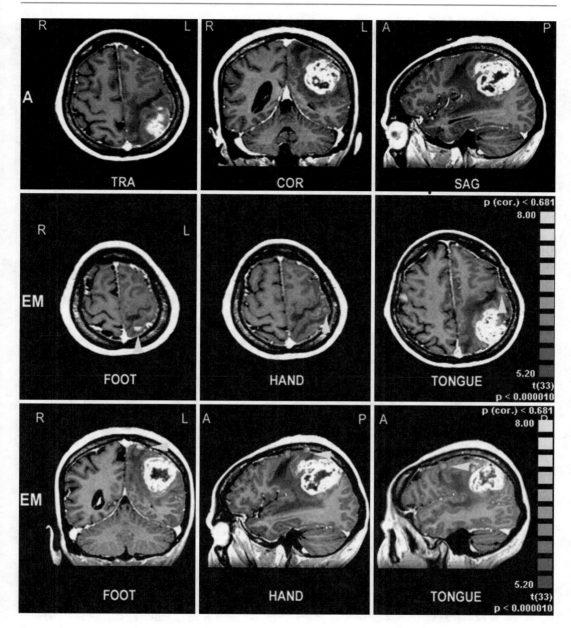

Fig. 15 Presurgical fMRI somatotopic mapping of the motor cortex. On morphological images, no Rolandic landmarks can be identified in the left hemisphere due to the mass effect of this large malignant glioma (*upper row, A* anatomy). Foot, hand, and tongue movements (*EM* executed movement) revealed robust fMRI activation of the respective primary motor cortex body representations (*yellow arrowheads*). Using functional landmarks the Rolandic anatomy (precentral gyrus, central sulcus, postcentral gyrus) can be easily identified in relation to the brain tumor. FMRI indicated a parietal localization of the contrast-enhancing glioma. Note the additional premotor activation (*red arrowhead*) localizing the ventral wall of the precentral gyrus/precentral sulcus

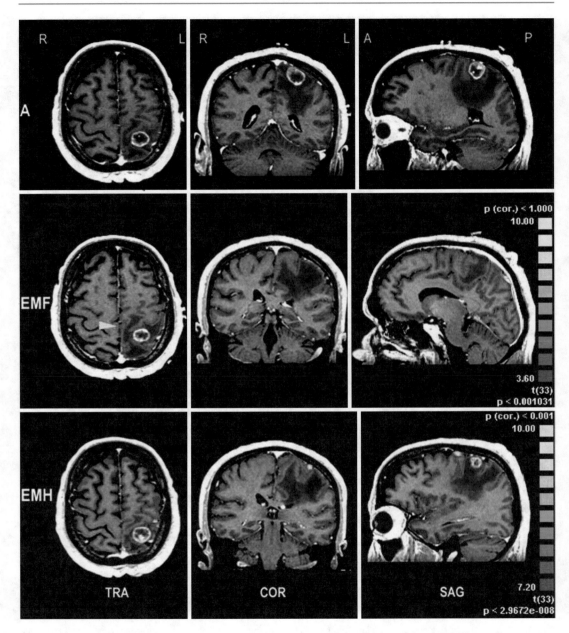

Fig. 16 Presurgical fMRI somatotopic mapping of the upper motor cortex in a left postcentral high-grade glioma. On morphological images, the compressed "precentral knob" can be identified in transverse and sagittal views. Foot (*EMF*) and hand (*EMH*) movements were associated with activation of the respective primary motor cortex representations, confirming the postcentral localization of the tumor

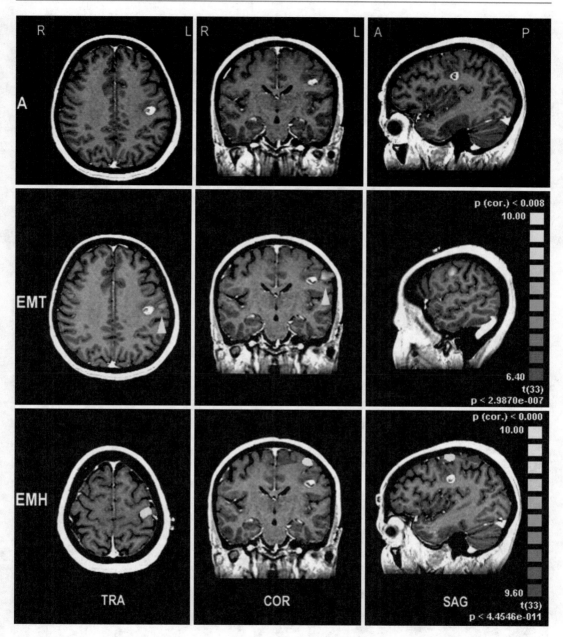

Fig. 17 Presurgical fMRI somatotopic mapping of the lower motor cortex in a left Rolandic cavernoma. On morphological images, the Rolandic anatomy was intact. Tongue (*MT*) and hand (*MH*) movements were driven by activation of the respective primary motor cortex representations, confirming the central localization of the tumor and a close spatial relationship to the tongue representation

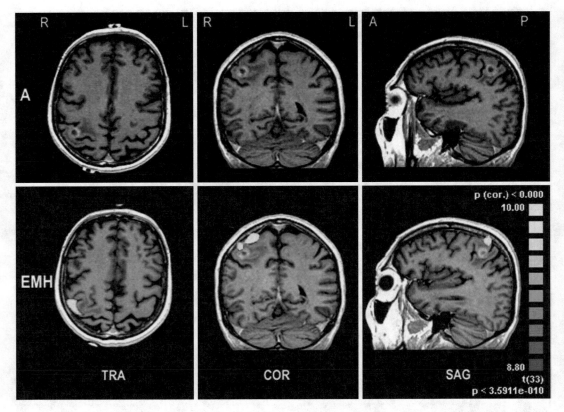

Fig. 18 Presurgical fMRI localization of the motor hand area. On morphological images, a Rolandic metastasis is visualized at the motor hand area, bridging the central sulcus towards the postcentral gyrus. fMRI confirmed a close spatial relationship between the primary motor hand rep- resentation and the tumor. Interestingly the center of grav- ity of the BOLD cluster was shifted upwards from the precentral knob towards the foot representation (see EMH, coronal view)

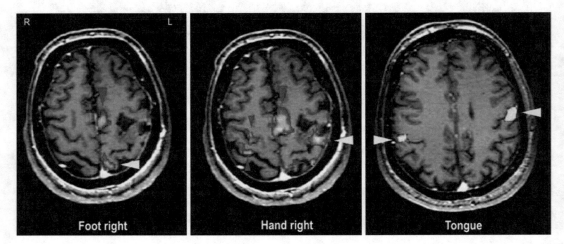

Fig. 19 Presurgical fMRI somatotopic mapping of the motor cortex in a hemiparetic patient with a recurrent left Rolandic astrocytoma prior to repeated surgery. Foot, hand, and tongue movements revealed robust fMRI acti- vation of the respective primary motor cortex body repre- sentation (*yellow arrowheads*). Note the increased activation of secondary areas (*red arrowheads*): in the supplementary motor area during toe and finger move- ments and in the whole cortical motor network in both hemispheres during finger movements, respectively

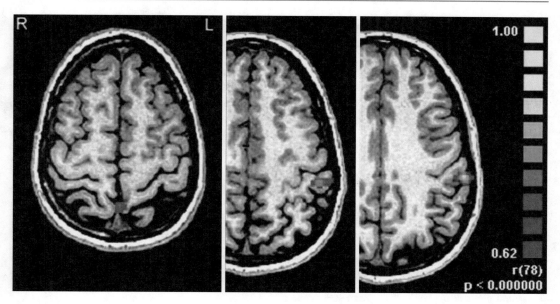

Fig. 20 fMRI primary somatosensory cortex somatotopy. *From left to right*: toe, finger, and lip representations. Stimulation: D1 and D2 right foot and right hand, upper and lower lips to the right side; stimulus frequency = 4 Hz, air pressure = 3 bar. Clinical standard fMRI protocols for somatosensory stimulation, conventional block design, stimulation vs. rest. (**a**) Primary somatosensory cortex (S1), six periods of rest alternating with five periods of stimulation, each of 6-s duration (Stippich et al. 2004). (**b**) Secondary somatosensory cortex (S2), four periods of rest alternating with three periods of stimulation, each of 15-s duration (Stippich et al. 2005). (Modified from Stippich et al. 1999, with permission)

somatosensory cortex only (Stippich et al. 2004) or 105 s for a robust primary and secondary somatosensory activation, respectively (Stippich et al. 2005). This presurgical fMRI protocol enables assessment of the spatial relationship between brain tumors and postcentral gyrus, facilitating the estimation of possible postoperative sensory deficits (Fig. 21).

Diagnostic information about the spatial relationship between the central sulcus or the precentral gyrus and precentral or frontal brain tumors can be indirectly obtained from somatosensory fMRI as both anatomical structures are situated directly anteriorly to the postcentral gyrus.

4.6 Localization of the Precentral Gyrus in Patients with Preexisting Paresis

This special protocol was designed in volunteers to help localizing the precentral gyrus in patients

with prominent contralateral paresis (Stippich et al. 2000). Its clinical application is not generally used and thus requires own validation. In these paretic patients, the primary motor cortex is commonly infiltrated by the tumor or severely compressed precluding both a reliable identification of the Rolandic anatomy on morphological images and proper performance of contralateral movements for presurgical fMRI. However, as a basic principle, residual contralateral motor function and passive somatosensory stimulation should be first used for the functional localization of the pre- and postcentral gyrus. As a further adjunct complex finger opposition of the nonparetic hand ipsilateral to the brain tumor can be used to activate the whole cortical motor network in both hemispheres, control condition is "resting." The premotor activation on the tumor's side may serve as an additional functional landmark for the precentral gyrus by localizing the anterior wall of the precentral gyrus near the junction of the precentral sulcus with the posterior part of the

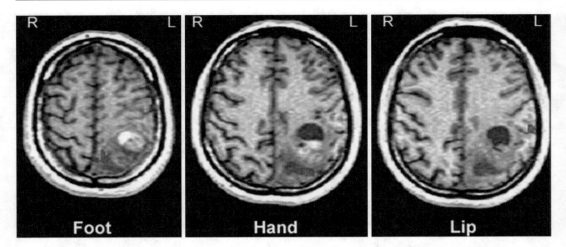

Fig. 21 Presurgical fMRI somatotopic mapping of the primary somatosensory cortex (S1) in a left parietal malignant glioma indicated compression of the upper postcentral gyrus at the level of the foot representation and tumor growth into the lower postcentral gyrus with dorsal displacement of the S1 hand representation. (Modified from Stippich et al. 1999, with permission)

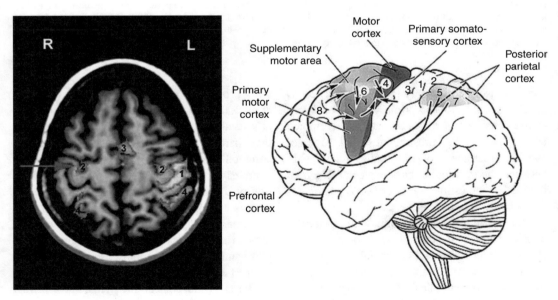

Fig. 22 Typical cortical activation pattern of complex finger opposition (*right hand*). Premotor activation ipsilateral to the moving hand (*red arrow*) serves as a functional landmark for the precentral gyrus in hemiparetic patients (a clinical case is presented in Figs. 23 and 24). Premotor activation is typically localized at the anterior wall of the precentral gyrus directly adjacent to the junction of the precentral sulcus with the superior frontal sulcus. It is important to note that this functional landmark does not localize the motor hand area! In the drawing of the cortical motor and somatosensory network (*right*), the numbers indicate the Brodmann areas. (Reprinted from Stippich et al. 2005, with permission)

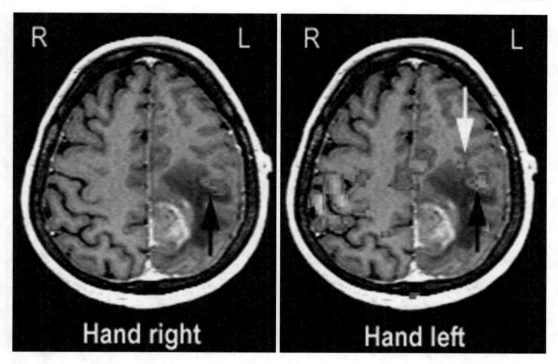

Fig. 23 Example of fMRI localization of the motor hand area in a hemiparetic patient with a left malignant glioma using contralateral and ipsilateral movements. Residual motor function of the paretic right hand (grade 3/5) is driven by residual activation of the contralateral motor hand area (*black arrow*). Complex finger opposition of the non-paretic left hand is associated with activation of the cortical motor network in both hemispheres. Robust ipsilateral primary motor coactivation (*black arrow*) confirms the localization of the motor hand area. Additional ipsilateral premotor activation (*white arrow*) indicates the ventral wall of the precentral gyrus

superior frontal sulcus (Figs. 22 and 23). Please note that the risk for postoperative related motor deficits cannot be estimated using premotor activation as a functional landmark! However, in healthy volunteers primary motor coactivation can frequently be observed in the motor hand area ipsilateral to the moving hand (Stippich et al. 2007a). Our clinical experience indicates that ipsilateral primary motor coactivation may also be supportive to localize the motor hand area on the tumor side in hemiparetic patients.

In general, the combination of presurgical motor fMRI with anisotropic diffusion-weighted MRI and diffusion tensor imaging (DTI)-tractography is highly recommended for the assessment of the effects of Rolandic brain tumors on the pyramidal tract (Stippich et al. 2003a; Rasmussen et al. 2007; Berntsen et al. 2010; González-Darder and González-López 2010; Nimsky 2011; Dimous et al. 2013; Jia et al. 2013; Kumar et al. 2014; Conti Nibali et al. 2019) (Figs. 24 and 25).

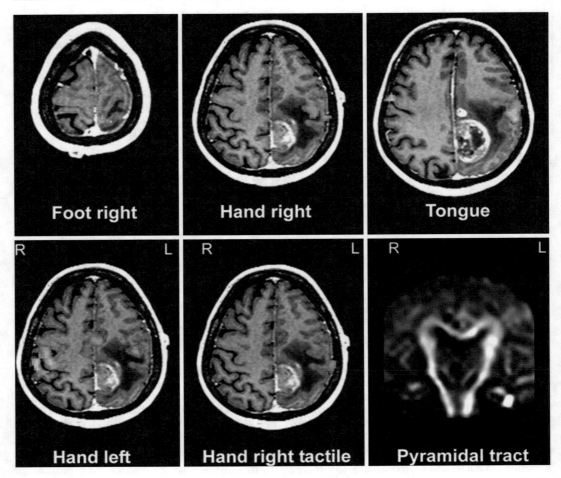

Fig. 24 Presurgical fMRI in Rolandic brain tumors— standard and special protocols. *Upper row* (standard protocol): Somatotopic mapping of the primary motor cortex indicated a parietal localization of the contrast-enhancing malignant glioma (same patient as in Fig. 23). *Lower row* (special protocols): Complex finger opposition of the nonparetic left hand (*left*) and fully automated tactile stimulation of the contralesional right hand (*middle*) localized the pre- and postcentral gyrus in relation to the brain tumor. This diagnostic information is equivalent to that available from contralateral hand movement (please compare *upper row, middle*) and can be obtained also in patients with complete loss of contralateral motor function. Anisotropic diffusion images of the pyramidal tract completed this presurgical MRI protocol. Diffusion tensor tractography could provide more detailed anatomical information. (Modified from Stippich et al. 2003a, with permission)

5 Presurgical fMRI of Language Function

The number of groups localizing language brain function preoperatively is ever growing—a larger collective study included 81 patients (Stippich et al. 2007b). The diagnostic aims of presurgical language fMRI according to the "classical model of language" include the localization of the Broca's and Wernicke's speech areas in relation to brain tumors or epileptogenic zones and the identification of the language-dominant hemisphere. In contrast to motor or somatosensory fMRI, the indication for presurgical language fMRI cannot be supported by morphological imaging alone. The latter provides

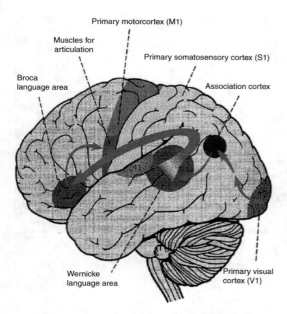

Primary motorcortex (M1)

Muscles for
articulation

Primary somatosensory cortex (S1)

Broca
language area

Association cortex

Wernicke
language area

Primary visual
cortex (V1)

Fig. 25 Schematic drawing of language areas in the left hemisphere according to the classical language model (Wernicke 1874). *Red arrows* indicate important anatomo-functional connections (e.g., arcuate fascicle). (Modified from Roche Lexikon Medizin, 4th edn, 1998, Urban and Fischer, Munich, p 1578)

only rough information about whether the potentially function-bearing gyri—namely, the left inferior frontal gyrus (Brodmann areas 44 and 45) or the left superior temporal gyrus (Brodmann area 22)—are affected by the tumor (Fig. 26) or not. However, it has been demonstrated that the classical language model (Lichtheim 1885; Geschwind 1971) is not sufficient to reflect the complexity of cortical language representations (Bookheimer 2002; Gabrieli et al. 1998; Grabowski 2000; Weems and Reggia 2006; Tremblay and Dick 2016). Moreover, the temporo-parietal junction is functionally critical to language, as is Geschwind's language area of the left supramarginal gyrus and adjacent parts of the angular gyrus (Geschwind 1972; Damasio and Geschwind 1984) or Dronkers' language area of the left frontal insula (Dronkers 1996; Dronkers et al. 2007; Flinker et al. 2015; Battistella et al.

2020). Hence, clinical and neuropsychological symptoms are ultimately decisive. Nevertheless, language fMRI can be very useful in the presurgical diagnostic situation (Tyndall et al. 2017; Benjamin et al. 2017; Agarwal et al. 2019a, b; Mark et al. 2021). Here, presurgical language fMRI protocols should always comprise several different paradigms. There is no such thing as one universal paradigm for fMRI language assessment!

Language fMRI is not used as frequently as motor fMRI in preoperative neuroimaging. This is partly due to the higher equipment load and personnel and logistical requirements, which make implementation of the procedure in the clinical routine more challenging. Moreover, most neurocenters have developed their own methodology, making fMRI results difficult to compare. This variability does affect not only the chosen stimulation paradigm, on which the examination results depend to a great extent, but also the way in which it is presented—visually or acoustically—as well as measurement and evaluation parameters. Even so, and on the basis of results from numerous validation studies using established reference procedures (EcoG, Wada test), it can be assumed that fMRI can reliably and noninvasively localize Broca's and Wernicke's language areas prior to brain surgery (Dym et al. 2011; Sharan et al. 2011; Janecek et al. 2013; Bohm et al. 2020; Massot-Tarrús et al. 2020; Meinhold et al. 2020). Determining language dominance with fMRI is possible, and in a meta-analysis a quite good sensitivity (83.5%) and specificity (88.1%) have been shown, when compared to the Wada test (Dym et al. 2011). However, the Wada test may still have value in the evaluation of epilepsy surgery candidates with atypical or bilateral language representation or when fMRI data are inconclusive (Sharan et al. 2011; Janecek et al. 2013; Wagner et al. 2012; Bauer et al. 2013) (for a more detailed description on this topic please refer to chapter "Presurgical Functional Localization Possibilities, Limitations and Validity."

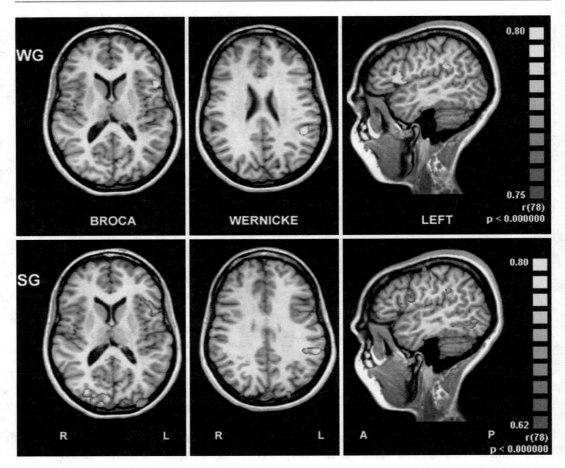

Fig. 26 Functional localization of Broca's and Wernicke's areas using the word-generation (*WG*) and sentence-generation (*SG*) paradigms. Note that the functional local-izations are congruent, but not perfectly identical. (Modified from Stippich et al. 2003b, with permission)

5.1   Review of Literature

In this paragraph, we will try to guide the reader through the complex and to a certain extent inho-mogeneous data published on presurgical lan-guage fMRI. Since in many studies patients with both brain tumors and epilepsy were included, it seemed not appropriate to distinguish between the two entities. Hence, this chapter covers also information relevant for chapter "Presurgical EEG-fMRI in Epilepsy."

Already 3 years after the first reports on fMRI, a preliminary study showed that the BOLD signal contrast obtained from simple tests of language and motor function was very similar between patients with epilepsy and normal controls, dem-onstrating the feasibility of the technique in patients with epilepsy (Morris 3rd et al. 1994). Since then, fMRI of language processing has become one of the most clinically relevant appli-cations in the field of epilepsy and also in patients with brain tumors prior to surgery. The main aim of the identification and interpretation of the complex language network is to predict and mini-mize postoperative language deficits. In patients with epilepsy considered for surgery—who are mainly patients with temporal lobe epilepsy (Hermann et al. 1999)—fMRI is predominantly used for language lateralization (i.e., determination of the hemispheric dominance) and only to a lesser extent for the intrahemispheric distribution of the eloquent cortex.

Numerous studies have demonstrated the high reliability of fMRI to identify the language-dominant hemisphere (Binder et al. 1995, 1996, 1997, 2000; Benson et al. 1996; Bahn et al. 1997; FitzGerald et al. 1997; Stapleton et al. 1997; Shaywitz et al. 1995; Cuenod et al. 1995; Hertz-Pannier et al. 1997; van der Kallen et al. 1998; Worthington et al. 1997; Frost et al. 1999; Szaflarski et al. 2002; Giussani et al. 2010; Dym et al. 2011; Sharan et al. 2011; Janecek et al. 2013; Lemée et al. 2019). However, the areas identified in different studies of language evaluation vary markedly, likely due to the use of different linguistic activation or control tasks, imaging, and post-processing techniques, among other factors (Dym et al. 2011). Again, there is no single fMRI paradigm that identifies "language cortex," as language is a complex process which involves many different components, including specialized sensory systems for speech, text, and object recognition; processing of whole-word information and word meaning; word syntax processing; and multiple mechanisms for written and spoken language production (Binder et al. 2002; Zacà et al. 2013; Barnett et al. 2014). Hence, the activation pattern is crucially dependent on the chosen fMRI task design.

Hearing words—whether the task involves passive listening, repeating, or categorizing—activates the superior temporal gyrus bilaterally compared to a resting condition (Binder et al. 2000; Price et al. 1996; Wise et al. 1991). The symmetry of this activation can be explained by the task contrast (complex sounds vs. no sounds). The rest condition does not contain any control for prelinguistic auditory processing which engages the auditory cortex in both superior temporal gyri. Brain areas associated with semantic word processing might be also activated during the resting state and hence reduce sensitivity for the activation task (Binder et al. 1999). Similar

problems occur in designs that oppose reading or naming tasks to a resting or visual fixation baseline. In a study performed on patients with primarily lateralized lesions, Benson et al. found that such protocols do neither reliably produce lateralized activation nor correlate with language dominance measured with the Wada test (Benson et al. 1999).

The most common types of tasks successfully used for the assessment of language lateralization are the word-generation tasks (also called verbal fluency tasks) and the semantic decision-making tasks, whereby the former tend to show relatively consistent activation of the anterior language areas and the latter a more widely distributed network including the anterior and posterior hemispheric regions (Binder et al. 1997).

In the word-generation tasks, the subjects or patients are confronted with a noun, a semantic category (e.g., animal, food), and are asked to retrieve a phonologically or semantically associated word. In the verb-generation tasks, the subject/patient generates a verb in response to seeing or hearing a noun. These tasks reliably activate the dominant inferior and dorsolateral frontal lobe including the prefrontal and premotor areas (Wise et al. 1991; Warburton et al. 1996; Raichle et al. 1994; Petersen et al. 1988). Many studies have shown that lateralization measures obtained from these frontal activations by fMRI agree well with Wada language lateralization (Bahn et al. 1997; Yetkin et al. 1998; Benson et al. 1999; Lehericy et al. 2000a; Janecek et al. 2013). There is evidence that semantic language tasks such as verb generation in response to nouns, noun categorization, or noun generation within specific categories may be more effective in language lateralization than phonologically based generation tasks such as concealed repetition (Lehericy et al. 2000a). In fMRI studies, word-generation tasks are usually performed silently to avoid movement artifacts. The resulting lack of proof of a proper task performance is usually not a problem when clear activation is observed, but bars the investigator from assessing poor task performance in cases of poor activation.

A semantic decision task was used by Springer and colleagues to address the issue of language dominance in patients with epilepsy (Springer et al. 1999). Fifty right-handed patients with epilepsy were compared with 100 right-handed normal controls. Language activation was accomplished by opposing a semantic decision task to a tone discrimination task. The latter was developed to control for nonlinguistic components of the task (e.g., attention, sound processing, manual response). Using a categorical dominance classification, 94% of the normal control subjects were considered left-hemispheric dominant, 6% had a bilateral language representation, and none of the subjects had a right-lateralized dominance. In the group of patients with epilepsy, there was a greater variability of language dominance, with 78% showing a left-hemisphere dominance, 16% showing a roughly symmetric pattern, and 6% showing a right-hemisphere dominance. Atypical language dominance in patients with epilepsy was associated with an earlier age onset of seizures and with a weaker right-handed dominance. The relatively high prevalence of atypical language representation in patients with epilepsy (Sharan et al. 2011) stresses the importance of the assessment of the hemispheric dominance before interventional procedures in areas potentially relevant for language in either cerebral hemisphere (Spreer et al. 2001).

Further studies with the paradigms described above were performed by Binder et al. (1995, 1996, 1997). The activation pattern was in general strongly left lateralized and involved both the prefrontal and posterior association areas. The activation correlated strongly with the language lateralization obtained from the Wada test (Binder et al. 1996). A similar result using a semantic word-decision task was observed by Desmond and colleagues. Seven postoperative patients with temporal lobe epilepsy were examined and the BOLD signal was compared with data from preoperative Wada test. In all cases, using a region of interest-based analysis looking only at the inferior frontal regions, the lateralization by fMRI

was the same as that observed by the Wada test (Desmond et al. 1995). An attractive feature of semantic word-decision tasks is that of the rating of the behavioral responses through a push-button system on response to stimuli, thereby permitting precise quantification of task performance to be precisely quantified.

As mentioned above, both word-generation and semantic word-decision tasks identify mainly the frontal lobe language areas but are less consistent activators for the temporal language regions. An fMRI paradigm with consistent temporal lobe activation was reported by Gaillard et al. (2002). The paradigm consisted of the silent pronunciation of items in response to a visualized item description. The authors found language lateralization in 27 of 30 patients with temporal lobe epilepsy. The fMRI dominance was consistent with the Wada test in 15 of 20 patients.

Word-generation tasks are also most frequently used in language fMRI studies on brain tumor patients (Latchaw et al. 1995; Herholz et al. 1997; Hirsch et al. 2000; Håberg et al. 2004; Hall et al. 2005; Van Westen et al. 2005). There is the general agreement that a combination of different tasks increases paradigm effectiveness (Zacà et al. 2013). Van Westen et al. used a combination of word generation and rhyming in 20 patients with tumors close to the sensorimotor or language areas in an fMRI study performed at 3 T and reported a paradigm effectiveness varying from 79% to 95% (Van Westen et al. 2005). In another study on a large group of patients (56 patients with lesions near language-relevant areas), the authors found activation of the Wernicke's area in 91% and of the Broca's area in 77% applying a combination of a silent word-generation task (picture naming) upon listening to spoken words. In the same study, language lateralization with fMRI and Wada test was congruent in all 13 patients examined (Hirsch et al. 2000).

Successful fMRI lateralization paradigms have also been reported on children as young as 6 years (Benson et al. 1996; Hertz-Pannier et al. 1997; Stapleton et al. 1997; Logan 1999;

Hertz-Pannier et al. 2002), and the hemodynamic response appears to be similar to that observed in adults (Benson et al. 1996; Hertz-Pannier et al. 1997). Word-generation tasks are the most commonly used tasks for the evaluation of pediatric epilepsy surgery candidates and, as in adults, show a general agreement with the Wada test and electrocortical stimulation (Hertz-Pannier et al. 1997; Stapleton et al. 1997; Logan 1999). There is some evidence that young children do activate more widespread than adults, at least in verbal fluency tasks (Gaillard et al. 2000b). fMRI studies on children with paradigms consisting of reading larger passages in the silent naming of a read description of an object (Gaillard et al. 2001b) have also been performed. Important issues such as the adequate choice of the suitable experimental and control conditions in children have been considered in more detail (Bookheimer 2000; Gaillard et al. 2001a).

A large study assessing language lateralization with fMRI and the Wada test on 229 patients with epilepsy revealed discordant results between the two techniques in 14% of patients. Even if the data of this study showed that fMRI may be more sensitive than the Wada test to right-hemisphere language processing, the data also showed a relevant discordance of the results between the two methods. This discordance mainly affected the patients categorized by either test as having a bilateral language representation (Janecek et al. 2013). To date it can be assumed that fMRI is the most appropriate initial examination to localize essential language areas in the preoperative diagnostic workup and is usually sufficient, if a typical language lateralization can be observed. However, in cases with atypical or bilateral language representation or when fMRI is not conclusive for other reasons, further information about language representation needs to be obtained by other, more invasive, methods (Sharan et al. 2011). Further, it should be kept in mind that the Wada test and fMRI do not provide the same information and are therefore complementary. Only the Wada test can simulate whether a specific function can be performed, if one particular part of the hemisphere is removed.

In contrast to the Wada test, fMRI has the potential to provide detailed maps of the intrahemispheric localization of critical language areas in addition to the information on lateralization (Sharan et al. 2011). There are a number of studies suggesting a close spatial relationship between fMRI activation and intraoperative electrocortical stimulation (FitzGerald et al. 1997; Yetkin et al. 1997; Ruge et al. 1999; Rutten et al. 1999; Schlosser et al. 1999; Lurito et al. 2000; Carpentier et al. 2001a, b; Ojemann et al. 2013). A study by Rutten et al. 2002c compared the results of fMRI quantitatively with intraoperative electrocortical stimulation mapping in 13 patients. In eight patients critical language areas were detected by electrocortical stimulation, and in seven of the eight patients, sensitivity of fMRI was 100% (i.e., fMRI correctly detected all critical language areas with a high spatial accuracy). This indicates that such areas could be safely resected without the need for intraoperative electrocortical stimulation. To obtain this high sensitivity, however, a combination of three different fMRI language paradigms (verb generation, picture naming, and sentence processing) was required. On the other hand, on average only 51% of fMRI activations were confirmed by electrocortical stimulation indicating a low specificity of fMRI. As mentioned before, both fMRI sensitivity and specificity are strongly dependent on the statistical threshold chosen for data evaluation. In this context, this study illustrates again the problems of basing clinical decisions (e.g., surgical strategies) on single fMRI activation maps alone. Different language-related paradigms activate a different set of brain regions, and a combination of different tasks is necessary to achieve a high sensitivity for the identification of the functionally relevant areas (Ramsey et al. 2001). Meanwhile, language fMRI is widely used in the presurgical setting with well-established paradigms, imaging, and data processing routines (Pillai and Zaca 2011; Sair et al. 2016; Benjamin et al. 2017; Black et al. 2017; Tyndall et al. 2017; Unadkat et al. 2019; Manan et al. 2020; Park et al. 2020).

Still, a generally accepted standard protocol for language fMRI has not been established yet. Further, the extent and pattern of activation also substantially depend on the applied statistical threshold (Pillai and Zaca 2011; Nadkarni et al. 2014) (for details see Sect. 3). Finally, the presence of fMRI activation in nonrelevant language areas limits the predictive value of fMRI for the detection of critical language areas. Some regions activated during language tasks obviously play a minor, supportive role for language function, and resection of these areas may not necessarily produce clinically relevant deficits. Because of such difficulties, the clinical role of fMRI in the identification of eloquent cortical areas of cognitive function is still limited. Thus, at this stage, fMRI can be considered as useful for the facilitation of intraoperative electrocortical stimulation, but can still not replace it (Deblaere et al. 2002; Ojemann et al. 2013; Metwali et al. 2019; Azad and Duffau 2020).

Another question is whether fMRI can replace the Wada test as the reference procedure for the determination of the language and memory dominance in candidates eligible for brain surgery. A meta-analysis overseeing more than 400 patients has shown a very high sensitivity and specificity of fMRI to determine language dominance as compared to the Wada test (Dym et al. 2011). If established as a valid and reliable technique, fMRI would either render the Wada test obsolete or at least reduce its dominant role and only make it indispensable when fMRI is not practical because of either technical issues or patient properties. The idea behind the Wada test is that the parts of one hemisphere supplied by the anterior circulation are transiently anesthetized using a bolus of short-acting barbiturates (amobarbital), allowing the contralateral hemisphere to be assessed independently (Wada and Rasmussen 1960; Sharan et al. 2011). The Wada test is invasive and carries significant risks, and the validity of its individual results can be compromised by acute drug effects, which may cause behavioral confounds of sedation and agitation. Although the Wada test is commonly designated by the reference procedure in language lateralization tests (Rausch et al. 1993), it is not a standardized procedure. Differences in almost every aspect of methodology and design can be found in the various Wada test protocols described in the literature (Simkins-Bullock 2000) and make between-center comparisons of the results difficult.

In a review of the literature by Baxendale (2002), 70 patients were found in the literature that had undergone both fMRI and Wada test (Desmond et al. 1995; Binder et al. 1996; Bahn et al. 1997; Hertz-Pannier et al. 1997; Worthington et al. 1997; Benbadis et al. 1998; Yetkin et al. 1998; Benson et al. 1999; Bazin et al. 2000; Lehericy et al. 2000a; Carpentier et al. 2001a). With the exception of only one study (Worthington et al. 1997), showing a comparatively low concordance of only 75% between the two techniques using a verbal fluency task in fMRI, all other studies reported an impressive high concordance between the two techniques despite the use of different language tasks and Wada test protocols. A study by Binder and colleagues correlated the assessment of language lateralization between the two techniques from the respective lateralization indices, whereby for the Wada test a continuous variable was used and for fMRI the asymmetry in the voxels activated in each hemisphere by a semantic word-decision task was considered (Binder et al. 1996). The correlation was extremely strong ($r = 0.96$, $p < 0.0001$) and all 22 subjects were classified as having the same lateralization by the two modalities. A concordance of almost 100% was also found in other studies employing categorical analyses for the classification of language representation (Benbadis et al. 1998; Yetkin et al. 1998). While these observations are promising, there are reasons to be cautious about replacing the Wada test by fMRI at this stage (Wagner et al. 2012; Bauer et al. 2013). In all comparative studies between Wada test and fMRI reviewed above, there were less than 35 collective patients with a reversed or atypical cerebral language dominance pattern as defined by the Wada test, an extremely small patient sample on which to base clinical decisions. As mentioned above, there is evidence of a greater variability of language dominance in patients with epilepsy compared to normal controls (Springer et al. 1999; Carpentier et al. 2001a; Janecek et al. 2013). An atypical language representation is perhaps the most important condition to detect, and the limited data currently available from language fMRI studies in patients with epilepsy do not allow to draw any firm conclusions about the sensitivity or specificity of the various fMRI tests (Spritzer et al. 2012). Moreover, the "true" incidence of a significant discrepancy between fMRI and Wada test for language lateralization assessment is not known, and the reasons for the occasional found inconsistencies have not been investigated systematically. For example, Hammeke and colleagues reported a significant discrepancy between fMRI and Wada lateralization indices in approximately one of ten patients (Hammeke et al. 2000). In particular, temporal tumors in the dominant hemisphere have been reported to cause a false-negative activation of the dominant hemisphere (Westerveld et al. 1999; Gaillard et al. 2000a).

Finally, it has to be emphasized that the Wada test is not only applied to determine language dominance (Simkins-Bullock 2000; Sharan et al. 2011), but also, and perhaps more importantly, to assess the ability of each hemisphere to sustain verbal memory. Nonetheless, at this stage more studies with a larger patient pool are required to assess whether fMRI can reliably substitute the Wada test, which so far has been repeatedly validated with respect to memory function, language representation, and prediction of both cognitive and seizure outcome (Binder et al. 2002; Simkins-Bullock 2000; Sharan et al. 2011). Moreover, acceptance of fMRI will largely depend on the perceived clinical need for the "lesion test" aspect of the Wada test, which undoubtedly provides more direct information about how well language and memory functions can be supported after

functional removal of the contralateral hemisphere (Sharan et al. 2011). Thus, at present, the diagnostic value of fMRI and the Wada test seems to be rather complementary (Sharan et al. 2011). Killgore et al. found that, when combined, fMRI and Wada test provided complementary data that resulted in an improved prediction of postoperative seizure control compared with either procedure alone (Killgore et al. 1999). Recent studies indicated that the Wada test may no longer be necessary, when prior fMRI yielded robust and reliable language or memory lateralization (Bohm et al. 2020; Massot-Tarrús et al. 2020).

5.2 Special Practical Issues in Presurgical fMRI of Language Function

In contrast to the easy-to-perform movement tasks in motor fMRI, assessment of cognitive brain function—and hereby language function—requires an even closer cooperation of the patient. Therefore, all patients have to be well prepared for the fMRI tasks. The individual patient training, that is required prior to any language fMRI study, can—depending on the degree of the pre-existing tumor-associated language or other cognitive deficit—take up to several hours. Such training should guarantee the best possible match between the fMRI paradigms used and the patient's linguistic ability in order to ensure robust functional localizations and BOLD signals. For these reasons, pre-fMRI training is ideally combined with neuropsychological testing, which also includes detailed documentation of language deficits. The problem of the objective assessment of task performance in cognitive paradigms is very difficult in a clinical MR setting. Particularly in non-vocalized paradigms, it is challenging to estimate the patient's performance during block-designed fMRI. Devices assessing the patient's response on the task used in non-clinical or research fMRI conditions can only be used in cooperative patients and are thus often unsuited to routine presurgical fMRI. The best guarantee for sufficient patient cooperation during clinical fMRI scanning remains the intensive training prior to the examination mentioned above. In addition, patients are asked to give their subjective appraisal of task success after each single measurement included in the whole examination. Online evaluation of fMRI data ("real-time fMRI") is an important aid offered by most MR manufacturers today, enabling immediate assessment of the examination success (Fernandez et al. 2001; Feigl et al. 2008). Hence, erroneous measurements can be immediately detected and repeated.

For the examination itself, the visual or acoustic stimulation unit must be installed and later dismantled within a short period of time to avoid unnecessary disruption of the daily workflow in clinical neuroimaging. If one assumes a time frame of 1 h for the entire fMRI examination, including assembly, dismantling, and adjustment of all stimulation devices, acquisition of a morphological contrast-enhanced T1-weighted 3D data set for neuronavigation, and possibly another two or three diagnostic neuroimaging sequences, approximately 20 min remains for the acquisition of fMRI data. Within this time, several different language paradigms (Hirsch et al. 2000; Ramsey et al. 2001; Rutten et al. 2002c; Van Westen et al. 2005; Pillai and Zaca 2011; Unadkat et al. 2019; Manan et al. 2020), preferably of varying degrees of difficulty and each with a repeated measurement to confirm functional localization, should be applied, indicating that each clinical language fMRI measurement cannot take much longer than 5 min. In contrast, preoperative motor fMRI is far easier to implement in the clinical workflow as the time needed for somatotopic mapping does usually not exceed 10 min including patient instruction and feedback. Setup of dedicated apparatus is not necessary.

5.3 Selection of Candidates for Presurgical Language fMRI

In contrast to patients with Rolandic brain tumors, the selection of suitable candidates for presurgical language fMRI among patients with frontal and temporoparietal tumors is made largely irrespective of detectable morphological changes in potentially functionally important anatomical structures due to the lack of unequivocal morphological landmarks and due to significant anatomic variations in important language areas. Clinical and neuropsychological symptoms are of key importance. In our opinion, presurgical fMRI for language-associated brain activation makes sense in the following scenarios:

- Patients presenting with tumor-associated language deficits—including tumors in the right hemisphere, since in this case atypical organization of the language-relevant cortical representations has to be assumed (see Fig. 32)
- Patients without language deficits, but with tumors located in the left hemisphere, that are by anatomical consideration in close proximity to the inferior frontal gyrus (Broca's area) and the adjacent dorsal middle frontal gyrus (Exner's area), the medial frontal insula (Dronkers' area), the superior temporal gyrus (Wernicke's area), and the supramarginal or angular gyri (Geschwind's area) (see Figs. 27, 28, and 29)
- Left-handed patients, including patients with right-sided brain tumors
- Multilingual patients

Note The selection criteria mentioned here are meant as suggestions arising from typical MR morphological and clinical findings in patients with frontal or temporoparietal brain tumors. It is currently not possible to make a medical indication for fMRI in the strict sense. This is due to the still limited number of controlled prospective studies demonstrating the clinical benefit of presurgical fMRI in terms of reduced postoperative morbidity or mortality.

5.4 Language Paradigms for Presurgical fMRI

Language is conveyed over an extensive network of multiple functional areas to the frontal, temporal, and parietal lobes in both cerebral

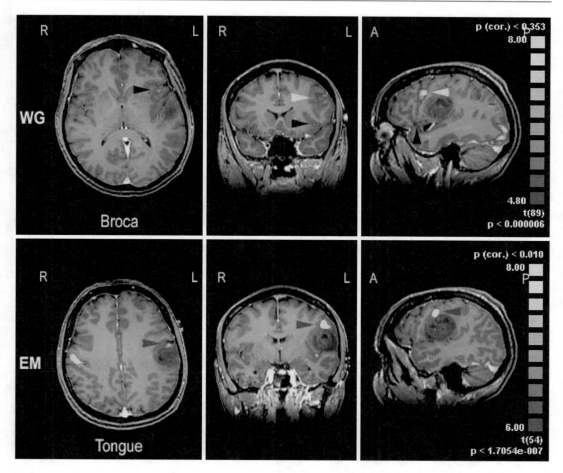

Fig. 27 Presurgical fMRI localization of Broca's area using the word-generation (*WG*) paradigm in a patient with a left inferior frontal astrocytoma as reflected by the typical activation of the inferior frontal gyrus, pars opercularis (*black arrowhead*). Note the additional strong language-associated activation (*yellow arrowhead*) at the upper edge of the inferior frontal gyrus (pars opercularis) / dorsal middle frontal gyrus (Exner's area). This activation can be distinguished clearly from primary motor tongue activation (*EM* executed movement) of the inferior precentral gyrus (*red arrowhead*)

hemispheres (see chapter "Functional Neuroanatomy"). As demonstrated above, language fMRI can be performed using various paradigms. For this reason no general recommendations can be made. The choice of clinically appropriate fMRI protocols should be made on the basis of the abovementioned diagnostic aims and within the framework of the clinical possibilities: To obtain reliable BOLD activations, paradigms need to be standardized and adjustable to the individual abilities of each patient. The language areas essential for intact speech (Broca's, Exner's, Dronkers', Wernicke's, Geschwind's) should be localized, whereas the importance of the identification of other secondary areas is not so clear in order to preserve them during surgery. A number of different word-generation tasks are suitable to this end, whereby language-associated memory, as well as other linguistic and cognitive processes, can also be assessed using task categories for free generation of several words per trigger (Bookheimer 2002). Sentence-generation tasks pose an even greater challenge (Just et al. 1996; Sakai et al. 2001), however, but can be easily standardized when a defined sentence is generated per trigger.

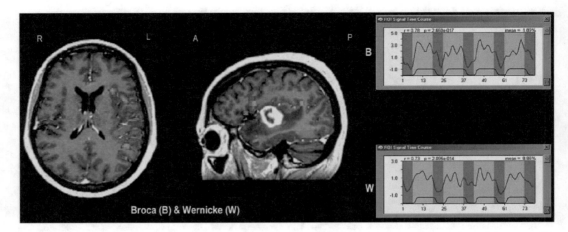

Fig. 28 Presurgical fMRI language localization and lateralization in a right-handed patient with a malignant glioma of the left superior temporal gyrus—critical to Wernicke's area by anatomical consideration. Sentence generation (SG) revealed clear left language dominance and localized Wernicke's area at the dorsal end of the superior temporal gyrus. BOLD signal time courses for Broca's area (B, r = 0.78, ΔS = 1.89%) and Wernicke's area (W, R = 0.73, ΔS = 0.86%). Note again the two BOLD activations in Broca's area (small cluster at the pars triangularis, larger cluster at the upper pars opercularis)

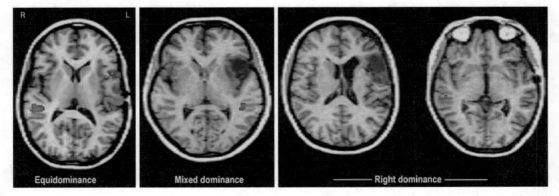

Fig. 29 Patterns of atypical language dominance as revealed by presurgical fMRI: equidominance between both hemispheres, mixed dominance (here with a right dominance for Broca's area and a normal left dominance for Wernicke's area), and pure right dominance for Broca's and Wernicke's areas

Clinical feasibility tests showed that the individual triggers must be structured as simple and unambiguous as possible in order to detect functional activity robustly. To this end the stimulus presentation frequency should be adjustable to the linguistic abilities of the individual patients, without changing the basic structure of the block design. Task-synchronous motion artifacts can be reduced by using non-vocalized language tasks (overt speech) (Hinke et al. 1993; Rueckert et al. 1994; Palmer et al. 2001), although the resulting brain activation is not identical to that derived from corresponding vocalized paradigms (Partovi et al. 2012b).

The examination protocol suggested here has been specifically designed to fulfill these clinical requirements (Stippich et al. 2003b). Within a measurement time of approximately 4 min (234 s) per paradigm, reliable functional localization of the Broca's and Wernicke's areas can be achieved, as well as of the anatomically homologous areas in the right hemisphere as a basis on which to calculate regional lateralization indices. Exner's (Roux et al. 2009), Geschwind's (Geschwind 1971, 1972) and Dronkers' (Dronkers 1996, 2007) activation may be observed in addition but is by definition not required according to the classical Wernicke-Lichtheim (Wernicke 1874) model of language (for historical reasons). At 1.5 T the physiological BOLD signals are quite robust in the abovementioned different functional language areas, with mean correlations between measured BOLD signals and a hemodynamic reference function ranging from $r = 0.55$ to $r = 0.80$, whereby BOLD signal intensities range typically from 1.5% to 2.5% (Fig. 27). Both paradigms (sentence and word generation) are visually triggered and can be adjusted to the linguistic ability of the patient by varying the trigger frequency. By using nonmagnetic, optically correctable reflective glasses with a slot for commercial optical lenses, it is possible to correct for ametropia (Stippich et al. 2007b). At the same time, visual stimulation prevents possible undesired superposition of language-associated activations in the Wernicke's speech area (BA21) onto activations in the directly adjacent auditory cortex (BA41, 42), as can occur with acoustic stimulation (Binder et al. 1995).

Of note, the American Society for Functional Neuroradiology has published a list of established clinical fMRI protocols from various larger neuro- and imaging centers throughout the USA to investigate language function in adults and children (https://www.asfnr.org; see also: Black et al. 2017; Benjamin et al. 2018; Agarwal et al. 2019a, b; Manan et al. 2020; Stopa et al. 2020). This information may also be helpful for investigators who wish to set up proper presurgical language fMRI studies at their institutions.

5.5 Presurgical fMRI of Language Function

In patients with brain tumors, presurgical language fMRI localizes the Broca's and Wernicke's areas in relation to the pathology and enables estimation of hemispheric dominance (Figs. 28 and 29). Benjamin and colleagues considered six critical languages relevant for preoperative fMRI (Benjamin et al. 2017). Besides providing essential functional landmarks for surgical decision-making and operative planning, different lateralization patterns of language activation can be identified, which may be roughly characterized by left dominance, right dominance, equidominance, mixed, or even reversed dominance. This information is available noninvasively and is more detailed as compared to the information obtained from the Wada test (Fig. 30) (Sharan et al. 2011). However, diagnostic results from different paradigms may differ (Fig. 31). Until now there is no clear rationale for the handling of this problem. Despite a high sensitivity of language fMRI to lateralize language (Dym et al. 2011), the available data to date on the reliability of fMRI for the determination of the language-dominant hemisphere is not fully clear (Janecek et al. 2013; Spritzer et al. 2012). Meanwhile, further validation studies have been performed on larger groups of patients in whom fMRI, reference techniques, and clinical and neuropsychological examinations were carried out in a standardized way (Giussani et al. 2010; Brennan et al. 2016; Meinhold et al. 2020). With regard to language lateralization, it appears acceptable to dispense with extensive invasive diagnostic examination in cases where, by using several paradigms, a typical left dominance is proven with fMRI (Sharan et al. 2011; Agarwal et al. 2019a, b). On the other hand, additional invasive validation tests should be performed in cases of conflicting results from various different fMRI paradigms and atypical language dominance (Figs. 32 and 33) (Cunningham et al. 2008; Janecek et al. 2013; Stopa et al. 2020).

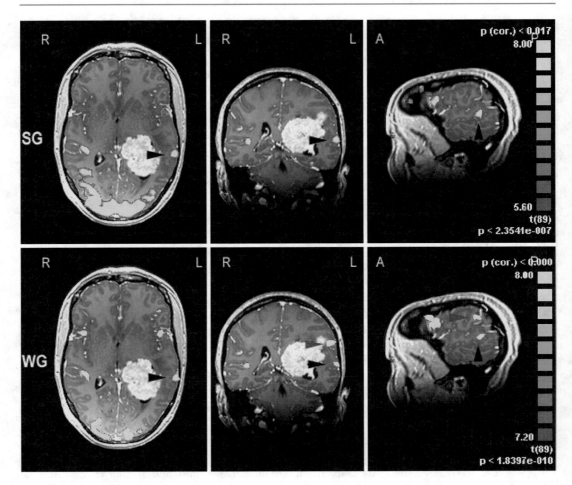

Fig. 30 Presurgical fMRI language localization and lateralization in a patient with a giant intraventricular meningioma using different paradigms. The diagnostic results are not identical but congruent and support each other. Sentence generation (*SG*) localized Wernicke's area in its typical localization of the left superior temporal gyrus adjacent to the superior temporal sulcus (*black arrow-head*) and revealed an equidominance. Word generation (*WG*) confirmed this finding, but localized a second language center in Wernicke's area in the left supramarginal gyrus (*red arrowhead*) that was also taken into consideration for operation planning and execution. Note the bilateral Broca's activation (also equidominant)

6 Diagnostic Capabilities and Limitations of Presurgical Task-Based fMRI

Traditionally, functional areas are electrophysiologically mapped intraoperatively to reliably assess the spatial relationship between the brain tumor and functional cortex (Ojemann et al. 1989; Ojemann 1991; Duffau et al. 1999, 2000, 2001, 2002b, 2003; Duffau 2001, 2005, 2006).

Intraoperative ECoG is considered very reliable, but comprises several disadvantages. Duration of surgery can be substantially prolonged and patients often need to be subjected to awake craniotomy. Furthermore, it only provides information from activations of the brain surface, while the by far larger portion of the cortex deep in the cerebral convolutions remains inaccessible (Cosgrove et al. 1996). Another significant disadvantage of ECoG is that the information is not available preoperatively and can therefore not be

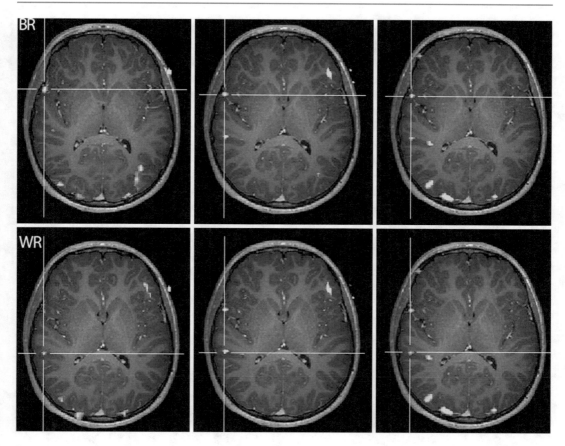

Fig. 31 Presurgical fMRI language lateralization (and localization) in a multilingual left-handed patient. Italian (*left*), French (*middle*), and German (*right*) language paradigms revealed reproducible right-hemispheric language dominance for the anatomical right homologues of Broca's (*BR*) and Wernicke's (*WR*) language areas. Awake craniotomy and intraoperative electrocorticography were performed during epilepsy surgery

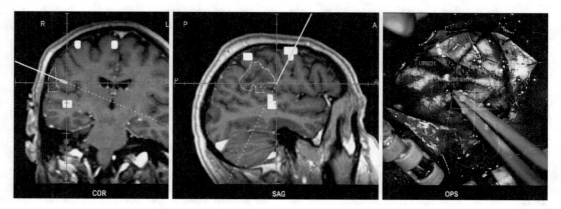

Fig. 32 Intraoperative validation of preoperative fMRI language localization in a right-handed male patient with a right parietal oligoastrocytoma (WHO II) and aphasic symptoms. Atypical right language dominance was diagnosed preoperatively using fMRI and the Wada test. Stimulation of the area that showed BOLD activation in the STG (WR) interrupted language production during awake craniotomy, confirming preoperative fMRI localization. *Yellow lines* indicate planned resection borders in neuronavigation. *Left*: Coronal (*COR*) and sagittal (*SAG*) views; functional activations (*white clusters*). *Right*: Operative site (*OPS*)

implemented in the pretherapeutic assessment of the operative indication and the planning of function-preserving surgery. Likewise, the Wada test as a reference procedure for speech lateralization and memory puts the patient under strain, involves all the risks of arterial catheter angiography, and is not standardized—test results can therefore vary (Wada and Rasmussen 1960; Rausch et al. 1993). After all, morphological imaging with MRI provides very detailed information on intracranial pathologies (Osborn 2012), but not on brain function. FMRI is capable to overcome these disadvantages of the "traditional diagnostic procedures" by visualizing the anatomy, pathology, and function noninvasively within a single examination already prior to sur-

gery (Black et al. 2019). In addition, the course of important WM tracts as the arcuate fascicle can be assessed preoperatively using DTI, and the acquired DTI data can be fused with fMRI in order to enhance pre- and intraoperative planning (Rasmussen et al. 2007; Archip et al. 2007; Berntsen et al. 2010; González-Darder and González-López 2010; Nimsky 2011; Dimous et al. 2013; Jia et al. 2013; Sang et al. 2018; Conti Nibali et al. 2019; Mancini et al. 2019).

When carried out in a standard way, fMRI is basically capable of providing a clinical "functional diagnosis" for individual patients (Thulborn 2006; Tyndall et al. 2017). Functional landmarks help to estimate possible therapy-related deficits and are thus particularly useful in

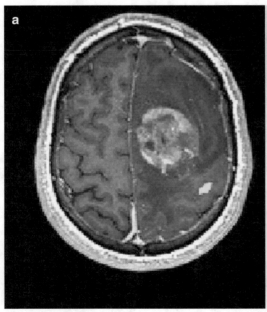
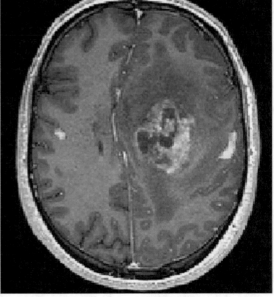

Fig. 33 (**a**) Presurgical somatotopic fMRI of motor function (**a**) provided detailed information on the spatial relationship between the primary motor hand and tongue representations to the left frontal glioblastoma involving the cingulum and corpus callosum. Language fMRI (**b**) revealed a left language dominance, with a marked activation of the right anatomical homologue of Broca's area, which may indicate tumor-associated neuroplasticity. This overt language paradigm confirmed the primary motor tongue representation on the left when compared to the prior motor study. (**b**) Integration of the relevant func-

tional activations (landmarks) of the Broca's, Wernicke's, and Geschwind's language areas; primary motor and premotor tongue representations; primary motor hand representation; and DTI-tractographies of the pyramidal tract and arcuate fascicle into the T1-weighted contrast-enhanced 3D-MRI used for neuronavigation during extended open biopsy. In these patients, fMRI makes it easier to verify the indication to operate, as well as to plan, function-sparing surgery, while taking atypical language representations or tumor-induced neuroplastic changes into consideration

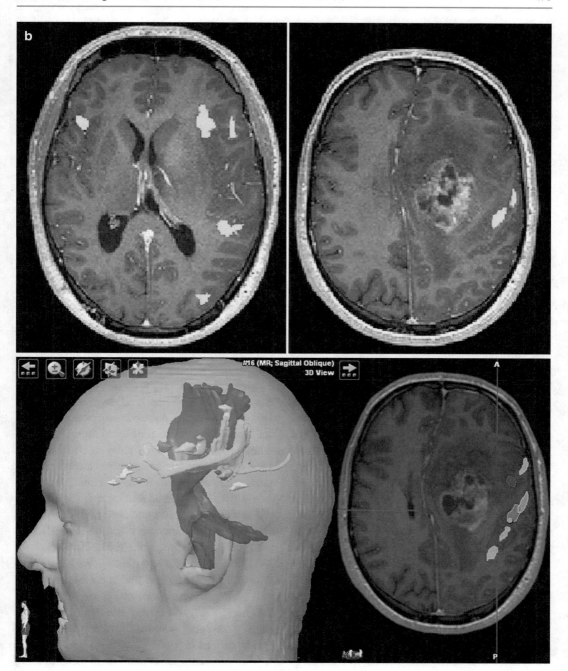

Fig. 33 (continued)

providing information on the lesion's location, verifying the indication, and selecting a function-sparing therapeutic procedure. Once the indication for surgery is made, careful planning and appropriate selection of incision, trepanation, surgical access, and resection margins are essential to function-preserving surgery. Intraoperatively, functional localizations facilitate surgical orientation, although inaccuracies resulting from displaced brain tissue, known as brain shift, need to be accounted for (Stippich et al. 2002a, 2003a; Rasmussen et al. 2007; Archip et al. 2007; González-Darder and González-López 2010; Kuhnt et al. 2012; Berkels et al. 2014). All these factors increase patient safety and help to minimize the risk of postoperative deficits which would further reduce the quality of life.

According to current knowledge, it can be assumed that presurgical fMRI is able to contribute to a reduction and more targeted selection of invasive diagnostic procedures both before and during neurosurgical interventions in patients with brain tumors or epileptogenic foci. FMRI can have a positive effect on surgery-related morbidity and disease-related mortality (Kundu et al. 2013; Bailey et al. 2015; Vysotski et al. 2018; Liouta et al. 2019). Available results evaluating the use of fMRI data for presurgical planning in relation to functional outcome approve the valuable information obtained by fMRI with respect to the risk of postoperative neurological dysfunction. However, there are also conflicting results published that showed fMRI to explain preoperative but not postoperative deficit. As mentioned before, it is assumed, in general, that a distance of at least 10 mm between tumor border and functional cortex should be respected for assuring a functionally good postsurgical outcome (Håberg et al. 2004; Krishnan et al. 2004; Berntsen et al. 2010). Assessment of the lesion-to-activation distance (LAD) and the language lateralization index (LI) has proved to be of value (Kundu et al. 2013; Voss et al. 2013) for evaluation of postoperative outcome. It has been shown that the proximity of the tumor to an activation area might also interact with how the language network is affected (Kundu et al. 2013). Moreover, the LAD to the primary sensorimotor cortex influences the occurrence of neurological deficits, in contrast to the LAD to the supplementary motor area (SMA) (Voss et al. 2013). Of note is, however, that such attempts should not put the surgeon in an unfounded security as distance measurements can solve the problem of neither ill-defined tumor margins especially in tumors of glial origin or in case of infiltrative tumor growth nor fMRI's

inability to define the exact extent of a functional area, which is arbitrary and given by the chosen statistical threshold during data evaluation. We consider defining "safe resection margins" in presurgical diagnostics on the basis of fMRI data alone as potentially unreliable, since the spatial extent of activated areas depends on the evaluation parameters chosen and can therefore vary. Furthermore, there is not enough data available that would allow to predict possible postsurgical deficits based on fMRI cerebral reorganization patterns, be it transient or permanent.

Preoperative fMRI has limitations imposed by patient-specific and methodological factors. Despite intensive patient training, optimized examination protocols, and appropriate head fixation, some patients cannot be examined due to poor cooperation or marked restlessness. When motor paradigms are used, undesirable continuation of movement during resting periods or undesirable and mostly uncontrolled and interspersed accompanying movements in other parts of the body can compromise the quality of the examination, even if individually adjusted evaluation is used to register the respective error precisely. In the end, after this time-consuming process, examination results often need to be discarded. The same applies to strong motion artifacts which cannot be corrected at later data processing stages. Stimulus-related motion artifacts can simulate activations, leading to false high BOLD signals or even to incorrect localization (Hajnal et al. 1994; Krings et al. 2001; Hoeller et al. 2002; Steger and Jackson 2004). With regard to motion artifacts, tongue and toe movements, as well as finger opposition tasks, are less critical than hand, foot, and lip movements. And for language paradigms non-vocalized are less critical than vocalized tasks.

The problems associated with investigating motor function in patients with tumor-related hemipareses have already been addressed (see Sect. 4.6). In most cases, functional localization of the pre- and postcentral gyrus can be achieved by using residual motor function in the affected extremities and applying special paradigms (Stippich et al. 2003a). Compared to motor fMRI,

BOLD signals are significantly weaker on tactile stimulation. Particularly in the lower extremities, tactile stimulation does not always achieve sufficient activation. This is accounted for by the lower number of receptors in toe tips, the comparatively small cortical toe representation, and—in our clinical fMRI setup—the ill-defined compressed air pulses when long pneumatic tubes are used. In this context resting-state fMRI provides valuable additional information, as patient cooperation is not required (Lee et al. 2013, 2016; Sair et al. 2016; Lemée et al. 2019; Park et al. 2020).

The success of language fMRI pivotally depends on patient training and optimal adjustment of the paradigm to suit language ability (Stippich et al. 2002a; Lit). If patients are over-tested, they perform only a portion of the required tasks leading to lower activation. The same is true of under-testing where too few triggers are given. Additionally, "free thinking" can then lead to uncontrolled activation, for example, when patients get bored, since, using our paradigms, neither of the sources of error can be controlled directly during fMRI. As a consequence, the paradigm parameters which were proven during pre-fMRI training to be optimal for each individual patient are always used for the preoperative measurement. To increase certainty, the patient is interviewed after each fMRI measurement about whether the task could be successfully accomplished. If this was not the case, the task is repeated. Training always takes place immediately prior to fMRI and lasts at least 20 min in order for the patients to master all four different language paradigms and to avoid interaction of learning effects on examination results. The training period can last longer in patients with limited linguistic ability.

Of note is that language lateralization—as determined by fMRI—depends on the "cerebral workload" associated with the applied tasks, as the activation in the left hemisphere increases with trigger frequency, whereas activation in the right hemisphere does not fully parallel this effect (Konrad et al. 2005). This implies that the strongest lateralization effect will be measured with paradigms that are optimally adapted to the patient's individual performance. More importantly brain tumors per se may modulate language lateralization by inducing neuroplastic changes and functional reorganization. In this instance, tumors most likely tend to reduce the activation in the affected hemisphere and may in addition induce an increase of activation in the unaffected hemisphere (Partovi et al. 2012a). This means that brain tumors of the left hemisphere that are critical to essential language areas modulate language lateralization towards the right side, which is in most cases the nondominant one (Holodny et al. 2002; Wellmer et al. 2009; Partovi et al. 2012a; Jansma et al. 2015). Consequently, the lateralization indices calculated in patients with brain tumors that affect language function have to be interpreted with special caution: Here, a right language dominance in the presurgical fMRI examination does not necessarily mean that the reduced activation in the left hemisphere is no longer essential to preserve language function, especially when the Broca's and/or Wernicke's areas are affected directly by the tumor. In this instance, the assumption that the right hemisphere is fully capable to functionally compensate for the left may be fatal. In contrast, such neuroplastic changes should be interpreted as the brain's attempts to cope with the pathology, and thus, the residual activation in the classical language areas should be considered as very essential, even if it is weaker than that on the unaffected side. Of note, fMRI activation may be critically affected by prior brain surgery and needs to be interpreted with special caution in the postoperative imaging setting (Peck et al. 2009).

In the case of uncooperative patients, resting-state fMRI has opened up a new field in the investigation of functionally important brain areas (Shimoni et al. 2009; Zhang et al. 2009; Lee et al. 2012; Manglore et al. 2013; Mitchell et al. 2013). Resting-state fMRI measures spontaneous, that is, intrinsic, BOLD fluctuations to identify eloquent areas in the brain without the need of task performance by the patients. Therefore, this method is very promising for measuring functional activity in sedated patients, in disabled or uncooperative patients, and in small children. However, until now this technique has been used mostly for group analysis in research studies. The results on clinical applications in individual patients are promising, but still limited. A clear advantage of resting-state fMRI is the reduced scanning time in comparison to task-based fMRI, as different neurofunctional systems can be assessed in a single scanning session. Activity correlation in motor regions has been shown to be quite similar between task-free and task-elicited fMRI (Liu et al. 2009). In one study, more specific analysis and less data variability were found for the motor cortex with resting-state fMRI compared with task-based fMRI (Shimoni et al. 2009). Already those initial reports underlined that resting-state fMRI may have a clinical potential in pretherapeutic assessment of eloquent areas in patients with brain tumors, vascular lesions, or epilepsy. Meanwhile, substantial work on presurgical resting-state fMRI has been done (Lee et al. 2016; Sparacia et al. 2019), including comparisons to task-based fMRI (Sair et al. 2016; Battistella et al. 2020; Park et al. 2020), invasive reference measures (Vakamudi et al. 2020), and pre/posttreatment effects (Sparacia et al. 2020). However, clinical application of resting-state fMRI is still limited and further investigation is required to define its role and potency in the clinical and pretherapeutical setting. A more detailed description on resting-state fMRI is given in chapter "Presurgical Resting-State fMRI."

Diffusion tensor imaging (DTI) provides visualization of white matter (WM) tracts and is applied in many centers for the assessment of the relationship between lesions, for example, tumors, and the course of functionally important WM tracts such as the pyramidal tract or the arcuate fascicle. This technique has been reported to be very useful both in the presurgical planning (Leclercq et al. 2011; Morita et al. 2011; Bertani et al. 2012; Hayashi et al. 2012; Abdullah et al. 2013; Potgieser et al. 2014) and for the prediction and evaluation of postoperative outcomes (Hayashi et al. 2012; Bailey et al. 2015; Henderson et al. 2020). A number of studies are available showing the integration of fMRI with DTI data (Smits et al. 2007) under stereotactic guidance in the intraoperative setting for identification of eloquent areas (Rasmussen et al. 2007; Archip et al. 2007; Berntsen et al. 2010; González-Darder and González-López 2010; Nimsky 2011; Kuhnt et al. 2012; Dimous et al. 2013; Jia et al. 2013; Kumar et al. 2014). Initial results demonstrate the impact of the combination of these two modalities on intraoperative strategies to avoid damaging of the eloquent cortex or WM tracts. Good tumor resection results with preservation of neurological function could be achieved, whereas a safe distance of at least 10 mm between the lesion's margins and the eloquent area should be maintained in order to avoid transient or permanent neurological deficits (Berntsen et al. 2010). fMRI has proven to be more beneficial for the localization of the functional important areas, whereas DTI data have been shown to be more useful for the resection itself (Rasmussen et al. 2007). Together both techniques show great promise in postsurgical outcomes (Dimous et al. 2013; Jia et al. 2013; Conti Nibali et al. 2019). Despite such promising results, additional technical inaccuracies must be taken into consideration in neuronavigation and referencing. At this stage further studies are necessary to more accurately define the limits of "safe" resections, especially considering intraoperative brain shift (Gil-Robles and Duffau 2010; González-Darder and González-López 2010).

The position of brain structures can change intraoperatively ("brain shift"), so that preoperatively obtained data no longer accurately reflect the intraoperative situation (Wirtz et al. 1997; Wittek et al. 2005; Nimsky et al. 2006; Kuhnt et al. 2012; Gerard et al. 2017; Fan et al. 2018). Effluent cerebrospinal fluid alone can lead to shifts of several millimeters after opening of the dura. Moreover, there is often a sharp shift in the position of the brain due to tissue resection. Also for these reasons, preoperative fMRI cannot replace intraoperative mapping of brain function completely. However, preoperatively acquired MRI data are useful as they can be intraoperatively updated with ultrasound hereby to some extent compensating for the brain shift phenomenon (Rasmussen et al. 2007). Intraoperative repetition of fMRI and DTI has also been established with proven value, but on the cost of relevantly longer operation times (Nimsky 2011). Other, investigator-dependent, inaccuracies occur in the manual superposition of the EPI data distorted by the method onto anatomical 3D data sets. As a precaution, a possible localization error of approximately 0.5 cm should always be assumed (Stippich et al. 2003a). Technical improvements include distortion corrections for EPI data sets (Weiskopf et al. 2005; Liu and Ogawa 2006; Priest et al. 2006; Lima Cardoso et al. 2017) enabling for automated superposition procedures, which helps to further reduce inaccuracies in the functional intraoperative localization of eloquent brain structures.

The BOLD signals based on fMRI originate mainly in the capillary bed of the activated brain area and downstream veins (Frahm et al. 1994; Menon et al. 1995). Thus, fMRI measures a hemodynamic secondary phenomenon and not neuronal activity directly. Possible localization errors due to BOLD signals from draining veins can be identified by superimposing functional image data onto contrast-enhanced anatomical T1-weighted image sequences (Krings et al. 1999). Careful analysis of the signal time curves of functional raw data helps to distinguish between parenchymatous and venous activation, since each of both rises at different rates (Krings et al. 2001). A reduced venous contribution to the BOLD signal could be observed at 7 T MR systems; however, for many reasons 7 T scanners are rarely used in clinical routine at this stage (Van der Zwaag et al. 2009; Lima Cardoso et al. 2017; Trattnig et al. 2018) and 9.4 T human MRI has to be considered experimental (Huber et al. 2018). By causing vessel compression, pathological changes in vascular autoregulation, and neurovascular coupling, brain tumors and vascular malformations can affect the localization, lateralization, and intensity of the BOLD signals mea-

sured (Holodny et al. 1999, 2000; Krings et al. 2002a; Ulmer et al. 2003, 2004a, b; Kim et al. 2005; Liu et al. 2005; Hou et al. 2006; Ludemann et al. 2006; Ben Bashat et al. 2012). Hence, brain tumors have the potential to alter neurovascular units, cause neurovascular uncoupling, and confound the interpretation of fMRI results (Agarwal et al. 2021). For this reason, activations within contrast-enhanced portions of brain tumors should be assumed as artifacts and not be used for risk assessment, surgery planning, or functional neuronavigation. The same applies to BOLD signals in strongly vascularized cerebral metastases or arteriovenous malformations (Lazar et al. 1997; Alkadhi et al. 2000; Lehericy et al. 2002; Ozdoba et al. 2002; Li et al. 2020). Cerebrovascular reactivity mapping enables to detect neurovascular uncoupling and complements presurgical BOLD fMRI also in low-grade gliomas (Pillai and Zaca 2011; Zaca et al. 2014).

In summary, for over 25 years task-based fMRI has proven validity and high sensitivity to localize different representations of the human body in the primary motor cortex, to localize essential language areas, and to lateralize language function prior to surgery in patients with brain tumors and epilepsy. Besides providing MR criteria for selecting, planning, and performing optimized function-preserving treatment tailored to individual patients, fMRI helps to better select patients who require additional pre- and intraoperative invasive diagnostic measures such as the Wada test or electrocorticography and furthermore to reduce the number of such invasive procedures needed through substitution. The method has, however, not reached the status of a fully standardized clinical application in MR neuroimaging, yet. To this end, further consensus on the performance, analysis, and medical appraisal of presurgical fMRI is warranted, as well as the specification of recommendations and guidelines by more assigned medical societies. Diffusion tensor imaging (DTI) is also of great value in the pre- and intraoperative setting, especially when combined with fMRI, by providing detailed information on functionally important white

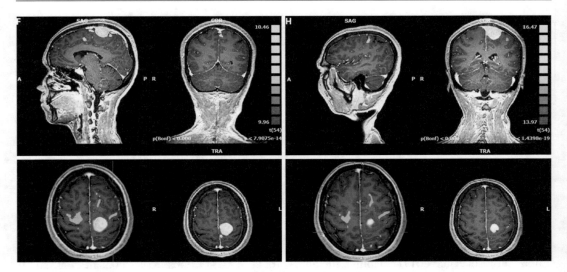

Fig. 34 Presurgical somatotopic motor fMRI and DTI-tractography in a left Rolandic meningioma for planning the best surgical access. fMRI localization of the primary motor foot representation (*F*, left image quartet) directly adjacent to the dorsal aspect of the tumor and of the motor hand representation (*H*, right image quartet). The functional localizations and DTI-tractography were implemented into the T1-weighted 3D data set for functional neuronavigation (*lower row, left* in each quartet)

matter connections such as the pyramidal tract or the arcuate fascicle (Fig. 34). Novel applications employing BOLD measurements of resting-state brain activity (rsfMRI) have successfully entered the arena of presurgical functional neuroimaging and complement task-based fMRI by providing additional diagnostic information on important neurofunctional networks and their connectivity even without active cooperation of the patient.

References

Abdullah KG, Lubelski D et al (2013) Use of diffusion tensor imaging in glioma resection. Neurosurg Focus 34(4):E1

Achten E, Jackson GD et al (1999) Presurgical evaluation of the motor hand area with functional MR imaging in patients with tumors and dysplastic lesions. Radiology 210(2):529–538

Agarwal S, Sair HI, Yahyavi-Firouz-Abadi N, Airan R, Pillai JJ (2016) Neurovascular uncoupling in resting state fMRI demonstrated in patients with primary brain gliomas. J Magn Reson Imaging 43(3):620–626. https://doi.org/10.1002/jmri.25012. Epub 2015 Jul 22

Agarwal S, Sair HI, Gujar S, Pillai JJ (2019a) Language mapping with fMRI: current standards and reproduc-ibility. Top Magn Reson Imaging 28(4):225–233. https://doi.org/10.1097/RMR.0000000000000216

Agarwal S, Sair HI, Gujar S, Hua J, Lu H, Pillai JJ (2019b) Functional magnetic resonance imaging activation optimization in the setting of brain tumor-induced neurovascular uncoupling using resting-state blood oxygen level-dependent amplitude of low frequency fluctuations. Brain Connect 9(3):241–250. https://doi.org/10.1089/brain.2017.0562. Epub 2019 Feb 28

Agarwal S, Sair HI, Pillai JJ (2021) The problem of neurovascular uncoupling. Neuroimaging Clin N Am 31(1):53–67. Review. https://doi.org/10.1016/j.nic.2020.09.003. Epub 2020 Oct 29

Akbar M, Stippich C, Aschoff A (2005) Magnetic resonance imaging and cerebrospinal fluid shunt valves. N Engl J Med 353(13):1413–1414

Alkadhi H, Kollias SS et al (2000) Plasticity of the human motor cortex in patients with arteriovenous malforma-tions: a functional MR imaging study. AJNR Am J Neuroradiol 21(8):1423–1433

Allendorfer JB, Hernando KA, Hossain S, Nenert R, Holland SK, Szaflarski JP (2016) Arcuate fasciculus asymmetry has a hand in language function but not handedness. Hum Brain Mapp 37(9):3297–3309. https://doi.org/10.1002/hbm.23241. Epub 2016 May 4

Andrews E, Frigau L, Voyvodic-Casabo C, Voyvodic J, Wright J (2013) Multilingualism and fMRI: lon-gitudinal study of second language acquisition. Brain Sci 3(2):849–876. https://doi.org/10.3390/brainsci3020849

Archip N, Clatz O et al (2007) Non-rigid alignment of pre-operative MRI, fMRI, and DT-MRI with intra-operative MRI for enhanced visualization and navigation in image-guided neurosurgery. NeuroImage 35(2):609–624

Atlas SW, Howard RS 2nd et al (1996) Functional magnetic resonance imaging of regional brain activity in patients with intracerebral gliomas: findings and implications for clinical management. Neurosurgery 38(2):329–338

Avila C, Barros-Loscertales A et al (2006) Memory lateralization with 2 functional MR imaging tasks in patients with lesions in the temporal lobe. AJNR Am J Neuroradiol 27(3):498–503

Azad TD, Duffau H (2020) Limitations of functional neuroimaging for patient selection and surgical planning in glioma surgery. Neurosurg Focus 48(2):E12. Review. https://doi.org/10.3171/2019.11.FOCUS19769

Baciu M, Le Bas JF et al (2003) Presurgical fMRI evaluation of cerebral reorganization and motor deficit in patients with tumors and vascular malformations. Eur J Radiol 46(2):139–146

Bahn MM, Lin W et al (1997) Localization of language cortices by functional MR imaging compared with intracarotid amobarbital hemispheric sedation. AJR Am J Roentgenol 169(2):575–579

Bailey PD, Zacà D, Basha MM, Agarwal S, Gujar SK, Sair HI, Eng J, Pillai JJ (2015) Presurgical fMRI and DTI for the prediction of perioperative motor and language deficits in primary or metastatic brain lesions. J Neuroimaging 25(5):776–784. https://doi.org/10.1111/jon.12273. Epub 2015 Jul 14

Balter S, Lin G, Leyden KM, Paul BM, McDonald CR (2019) Neuroimaging correlates of language network impairment and reorganization in temporal lobe epilepsy. Brain Lang 193:31–44. https://doi.org/10.1016/j.bandl.2016.06.002. Epub 2016 Jul 5

Banan R, Hartmann C (2017) The new WHO 2016 classification of brain tumors—what neurosurgeons need to know. Acta Neurochir (Wien) 159(3):403–418. Review. https://doi.org/10.1007/s00701-016-3062-3. Epub 2017 Jan 17

Bandettini PA, Wong EC et al (1992) Time course EPI of human brain function during task activation. Magn Reson Med 25(2):390–397

Barnett A, Marty-Dugas J, McAndrews MP (2014) Advantages of sentence-level fMRI language tasks in presurgical language mapping for temporal lobe epilepsy. Epilepsy Behav 32:114–120

Batson MA, Petridou N, Klomp DW, Frens MA, Neggers SF (2015) Single session imaging of cerebellum at 7 Tesla: obtaining structure and function of multiple motor subsystems in individual subjects. PLoS One 10(8):e0134933, eCollection 2015. https://doi.org/10.1371/journal.pone.0134933

Battistella G, Borghesani V, Henry M, Shwe W, Lauricella M, Miller Z, Deleon J, Miller BL, Dronkers N, Brambati SM, Seeley WW, Mandelli ML, Gorno-Tempini ML (2020) Task-free functional language networks: reproducibility and clinical application. J Neurosci 40(6):1311–1320. https://doi.org/10.1523/JNEUROSCI.1485-19.2019. Epub 2019 Dec 18

Baudendistel K, Schad LR et al (1996) Monitoring of task performance during functional magnetic resonance imaging of sensorimotor cortex at 1.5 T. Magn Reson Imaging 14(1):51–58

Bauer PR, Reitsma JB et al (2013) Can fMRI safely replace the Wada test for preoperative assessment of language lateralisation? A meta-analysis and systematic review. J Neurol Neurosurg Psychiatry 85(5):581–588

Baumann SB, Noll DC et al (1995) Comparison of functional magnetic resonance imaging with positron emission tomography and magnetoencephalography to identify the motor cortex in a patient with an arteriovenous malformation. J Image Guid Surg 1(4):191–197

Baxendale S (2002) The role of functional MRI in the presurgical investigation of temporal lobe epilepsy patients: a clinical perspective and review. J Clin Exp Neuropsychol 24(5):664–676

Bazin B, Cohen L et al (2000) Study of hemispheric lateralization of language regions by functional MRI. Validation with the Wada test. Rev Neurol (Paris) 156(2):145–148

Beckett AJS, Dadakova T, Townsend J, Huber L, Park S, Feinberg DA (2020) Comparison of BOLD and CBV using 3D EPI and 3D GRASE for cortical layer functional MRI at 7 T. Magn Reson Med 84(6):3128–3145. https://doi.org/10.1002/mrm.28347. Epub 2020 Jun 18

Beisteiner R (2017) Can functional magnetic resonance imaging generate valid clinical neuroimaging reports? Front Neurol 8:237, eCollection 2017. https://doi.org/10.3389/fneur.2017.00237

Beisteiner R, Robinson S, Wurnig M, Hilbert M, Merksa K, Rath J, Höllinger I, Klinger N, Marosi C, Trattnig S, Geissler A (2011) Clinical fMRI: evidence for a 7T benefit over 3T. NeuroImage 57(3):1015–1021. https://doi.org/10.1016/j.neuroimage.2011.05.010. Epub 2011 May 17

Belliveau JW, Kennedy DN Jr et al (1991) Functional mapping of the human visual cortex by magnetic resonance imaging. Science 254(5032):716–719

Bello L, Acerbi F et al (2006) Intraoperative language localization in multilingual patients with gliomas. Neurosurgery 59(1):115–125; discussion 115–125

Ben Bashat D, Artzi M, Ben Ami H, Aizenstein O, Blumenthal DT, Bokstein F, Corn BW, Ram Z, Kanner AA, Lifschitz-Mercer B, Solar I, Kolatt T, Palmon M, Edrei Y, Abramovitch R (2012) Hemodynamic response imaging: a potential tool for the assessment of angiogenesis in brain tumors. PLoS One 7(11):e49416. https://doi.org/10.1371/journal.pone.0049416. Epub 2012 Nov 27

Benbadis SR, Binder JR et al (1998) Is speech arrest during Wada testing a valid method for determining hemispheric representation of language? Brain Lang 65(3):441–446

Benjamin CF, Walshaw PD, Hale K, Gaillard WD, Baxter LC, Berl MM, Polczynska M, Noble S, Alkawadri R, Hirsch LJ, Constable RT, Bookheimer SY (2017) Presurgical language fMRI: Mapping of six critical regions. Hum Brain Mapp 38(8):4239–4255. https://doi.org/10.1002/hbm.23661. Epub 2017 May 23

Benjamin CFA, Li AX, Blumenfeld H, Constable RT, Alkawadri R, Bickel S, Helmstaedter C, Meletti S, Bronen R, Warfield SK, Peters JM, Reutens D, Połczyńska M, Spencer DD, Hirsch LJ (2018) Presurgical language fMRI: clinical practices and patient outcomes in epilepsy surgical planning. Hum Brain Mapp 39(7):2777–2785. Published online 2018 Mar 12. https://doi.org/10.1002/hbm.24039

Benson RR, Logan WJ et al (1996) Functional MRI localization of language in a 9-year-old child. Can J Neurol Sci 23(3):213–219

Benson RR, FitzGerald DB et al (1999) Language dominance determined by whole brain functional MRI in patients with brain lesions. Neurology 52(4):798–809

Berger H (1929) Über das Elektroenzephalogramm des Menschen. Arch Psychiatr Nervenk 87:527–570

Berkels B, Cabrilo I et al (2014) Co-registration of intra-operative brain surface photographs and pre-operative MR images. Int J Comput Assist Radiol Surg 9(3):387–400

Berntsen EM, Gulati S et al (2010) Functional magnetic resonance imaging and diffusion tensor tractography incorporate into an intraoperative 3-dimensional ultrasound-based neuronavigation system: impact on therapeutic strategies, extent of resection, and clinical outcome. Neurosurgery 67(2):251–264

Bertani G, Carrabba G et al (2012) Predictive value of inferior fronto-occipital fasciculus (IFO) DTI-fiber tracking for determining the extent of resection for surgery of frontal and temporal gliomas preoperatively. J Neurosurg Sci 56(2):137–143

Binder JR, Rao SM et al (1995) Lateralized human brain language systems demonstrated by task subtraction functional magnetic resonance imaging. Arch Neurol 52(6):593–601

Binder JR, Swanson SJ et al (1996) Determination of language dominance using functional MRI: a comparison with the Wada test. Neurology 46(4):978–984

Binder JR, Frost JA et al (1997) Human brain language areas identified by functional magnetic resonance imaging. J Neurosci 17(1):353–362

Binder JR, Frost JA et al (1999) Conceptual processing during the conscious resting state. A functional MRI study. J Cogn Neurosci 11(1):80–95

Binder JR, Frost JA et al (2000) Human temporal lobe activation by speech and nonspeech sounds. Cereb Cortex 10(5):512–528

Binder JR, Achten E et al (2002) Functional MRI in epilepsy. Epilepsia 43(Suppl 1):51–63

Bittar RG, Olivier A et al (1999a) Localization of somatosensory function by using positron emission tomography scanning: a comparison with intraoperative cortical stimulation. J Neurosurg 90(3):478–483

Bittar RG, Olivier A et al (1999b) Presurgical motor and somatosensory cortex mapping with functional magnetic resonance imaging and positron emission tomography. J Neurosurg 91(6):915–921

Bittar RG, Olivier A et al (2000) Cortical motor and somatosensory representation: effect of cerebral lesions. J Neurosurg 92(2):242–248

Black DF, Vachha B, Mian A, Faro SH, Maheshwari M, Sair HI, Petrella JR, Pillai JJ, Welker K (2017) American Society of Functional Neuroradiology— Recommended fMRI paradigm algorithms for presurgical language assessment. AJNR Am J Neuroradiol 38(10):E65–E73. https://doi.org/10.3174/ajnr.A5345. Epub 2017 Aug 31

Black DF, Little JT, Johnson DR (2019) Neuroanatomical considerations in preoperative functional brain mapping. Top Magn Reson Imaging 28(4):213–224. https://doi.org/10.1097/RMR.0000000000000213

Blatow M, Nennig E et al (2007) FMRI reflects functional connectivity of human somatosensory cortex. NeuroImage 37(3):927–936

Bogen JE (1976) Wernicke's region—where is it? Ann N Y Acad Sci 290:834–843

Bogomolny DL, Petrovich NM et al (2004) Functional MRI in the brain tumor patient. Top Magn Reson Imaging 15(5):325–335

Bohm P, McKay J, Lucas J, Sabsevitz D, Feyissa AM, Ritaccio T, Grewal SS, Wharen RE, Gupta V, Tatum WO (2020) Wada testing and fMRI in a polyglot evaluated for epilepsy surgery. Epileptic Disord 22(2):207–213. https://doi.org/10.1684/epd.2020.1145

Bookheimer SY (2000) Methodological issues in pediatric neuroimaging. Ment Retard Dev Disabil Res Rev 6(3):161–165

Bookheimer S (2002) Functional MRI of language: new approaches to understanding the cortical organization of semantic processing. Annu Rev Neurosci 25:151–188

Bowring A, Maumet C, Nichols TE (2019) Exploring the impact of analysis software on task fMRI results. Hum Brain Mapp 40(11):3362–3384. https://doi.org/10.1002/hbm.24603. Epub 2019 May 2

Brennan NP, Peck KK, Holodny A (2016) Language mapping using fMRI and direct cortical stimulation for brain tumor surgery: the good, the bad, and the questionable. Top Magn Reson Imaging 25(1):1–10. https://doi.org/10.1097/RMR.0000000000000074

Briganti C, Sestieri C et al (2012) Reorganization of functional connectivity of the language network in patients with brain gliomas. AJNR Am J Neuroradiol 33(10):1983–1990

Brindle KM, Izquierdo-García JL, Lewis DY, Mair RJ, Wright AJ (2017) Brain tumor imaging. J Clin

Oncol 35(21):2432–2438. https://doi.org/10.1200/JCO.2017.72.7636. Epub 2017 Jun 22

Buckner RL, Bandettini PA et al (1996) Detection of cortical activation during averaged single trials of a cognitive task using functional magnetic resonance imaging. Proc Natl Acad Sci U S A 93(25):14878–14883

Carpentier A, Pugh KR et al (2001a) Functional MRI of language processing: dependence on input modality and temporal lobe epilepsy. Epilepsia 42(10):1241–1254

Carpentier AC, Constable RT et al (2001b) Patterns of functional magnetic resonance imaging activation in association with structural lesions in the Rolandic region: a classification system. J Neurosurg 94(6):946–954

Cedzich C, Taniguchi M et al (1996) Somatosensory evoked potential phase reversal and direct motor cortex stimulation during surgery in and around the central region. Neurosurgery 38(5):962–970

Centeno M, Koepp MJ, Vollmar C, Stretton J, Sidhu M, Michallef C, Symms MR, Thompson PJ, Duncan JS (2014) Language dominance assessment in a bilingual population: validity of fMRI in the second language. Epilepsia 55(10):1504–1511. https://doi.org/10.1111/epi.12757. Epub 2014 Sept 2

Choudhri AF, Narayana S et al (2013) Same day trimodality functional brain mapping prior to resection of a lesion involving eloquent cortex: technical feasibility. Neuroradiol J 26(5):548–554

Cirillo S, Caulo M, Pieri V, Falini A, Castellano A (2019) Role of functional imaging techniques to assess motor and language cortical plasticity in glioma patients: a systematic review. Neural Plast 2019:4056436, eCollection 2019. https://doi.org/10.1155/2019/4056436

Conti Nibali M, Rossi M, Sciortino T, Riva M, Gay LG, Pessina F, Bello L (2019) Preoperative surgical planning of glioma: limitations and reliability of fMRI and DTI tractography. J Neurosurg Sci 63(2):127–134. Review. https://doi.org/10.23736/S0390-5616.18.04597-6. Epub 2018 Oct 2

Cordella R, Acerbi F (2013) Intraoperative neurophysiological monitoring of the cortico-spinal tract in image-guided mini-invasive neurosurgery. Clin Neurophysiol 124(6):1244–1254

Cosgrove GR, Buchbinder BR, Jiang H (1996) Functional magnetic resonance imaging for intracranial navigation. Neurosurg Clin N Am 7(2):313–322

Cox RW (1996) AFNI: software for analysis and visualization of functional magnetic resonance neuroimages. Comput Biomed Res 29(3):162–173

Csaba J (2003) Positron emission tomography in presurgical localization of epileptic foci. Ideggyogy Sz 56(7–8):249–254

Cuenod CA, Bookheimer SY et al (1995) Functional MRI during word generation, using conventional equipment: a potential tool for language localization in the clinical environment. Neurology 45(10):1821–1827

Cunningham JM, Morris GL III et al (2008) Unexpected right hemisphere language representation identified by the intracarotid procedure in right-handed epilepsy surgery candidates. Epilepsy Behav 13(1):139–143

Damasio AR, Geschwind N (1984) The neural basis of language. Annu Rev Neurosci 7:127–147. https://doi.org/10.1146/annurev.ne.07.030184.001015

Deblaere K, Backes WH et al (2002) Developing a comprehensive presurgical functional MRI protocol for patients with intractable temporal lobe epilepsy: a pilot study. Neuroradiology 44(8):667–673

Delfanti RL, Piccioni DE, Handwerker J, Bahrami N, Krishnan A, Karunamuni R, Hattangadi-Gluth JA, Seibert TM, Srikant A, Jones KA, Snyder VS, Dale AM, White NS, McDonald CR, Farid N (2017) Imaging correlates for the 2016 update on WHO classification of grade II/III gliomas: implications for IDH, 1p/19q and ATRX status. J Neuro-Oncol 135(3):601–609. https://doi.org/10.1007/s11060-017-2613-7. Epub 2017 Sept 4

DeMonte F, Gilbert MR et al (2007) Tumors of the brain and spine. In: MD Anderson cancer care series. Springer, New York, XII, 364 p

Deng X, Xu L, Zhang Y, Wang B, Wang S, Zhao Y, Cao Y, Zhang D, Wang R, Ye X, Wu J, Zhao J (2016) Difference of language cortex reorganization between cerebral arteriovenous malformations, cavernous malformations, and gliomas: a functional MRI study. Neurosurg Rev 39(2):241–9; discussion 249. https://doi.org/10.1007/s10143-015-0682-7. Epub 2015 Nov 13

Desmond JE, Sum JM et al (1995) Functional MRI measurement of language lateralization in Wada-tested patients. Brain 118(Pt 6):1411–1419

Deverdun J, van Dokkum LEH, Le Bars E, Herbet G, Mura T, D'agata B, Picot MC, Menjot N, Molino F, Duffau H, Moritz GS (2020) Language reorganization after resection of low-grade gliomas: an fMRI task based connectivity study. Brain Imaging Behav 14(5):1779–1791. https://doi.org/10.1007/s11682-019-00114-7

Diciotti S, Gavazzi C, Della Nave R, Boni E, Ginestroni A, Paoli L, Cecchi P, De Stefano N, Mascalchi M (2007) Self-paced frequency of a simple motor task and brain activation. An fMRI study in healthy subjects using an on-line monitor device. NeuroImage 38(3):402–412. https://doi.org/10.1016/j.neuroimage.2007.07.045. Epub 2007 Aug 11

Dimous S, Battisti RA et al (2013) A systematic review of functional magnetic resonance imaging and diffusion tensor imaging modalities used in presurgical planning of brain tumour resection. Neurosurg Rev 36(2):205–214

Dorfer C, Rydenhag B, Baltuch G, Buch V, Blount J, Bollo R, Gerrard J, Nilsson D, Roessler K, Rutka J, Sharan A, Spencer D, Cukiert A (2020) How technology is driving the landscape of epilepsy surgery.

Epilepsia 61(5):841–855. https://doi.org/10.1111/epi.16489. Epub 2020 Mar 29

Drake LR, Hillmer AT, Cai Z (2020) Approaches to PET imaging of glioblastoma. Molecules 25(3):568. https://doi.org/10.3390/molecules25030568

Dronkers NF (1996) A new brain region for coordinating speech articulation. Nature 384(6605):159–161. https://doi.org/10.1038/384159a0

Dronkers NF, Plaisant O, Iba-Zizen MT, Cabanis EA (2007) Paul Broca's historic cases: high resolution MR imaging of the brains of Leborgne and Lelong. Brain 130(Pt 5):1432–1441. https://doi.org/10.1093/brain/awm042. Epub 2007 Apr 2

Duffau H (2001) Acute functional reorganisation of the human motor cortex during resection of central lesions: a study using intraoperative brain mapping. J Neurol Neurosurg Psychiatry 70(4):506–513

Duffau H (2005) Lessons from brain mapping in surgery for low-grade glioma: insights into associations between tumour and brain plasticity. Lancet Neurol 4(8):476–486

Duffau H (2006) New concepts in surgery of WHO grade II gliomas: functional brain mapping, connectionism and plasticity—a review. J Neuro-Oncol 79(1):77–115

Duffau H, Capelle L et al (1999) Intra-operative direct electrical stimulations of the central nervous system: the Salpetriere experience with 60 patients. Acta Neurochir 141(11):1157–1167

Duffau H, Sichez JP, Lehericy S (2000) Intraoperative unmasking of brain redundant motor sites during resection of a precentral angioma: evidence using direct cortical stimulation. Ann Neurol 47(1):132–135

Duffau H, Bauchet L et al (2001) Functional compensation of the left dominant insula for language. Neuroreport 12(10):2159–2163

Duffau H, Capelle L et al (2002a) Intraoperative mapping of the subcortical language pathways using direct stimulations. An anatomo-functional study. Brain 125(Pt 1):199–214

Duffau H, Denvil D, Capelle L (2002b) Long term reshaping of language, sensory, and motor maps after glioma resection: a new parameter to integrate in the surgical strategy. J Neurol Neurosurg Psychiatry 72(4):511–556

Duffau H, Capelle L et al (2003) Usefulness of intraoperative electrical subcortical mapping during surgery for low-grade gliomas located within eloquent brain regions: functional results in a consecutive series of 103 patients. J Neurosurg 98(4):764–778

Dym RJ, Burns J et al (2011) Is functional MR imaging assessment of hemispheric language dominance as good as the WADA test? A meta-analysis. Radiology 261(2):446–455

Dymarkowski S, Sunaert S et al (1998) Functional MRI of the brain: localisation of eloquent cortex in focal brain lesion therapy. Eur Radiol 8(9):1573–1580

Ellis DG, White ML, Hayasaka S, Warren DE, Wilson TW, Aizenberg MR (2020) Accuracy analysis of fMRI and MEG activations determined by intraoperative mapping. Neurosurg Focus 48(2):E13. https://doi.org/10.3171/2019.11.FOCUS19784

Esposito F, Seifritz E, Formisano E, Morrone R, Scarabino T, Tedeschi G, Cirillo S, Goebel R, Di Salle F (2003) Real-time independent component analysis of fMRI time-series. NeuroImage 20(4):2209–2224. https://doi.org/10.1016/j.neuroimage.2003.08.012

Fakhri M, All Oghablan M et al (2013) Atypical language lateralization: an fMRI study in patients with cerebral lesions. Funct Neurol 28(1):55–61

Fan X, Roberts DW, Olson JD, Ji S, Schaewe TJ, Simon DA, Paulsen KD (2018) Image updating for brain shift compensation during resection. Oper Neurosurg (Hagerstown) 14(4):402–411. https://doi.org/10.1093/ons/opx123

Fandino J, Kollias SS et al (1999) Intraoperative validation of functional magnetic resonance imaging and cortical reorganization patterns in patients with brain tumors involving the primary motor cortex. J Neurosurg 91(2):238–250

Farrens AJ, Zonnino A, Erwin A, O'Malley MK, Johnson CL, Ress D, Sergi F (2018) Quantitative testing of fMRI-compatibility of an electrically active mechatronic device for robot-assisted sensorimotor protocols. IEEE Trans Biomed Eng 65(7):1595–1606. https://doi.org/10.1109/TBME.2017.2741346. Epub 2017 Aug 17

Feigl GC, Safavi-Abbasi S, Gharabaghi A, Gonzalez-Felipe V, El Shawarby A, Freund HJ, Samii M (2008) Real-time 3T fMRI data of brain tumour patients for intra-operative localization of primary motor areas. Eur J Surg Oncol 34(6):708–715. https://doi.org/10.1016/j.ejso.2007.06.011. Epub 2007 Sept 29

Fernandez G, de Greiff A et al (2001) Language mapping in less than 15 minutes: real-time functional MRI during routine clinical investigation. NeuroImage 14(3):585–594

Fesl G, Moriggl B et al (2003) Inferior central sulcus: variations of anatomy and function on the example of the motor tongue area. NeuroImage 20(1):601–610

Findley AM, Ambrose JB et al (2012) Dynamics of hemispheric dominance for language assessed by magnetoencephalographic imaging. Ann Neurol 71(5):668–686

Fink JR, Muzi M, Peck M, Krohn KA (2015) Multimodality brain tumor imaging: MR imaging, PET, and PET/MR imaging. J Nucl Med 56(10):1554–1561. https://doi.org/10.2967/jnumed.113.131516. Epub 2015 Aug 20

Fisicaro RA, Jiao RX, Stathopoulos C, Petrovich Brennan NM, Peck KK, Holodny AI (2015) Challenges in identifying the foot motor region in patients with brain tumor on routine MRI: advantages of fMRI. AJNR Am J Neuroradiol 36(8):1488–1493. https://doi.org/10.3174/ajnr.A4292. Epub 2015 Apr 16

FitzGerald DB, Cosgrove GR et al (1997) Location of language in the cortex: a comparison between functional MR imaging and electrocortical stimulation. AJNR Am J Neuroradiol 18(8):1529–1539

Flinker A, Korzeniewska A, Shestyuk AY, Franaszczuk PJ, Dronkers NF, Knight RT, Crone NE (2015) Redefining the role of Broca's area in speech. Proc Natl Acad Sci U S A 112(9):2871–2875. https://doi.org/10.1073/pnas.1414491112. Epub 2015 Feb 17

Fox PT, Mintun MA et al (1986) Mapping human visual cortex with positron emission tomography. Nature 323(6091):806–809

Frahm J, Merboldt KD et al (1994) Brain or vein—oxygenation or flow? On signal physiology in functional MRI of human brain activation. NMR Biomed 7(1–2):45–53

Friston K (1996) Statistical parametric mapping and other analyses of functional imaging data. In: Mazziotta J, Toga AW (eds) Brain mapping: the methods. Academic, New York, pp 363–386

Frost JA, Binder JR et al (1999) Language processing is strongly left lateralized in both sexes. Evidence from functional MRI. Brain 122(Pt 2):199–208

Gabrieli JD, Poldrack RA, Desmond JE (1998) The role of left prefrontal cortex in language and memory. Proc Natl Acad Sci U S A 95(3):906–913

Gaillard WD, Bookheimer SY, Cohen M (2000a) The use of fMRI in neocortical epilepsy. Adv Neurol 84:391–404

Gaillard WD, Hertz-Pannier L et al (2000b) Functional anatomy of cognitive development: fMRI of verbal fluency in children and adults. Neurology 54(1):180–185

Gaillard WD, Grandin GB, Xu B (2001a) Developmental aspects of pediatric fMRI: considerations for image acquisition, analysis, and interpretation. NeuroImage 13(2):239–249

Gaillard WD, Pugliese M et al (2001b) Cortical localization of reading in normal children: an fMRI language study. Neurology 57(1):47–54

Gaillard WD, Balsamo L et al (2002) Language dominance in partial epilepsy patients identified with an fMRI reading task. Neurology 59(2):256–265

García-Eulate R, García-García D et al (2011) Functional bold MRI: advantages of the 3 T vs. the 1.5 T. Clin Imaging 35(3):236–241

Garin CM, Nadkarni NA, Landeau B, Chételat G, Picq JL, Bougacha S, Dhenain M (2021) Resting state functional atlas and cerebral networks in mouse lemur primates at 11.7 Tesla. NeuroImage 226:117589. https://doi.org/10.1016/j.neuroimage.2020.117589. Epub 2020 Nov 26

Gasser T, Ganslandt O et al (2005) Intraoperative functional MRI: implementation and preliminary experience. NeuroImage 26(3):685–693

Gene M, Brennan NP, Holodny AI (2021) Patient preparation and paradigm design in fMRI. Neuroimaging Clin N Am 31(1):11–21. https://doi.org/10.1016/j.nic.2020.09.007. Epub 2020 Oct 29

Georgi JC, Stippich C et al (2004) Active deep brain stimulation during MRI: a feasibility study. Magn Reson Med 51(2):380–388

Gerard IJ, Kersten-Oertel M, Petrecca K, Sirhan D, Hall JA, Collins DL (2017) Brain shift in neuronavigation of brain tumors: a review. Med Image Anal 35:403–420. Review. https://doi.org/10.1016/j.media.2016.08.007. Epub 2016 Aug 24

Geschwind N (1971) Current concepts: aphasia. N Engl J Med 284(12):654–656

Geschwind N (1972) Language and the brain. Sci Am 226(4):76–83. https://doi.org/10.1038/scientificamerican0472-76

Gevins A (1995) High-resolution electroencephalographic studies of cognition. Adv Neurol 66:181–195; discussion 195–198

Gevins A, Leong H et al (1995) Mapping cognitive brain function with modern high-resolution electroencephalography. Trends Neurosci 18(10):429–436

Gil-Robles S, Duffau H (2010) Surgical management of World Health Organization Grade II gliomas in eloquent areas: the necessity of preserving a margin around functional structures. Neurosurg Focus 28(2):E8

Giussani C, Roux FE, Ojemann J, Sganzerla EP, Pirillo D, Papagno C (2010) Is preoperative functional magnetic resonance imaging reliable for language areas mapping in brain tumor surgery? Review of language functional magnetic resonance imaging and direct cortical stimulation correlation studies. Neurosurgery 66(1):113–120. https://doi.org/10.1227/01.NEU.0000360392.15450.C9

Golaszewski SM, Zschiegner F et al (2002) A new pneumatic vibrator for functional magnetic resonance imaging of the human sensorimotor cortex. Neurosci Lett 324(2):125–128

Golaszewski SM, Siedentopf CM et al (2004) Modulatory effects on human sensorimotor cortex by whole-hand afferent electrical stimulation. Neurology 62(12):2262–2269

Golaszewski SM, Siedentopf CM et al (2006) Human brain structures related to plantar vibrotactile stimulation: a functional magnetic resonance imaging study. NeuroImage 29(3):923–929

Gold S, Christian B et al (1998) Functional MRI statistical software packages: a comparative analysis. Hum Brain Mapp 6(2):73–84

González-Darder JM, González-López P (2010) Multimodal navigation in the functional microsurgical resection of intrinsic brain tumors located in eloquent motor areas: role of tractography. Neurosurg Focus 28(2):E5

Grabowski TJ (2000) Investigating language with functional neuroimaging. In: Mazziotta J, Toga AW (eds) Brain mapping: the systems. Academic, San Diego, pp 425–461

Grummich P, Nimsky C et al (2006) Combining fMRI and MEG increases the reliability of presurgical language localization: a clinical study on the difference between and congruence of both modalities. NeuroImage 32(4):1793–1803

Håberg A, Kvistad KA et al (2004) Preoperative blood oxygen level-dependent functional magnetic resonance imaging in patients with primary brain tumors: clinical application and outcome. Neurosurgery 54(4):902–914; discussion 914–915

Hajnal JV, Myers R et al (1994) Artifacts due to stimulus correlated motion in functional imaging of the brain. Magn Reson Med 31(3):283–291

Hall WA, Liu H, Truwit CL (2005) Functional magnetic resonance imaging-guided resection of low-grade gliomas. Surg Neurol 64(1):20–27; discussion 27

Hämäläinen M, Ilmoniemi RJ, Knuutila J, Lounasmaa OV (1993) Magnetoencephalography—theory, instrumentation and applications to noninvasive studies of the working human brain. Rev Mod Phys 65:413–487

Hammeke TA, Yetkin FZ et al (1994) Functional magnetic resonance imaging of somatosensory stimulation. Neurosurgery 35(4):677–681

Hammeke TA, Bellgowan PS, Binder JR (2000) fMRI: methodology—cognitive function mapping. Adv Neurol 83:221–233

Hari R, Ilmoniemi RJ (1986) Cerebral magnetic fields. Crit Rev Biomed Eng 14(2):93–126

Hasegawa M, Carpenter PA, Just MA (2002) An fMRI study of bilingual sentence comprehension and workload. NeuroImage 15(3):647–660

Hayashi Y, Kinoshita M et al (2012) Correlation between language function and the left arcuate fasciculus detected by diffusion tensor imaging tractography. J Neurosurg 117(5):839–843

Hazzaa NM, Mancini L, Thornton J, Yousry TA (2019) Somatotopic organization of corticospinal/corticobulbar motor tracts in controls and patients with tumours: A combined fMRI-DTI study. Neuroimage Clin 23:101910. https://doi.org/10.1016/j.nicl.2019.101910. Epub 2019 Jun 26

Henderson F, Abdullah KG, Verma R, Brem S (2020) Tractography and the connectome in neurosurgical treatment of gliomas: the premise, the progress, and the potential. Neurosurg Focus 48(2):E6. https://doi.org/10.3171/2019.11.FOCUS19785

Herholz K, Reulen HJ et al (1997) Preoperative activation and intraoperative stimulation of language-related areas in patients with glioma. Neurosurgery 41(6):1253–1260; discussion 1260–1262

Hermann BP, Perrine K et al (1999) Visual confrontation naming following left anterior temporal lobectomy: a comparison of surgical approaches. Neuropsychology 13(1):3–9

Hernandez AE, Dapretto M et al (2001) Language switching and language representation in Spanish-English bilinguals: an fMRI study. NeuroImage 14(2):510–520

Hertz-Pannier L, Gaillard WD et al (1997) Noninvasive assessment of language dominance in children and adolescents with functional MRI: a preliminary study. Neurology 48(4):1003–1012

Hertz-Pannier L, Chiron C et al (2002) Late plasticity for language in a child's non-dominant hemisphere: a pre- and post-surgery fMRI study. Brain 125(Pt 2):361–372

Hinke RM, Hu X et al (1993) Functional magnetic resonance imaging of Broca's area during internal speech. Neuroreport 4(6):675–678

Hirsch J, Ruge MI et al (2000) An integrated functional magnetic resonance imaging procedure for preoperative mapping of cortical areas associated with tactile,

motor, language, and visual functions. Neurosurgery 47(3):711–721; discussion 721–722

Hoeller M, Krings T et al (2002) Movement artefacts and MR BOLD signal increase during different paradigms for mapping the sensorimotor cortex. Acta Neurochir (Wien) 144(3):279–284; discussion 284

Holman BL, Devous MD Sr (1992) Functional brain SPECT: the emergence of a powerful clinical method. J Nucl Med 33(10):1888–1904

Holodny AI, Schulder M et al (1999) Decreased BOLD functional MR activation of the motor and sensory cortices adjacent to a glioblastoma multiforme: implications for image-guided neurosurgery. AJNR Am J Neuroradiol 20(4):609–612

Holodny AI, Schulder M et al (2000) The effect of brain tumors on BOLD functional MR imaging activation in the adjacent motor cortex: implications for image-guided neurosurgery. AJNR Am J Neuroradiol 21(8):1415–1422

Holodny AI, Schwartz TH et al (2001) Tumor involvement of the corticospinal tract: diffusion magnetic resonance tractography with intraoperative correlation. J Neurosurg 95(6):1082

Holodny AI, Schulder M, Ybasco A, Liu WC (2002) Translocation of Broca's area to the contralateral hemisphere as the result of the growth of a left inferior frontal glioma. J Comput Assist Tomogr 26(6):941–943. https://doi.org/10.1097/00004728-200211000-00014

Holodny AI, Shevzov-Zebrun N, Brennan N, Peck KK (2011) Motor and sensory mapping. Neurosurg Clin N Am 22(2):207–218., viii. Review. https://doi.org/10.1016/j.nec.2010.11.003

Hou BL, Bradbury M et al (2006) Effect of brain tumor neovasculature defined by rCBV on BOLD fMRI activation volume in the primary motor cortex. NeuroImage 32(2):489–497

Hsu CC, Wu MT, Lee C (2001) Robust image registration for functional magnetic resonance imaging of the brain. Med Biol Eng Comput 39(5):517–524

Huber L, Tse DHY, Wiggins CJ, Uludağ K, Kashyap S, Jangraw DC, Bandettini PA, Poser BA, Ivanov D (2018) Ultra-high resolution blood volume fMRI and BOLD fMRI in humans at 9.4 T: capabilities and challenges. NeuroImage 178:769–779. https://doi.org/10.1016/j.neuroimage.2018.06.025. Epub 2018 Jun 8

Hulvershorn J, Bloy L et al (2005a) Spatial sensitivity and temporal response of spin echo and gradient echo bold contrast at 3 T using peak hemodynamic activation time. NeuroImage 24(1):216–223

Hulvershorn J, Bloy L et al (2005b) Temporal resolving power of spin echo and gradient echo fMRI at 3 T with apparent diffusion coefficient compartmentalization. Hum Brain Mapp 25(2):247–258

Humbert O, Bourg V, Mondot L, Gal J, Bondiau PY, Fontaine D, Saada-Bouzid E, Paquet M, Chardin D, Almairac F, Vandenbos F, Darcourt J (2019) (18) F-DOPA PET/CT in brain tumors: impact on multidisciplinary brain tumor board decisions. Eur J Nucl Med

Mol Imaging 46(3):558–568. https://doi.org/10.1007/s00259-018-4240-8. Epub 2019 Jan 5

Illes J, Francis WS et al (1999) Convergent cortical representation of semantic processing in bilinguals. Brain Lang 70(3):347–363

Iv M, Bisdas S (2021) Neuroimaging in the era of the evolving WHO classification of brain tumors, from the AJR special series on cancer staging. AJR Am J Roentgenol. https://doi.org/10.2214/AJR.20.25246. Online ahead of print

Jack CR Jr, Thompson PM et al (1994) Sensory motor cortex: correlation of presurgical mapping with functional MR imaging and invasive cortical mapping. Radiology 190(1):85–92

Jacobs AH, Kracht LW et al (2005) Imaging in neuro-oncology. NeuroRx 2(2):333–347

Janecek JK, Swanson SJ et al (2013) Language lateralization by fMRI and WADA testing in 229 patients with epilepsy: rates and predictors of discordance. Epilepsia 54(2):314–322

Jansma JM, Ramsey N, Rutten GJ (2015) A comparison of brain activity associated with language production in brain tumor patients with left and right sided language laterality. J Neurosurg Sci 59(4):327–335. Epub 2015 Sep 3

Jia XX, Yu Y et al (2013) FMRI-driven DTT-assessment of corticospinal tracts prior to cortex resection. Can J Neurol Sci 40(4):558–563

Jiang Z, Krainik A (2010) Impaired fMRI activation in patients with primary brain tumors. NeuroImage 52(2):538–548

Johnson DR, Guerin JB, Giannini C, Morris JM, Eckel LJ, Kaufmann TJ (2017) 2016 Updates to the WHO brain tumor classification system: what the radiologist needs to know. Radiographics 37(7):2164–2180. Review. https://doi.org/10.1148/rg.2017170037. Epub 2017 Oct 13

Jovčevska I, Kočevar N, Komel R (2013) Glioma and glioblastoma—how much do we (not) know? Mol Clin Oncol 1(6):935–941

Just MA, Carpenter PA et al (1996) Brain activation modulated by sentence comprehension. Science 274(5284):114–116

Kampe KK, Jones RA, Auer DP (2000) Frequency dependence of the functional MRI response after electrical median nerve stimulation. Hum Brain Mapp 9(2):106–114

Kasprian G, Seidel S (2010) Modern neuroimaging of brain plasticity. Radiologe 50(2):136–143

Kaye AH, Laws ER (2011) Brain tumors: an encyclopedic approach, expert consult—online and print, 3rd edn. Saunders, St. Louis

Killgore WD, Glosser G et al (1999) Functional MRI and the Wada test provide complementary information for predicting post-operative seizure control. Seizure 8(8):450–455

Kim KH, Relkin NR et al (1997) Distinct cortical areas associated with native and second languages. Nature 388(6638):171–174

Kim MJ, Holodny AI et al (2005) The effect of prior surgery on blood oxygen level-dependent functional MR imaging in the preoperative assessment of brain tumors. AJNR Am J Neuroradiol 26(8):1980–1985

Klein D, Milner B et al (1995) The neural substrates underlying word generation: a bilingual functional-imaging study. Proc Natl Acad Sci U S A 92(7):2899–2903

Kober H, Nimsky C et al (2001) Correlation of sensorimotor activation with functional magnetic resonance imaging and magnetoencephalography in presurgical functional imaging: a spatial analysis. NeuroImage 14(5):1214–1228

Kokkonen SM, Kiviniemi V et al (2005) Effect of brain surgery on auditory and motor cortex activation: a preliminary functional magnetic resonance imaging study. Neurosurgery 57(2):249–256; discussion 249–256

Kong NW, Gibb WR, Badhe S, Liu BP, Tate MC (2020) Plasticity of the primary motor cortex in patients with primary brain tumors. Neural Plast 2020:3648517, eCollection 2020. https://doi.org/10.1155/2020/3648517

Konrad F, Nennig E et al (2005) Does the individual adaptation of standardized speech paradigms for clinical functional magnetic resonance imaging (fMRI) effect the localization of the language-dominant hemisphere and of Broca's and Wernicke's areas. Rofo 177(3):381–385

Krainik A, Lehericy S et al (2001) Role of the supplementary motor area in motor deficit following medial frontal lobe surgery. Neurology 57(5):871–878

Krainik A, Lehericy S et al (2003) Postoperative speech disorder after medial frontal surgery: role of the supplementary motor area. Neurology 60(4):587–594

Krainik A, Duffau H et al (2004) Role of the healthy hemisphere in recovery after resection of the supplementary motor area. Neurology 62(8):1323–1332

Krasnow B, Tamm L et al (2003) Comparison of fMRI activation at 3 T and 1.5 T during perceptual, cognitive, and effective processing. NeuroImage 18(4):813–826

Krings T, Buchbinder BR et al (1997) Functional magnetic resonance imaging and transcranial magnetic stimulation: complementary approaches in the evaluation of cortical motor function. Neurology 48(5):1406–1416

Krings T, Reul J et al (1998) Functional magnetic resonance mapping of sensory motor cortex for image-guided neurosurgical intervention. Acta Neurochir (Wien) 140(3):215–222

Krings T, Erberich SG et al (1999) MR blood oxygenation level-dependent signal differences in parenchymal and large draining vessels: implications for functional MR imaging. AJNR Am J Neuroradiol 20(10):1907–1914

Krings T, Reinges MH et al (2001) Functional MRI for presurgical planning: problems, artefacts, and solution strategies. J Neurol Neurosurg Psychiatry 70(6):749–760

Krings T, Reinges MH et al (2002a) Factors related to the magnitude of T2* MR signal changes during functional imaging. Neuroradiology 44(6):459–466

Krings T, Topper R et al (2002b) Activation in primary and secondary motor areas in patients with CNS neoplasms and weakness. Neurology 58(3): 381–390

Krishnan R, Raabe A et al (2004) Functional magnetic resonance imaging-integrated neuronavigation: correlation between lesion-to-motor cortex distance and outcome. Neurosurgery 55(4):904–914; discusssion 914–915

Kuhnt D, Bauer MH, Nimsky C (2012) Brain shift compensation and neurosurgical image fusion using intraoperative MRI: current status and future challenges. Crit Rev Biomed Eng 40(3):175–185. Review. https://doi.org/10.1615/critrevbiomedeng.v40.i3.20

Kumar A, Chandra PS et al (2014) The role of neuronavigation-guided functional MRI and diffusion tensor tractography along with cortical stimulation in patients with eloquent cortex lesions. Br J Neurosurg 28(2):226–233

Kundu B, Penwarden A, Wood JM, Gallagher TA, Andreoli MJ, Voss J, Meier T, Nair VA, Kuo JS, Field AS, Moritz C, Meyerand ME, Prabhakaran V (2013) Association of functional magnetic resonance imaging indices with postoperative language outcomes in patients with primary brain tumors. Neurosurg Focus 34(4):E6. https://doi.org/10.3171/2013.2.FOCUS12413

Kundu B, Rolston JD, Grandhi R (2019) Mapping language dominance through the lens of the Wada test. Neurosurg Focus 47(3):E5. https://doi.org/10.3171/2019.6.FOCUS19346

Kurth R, Villringer K et al (1998) fMRI assessment of somatotopy in human Brodmann area 3b by electrical finger stimulation. Neuroreport 9(2):207–212

Kwong KK, Belliveau JW et al (1992) Dynamic magnetic resonance imaging of human brain activity during primary sensory stimulation. Proc Natl Acad Sci U S A 89(12):5675–5679

la Fougère C, Rominger A et al (2009) PET and SPECT in epilepsy: a critical review. Epilepsy Behav 15(1):50–55

Landis SH, Murray T et al (1999) Cancer statistics, 1999. CA Cancer J Clin 49(1):8–31, 1

Latchaw RE, Ugurbil K, Hu X (1995) Functional MR imaging of perceptual and cognitive functions. Neuroimaging Clin N Am 5(2):193–205

Lazar RM, Marshall RS et al (1997) Anterior translocation of language in patients with left cerebral arteriovenous malformation. Neurology 49(3): 802–808

Leclercq D, Delmaire C, de Champfleur NM, Chiras J, Lehéricy S (2011) Diffusion tractography: methods, validation and applications in patients with neurosurgical lesions. Neurosurg Clin N Am 22(2):253–268., ix. Review. https://doi.org/10.1016/j.nec.2010.11.004

Lee CC, Jack CR Jr et al (1996) Real-time adaptive motion correction in functional MRI. Magn Reson Med 36(3):436–444

Lee CC, Grimm RC et al (1998a) A prospective approach to correct for inter-image head rotation in fMRI. Magn Reson Med 39(2):234–243

Lee CC, Jack CR Jr, Riederer SJ (1998b) Mapping of the central sulcus with functional MR: active versus passive activation tasks. AJNR Am J Neuroradiol 19(5):847–852

Lee CC, Jack CR Jr et al (1998c) Real-time reconstruction and high-speed processing in functional MR imaging. AJNR Am J Neuroradiol 19(7):1297–1300

Lee CC, Ward HA et al (1999) Assessment of functional MR imaging in neurosurgical planning. AJNR Am J Neuroradiol 20(8):1511–1519

Lee MH, Smyser CD, Shimony JS (2012) Resting-state fMRI: a review of methods and clinical applications. AJNR Am J Neuroradiol 34(10):1866–1872

Lee MH, Smyser CD, Shimony JS (2013) Resting-state fMRI: a review of methods and clinical applications. AJNR Am J Neuroradiol 34(10):1866–1872. https://doi.org/10.3174/ajnr.A3263. Epub 2012 Aug 30

Lee MH, Miller-Thomas MM, Benzinger TL, Marcus DS, Hacker CD, Leuthardt EC, Shimony JS (2016) Clinical resting-state fMRI in the preoperative setting: are we ready for prime time? Top Magn Reson Imaging 25(1):11–18. https://doi.org/10.1097/RMR.0000000000000075

Lehericy S, Cohen L et al (2000a) Functional MR evaluation of temporal and frontal language dominance compared with the Wada test. Neurology 54(8): 1625–1633

Lehericy S, Duffau H et al (2000b) Correspondence between functional magnetic resonance imaging somatotopy and individual brain anatomy of the central region: comparison with intraoperative stimulation in patients with brain tumors. J Neurosurg 92(4):589–598

Lehericy S, Biondi A et al (2002) Arteriovenous brain malformations: is functional MR imaging reliable for studying language reorganization in patients? Initial observations. Radiology 223(3):672–682

Lemée JM, Berro DH, Bernard F, Chinier E, Leiber LM, Menei P, Ter Minassian A (2019) Resting-state functional magnetic resonance imaging versus task-based activity for language mapping and correlation with perioperative cortical mapping. Brain Behav 9(10):e01362. https://doi.org/10.1002/brb3.1362. Epub 2019 Sept 30

Leung LWL, Unadkat P, Bertotti MM, Bi WL, Essayed W, Bunevicius A, Chavakula V, Rigolo L, Fumagalli L, Tie Z, Golby AJ, Tie Y (2020) Clinical utility of preoperative bilingual language fMRI mapping in patients with brain tumors. J Neuroimaging 30(2):175–183. https://doi.org/10.1111/jon.12690. Epub 2020 Feb 10

Lewis MA, Ganeshan B, Barnes A, Bisdas S, Jaunmuktane Z, Brandner S, Endozo R, Groves A, Thust SC (2019) Filtration-histogram based magnetic resonance texture analysis (MRTA) for glioma IDH and 1p19q genotyping. Eur J Radiol 113:116–123. https://

doi.org/10.1016/j.ejrad.2019.02.014. Epub 2019 Feb 13

Li M, Jiang P, Wu J, Guo R, Deng X, Cao Y, Wang S (2020) Altered brain structural networks in patients with brain arteriovenous malformations located in broca's area. Neural Plast 24;2020:8886803. https://doi.org/10.1155/2020/8886803

Lichtheim L (1885) On aphasia. Brain 7:433–484

Lima Cardoso P, Fischmeister FPS, Dymerska B, Geißler A, Wurnig M, Trattnig S, Beisteiner R, Robinson SD (2017) Robust presurgical functional MRI at 7 T using response consistency. Hum Brain Mapp 38(6):3163–3174. https://doi.org/10.1002/hbm.23582. Epub 2017 Mar 21

Liouta E, Katsaros VK, Stranjalis G, Leks E, Klose U, Bisdas S (2019) Motor and language deficits correlate with resting state functional magnetic resonance imaging networks in patients with brain tumors. J Neuroradiol 46(3):199–206. https://doi.org/10.1016/j.neurad.2018.08.002. Epub 2018 Sept 1

Liu G, Ogawa S (2006) EPI image reconstruction with correction of distortion and signal losses. J Magn Reson Imaging 24(3):683–689

Liu H, Hall WA, Truwit CL (2003) The roles of functional MRI in MR-guided neurosurgery in a combined 1.5 Tesla MR-operating room. Acta Neurochir Suppl 85:127–135

Liu WC, Feldman SC et al (2005) The effect of tumour type and distance on activation in the motor cortex. Neuroradiology 47(11):813–819

Liu H, Buckner RL et al (2009) Task-free presurgical mapping using functional magnetic resonance imaging intrinsic activity. J Neurosurg 111(4):746–754

Liu F, Wang L, Lou Y, Li RC, Purdon PL (2021) Probabilistic structure learning for EEG/MEG source imaging with hierarchical graph priors. IEEE Trans Med Imaging 40(1):321–334. https://doi.org/10.1109/TMI.2020.3025608. Epub 2020 Dec 29

Logan WJ (1999) Functional magnetic resonance imaging in children. Semin Pediatr Neurol 6(2):78–86

Logothetis NK (2002) The neural basis of the blood-oxygen-level-dependent functional magnetic resonance imaging signal. Philos Trans R Soc Lond B Biol Sci 357(1424):1003–1037

Logothetis NK (2003) The underpinnings of the BOLD functional magnetic resonance imaging signal. J Neurosci 23(10):3963–3971

Logothetis NK, Pfeuffer J (2004) On the nature of the BOLD fMRI contrast mechanism. Magn Reson Imaging 22(10):1517–1531

Logothetis NK, Wandell BA (2004) Interpreting the BOLD signal. Annu Rev Physiol 66:735–769

Logothetis NK, Pauls J et al (2001) Neurophysiological investigation of the basis of the fMRI signal. Nature 412(6843):150–157

Louis DN, Ohgaki H et al (2007) The 2007 WHO classification of tumours of the central nervous system. Acta Neuropathol 114(2):97–109

Louis DN, Perry A, Reifenberger G, von Deimling A, Figarella-Branger D, Cavenee WK, Ohgaki H, Wiestler OD, Kleihues P, Ellison DW (2016) The 2016 World Health Organization classification of tumors of the central nervous system: a summary. Acta Neuropathol 131(6):803–20. Review. https://doi.org/10.1007/s00401-016-1545-1. Epub 2016 May 9

Ludemann L, Forschler A et al (2006) BOLD signal in the motor cortex shows a correlation with the blood volume of brain tumors. J Magn Reson Imaging 23(4):435–443

Lührs M, Sorger B, Goebel R, Esposito F (2017) Automated selection of brain regions for real-time fMRI brain-computer interfaces. J Neural Eng 14(1):016004. https://doi.org/10.1088/1741-2560/14/1/016004. Epub 2016 Nov 30

Lurito JT, Lowe MJ et al (2000) Comparison of fMRI and intraoperative direct cortical stimulation in localization of receptive language areas. J Comput Assist Tomogr 24(1):99–105

Majos A, Tybor K et al (2005) Cortical mapping by functional magnetic resonance imaging in patients with brain tumors. Eur Radiol 15(6):1148–1158

Manan HA, Franz EA, Yahya N (2020) Utilization of functional MRI language paradigms for pre-operative mapping: a systematic review. Neuroradiology 62(3):353–367. https://doi.org/10.1007/s00234-019-02322-w. Epub 2019 Dec 4

Mancini M, Vos SB, Vakharia VN, O'Keeffe AG, Trimmel K, Barkhof F, Dorfer C, Soman S, Winston GP, Wu C, Duncan JS, Sparks R, Ourselin S (2019) Automated fiber tract reconstruction for surgery planning: extensive validation in language-related white matter tracts. Neuroimage Clin 23:101883. https://doi.org/10.1016/j.nicl.2019.101883. Epub 2019 May 28

Manglore S, Dawn Bharath RD et al (2013) Utility of resting fMRI and connectivity in patients with brain tumor. Neurol India 61(2):144–151

Mark IT, Black DF, DeLone DR, Passe TJ, Witte RJ, Little JT, Ho ML, Fagan AJ, Parney IF, Burns TC, Welker KM (2021) Higher temporal resolution multiband fMRI provides improved presurgical language maps. Neuroradiology 63(3):439–445. https://doi.org/10.1007/s00234-020-02569-8. Epub 2020 Oct 6

Massot-Tarrús A, White KP, Mousavi SR, Hayman-Abello S, Hayman-Abello B, Mirsattari SM (2020) Concordance between fMRI and Wada test for memory lateralization in temporal lobe epilepsy: a meta-analysis and systematic review. Epilepsy Behav 107:107065. https://doi.org/10.1016/j.yebeh.2020.107065. Epub 2020 Apr 7

Mazziotta JC, Phelps ME et al (1982) Tomographic mapping of human cerebral metabolism: auditory stimulation. Neurology 32(9):921–937

McKinney PA (2004) Brain tumours: incidence, survival, and aetiology. J Neurol Neurosurg Psychiatry 75(Suppl II):ii12–ii17

Meinhold T, Hofer W, Pieper T, Kudernatsch M, Staudt M (2020) Presurgical language fMRI in children, adolescents and young adults: a validation study. Clin Neuroradiol 30(4):691–704. https://doi.org/10.1007/s00062-019-00852-7. Epub 2020 Jan 20

Menon RS, Ogawa S et al (1995) BOLD based functional MRI at 4 Tesla includes a capillary bed contribution: echoplanar imaging correlates with previous optical imaging using intrinsic signals. Magn Reson Med 33(3):453–459

Metwali H, Raemaekers M, Kniese K, Kardavani B, Fahlbusch R, Samii A (2019) Reliability of functional magnetic resonance imaging in patients with brain tumors: a critical review and meta-analysis. World Neurosurg 125:183–190. https://doi.org/10.1016/j.wneu.2019.01.194. Epub 2019 Feb 8

Mitchell TJ, Hacker CD et al (2013) A novel data-driven approach to preoperative mapping of functional cortex using resting-state functional magnetic resonance imaging. Neurosurgery 73(6):969–982

Moller M, Freund M et al (2005) Real time fMRI: a tool for the routine presurgical localisation of the motor cortex. Eur Radiol 15(2):292–295

Morita N, Wang S et al (2011) Diffusion tensor imaging of the corticospinal tract in patients with brain neoplasms. Magn Reson Med Sci 10(4):239–243

Morris GL 3rd, Mueller WM et al (1994) Functional magnetic resonance imaging in partial epilepsy. Epilepsia 35(6):1194–1198

Mueller WM, Yetkin FZ et al (1996) Functional magnetic resonance imaging mapping of the motor cortex in patients with cerebral tumors. Neurosurgery 39(3):515–520; discussion 520–521

Müller RA, Rothermel RD et al (1998) Determination of language dominance by [^{15}O]-water PET in children and adolescents: a comparison with the Wada test. J Epilepsy 11(3):152–161

Nadkarni TN, Andreoli MJ, Nair VA, Yin P, Young BM, Kundu B, Pankratz J, Radtke A, Holdsworth R, Kuo JS, Field AS, Baskaya MK, Moritz CH, Meyerand ME, Prabhakaran V (2014) Usage of fMRI for pre-surgical planning in brain tumor and vascular lesion patients: task and statistical threshold effects on language lateralization. Neuroimage Clin 7:415–423, eCollection 2015. https://doi.org/10.1016/j.nicl.2014.12.014

Naidich TP, Hof PR et al (2001) Anatomic substrates of language: emphasizing speech. Neuroimaging Clin N Am 11(2):305–341, ix

Nenert R, Allendorfer JB, Martin AM, Banks C, Vannest J, Holland SK, Szaflarski JP (2017) Age-related language lateralization assessed by fMRI: the effects of sex and handedness. Brain Res 1674:20–35. https://doi.org/10.1016/j.brainres.2017.08.021. Epub 2017 Aug 19

Newton JM, Dong Y, Hidler J, Plummer-D'Amato P, Marehbian J, Albistegui-Dubois RM, Woods RP, Dobkin BH (2008) Reliable assessment of lower limb motor representations with fMRI: use of a novel MR compatible device for real-time monitoring of ankle, knee and hip torques. NeuroImage 43(1):136–146. https://doi.org/10.1016/j.neuroimage.2008.07.001. Epub 2008 Jul 15

Nimsky C (2011) Intraoperative acquisition of fMRI and DTI. Neurosurg Clin N Am 22(2):269–277, ix. https://doi.org/10.1016/j.nec.2010.11.005

Nimsky C, Ganslandt O et al (2006) Intraoperative visualization for resection of gliomas: the role of functional neuronavigation and intraoperative 1.5 T MRI. Neurol Res 28(5):482–487

Nitschke MF, Melchert UH et al (1998) Preoperative functional magnetic resonance imaging (fMRI) of the motor system in patients with tumours in the parietal lobe. Acta Neurochir (Wien) 140(12):1223–1229

Niu C, Zhang M, Min Z, Rana N, Zhang Q, Liu X, Li M, Lin P (2014) Motor network plasticity and low-frequency oscillations abnormalities in patients with brain gliomas: a functional MRI study. PLoS One 9(5):e96850, eCollection 2014. https://doi.org/10.1371/journal.pone.0096850

Oda K, Yamaguchi F, Enomoto H, Higuchi T, Morita A (2018) Prediction of recovery from supplementary motor area syndrome after brain tumor surgery: preoperative diffusion tensor tractography analysis and postoperative neurological clinical course. Neurosurg Focus 44(6):E3. https://doi.org/10.3171/2017.12.FOCUS17564

Ogawa S, Lee TM et al (1990a) Brain magnetic resonance imaging with contrast dependent on blood oxygenation. Proc Natl Acad Sci U S A 87(24):9868–9872

Ogawa S, Lee TM et al (1990b) Oxygenation-sensitive contrast in magnetic resonance image of rodent brain at high magnetic fields. Magn Reson Med 14(1):68–78

Ogawa S, Tank DW et al (1992) Intrinsic signal changes accompanying sensory stimulation: functional brain mapping with magnetic resonance imaging. Proc Natl Acad Sci U S A 89(13):5951–5955

Ogawa S, Menon RS et al (1993) Functional brain mapping by blood oxygenation level-dependent contrast magnetic resonance imaging. A comparison of signal characteristics with a biophysical model. Biophys J 64(3):803–812

Ohgaki H (2009) Epidemiology of brain tumors. In: Methods of molecular biology, cancer biology, vol 472. Humana Press, Totowa, pp 323–341

Ojemann GA (1991) Cortical organization of language. J Neurosci 11(8):2281–2287

Ojemann G, Ojemann J et al (1989) Cortical language localization in left, dominant hemisphere. An electrical stimulation mapping investigation in 117 patients. J Neurosurg 71(3):316–326

Ojemann GA, Ojemann J, Ramsey NF (2013) Relation between functional magnetic resonance imaging (fMRI) and single neuron, local field potential (LFP) and electrocorticography (ECoG) activity in human cortex. Front Hum Neurosci 7:34, eCollection 2013. https://doi.org/10.3389/fnhum.2013.00034

Osborn AG (2012) Osborn's brain: imaging, pathology, and anatomy, 1st edn. Lippincott Williams & Wilkins, London

Osborn AG, Salzman KL, Barkovich AJ (2010) Diagnostic imaging—brain, 2nd edn. Lippincott Williams & Wilkins, Philadelphia

Ostrom QT, Barnholtz-Sloan JS (2011) Current state of our knowledge on brain tumor epidemiology. Curr Neurol Neurosci Rep 11(3):329–335

Ozdoba C, Nirkko AC et al (2002) Whole-brain functional magnetic resonance imaging of cerebral arteriovenous malformations involving the motor pathways. Neuroradiology 44(1):1–10

Pak RW, Hadjiabadi DH, Senarathna J, Agarwal S, Thakor NV, Pillai JJ, Pathak AP (2017) Implications of neurovascular uncoupling in functional magnetic resonance imaging (fMRI) of brain tumors. J Cereb Blood Flow Metab 37(11):3475–3487. https://doi.org/10.1177/027 1678X17707398. Epub 2017 May 11

Palmer ED, Rosen HJ et al (2001) An event-related fMRI study of overt and covert word stem completion. NeuroImage 14(1 Pt 1):182–193

Park KY, Lee JJ, Dierker D, Marple LM, Hacker CD, Roland JL, Marcus DS, Milchenko M, Miller-Thomas MM, Benzinger TL, Shimony JS, Snyder AZ, Leuthardt EC (2020) Mapping language function with task-based vs. resting-state functional MRI. PLoS One 15(7):e0236423, eCollection 2020. https://doi.org/10.1371/journal.pone.0236423

Parkin DM, Muir CS (1992) Cancer incidence in five continents. Comparability and quality of data. IARC Sci Publ 120:45–173

Parmar H, Sitoh YY, Yeo TT (2004) Combined magnetic resonance tractography and functional magnetic resonance imaging in evaluation of brain tumors involving the motor system. J Comput Assist Tomogr 28(4):551–556

Partovi S, Jacobi B, Rapps N, Zipp L, Karimi S, Rengier F, Lyo JK, Stippich C (2012a) Clinical standardized fMRI reveals altered language lateralization in patients with brain tumor. AJNR Am J Neuroradiol 33(11):2151–2157. Epub 2012 May 17

Partovi S, Konrad F, Karimi S, Rengier F, Lyo JK, Zipp L, Nennig E, Stippich C (2012b) Effects of covert and overt paradigms in clinical language fMRI. Acad Radiol 19(5):518–525

Peck KK, Holodny AI (2007) fMRI clinical applications. In: Reiser MF, Semmler W, Hricak H (eds) Magnetic resonance tomography. Springer, Berlin, pp 1308–1331

Peck KK, Bradbury M, Petrovich N, Hou BL, Ishill N, Brennan C, Tabar V, Holodny AI (2009) Presurgical evaluation of language using functional magnetic resonance imaging in brain tumor patients with previous surgery. Neurosurgery 64(4):644–652; discussion 652–3. https://doi.org/10.1227/01.NEU.0000339122.01957.0A.

Penfield W (1937) Somatic motor and sensory representation in the cerebral cortex of man as studied by electrical stimulation. Brain 60:389–443

Penfield W (1950) The cerebral cortex of man. MacMillan, New York, 57 ff

Pernet C, Poline JB (2015) Improving functional magnetic resonance imaging reproducibility. Gigascience 4:15, eCollection 2015. https://doi.org/10.1186/s13742-015-0055-8

Pernet CR, Gorgolewski KJ, Job D, Rodriguez D, Storkey A, Whittle I, Wardlaw J (2016) Evaluation of a presurgical functional MRI workflow: from data acquisition to reporting. Int J Med Inform 86:37–42. https://doi.org/10.1016/j.ijmedinf.2015.11.014. Epub 2015 Nov 30

Petersen SE, Fox PT et al (1988) Positron emission tomographic studies of the cortical anatomy of single-word processing. Nature 331(6157):585–589

Petrovich NM, Holodny AI et al (2004) Isolated translocation of Wernicke's area to the right hemisphere in a 62-year-man with a temporo-parietal glioma. AJNR Am J Neuroradiol 25(1):130–133

Pillai JJ, Mikulis DJ (2015) Cerebrovascular reactivity mapping: an evolving standard for clinical functional imaging. AJNR Am J Neuroradiol 36(1):7–13. https://doi.org/10.3174/ajnr.A3941. Epub 2014 Apr 30

Pillai JJ, Zaca D (2011) Relative utility for hemispheric lateralization of different clinical fMRI activation tasks within a comprehensive language paradigm battery in brain tumor patients as assessed by both threshold-dependent and threshold-independent analysis methods. NeuroImage 54(Suppl 1):S136–S145. https://doi.org/10.1016/j.neuroimage.2010.03.082. Epub 2010 Apr 7

Pillai JJ, Zaca D (2012) Comparison of BOLD cerebrovascular reactivity mapping and DSC MR perfusion imaging for prediction of neurovascular uncoupling potential in brain tumors. Technol Cancer Res Treat 11(4):361–374. https://doi.org/10.7785/tcrt.2012.500284. Epub 2012 Mar 1

Potgieser AR, Wagemakers M, van Hulzen AL, de Jong BM, Hoving EW, Groen RJ (2014) The role of diffusion tensor imaging in brain tumor surgery: a review of the literature. Clin Neurol Neurosurg 124:51–8. Review. https://doi.org/10.1016/j.clineuro.2014.06.009. Epub 2014 Jun 17

Pouratian N, Bookheimer SY et al (2002) Utility of preoperative functional magnetic resonance imaging for identifying language cortices in patients with vascular malformations. J Neurosurg 97(1):21–32

Price CJ (2000) The anatomy of language: contributions from functional neuroimaging. J Anat 197(Pt 3):335–359

Price CJ, Wise RJ et al (1996) Hearing and saying. The functional neuro-anatomy of auditory word processing. Brain 119(Pt 3):919–931

Priest AN, De Vita E et al (2006) EPI distortion correction from a simultaneously acquired distortion map using TRAIL. J Magn Reson Imaging 23(4):597–603

Puce A, Constable RT et al (1995) Functional magnetic resonance imaging of sensory and motor cortex:

comparison with electrophysiological localization. J Neurosurg 83(2):262–270

Pujol J, Conesa G et al (1996) Presurgical identification of the primary sensorimotor cortex by functional magnetic resonance imaging. J Neurosurg 84(1):7–13

Pujol J, Conesa G et al (1998) Clinical application of functional magnetic resonance imaging in presurgical identification of the central sulcus. J Neurosurg 88(5):863–869

Raichle ME (1983) Positron emission tomography. Annu Rev Neurosci 6:249–267

Raichle ME, Fiez JA et al (1994) Practice-related changes in human brain functional anatomy during nonmotor learning. Cereb Cortex 4(1):8–26

Ramsey NF, Sommer IE et al (2001) Combined analysis of language tasks in fMRI improves assessment of hemispheric dominance for language functions in individual subjects. NeuroImage 13(4):719–733

Rasmussen IA, Lindseth F et al (2007) Functional neuronavigation combined with intra-operative 3D ultrasound: initial experiences during surgical resections close to eloquent brain areas and future direction in automatic brain shift compensation of preoperative data. Acta Neurochir 149(4):365–378

Rausch R, Silfvenious H et al (1993) Intra-arterial amobarbital procedures. In: Engel JJ (ed) Surgical treatment of the epilepsies. Raven Press, New York, pp 341–357

Reinges MH, Krings T et al (2004) Preoperative mapping of cortical motor function: prospective comparison of functional magnetic resonance imaging and [^{15}O]-H$_2$O-positron emission tomography in the same co-ordinate system. Nucl Med Commun 25(10):987–997

Reinges MH, Krings T et al (2005) Prospective demonstration of short-term motor plasticity following acquired central pareses. NeuroImage 24(4):1248–1255

Roberts TP (2003) Functional magnetic resonance imaging (fMRI) processing and analysis. ASNR Electronic Learning Center Syllabus, pp 1–23

Robertson FC, Ullrich NJ, Manley PE, Al-Sayegh H, Ma C, Goumnerova LC (2019) The impact of intraoperative electrocorticography on seizure outcome after resection of pediatric brain tumors: a cohort study. Neurosurgery 85(3):375–383. https://doi.org/10.1093/neuros/nyy342

Roessler K, Donat M et al (2005) Evaluation of preoperative high magnetic field motor functional MRI (3 Tesla) in glioma patients by navigated electrocortical stimulation and postoperative outcome. J Neurol Neurosurg Psychiatry 76(8):1152–1157

Roessler K, Heynold E, Buchfelder M, Stefan H, Hamer HM (2019) Current value of intraoperative electrocorticography (iopECoG). Epilepsy Behav 91:20–24. Review. https://doi.org/10.1016/j.yebeh.2018.06.053. Epub 2018 Nov 9

Rösler J, Niraula B et al (2014) Language mapping in healthy volunteers and brain tumor patients with a novel navigated TMS system: evidence of tumor-induced plasticity. Clin Neurophysiol 125(3):526–536

Roux FE, Tremoulet M (2002) Organization of language areas in bilingual patients: a cortical stimulation study. J Neurosurg 97(4):857–864

Roux FE, Ranjeva JP et al (1997) Motor functional MRI for presurgical evaluation of cerebral tumors. Stereotact Funct Neurosurg 68(1–4 Pt 1):106–111

Roux FE, Boulanouar K et al (1999a) Cortical intraoperative stimulation in brain tumors as a tool to evaluate spatial data from motor functional MRI. Investig Radiol 34(3):225–229

Roux FE, Boulanouar K et al (1999b) Usefulness of motor functional MRI correlated to cortical mapping in Rolandic low-grade astrocytomas. Acta Neurochir (Wien) 141(1):71–79

Roux FE, Boulanouar K et al (2000) Functional MRI and intraoperative brain mapping to evaluate brain plasticity in patients with brain tumours and hemiparesis. J Neurol Neurosurg Psychiatry 69(4):453–463

Roux FE, Ibarrola D et al (2001) Methodological and technical issues for integrating functional magnetic resonance imaging data in a neuronavigational system. Neurosurgery 49(5):1145–1156; discussion 1156–1157

Roux FE, Boulanouar K et al (2003) Language functional magnetic resonance imaging in preoperative assessment of language areas: correlation with direct cortical stimulation. Neurosurgery 52(6):1335–1345; discussion 1345–1347

Roux FE, Dufor O, Giussani C, Wamain Y, Draper L, Longcamp M, Démonet JF (2009) The graphemic/motor frontal area Exner's area revisited. Ann Neurol 66(4):537–545. https://doi.org/10.1002/ana.21804

Rueckert L, Appollonio I et al (1994) Magnetic resonance imaging functional activation of left frontal cortex during covert word production. J Neuroimaging 4(2):67–70

Ruge MI, Victor J et al (1999) Concordance between functional magnetic resonance imaging and intraoperative language mapping. Stereotact Funct Neurosurg 72(2–4):95–102

Rutten GJ, van Rijen PC et al (1999) Language area localization with three-dimensional functional magnetic resonance imaging matches intrasulcal electrostimulation in Broca's area. Ann Neurol 46(3):405–408

Rutten GJ, Ramsey NF et al (2002a) FMRI-determined language lateralization in patients with unilateral or mixed language dominance according to the Wada test. NeuroImage 17(1):447–460

Rutten GJ, Ramsey NF et al (2002b) Interhemispheric reorganization of motor hand function to the primary motor cortex predicted with functional magnetic resonance imaging and transcranial magnetic stimulation. J Child Neurol 17(4):292–297

Rutten GJ, Ramsey NF et al (2002c) Development of a functional magnetic resonance imaging protocol for intraoperative localization of critical temporoparietal language areas. Ann Neurol 51(3):350–360

Rutten GJ, Ramsey NF et al (2002d) Reproducibility of fMRI-determined language lateralization in individual subjects. Brain Lang 80(3):421–437

Sair HI, Yahyavi-Firouz-Abadi N, Calhoun VD, Airan RD, Agarwal S, Intrapiromkul J, Choe AS, Gujar SK, Caffo B, Lindquist MA, Pillai JJ (2016) Presurgical brain mapping of the language network in patients with brain tumors using resting-state fMRI: comparison with task fMRI. Hum Brain Mapp 37(3):913–923. https://doi.org/10.1002/hbm.23075. Epub 2015 Dec 10

Sakai KL, Hashimoto R, Homae F (2001) Sentence processing in the cerebral cortex. Neurosci Res 39(1):1–10

Sang S, Wanggou S, Wang Z, Lin X, Jiang N, Ye N, Li X (2018) Clinical long-term follow-up evaluation of functional neuronavigation in adult cerebral gliomas. World Neurosurg 119:e262–e271. https://doi.org/10.1016/j.wneu.2018.07.127. Epub 2018 Jul 25

Scarabino T, Giannatempo GM, Popolizio T, Tosetti M, d'Alesio V, Esposito F, Di Salle F, Di Costanzo A, Bertolino A, Maggialetti A, Salvolini U (2007) 3.0-T functional brain imaging: a 5-year experience. Radiol Med 112(1):97–112. https://doi.org/10.1007/s11547-007-0124-x. Epub 2007 Feb 22

Schaechter JD, Stokes C, Connell BD, Perdue K, Bonmassar G (2006) Finger motion sensors for fMRI motor studies. NeuroImage 31(4):1549–1559. https://doi.org/10.1016/j.neuroimage.2006.02.029. Epub 2006 Apr 19

Schiffbauer H, Berger MS et al (2003) Preoperative magnetic source imaging for brain tumor surgery: a quantitative comparison with intraoperative sensory and motor mapping. Neurosurg Focus 15(1):E7

Schlaggar BL, Brown TT et al (2002) Functional neuroanatomical differences between adults and school-age children in the processing of single words. Science 296(5572):1476–1479

Schlosser MJ, McCarthy G et al (1997) Cerebral vascular malformations adjacent to sensorimotor and visual cortex. Functional magnetic resonance imaging studies before and after therapeutic intervention. Stroke 28(6):1130–1137

Schlosser MJ, Luby M et al (1999) Comparative localization of auditory comprehension by using functional magnetic resonance imaging and cortical stimulation. J Neurosurg 91(4):626–635

Schmid E, Thomschewski A, Taylor A, Zimmermann G, Kirschner M, Kobulashvili T, Brigo F, Rados M, Helmstaedter C, Braun K, Trinka E, E-PILEPSY Consortium (2018) Diagnostic accuracy of functional magnetic resonance imaging, Wada test, magnetoencephalography, and functional transcranial Doppler sonography for memory and language outcome after epilepsy surgery: a systematic review. Epilepsia 59(12):2305–2317. https://doi.org/10.1111/epi.14588. Epub 2018 Oct 30

Schreiber A, Hubbe U et al (2000) The influence of gliomas and nonglial space-occupying lesions on blood-oxygen-level-dependent contrast enhancement. AJNR Am J Neuroradiol 21(6):1055–1063

Schulder M, Maldjian JA et al (1998) Functional image-guided surgery of intracranial tumors located in or near the sensorimotor cortex. J Neurosurg 89(3):412–418

Schwindack C, Siminotto E et al (2005) Real-time functional magnetic resonance imaging (rt-fMRI) in patients with brain tumours: preliminary findings using motor and language paradigms. Br J Neurosurg 19(1):25–32

Seto E, Sela G, McIlroy WE, Black SE, Staines WR, Bronskill MJ, McIntosh AR, Graham SJ (2001) Quantifying head motion associated with motor tasks used in fMRI. NeuroImage 14(2):284–297. https://doi.org/10.1006/nimg.2001.0829

Shahar T, Rozovski U et al (2014) Preoperative imaging to predict intraoperative changes in tumor-to-corticospinal tract distance: an analysis of 45 cases using high-field intraoperative magnetic resonance imaging. Neurosurgery 75(1):23–30

Sharan A, Cher Ooi Y et al (2011) Intracarotid amobarbital procedure for epilepsy surgery. Epilepsy Behav 20(2):209–213

Sharma A, Kumar R (2020) Metabolic imaging of brain tumor recurrence. AJR Am J Roentgenol 215(5):1199–1207. Review. https://doi.org/10.2214/AJR.19.22624. Epub 2020 Sept 22

Shaywitz BA, Shaywitz SE et al (1995) Sex differences in the functional organization of the brain for language. Nature 373(6515):607–609

Shimoni JS, Zhang D et al (2009) Resting state fluctuations in brain activity: a new paradigm for presurgical planning using fMRI. Acad Radiol 16(5):578–583

Shinoura N, Yamada R et al (2005) Preoperative fMRI, tractography and continuous task during awake surgery for maintenance of motor function following surgical resection of metastatic tumor spread to the primary motor area. Minim Invasive Neurosurg 48(2):85–90

Shinoura N, Suzuki Y, Yamada R, Kodama T, Takahashi M, Yagi K (2006) Restored activation of primary motor area from motor reorganization and improved motor function after brain tumor resection. AJNR Am J Neuroradiol 27(6):1275–1282

Shinoura N, Suzuki Y, Yamada R, Tabei Y, Saito K, Yagi K (2009) Marked and rapid recovery of motor strength in premotor area compared with primary motor area in surgery for brain tumors. Br J Neurosurg 23(3):309–314. https://doi.org/10.1080/02688690802638166

Shinoura N, Yoshida M, Yamada R, Tabei Y, Saito K, Suzuki Y, Yagi K (2010) Combined damage to the right hemispheric hand area in the primary motor and sensory area plays a critical role in motor hemineglect. Eur Neurol 63(1):17–23. https://doi.org/10.1159/000258636. Epub 2009 Nov 14

Shriver S, Knierim KE, O'Shea JP, Glover GH, Golby AJ (2013) Pneumatically driven finger movement: a novel passive functional MR imaging technique for presurgical motor and sensory mapping. AJNR Am J Neuroradiol 34(1):E5–E7. https://doi.org/10.3174/ajnr.A2626. Epub 2011 Jul 21

Sidhu MK, Duncan JS, Sander JW (2018) Neuroimaging in epilepsy. Curr Opin Neurol 31(4):371–378. Review. https://doi.org/10.1097/WCO.0000000000000568

Siero JC, Hermes D, Hoogduin H, Luijten PR, Ramsey NF, Petridou N (2014) BOLD matches neuronal activity at the mm scale: a combined 7T fMRI and ECoG study in human sensorimotor cortex. NeuroImage 101:177–184.	https://doi.org/10.1016/j.neuroimage.2014.07.002. Epub 2014 Jul 12

Simkins-Bullock J (2000) Beyond speech lateralization: a review of the variability, reliability, and validity of the intracarotid amobarbital procedure and its nonlanguage uses in epilepsy surgery candidates. Neuropsychol Rev 10(1):41–74

Smits M, Vernooij MW et al (2007) Incorporating functional MR imaging into diffusion tensor tractography in the preoperative assessment of the corticospinal tract in patients with brain tumors. AJNR Am J Neuroradiol 28(7):1354–1361

Sorger B, Goebel R (2020) Real-time fMRI for brain-computer interfacing. Handb Clin Neurol 168:289–302. https://doi.org/10.1016/B978-0-444-63934-9.00021-4

Sparacia G, Parla G, Cannella R, Perri A, Lo Re V, Mamone G, Miraglia R, Torregrossa F, Grasso G (2019) Resting-state functional magnetic resonance imaging for brain tumor surgical planning: feasibility in clinical setting. World Neurosurg 131:356–363. https://doi.org/10.1016/j.wneu.2019.07.022

Sparacia G, Parla G, Lo Re V, Cannella R, Mamone G, Carollo V, Midiri M, Grasso G (2020) Resting-state functional connectome in patients with brain tumors before and after surgical resection. World Neurosurg 141:e182–e194. https://doi.org/10.1016/j.wneu.2020.05.054. Epub 2020 May 16

Spreer J, Quiske A et al (2001) Unsuspected atypical hemispheric dominance for language as determined by fMRI. Epilepsia 42(7):957–959

Springer JA, Binder JR et al (1999) Language dominance in neurologically normal and epilepsy subjects: a functional MRI study. Brain 122(Pt 11):2033–2046

Springer E, Dymerska B, Cardoso PL, Robinson SD, Weisstanner C, Wiest R, Schmitt B, Trattnig S (2016) Comparison of routine brain imaging at 3 T and 7 T. Investig Radiol 51(8):469–482. https://doi.org/10.1097/RLI.0000000000000256

Spritzer SD, Hoerth MT et al (2012) Determination of hemispheric language dominance in the surgical epilepsy patient. Neurologist 18(5):329–331

Stapleton SR, Kiriakopoulos E et al (1997) Combined utility of functional MRI, cortical mapping, and frameless stereotaxy in the resection of lesions in eloquent areas of brain in children. Pediatr Neurosurg 26(2):68–82

Stefanowicz J, Iżycka-Świeszewska E et al (2011) Brain metastases in paediatric patients: characteristics of a patient series and review of the literature. Folia Neuropathol 49(4):271–281

Steger TR, Jackson EF (2004) Real-time motion detection of functional MRI data. J Appl Clin Med Phys 5(2):64–70

Stippich C (2005) Clinical functional magnetic resonance imaging: basic principles and clinical applications. Radiol Up2date 5:317–336

Stippich C (2010) Prächirurgische funktionelle Magnetresonanztomographie [Presurgical functional magnetic resonance imaging]. Radiologe 50(2):110–122. German. https://doi.org/10.1007/s00117-009-1893-0

Stippich C, Hofmann R et al (1999) Somatotopic mapping of the human primary somatosensory cortex by fully automated tactile stimulation using functional magnetic resonance imaging. Neurosci Lett 277(1):25–28

Stippich C, Kapfer D et al (2000) Robust localization of the contralateral precentral gyrus in hemiparetic patients using the unimpaired ipsilateral hand: a clinical functional magnetic resonance imaging protocol. Neurosci Lett 285(2):155–159

Stippich C, Heiland S et al (2002a) Functional magnetic resonance imaging: physiological background, technical aspects and prerequisites for clinical use. Rofo 174(1):43–49

Stippich C, Ochmann H, Sartor K (2002b) Somatotopic mapping of the human primary sensorimotor cortex during motor imagery and motor execution by functional magnetic resonance imaging. Neurosci Lett 331(1):50–54

Stippich C, Kress B et al (2003a) Preoperative functional magnetic resonance tomography (FMRI) in patients with Rolandic brain tumors: indication, investigation strategy, possibilities and limitations of clinical application. Rofo 175(8):1042–1050

Stippich C, Mohammed J et al (2003b) Robust localization and lateralization of human language function: an optimized clinical functional magnetic resonance imaging protocol. Neurosci Lett 346(1–2):109–113

Stippich C, Romanowski A et al (2004) Fully automated localization of the human primary somatosensory cortex in one minute by functional magnetic resonance imaging. Neurosci Lett 364(2):90–93

Stippich C, Romanowski A et al (2005) Time-efficient localization of the human secondary somatosensory cortex by functional magnetic resonance imaging. Neurosci Lett 381(3):264–268

Stippich C, Blatow M, Durst A, Dreyhaupt J, Sartor K (2007a) Global activation of primary motor cortex during voluntary movements in man. NeuroImage 34(3):1227–1237. https://doi.org/10.1016/j.neuroimage.2006.08.046. Epub 2006 Nov 28

Stippich C, Rapps N et al (2007b) Feasibility of routine preoperative functional magnetic resonance imaging for localizing and lateralizing language in 81 consecutive patients with brain tumors. Radiology 243:828–836

Stopa BM, Senders JT, Broekman MLD, Vangel M, Golby AJ (2020) Preoperative functional MRI use in neurooncology patients: a clinician survey. Neurosurg Focus 48(2):E11. https://doi.org/10.3171/2019.11.FOCUS19779

Szaflarski JP, Binder JR et al (2002) Language lateralization in left-handed and ambidextrous people: fMRI data. Neurology 59(2):238–244

Tarapore PE, Matthew CT (2012) Preoperative multimodal motor mapping: a comparison of magnetoencephalography imaging, navigated transcranial magnetic stimulation, and direct cortical stimulation. J Neurosurg 117(2):354–362

Ternovoi SK, Sinitsyn VE et al (2004) Localization of the motor and speech zones of the cerebral cortex by functional magnetic resonance tomography. Neurosci Behav Physiol 34(5):431–437

Thulborn K (2006) Clinical functional magnetic resonance imaging. In: Haacke EM (ed) Current protocols in magnetic resonance imaging. Wiley, New York. Last Update: 20 Aug 2013. ISBN: 978-0-471-35345-4

Thulborn KR, Shen GX (1999) An integrated head immobilization system and high-performance RF coil for fMRI of visual paradigms at 1.5 T. J Magn Reson 139(1):26–34

Tie Y, Suarez RO, Whalen S, Radmanesh A, Norton IH, Golby AJ (2009) Comparison of blocked and event-related fMRI designs for pre-surgical language mapping. NeuroImage 47(Suppl 2):T107–T115. https://doi.org/10.1016/j.neuroimage.2008.11.020. Epub 2008 Dec 6

Todd N, Josephs O, Callaghan MF, Lutti A, Weiskopf N (2015) Prospective motion correction of 3D echo-planar imaging data for functional MRI using optical tracking. NeuroImage 113:1–12. https://doi.org/10.1016/j.neuroimage.2015.03.013. Epub 2015 Mar 14

Towle VL, Khorasani L et al (2003) Noninvasive identification of human central sulcus: a comparison of gyral morphology, functional MRI, dipole localization, and direct cortical mapping. NeuroImage 19(3):684–697

Tozakidou M, Wenz H et al (2013) Primary motor cortex activation and lateralization in patients with tumors of the central region. NeuroImage Clin 2:221–228

Trattnig S, Springer E, Bogner W, Hangel G, Strasser B, Dymerska B, Cardoso PL, Robinson SD (2018) Key clinical benefits of neuroimaging at 7T. NeuroImage 168:477–489. https://doi.org/10.1016/j.neuroimage.2016.11.031. Epub 2016 Nov 13

Tremblay P, Dick AS (2016) Broca and Wernicke are dead, or moving past the classic model of language neurobiology. Brain Lang 162:60–71. https://doi.org/10.1016/j.bandl.2016.08.004. Epub 2016 Aug 30

Tuntiyatorn L, Wuttiplakorn L, Laohawiriyakamol K (2011) Plasticity of the motor cortex in patients with brain tumors and arteriovenous malformations: a functional MR study. J Med Assoc Thail 94(9):1134–1140

Tyndall AJ, Reinhardt J, Tronnier V, Mariani L, Stippich C (2017) Presurgical motor, somatosensory and language fMRI: technical feasibility and limitations in 491 patients over 13 years. Eur Radiol 27(1):267–278. https://doi.org/10.1007/s00330-016-4369-4. Epub 2016 May 19

Ulmer JL, Krouwer HG, Mueller WM, Ugurel MS, Kocak M, Mark LP (2003) Pseudo-reorganization of language cortical function at fMR imaging: a consequence of tumor-induced neurovascular uncoupling. AJNR Am J Neuroradiol 24(2):213–217

Ulmer JL, Salvan CV et al (2004a) The role of diffusion tensor imaging in establishing the proximity of tumor borders to functional brain systems: implications for preoperative risk assessments and postoperative outcomes. Technol Cancer Res Treat 3(6):567–576

Ulmer JL, Hacein-Bey L, Mathews VP, Mueller WM, DeYoe EA, Prost RW, Meyer GA, Krouwer HG, Schmainda KM (2004b) Lesion-induced pseudo-dominance at functional magnetic resonance imaging: implications for preoperative assessments. Neurosurgery 55(3):569–579.; discussion 580-1. https://doi.org/10.1227/01.neu.0000134384.94749.b2

Unadkat P, Fumagalli L, Rigolo L, Vangel MG, Young GS, Huang R, Mukundan S Jr, Golby A, Tie Y (2019) Functional MRI task comparison for language mapping in neurosurgical patients. J Neuroimaging 29(3):348–356. https://doi.org/10.1111/jon.12597. Epub 2019 Jan 16

Vakamudi K, Posse S, Jung R, Cushnyr B, Chohan MO (2020) Real-time presurgical resting-state fMRI in patients with brain tumors: quality control and comparison with task-fMRI and intraoperative mapping. Hum Brain Mapp 41(3):797–814. https://doi.org/10.1002/hbm.24840. Epub 2019 Nov 6

van der Kallen BF, Morris GL et al (1998) Hemispheric language dominance studied with functional MR: preliminary study in healthy volunteers and patients with epilepsy. AJNR Am J Neuroradiol 19(1):73–77

van der Zwaag W, Susan F et al (2009) FMRI at 1.5, 3 and 7 T: characterising BOLD signal changes. NeuroImage 47(4):1425–1434

Van Westen D, Skagerberg G et al (2005) Functional magnetic resonance imaging at 3 T as a clinical tool in patients with intracranial tumors. Acta Radiol 46(6):599–609

Villanueva-Meyer JE, Mabray MC, Cha S (2017) Current clinical brain tumor imaging. Neurosurgery 81(3):397–415. https://doi.org/10.1093/neuros/nyx103

Voss J, Meier TB et al (2013) The role of secondary motor and language cortices in morbidity and mortality: a retrospective functional MRI study of surgical planning for patients with intracranial tumours. Neurosurg Focus 34(4):E7

Vysotski S, Madura C, Swan B, Holdsworth R, Lin Y, Rio AMD, Wood J, Kundu B, Penwarden A, Voss

J, Gallagher T, Nair VA, Field A, Garcia-Ramos C, Meyerand EM, Baskaya M, Prabhakaran V, Kuo JS (2018) Preoperative FMRI associated with decreased mortality and morbidity in brain tumor patients. Interdiscip Neurosurg 13:40–45. https://doi.org/10.1016/j.inat.2018.02.001. Epub 2018 Feb 14

Wada J, Rasmussen T (1960) Intracarotid injection of sodium amytal for the lateralization of cerebral speech dominance. Experimental and clinical observations. J Neurosurg 17:266–282

Wagner K, Hader C et al (2012) Who needs a Wada test? Present clinical indications for amobarbital procedures. J Neurol Neurosurg Psychiatry 83(5): 503–509

Warburton E, Wise RJ et al (1996) Noun and verb retrieval by normal subjects. Studies with PET. Brain 119(Pt 1):159–179

Weems SA, Reggia JA (2006) Simulating single word processing in the classic aphasia syndromes based on the Wernicke-Lichtheim-Geschwind theory. Brain Lang 98(3):291–309. https://doi.org/10.1016/j.bandl.2006.06.001. Epub 2006 Jul 7

Weiskopf N, Veit R et al (2003) Physiological self-regulation of regional brain activity using real-time functional magnetic resonance imaging (fMRI): methodology and exemplary data. NeuroImage 19(3):577–586

Weiskopf N, Scharnowski F et al (2004) Self-regulation of local brain activity using real-time functional magnetic resonance imaging (fMRI). J Physiol Paris 98(4–6):357–373

Weiskopf N, Klose U et al (2005) Single-shot compensation of image distortions and BOLD contrast optimization using multi-echo EPI for real-time fMRI. NeuroImage 24(4):1068–1079

Weiskopf N, Sitaram R, Josephs O, Veit R, Scharnowski F, Goebel R, Birbaumer N, Deichmann R, Mathiak K (2007) Real-time functional magnetic resonance imaging: methods and applications. Magn Reson Imaging 25(6):989–1003. https://doi.org/10.1016/j.mri.2007.02.007. Epub 2007 Apr 23

Wellmer J, Weber B, Urbach H, Reul J, Fernandez G, Elger CE (2009) Cerebral lesions can impair fMRI-based language lateralization. Epilepsia 50(10):2213–2224. https://doi.org/10.1111/j.1528-1167.2009.02102.x. Epub 2009 Apr 27

Wengenroth M, Blatow M, Guenther J, Akbar M, Tronnier VM, Stippich C (2011) Diagnostic benefits of presurgical fMRI in patients with brain tumours in the primary sensorimotor cortex. Eur Radiol 21(7):1517–1525

Wernicke C (1874) Der aphasische Symptomenkomplex. Eine psychologische Studie auf anatomischer Basis. Breslau: M. Cohn & Weigert

Westerveld K, Stoddard K, McCarthy K (1999) Case report of false lateralization using fMRI: comparison of language localization, Wada testing, and cortical stimulation. Arch Clin Neuropsychol 14:162–163

Wiberg A, Ng M, Al Omran Y, Alfaro-Almagro F, McCarthy P, Marchini J, Bennett DL, Smith S, Douaud G, Furniss D (2019) Handedness, language areas and neuropsychiatric diseases: insights from brain imaging and genetics. Brain 142(10):2938–2947. https://doi.org/10.1093/brain/awz257

Wienbruch C, Candia V et al (2006) A portable and low-cost fMRI compatible pneumatic system for the investigation of the somatosensory system in clinical and research environments. Neurosci Lett 398(3): 183–188

Wilkins KB, Yao J, Owen M, Karbasforoushan H, Carmona C, Dewald JPA (2020) Limited capacity for ipsilateral secondary motor areas to support hand function post-stroke. J Physiol 598(11):2153–2167. https://doi.org/10.1113/JP279377. Epub 2020 Apr 26

Wirtz CR, Tronnier VM et al (1997) Image-guided neurosurgery with intraoperative MRI: update of frameless stereotaxy and radicality control. Stereotact Funct Neurosurg 68(1–4 Pt 1):39–43

Wise R, Chollet F et al (1991) Distribution of cortical neural networks involved in word comprehension and word retrieval. Brain 114(Pt 4):1803–1817

Wittek A, Kikinis R et al (2005) Brain shift computation using a fully nonlinear biomechanical model. Med Image Comput Comput Assist Interv 8(Pt 2):583–590

Woolsey CN, Erickson TC, Gilson WE (1979) Localization in somatic sensory and motor areas of human cerebral cortex as determined by direct recording of evoked potentials and electrical stimulation. J Neurosurg 51(4):476–506

Worthington C, Vincent DJ et al (1997) Comparison of functional magnetic resonance imaging for language localization and intracarotid speech amytal testing in presurgical evaluation for intractable epilepsy. Preliminary results. Stereotact Funct Neurosurg 69(1–4 Pt 2):197–201

Wunderlich G, Knorr U et al (1998) Precentral glioma location determines the displacement of cortical hand representation. Neurosurgery 42(1):18–26; discussion 26–27

Yetkin FZ, Mueller WM et al (1997) Functional MR activation correlated with intraoperative cortical mapping. AJNR Am J Neuroradiol 18(7):1311–1315

Yetkin FZ, Swanson S et al (1998) Functional MR of frontal lobe activation: comparison with Wada language results. AJNR Am J Neuroradiol 19(6):1095–1098

Yousry TA, Schmid UD et al (1995) Topography of the cortical motor hand area: prospective study with functional MR imaging and direct motor mapping at surgery. Radiology 195(1):23–29

Yousry TA, Schmid UD et al (1996) The central sulcal vein: a landmark for identification of the central sulcus using functional magnetic resonance imaging. J Neurosurg 85(4):608–617

Yousry TA, Schmid UD et al (1997) Localization of the motor hand area to a knob on the precentral gyrus. A new landmark. Brain 120(Pt 1):141–157

Yousry I, Naidich TP, Yousry TA (2001) Functional magnetic resonance imaging: factors modulating the cortical activation pattern of the motor system. Neuroimaging Clin N Am 11(2):195–202, viii

Zaca D, Hua J, Pillai JJ (2011) Cerebrovascular reactivity mapping for brain tumor presurgical planning. World J Clin Oncol 2(7):289–298. https://doi.org/10.5306/wjco.v2.i7.289

Zacà D, Jarso S, Pillai JJ (2013) Role of semantic paradigms for optimization of language mapping in clinical FMRI studies. AJNR Am J Neuroradiol 34(10):1966–1971

Zacà D, Jovicich J, Nadar SR, Voyvodic JT, Pillai JJ (2013) Cerebrovascular reactivity mapping in patients with low grade gliomas undergoing presurgical sensorimotor mapping with BOLD fMRI. J Magn Reson Imaging 40(2):383–390. https://doi.org/10.1002/jmri.24406. Epub 2013 Nov 4

Zaca D, Agarwal S, Gujar SK, Sair HI, Pillai JJ (2014) Special considerations/technical limitations of blood-oxygen-leveldependent functional magnetic resonance imaging. Neuroimaging Clin N Am 24(4):705–715.

https://doi.org/10.1016/j.nic.2014.07.006. Epub 2014 Sep 2

Zhang D, Johnston JM et al (2009) Preoperative sensorimotor mapping in brain tumor patients using spontaneous fluctuations in neuronal activity imaged with fMRI: initial experience. Neurosurgery 65(6 Suppl):226–236

Zimmermann M, Rössler K, Kaltenhäuser M, Grummich P, Brandner N, Buchfelder M, Dörfler A, Kölble K, Stadlbauer A (2019) Comparative fMRI and MEG localization of cortical sensorimotor function: bimodal mapping supports motor area reorganization in glioma patients. PLoS One 14(3):e0213371, eCollection 2019. https://doi.org/10.1371/journal.pone.0213371

Zimmermann M, Rössler K, Kaltenhäuser M, Grummich P, Yang B, Buchfelder M, Doerfler A, Kölble K, Stadlbauer A (2020) Refined functional magnetic resonance imaging and magnetoencephalography mapping reveals reorganization in language-relevant areas of lesioned brains. World Neurosurg 136:e41–e59. https://doi.org/10.1016/j.wneu.2019.10.014. Epub 2019 Oct 10

Presurgical Resting-State fMRI

Joshua S. Shimony, John J. Lee,
Benjamin A. Seitzman, Patrick Luckett,
and Eric C. Leuthardt

Contents

J. S. Shimony (✉) · J. J. Lee · B. A. Seitzman ·
P. Luckett · E. C. Leuthardt
Washington University School of Medicine,
Saint Louis, MO, USA
e-mail: shimonyj@wustl.edu; jjlee@wustl.edu;
seitzman@wustl.edu; luckett.patrick@wustl.edu;
leuthardte@wustl.edu

Abstract

Purpose: Task functional MRI (fMRI) has traditionally been used to locate eloquent regions of the brain that are relevant to specific cognitive tasks, such as motor and language. This information is routinely used for pre-surgical planning. Resting-state fMRI uses alternative

© The Author(s), under exclusive license to Springer Nature Switzerland AG 2022
C. Stippich (ed.), *Clinical Functional MRI*, Medical Radiology Diagnostic Imaging,
https://doi.org/10.1007/978-3-030-83343-5_5

methods to find networks, but does not require any task performance by a patient.

Materials and methods: Resting-state fMRI uses correlations in the blood oxygen level-dependent (BOLD) signal to identify connected regions across the brain that form networks. Several methods of analyzing the data have been applied to calculate resting-state networks. In particular, seed-based correlation mapping and independent component analysis are two commonly used techniques.

Results: Multiple studies using these analysis techniques are described in this chapter. Resting-state data has been compared successfully with task fMRI and electrocortical stimulation mapping. Resting-state fMRI has been used as an adjunct to task fMRI in patients with brain tumors and epilepsy.

Conclusions: Resting-state fMRI has been compared favorably to other methods of determining functional connectivity, including task fMRI and electrocortical stimulation. These results demonstrate great promise for the future of resting-state fMRI in pre-surgical planning.

1 Introduction

1.1 Background

Localization of function within the brain using fMRI has been traditionally performed by presenting stimuli or imposing tasks (such as finger tapping or object naming) to elicit neuronal responses (Posner and Marcus 1994; Spitzer et al. 1995). This type of experiment has been very effective, as evidenced by the many thousands of manuscripts published utilizing task-based functional MRI (fMRI). fMRI detects changes in the blood oxygen level-dependent (BOLD) signal that reflect the neurovascular response to neural activity. Thus, task fMRI is able to identify regions in the brain associated with a given task.

Since the earliest days of fMRI, it has been recognized that the BOLD signal exhibits spontaneous fluctuations (Purdon and Weisskoff 1998). These fluctuations were initially regarded as noise to be averaged out over many trials or task blocks (Triantafyllou et al. 2005). More recent studies have shown that these spontaneous fluctuations reflect the brain's functional organization. The human brain is a disproportionate consumer of metabolic energy relative to its weight: 20% of total energy utilization but only 2% of body weight (Clark and Sokoloff 1999). This energy appears to be largely used for signaling (Shulman et al. 2004; Attwell and Laughlin 2001; Ames et al. 1992; Lennie 2003; Raichle and Mintun 2006). However, task performance only minimally increases energy consumption in the brain (Raichle and Mintun 2006). Therefore, task-based experiments ignore the overwhelming preponderance of the brain's energy consumption and activity. Biswal and colleagues first suggested that intrinsic brain activity could be utilized for functional localization and demonstrated that BOLD fluctuations observed in the resting state are correlated within the somatomotor system (Biswal et al. 1995). Correlated intrinsic activity currently is referred to as functional connectivity MRI or resting-state fMRI (rsfMRI). The development of these methods has opened up many exciting possibilities for future neurocognitive research as well as clinical applications, including pre-surgical planning, which is the subject of this chapter. rsfMRI has advantages over task fMRI in a clinical setting: the measurement is logistically simpler and there is no need for the patient to actively perform a task.

In this chapter, we focus on techniques that can assist in pre-surgical planning; however, a review of several other methods of analysis of rsfMRI can be found in the work of Lv et al. (2018).

1.2 Resting-State Networks

The topographies of functionally connected regions across the brain are known as resting-state networks (RSNs; equivalently, intrinsic connectivity networks) (Seeley et al. 2007). Resting-state fMRI scans are generally acquired while the subject is in a state of quiet wakefulness (Fox and Raichle 2007). The importance of RSNs lies in the fact that their topography closely corresponds to responses elicited by a wide variety of sensory, motor, and cognitive tasks (Smith et al. 2009). Intrinsic activity persists, albeit in a somewhat modified form, during sleep (Samann et al. 2010; Larson-Prior et al. 2009) or even under sedation (Mhuircheartaigh et al. 2010). The persistence of spontaneous fluctuations during states of reduced awareness suggests that intrinsic neuronal activity plays a role in the maintenance of the brain's functional integrity (Pizoli et al. 2011). Spontaneous BOLD activity has been detected in all mammalian species investigated thus far (Hutchison et al. 2012; Schwarz et al. 2013; Nasrallah et al. 2013), which reinforces the notion that this phenomenon is physiologically important. However, the full range of physiologi-cal functions performed by this intrinsic activity remains unclear.

Figure 1 (modified from Seitzman et al. 2019) presents the typical location of multiple RSNs in a group average (Power et al. 2011; Seitzman et al. 2020), although substantial differences between individuals have been documented (Gordon et al. 2017). Perhaps the most fundamental RSN is the default mode network (DMN), first identified by a meta-analysis of task-based functional neuroimaging experiments performed with positron-emission tomography (PET) (Shulman et al. 1997; Gusnard et al. 2001). The defining property of the DMN is that it is more active at rest than during performance of goal-directed tasks. The DMN was first identified using rsfMRI by Greicius et al. (2003), a finding that has since been replicated many times over using a variety of analysis methods (Beckmann et al. 2005; De Luca et al. 2006; Power et al. 2011; Smith et al. 2009; Yeo et al. 2011; Damoiseaux et al. 2006; Van Den Heuvel et al.

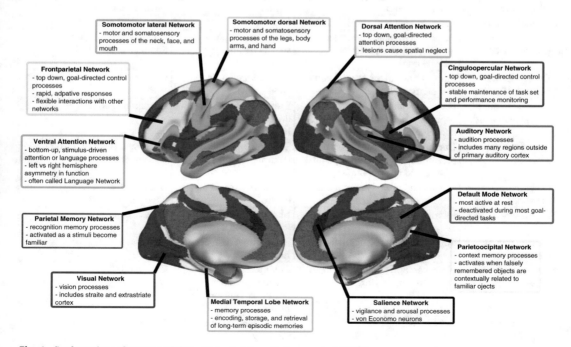

Fig. 1 Surface plots of common RSNs. (Adapted from Seitzman et al. 2019)

2008; Lee et al. 2012a). Notably, the existence of the DMN was not suspected, despite its large size on the brain cortex, until it was revealed by functional neuroimaging.

The primary sensory and motor RSNs are of great interest to the neurosurgeon since injury to these networks can lead to patient morbidity. The somatomotor (SMN) network, first identified by Biswal and colleagues (Biswal et al. 1995), encompasses primary and higher order motor and sensory areas. The visual (VIS) network spans much of the occipital cortex (Beckmann et al. 2005; De Luca et al. 2006; Power et al. 2011; Smith et al. 2009; Yeo et al. 2011) and the auditory network includes Heschl's gyrus, the superior temporal gyrus, and the posterior insula (Smith et al. 2009). The language network (also called the ventral attention network), which is critical for pre-surgical planning, includes Broca's and Wernicke's areas but also extends to prefrontal, temporal, parietal, and subcortical regions (Tomasi and Volkow 2012; Lee et al. 2012b; Hacker et al. 2013). The language network has large areas of overlap with the ventral attention network that is responsible for bottom-up, stimulus-driven attention processes.

Multiple other RSNs have been identified as association networks and are detailed in Table 1. These RSNs show more variability across individuals and map onto higher level cognitive functions; however, traditionally these regions of the brain have rarely been considered as "eloquent" cortex. Many of the networks are involved in essential aspects of human life, such as executive task control, forming memories, and attending to our environment. Further research on the clinical consequences of disruptions in these networks will be necessary to improve patient outcomes.

Table 1 Commonly defined RSNs

Name	Location	Function	References
Somatomotor network (SMN)	Pre- and post-central gyrus/ sulcus, supplementary motor area	Motor and sensory	Biswal et al. (1995)
Visual network	Occipital cortex	Vision	Buckner and Yeo (2014)
Auditory network	Superior temporal gyrus, insula	Hearing	Sadaghiani et al. (2009)
Default mode network (DMN)	Posterior cingulate, precuneus, medial prefrontal, inferior parietal cortices	Memory, prospection, social cognition	Greicius et al. (2003), Shulman et al. (1997)
Dorsal attention network (DAN)	Intraparietal sulcus, frontal and secondary eye fields	Top-down goal-directed attention	Corbetta and Shulman (2002)
Ventral attention/ language network	Broca, Wernicke, middle and superior temporal, supramarginal, and angular gyri	Bottom-up stimulus-driven attention, language	Benjamin et al. (2017)
Frontoparietal network	Dorsolateral and dorsomedial prefrontal cortex, inferior parietal lobule, middle temporal gyrus	Top-down goal-directed control processes	Power and Petersen (2013), Vincent et al. (2008)
Cingulo-opercular network	Frontal and orbital operculum, anterior cingulate, and insula	Sustained aspects of control	Dosenbach et al. (2006), Seeley et al. (2007)
Salience network	Inferior anterior insula, anterior cingulate cortex	Maintenance of vigilance and arousal	Power et al. (2011)
Parietal memory network	Superior parieto-occipital fissure, posterior cingulate	Recognition memory functions	Gilmore et al. (2015)
Medial temporal lobe network	Hippocampus, parahippocampal and entorhinal cortex	Long-term memory encoding, storage, retrieval of episodic memory	Corkin (2002)
Parieto-occipital network	Parahippocampal cortex, retrosplenial cortex, portions of the precuneus and angular gyrus	Visual contextual memory	Bar and Aminoff (2003)

2 Methods

2.1 Data Acquisition

Resting-state fMRI data can be acquired using pulse sequences similar to those used for task fMRI. This is typically done on a 3T scanner using a T2* echo planar imaging (EPI) sequence. Resolution is typically 3 mm cubic voxels, echo time (TE) is approximately 30 ms, and repetition time (TR) is usually between 2 and 3 s, but there is wide variability between different studies and different scanners. We typically instruct patients to remain still and fixate on a visual crosshair without falling asleep. Some minor differences have been demonstrated between RSNs with eyes open versus eyes closed (Laumann et al. 2017) and between awake and asleep states (Mitra et al. 2016). In practice, we find that there is less tendency to fall asleep when eyes are kept open. Long acquisition lengths are typically divided into runs of approximately 6 min each in order to give subjects periodic short breaks. Anatomic imaging is essential for registration of data to atlas space and typically includes high-resolution (1.0 mm cubic) T1-weighted magnetization prepared-rapid acquisition gradient echo (MP-RAGE) and a T2-weighted fast spin echo sequence.

Recent developments in scanner technology have provided significant improvements to the methods described above. One such improvement is simultaneous multi-slice imaging using multiband (MB) excitation (Feinberg and Setsompop 2013), which has enabled a significant reduction in the acquisition time of multi-slice EPI, reducing the TR by up to an order of magnitude. This method has improved our ability to filter noise and to define RSNs. A second recent development is multi-echo (ME) fMRI (Kundu et al. 2017), which acquires multiple-echo images per slice, allowing T2* decay to be modeled at every voxel with detailed temporal resolution. This improves our ability to separate artifact from signal, further improving fidelity of the rsfMRI signal. A third recent development is the availability of clinically approved 7T MRI scanners, which provide increased signal-to-noise ratio over 3T magnets (Shmuel et al. 2007). All these improvements have their respective drawbacks and require careful tuning to optimize image characteristics.

2.2 Overview of Processing Methods

Methodologies for identifying RSNs are dominated by two complementary strategies, spatial independent component analysis (sICA) (Beckmann et al. 2005) and seed-based correlation mapping (Biswal et al. 1995). Both strategies depend on spontaneous neural activities correlating (coherently) across widely distributed regions of the brain. Both strategies yield highly reproducible results at the group level (Damoiseaux et al. 2006; Shehzad et al. 2009). sICA decomposes resting-state fMRI data into a sum of components, each component corresponding to a spatial topography and a time course. In contrast, seed-based correlation mapping is computed by voxel-wise evaluation of the Pearson correlation between time courses of a targeted region of interest (ROI) and all other voxels in the brain (Fox et al. 2009). The principal advantage of sICA is that it provides decompositions of BOLD signals into those likely to be of neural origin and those which may be artifacts; however identification of neural components and separation of artifacts typically require observer expertise. The results obtained using sICA may vary substantially depending on processing parameters (e.g., number of requested components). Thus, sICA can be difficult to use in the investigation of targeted RSNs, especially in single subjects. In contrast, targeting of selected RSNs is built-in to seed-based correlation mapping. The principal difficulty of using seed-based correlation mapping is excluding nonneural artifacts, which is typically accomplished using regression techniques (Fox et al. 2009; Jo et al. 2010; Vincent et al. 2006).

sICA and seed-based correlation mapping both represent strategies for assigning brain voxels to RSNs. Since sICA makes no a priori assumptions regarding the topography of the obtained components, this method exemplifies unsupervised classification. In contrast, seed-based correlation mapping depends on prior knowledge, and so exemplifies supervised classification. For additional discussion of the distinction between supervised and unsupervised methodologies see Hacker et al. (2013).

2.3 General Preprocessing

Preprocessing of fMRI data varies across laboratories. The following describes the procedures used at Washington University School of Medicine (Shulman et al. 2010). Briefly, these include compensation for slice-dependent time shifts, elimination of systematic odd-even slice intensity differences due to interleaved acquisition, and rigid body correction for head movement within and across runs. The fMRI data are intensity scaled (one multiplicative factor applied to all voxels of all frames within each run) (Ojemann et al. 1997). This scaling facilitates assessment of voxel-wise variance for purposes of quality assessment without computed correlations. Atlas transformation is achieved by composition of linear (affine) transforms connecting fMRI volumes with T1- and T2-weighed structural images. Head movement correction is included in a single resampling to generate a volumetric time series in a 3 mm cubic atlas space.

2.4 Preprocessing in Preparation for Seed-Based Correlation Mapping

Additional preprocessing in the preparation for seed-based correlation mapping includes the following standard procedures: (1) spatial smoothing with 6 mm full-width half-maximum isotropic Gaussian filtering; (2) voxel-wise removal of linear trends estimated by regression over each run; (3) temporal low-pass filtering to retain frequencies <0.1 Hz; and (4) reduction of spurious variance by regression of nuisance waveforms derived from head motion correction

and extraction of the time series from regions of noninterest in white matter and CSF. This last step is further improved by using anatomic segmentation software such as FreeSurfer (Fischl 2012). In our lab, this step includes regression of the global signal averaged over the whole brain (Buckner et al. 2005; Fox et al. 2009). A consequence of global signal regression is that all subsequently computed correlations are effectively partial correlations of first-order controlling for a widely shared variance. As global signal regression (GSR) continues to be a contentious maneuver this topic is considered further in the next section.

2.5 Global Signal Regression

Global signal regression (GSR) prior to correlation mapping is a highly effective means of reducing widely shared variance and thereby improving the spatial specificity of computed maps (Fox et al. 2009; Aguirre et al. 1998; Macey et al. 2004). Some part of the global signal undoubtedly is of neural origin (Scholvinck et al. 2010). However, much of the global signal represents nonneural artifact attributable to physical effects of head motion (Friston et al. 1996; Yan et al. 2013; Power et al. 2012; Satterthwaite et al. 2012) and variations in the partial pressure of arterial carbon dioxide (Wise et al. 2004). Absent GSR, all parts of the brain appear to be strongly positively correlated (Lowe et al. 1998; Vincent et al. 2006; Joel et al. 2011; Chai et al. 2012). GSR causes all subsequently computed correlation maps to be approximately zero centered; in other words, positive and negative values are approximately balanced over the whole brain (Fox et al. 2009). Thus, GSR negatively biases all computed correlations, but preserves relative correlations, i.e., map topographies. This negative bias has caused some to criticize GSR on grounds that it induces artifactual anticorrelations (Anderson et al. 2011; Murphy et al. 2009). This objection to GSR has largely dissipated following the demonstration that some parts of the brain appear to be truly anticorrelated in the resting state, as demonstrated using sICA (Liao et al. 2010; Zuo et al. 2010). More recent objections to GSR focus on the possibility that it can distort quantitative functional connectivity differences across diagnostic groups (Saad et al. 2012). However, this objection to GSR is irrelevant in the context of using rsfMRI for purposes of RSN mapping in individuals.

2.6 Seed-Based Correlation Mapping

Seed-based correlation mapping is one of the most widely adopted techniques for studying cofluctuations in intrinsic neuronal activity, or functional connectivity (Cordes et al. 2000; Shehzad et al. 2009). The high adoption rate of the seed-based approach is partly attributable to simplicity of implementation, and to the ease with which the results can be interpreted. Biswal et al. used this method to first demonstrate the feasibility of

using fMRI to detect spatially distributed networks (Biswal et al. 1995).

Pearson product-moment correlation is the most widely used measure of functional connectivity (Biswal et al. 1995; Fox et al. 2005; Lowe et al. 1998; Xiong et al. 1999; Cordes et al. 2000; Greicius et al. 2003). Seed-based analyses require prior knowledge of the locations of regions of interest (ROI) and these can be obtained from previously determined atlas coordinates or from task-based fMRI data. For instance, a simple motor paradigm may be used to generate data involving the motor network. The activation data is then analyzed, and the voxel that is associated with the strongest activation is used as a "seed" region to then study the resting-state data. Once the coordinates of the seed region have been identified, the resting-state time courses from the rest of the brain are compared with this region, and a correlation map is generated. An example of multiple RSNs derived using the seed-based approach is presented in Fig. 2 (Zhang and Raichle 2010).

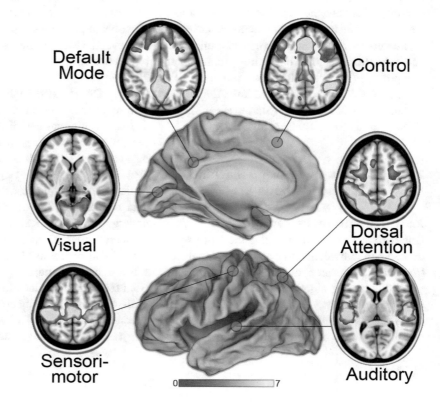

Fig. 2 Examples of multiple RSNs generated using a seed-based approach (blue circles in the figure) (Zhang and Raichle 2010). Six of the major networks are illustrated: visual, sensorimotor, auditory, default mode, dorsal attention, and frontoparietal executive control. The scale numbered 0–7 indicates relative correlation strength

2.7 Independent Component Analysis

Unsupervised data-driven approaches are of interest to researchers looking to analyze resting-state data without a priori assumptions. sICA is the most widely used data-driven approach to analyze resting-state data (De Luca 2005; Goldman 2003; Beckmann and Smith 2004; Greicius et al. 2004). sICA decomposes resting-state fMRI data (space × time) into spatial components that are maximally independent. Each spatial component is associated with a particular time course. The components are useful for distinguishing noise from physiological data through identifying statistically independent systems. Comparison studies between seed-based correlation maps and spatial patterns determined by sICA have found similar spatial patterns (Beckmann et al. 2005; Rosazza et al. 2012). A recent review of sICA methods is provided by Bijsterbosch et al. (2017).

Although the sICA approach eliminates the need for a priori seed identification, the user is required to choose the initial number of components as well as to select which components represent noise and which represent functional networks. Some studies have aimed to automate this process (Lu et al. 2017) and use sICA as a method for identifying and eliminating noise within the BOLD signal (Starck et al. 2010; Thomas et al. 2002; Tohka et al. 2008).

2.8 RSN Mapping Using Machine Learning Methods

2.8.1 Multilayer Perceptron

One current method for mapping the topography of RSNs in individuals uses a multilayer perceptron (MLP) (Hacker et al. 2013). Perceptrons are machine learning algorithms that can be trained to associate arbitrary input patterns with discrete output labels (Rumelhart et al. 1986). For example, perceptrons can be trained to read hand-written digits, e.g., zip codes on addressed letters (Lecun et al. 1989). With RSNs, an MLP is trained to classify seed-based correlation maps with particular RSNs. Running the trained MLP on correlation maps corresponding to all voxels in the brain generates voxel-wise RSN membership estimates. Thus, RSN mapping using a trained MLP exemplifies supervised classification. An example of the RSN produced by the MLP algorithm in three normal subjects is presented in Fig. 3. It is critical to note that our MLP assigns RSN membership to rsfMRI correlation maps, thus providing a voxel-by-voxel map which can better accommodate individual variability. Our implementation of MLP-based RSN mapping utilizes the same preprocessing steps described above in connection with seed-based correlation mapping (Sects. 2.2–2.6).

The MLP accurately generates RSN topography estimates for individuals. The results are consistent with previous studies, even in brain regions not represented in the training data, and can be used for generating individualized RSN maps. Based on these results, the MLP has been used as an adjunct to task fMRI for localization of RSNs in pre-surgical planning at our institute for several years. Some case examples are presented below.

2.8.2 Deep Learning

In a more recent development, we trained a 3D deep convolutional neural network (3DCNN) to recognize the language network using rsfMRI data acquired in >2700 normal subjects (Luckett et al. 2020). We tested, at a group level, the localization of the language network on unseen test data obtained in 35 patients with brain tumors undergoing pre-surgical evaluation. We directly compared inferred language networks with task fMRI for an expressive language paradigm which was also acquired during pre-surgical evaluation. Both fMRI methods localized major components of the language system such as Broca's area and Wernicke's area (Fig. 4). The word-stem completion task fMRI strongly activated Broca's area

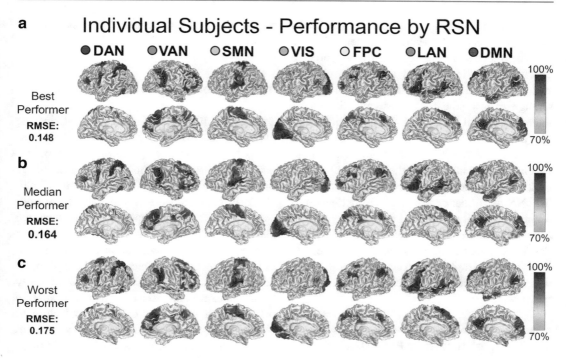

Fig. 3 Single subject, voxel estimation of RSNs using the trained MLP in three subjects. The results are from the best (**a**), median (**b**), and worst (**c**) performers as determined by root mean square error. MLP output was converted to a percentile scale and sampled onto each subject's cortical surface (Hacker et al. 2013)

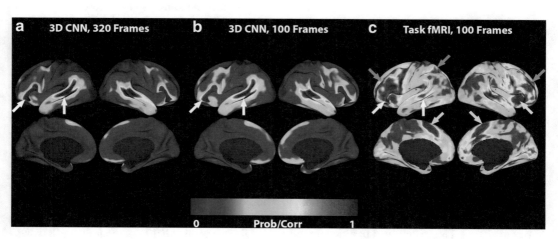

Fig. 4 Probability maps for the language network. All rsfMRI and task fMRI results are averages over 35 patients. Surface plots show probabilities >0.02 for clarity. (**a**) Maps from the 3DCNN after training with the full input data set of 320 frames per patient, (**b**) maps from the 3DCNN after training with reduced data set of 100 frames per patient, (**c**) maps from the task fMRI. White arrows indicate Broca's and Wernicke's areas. Yellow arrows indicate task responses in the right anterior insula and rostral cingulate zone (core task-control regions). Orange arrows indicate task responses in anterolateral prefrontal cortex and superior parietal lobule (dorsal attention network). (Modified from Luckett et al. 2020)

but also several task-general areas not specific to language. In Fig. 4, white arrows indicate Broca's and Wernicke's areas. Yellow arrows indicate task responses in the right anterior insula and rostral cingulate zone (core task-control regions). Orange arrows indicate task responses in antero-lateral prefrontal cortex and superior parietal lobule (dorsal attention network). As can be seen in the figure, the 3DCNN method provided a more specific representation of the language system with better defined margins. Additionally, 3DCNN performance was remarkably tolerant to a limited quantity of rsfMRI data. No significant differences are evident between Fig. 4a and b, despite the latter using only one-third of the data frames of the former. In conclusion, a 3DCNN was able to accurately localize the language network.

3   Application to Pre-surgical Planning

3.1   Introduction

Multiple studies have demonstrated that maximal resection of a brain tumor while sparing nearby eloquent cortex leads to improved outcomes, with reduced morbidity (Keles et al. 2001, 2006; Lacroix et al. 2001; McGirt et al. 2009; Sanai et al. 2008). Historically, neurosurgeons have been concerned with localization of the motor and language system on the assumption that these parts of the brain ("eloquent" cortex) instantiate critical functionality. However, a broader understanding of brain function suggests that all parts of the brain contribute to functionality (Golland et al. 2008; Hacker et al. 2013; Lee et al. 2012a; Yeo et al. 2011). Thus, improved functional mapping of multiple RSNs beyond motor and language could lead to further improvements in patient outcomes.

Multiple prior publications have explored localization of motor and language RSNs for use in pre-surgical planning for both tumor and epilepsy surgery. A review of this literature is presented below with some case examples from our institute.

3.2   Prior Studies: Motor System

The earliest literature focused on localizing the motor system. An early case report demonstrating rsfMRI for localizing the motor cortex in a patient with a brain tumor was presented by Shimony et al. (2009). Kokkonen et al. (2009) similarly compared motor task data to resting-state data and showed that the motor functional network could be localized on the basis of resting-state data in eight tumor patients as well as ten healthy control subjects. Seed-based methods were used by Liu et al. (2009) to successfully locate sensorimotor areas by using rsfMRI in patients with tumors or epileptic foci close to sensorimotor areas. They found agreement between rsfMRI, task-based fMRI, and intraoperative cortical stimulation data.

Zhang et al. (2009) described their initial experience in using rsfMRI brain mapping for pre-surgical planning of tumor resections in four tumor patients. The tumors in all four patients were adjacent to the motor and sensory cortices, thus necessitating accurate localization prior to surgery to minimize postoperative deficits. Each of the patients was scanned using rsfMRI and again using task-based fMRI while performing a block design finger-tapping task. The four tumor patients were mapped individually using task fMRI and using rsfMRI following the placement of a motor seed region on the contralateral side of the brain. The motor system was reliably identified on the ipsilesional side and compared well with the task fMRI localization.

Dierker et al. (2017) compared the localization of the SMN in 38 patients with brain tumors using finger-tapping task fMRI versus MLP analysis of rsfMRI. The comparison was anatomic information obtained from two different registration schemes. In agreement with prior publications, both methods provided accurate representations of the SMN region, with the resting-state representation covering a larger portion of the somatomotor system. The authors concluded that either method can provide the information necessary for appropriate presurgical planning, provided that the differences between the two methods are appropriately considered. Yahyavi-Firouz-Abadi et al. (2017) compared the localization of the ventral SMN in 26 patients with brain tumors using both task fMRI and ICA-based rsfMRI. They concluded that in most patients the ventral SMN can be identified using ICA methods but with variable concordance compared to task fMRI.

3.3 Prior Studies: Language System

Tie et al. (2014) used ICA on a training group of 14 healthy subjects to identify the language network from the rsfMRI data. The result of that analysis was then used to identify the language network in a second group of 18 healthy subjects at the individual level. They further proposed an automated system for determining the language network in individual patients using sICA. A more detailed presentation of our institution's experience using rsfMRI for pre-surgical mapping with both seed-based and MLP approaches follows in the next sections. Sair et al. (2016) compared the localization of the language system using task fMRI and ICA-analyzed rsfMRI in 49 tumor patients. They reported moderate group-level concordance between the methods, but with substantial subject-level variability.

Branco et al. (2016) and Parker Jones et al. (2017) demonstrated with different techniques that the language system can be reliably identified using rsfMRI in patients with brain tumors. Park et al. (2020) compared the localization of the SMN in 35 patients with brain tumors using a word-stem completion task fMRI versus MLP analysis of rsfMRI data. Both methods localized the major components of the language system although not with equal intersubject consistency. The authors emphasized differences between the

two methods, specifically that the task fMRI method activated several task-general areas not specific to language (Fig. 4).

3.4 Prior Studies: Comparison with Cortical Stimulation Mapping

A series of studies have compared the localization of the motor and language systems using rsfMRI with direct intraoperative electrocortical stimulation (ECS) mapping. Mitchell and colleagues reported application of MLP-based RSN mapping to pre-surgical planning in six patients with intractable epilepsy and seven patients with brain tumors (Mitchell et al. 2013). Epilepsy patients underwent electrocorticographic monitoring to localize the epileptogenic zone of seizure onset and to perform functional mapping with ECS. Patients with tumors underwent intraoperative ECS mapping prior to resection of the tumor mass. MLP-based RSN mapping robustly identified the motor and language networks in all patients, including those with distorted anatomy attributable to mass effect. These findings demonstrated that the MLP-defined RSNs can reliably identify areas of eloquent cortex.

Rosazza et al. (2014) and Qiu et al. (2014) compared the localization of the SMN using task fMRI, rsfMRI methods, and direct ECS. Rosazza reported comparable but not equivalent results between the methods, concluding that rsfMRI can be considered a possible alternative to task fMRI. Qiu reported overall higher sensitivity/specificity for SMN localization for rsfMRI over task fMRI as compared to ECS as a gold standard. Cochereau et al. (2016) evaluated the accuracy of rsfMRI in surgical planning by assessing the overlap between ICA language-identified regions and intraoperative ECS mapping. They concluded that ICA partly succeeded in distinguishing eloquent versus surgically removable areas and could be used as a complementary tool to intraoperative ECS. Lu et al. (2017) successfully used an advanced ICA method which automatically identified the language components and compared it with intraoperative ECS mapping. They demonstrated that the former was more sensitive in detecting the language system compared to seed-based correlation. Lemee et al. (2019) compared language areas identified with task fMRI, rsfMRI, and ECS in 50 adults with brain lesions. They reported that rsfMRI was able to detect the language areas with 100% sensitivity compared to ECS, and is thus significantly better than task fMRI.

3.5 Prior Studies: General

Leuthardt et al. (2018) reported on our experience with the integration of rsfMRI for presurgical planning into the workflow of a large institute. The rsfMRI data processing was done using an automated imaging pipeline using the MLP algorithm reported earlier and the output was integrated into the intraoperative stereotactic navigation system. Task fMRI data was processed using traditional clinical tools. Statistics from $N = 191$ consecutive patients seen during a period of 18 months were collected. The failure rate was 13% for rsfMRI analysis and 38.5% for task fMRI, a significant improvement for rsfMRI. This study demonstrated that rsfMRI can be used successfully in a busy practice as an adjunct to task fMRI.

The study by Hart et al. (2017) was unique in that the authors used rsfMRI to successfully evaluate eight different RSNs in each of their tumor patients. This study highlights an additional advantage of rsfMRI in that multiple RSNs can be extracted from a single acquisition which can expand the scope of network mapping beyond just the motor and language systems.

3.6 Clinical Cases

3.6.1 Case 1

A 57-year-old man with a history of rectal adenocarcinoma presented with persistent headache and blurred vision. Brain MRI examination demonstrated an enhancing left frontoparietal mass,

initially favored to represent metastasis. Preoperative rsfMR imaging showed that the left motor activation center was located superior to the tumor, abutting the peri-tumor edema with minimal displacement (Fig. 5a). Broca's area was located anterior to the peri-tumor edema, while Wernicke's area abutted the inferior portion of left frontoparietal junction mass (Fig. 5b). Given the close proximity of the mass with respect to the motor and language centers, it was decided that an awake craniotomy would be performed with electrocortical stimulation.

In the operating room, the patient was noted to have significant aspiration. Consequently, awake craniotomy and brain mapping were deemed to be of high risk. After consulting the patient's family, it was decided to proceed with surgical resection based on the preoperative rsfMRI assuming that resection could offer therapeutic benefit albeit with an increased risk of developing permanent speech or motor deficits. The rsfMRI helped define the spatial relationship between the motor and language centers and the mass, supporting a path through the parietal lobe for tumor resection. A standard craniotomy was then performed and continued stereotactic navigation was used to visualize the optimal gyrus for surgical approach. This surgical path was posterior and oblique relative to where the tumor was located and a nonintuitive cortical entry from anatomical landmarks alone. Along this deeper track, the tumor was subsequently resected. Adequate resection of the tumor was confirmed with intraoperative MRI. The patient's postoperative course was unremarkable with no new speech or motor deficits. Following the tumor resection, the patient experienced complete resolution of headache and blurred vision. Surgical pathology results were consistent with grade 4 glioblastoma (modified from Kamran et al. 2014).

3.6.2 Case 2

A 47-year-old man with left frontal lobe anaplastic oligodendroglioma undergoing chemotherapy treatment, status post-partial surgical resection and post-fractionated radiation treatment, was found to have new mass-like nodular areas of

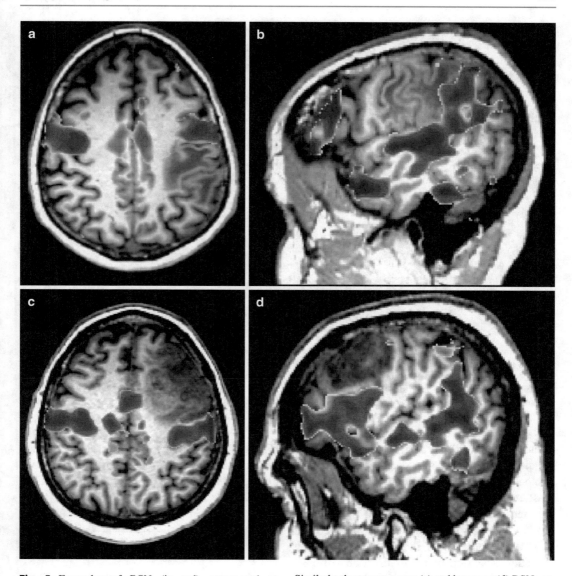

Fig. 5 Examples of RSN (in red) superposed on T1-weighted images in two case examples. The somatomotor (**a**) and language (**b**) RSNs are shown for case 1. Similarly, the somatomotor (**c**) and language (**d**) RSNs are shown for case 2. See text for more detail. (Adapted from Kamran et al. 2014)

enhancement at the tumor resection site at the 1-year follow-up brain MRI examination. These imaging findings were regarding tumor recurrence. The patient had profound expressive aphasia at the time of presentation. rsfMRI demonstrated Broca's area less than 1 cm from the edge of the previous resection cavity and abutting the edematous parenchyma surrounding the new foci of enhancement (Fig. 5d). Regions related to motor and Wernicke's area were not in close proximity to the recurrent tumor and were therefore of less concern from a neurosurgical standpoint (Fig. 5c). Consensus decision was to perform a repeat awake craniotomy and resect the recurrent tumor. During the standard awake craniotomy procedure, once the brain was exposed and the patient was roused, he was extremely combative and could not adequately follow the commands despite repeated attempts of inducing mild sedation using narcotics to

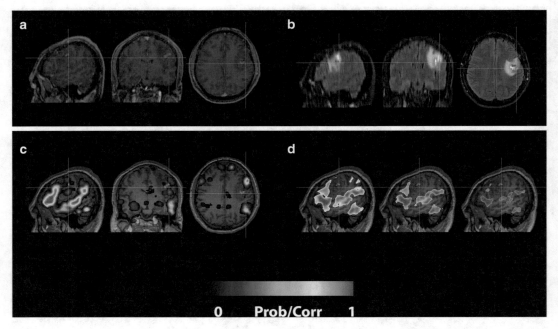

Fig. 6 Patient with high-grade glioma with anaplastic features in the subcortical left frontal lobe. (**a**) Contrast-enhanced T1 and (**b**) fluid-attenuated inversion recovery demonstrating the tumor and surrounding edema. (**c**) Probability map of language network from 3DCNN with mild overlap of the tumor and (**d**) probability map of language from the task fMRI also showing mild overlap over the tumor. Deep learning results show probabilities >0.02 for clarity. Task fMRI thresholds are varied in accordance with clinical practice. (Modified from Luckett et al. 2020)

reduce pain and discomfort. Given the patient's condition, mapping could not be accomplished. A block of tissue corresponding to the enhancing mass noted on the prior MRI examination was resected, furthest away from the speech and motor areas identified on preoperative rsfMRI. Postoperatively, there was no worsening of patient's speech or motor functions. Biopsy results for the resected tissue were consistent with radiation necrosis with no evidence of tumor recurrence (modified from Kamran et al. 2014).

3.6.3 Case 3

Images from a 24-year-old right-handed male with anaplastic glioma in the subcortical left frontal lobe are presented in Fig. 6. Figure 6a, b displays the anatomy with postcontrast T1-weighted and FLAIR images. Figure 6c, d displays the language localization information from the 3DCNN and task fMRI overlying the anatomical images. The sagittal views of the two methods are very similar, although the 3DCNN

(Fig. 6c) demonstrates more overlap of the language localization with the tumor as compared to the task fMRI (Fig. 6d) (modified from Luckett et al. 2020).

4   Conclusion

This chapter presents an introduction to rsfMRI and to common RSNs that are identified across the brain. We briefly discussed data acquisition parameters and different data processing methods to preprocess and filter the noisy raw data. A literature review presented multiple studies that have used resting state for the localization of RSNs for pre-surgical planning and compared rsfMRI with task fMRI and direct ECS mapping. Finally, we reviewed three case examples of our experience on how using rsfMRI techniques can provide useful clinical information.

As these results demonstrate, RSNs mapped from rsfMRI data are useful for pre-surgical planning with the objective of decreasing morbidity while maximizing complete resection of pathological tissue. Despite progress, further research is necessary to improve these tools and make them available in the operating room. Additional research is needed to explore the differences between rsfMRI, task fMRI, and the gold standard of ECS mapping, and to better understand the clinical consequences of disrupted RSNs beyond just the motor and language systems. Related engineering developments should incorporate the pre-surgical MRI results into intraoperative neuro-navigation systems, including the rsfMRI results in conjunction with white matter fiber bundle anatomy derived from diffusion imaging.

Acknowledgements We wish to thank the National Institute of Health for its generous support of this project via NIH R01 CA203861. Dr. Shimony is additionally supported by the Eunice Kennedy Shriver National Institute of Child Health and Human Development of the National Institutes of Health under Award Number U54 HD087011 to the Intellectual and Developmental Disabilities Research Center at Washington University. Dr. Snyder is supported by P30 NS098577-01. Dr. Leuthardt is additionally supported by the Christopher Davidson Foundation.

References

Aguirre GK, Zarahn E, D'Esposito M (1998) The inferential impact of global signal covariates in functional neuroimaging analyses. NeuroImage 8:302–306

Ames A 3rd, Li YY, Heher EC, Kimble CR (1992) Energy metabolism of rabbit retina as related to function: high cost of Na+ transport. J Neurosci 12:840–853

Anderson JS, Druzgal TJ, Lopez-Larson M, Jeong EK, Desai K, Yurgelun-Todd D (2011) Network anticorrelations, global regression, and phase-shifted soft tissue correction. Hum Brain Mapp 32:919–934

Attwell D, Laughlin SB (2001) An energy budget for signaling in the grey matter of the brain. J Cereb Blood Flow Metab 21:1133–1145

Bar M, Aminoff E (2003) Cortical analysis of visual context. Neuron 38:347–358

Beckmann CF, Smith SM (2004) Probabilistic independent component analysis for functional magnetic resonance imaging. IEEE Trans Med Imaging 23:137–152

Beckmann CF, Deluca M, Devlin JT, Smith SM (2005) Investigations into resting-state connectivity using independent component analysis. Philos Trans R Soc Lond B Biol Sci 360:1001–1013

Benjamin CF, Walshaw PD, Hale K, Gaillard WD, Baxter LC, Berl MM, Polczynska M, Noble S, Alkawadri R, Hirsch LJ, Constable RT, Bookheimer SY (2017) Presurgical language fMRI: mapping of six critical regions. Hum Brain Mapp 38:4239–4255

Bijsterbosch J, Smith SM, Beckmann CF (2017) Introduction to resting state fMRI functional connectivity. Oxford University Press, Oxford

Biswal B, Yetkin FZ, Haughton VM, Hyde JS (1995) Functional connectivity in the motor cortex of resting human brain using echo-planar MRI. Magn Reson Med 34:537–541

Branco P, Seixas D, Deprez S, Kovacs S, Peeters R, Castro SL, Sunaert S (2016) Resting-state functional magnetic resonance imaging for language preoperative planning. Front Hum Neurosci 10:11

Buckner RL, Yeo BT (2014) Borders, map clusters, and supra-areal organization in visual cortex. NeuroImage 93(Pt 2):292–297

Buckner RL, Snyder AZ, Shannon BJ, Larossa G, Sachs R, Fotenos AF, Sheline YI, Klunk WE, Mathis CA, Morris JC, Mintun MA (2005) Molecular, structural, and functional characterization of Alzheimer's disease: evidence for a relationship between default activity, amyloid, and memory. J Neurosci 25:7709–7717

Chai XJ, Castanon AN, Ongur D, Whitfield-Gabrieli S (2012) Anticorrelations in resting state networks without global signal regression. NeuroImage 59:1420–1428

Clark DD, Sokoloff L (1999) Circulation and energy metabolism of the brain. In: Siegel GJ, Agranoff BW (eds) Basic neurochemistry. Molecular, cellular and medical aspects. Lippincott-Raven, Philadelphia

Cochereau J, Deverdun J, Herbet G, Charroud C, Boyer A, Moritz-Gasser S, Le Bars E, Molino F, Bonafe A, Menjot De Champfleur N, Duffau H (2016) Comparison between resting state fMRI networks and responsive cortical stimulations in glioma patients. Hum Brain Mapp 37:3721–3732

Corbetta M, Shulman GL (2002) Control of goal-directed and stimulus-driven attention in the brain. Nat Rev Neurosci 3:201–215

Cordes D, Haughton VM, Arfanakis K, Wendt GJ, Turski PA, Moritz CH, Quigley MA, Meyerand ME (2000) Mapping functionally related regions of brain with functional connectivity MR imaging. AJNR Am J Neuroradiol 21:1636–1644

Corkin S (2002) What's new with the amnesic patient H.M.? Nat Rev Neurosci 3:153–160

Damoiseaux JS, Rombouts SA, Barkhof F, Scheltens P, Stam CJ, Smith SM, Beckmann CF (2006) Consistent resting-state networks across healthy subjects. Proc Natl Acad Sci U S A 103:13848–13853

De Luca M (2005) Low frequency signals in fMRI. University of Oxford, Oxford

De Luca M, Beckmann CF, De Stefano N, Matthews PM, Smith SM (2006) fMRI resting state networks define distinct modes of long-distance interactions in the human brain. NeuroImage 29:1359–1367

Dierker D, Roland JL, Kamran M, Rutlin J, Hacker CD, Marcus DS, Milchenko M, Miller-Thomas MM, Benzinger TL, Snyder AZ, Leuthardt EC, Shimony JS (2017) Resting-state functional magnetic resonance imaging in presurgical functional mapping: sensorimotor localization. Neuroimaging Clin N Am 27:621–633

Dosenbach NU, Visscher KM, Palmer ED, Miezin FM, Wenger KK, Kang HC, Burgund ED, Grimes AL, Schlaggar BL, Petersen SE (2006) A core system for the implementation of task sets. Neuron 50: 799–812

Feinberg DA, Setsompop K (2013) Ultra-fast MRI of the human brain with simultaneous multi-slice imaging. J Magn Reson 229:90–100

Fischl B (2012) FreeSurfer. NeuroImage 62:774–781

Fox MD, Raichle ME (2007) Spontaneous fluctuations in brain activity observed with functional magnetic resonance imaging. Nat Rev Neurosci 8:700–711

Fox MD, Snyder AZ, Vincent JL, Corbetta M, Van Essen DC, Raichle ME (2005) The human brain is intrinsically organized into dynamic, anticorrelated functional networks. Proc Natl Acad Sci U S A 102:9673–9678

Fox MD, Zhang D, Snyder AZ, Raichle ME (2009) The global signal and observed anticorrelated resting state brain networks. J Neurophysiol 101:3270–3283

Friston KJ, Williams S, Howard R, Frackowiak RS, Turner R (1996) Movement-related effects in fMRI time-series. Magn Reson Med 35:346–355

Gilmore AW, Nelson SM, McDermott KB (2015) A parietal memory network revealed by multiple MRI methods. Trends Cogn Sci 19:534–543

Goldman RCM (2003) Tomographic distribution of resting alpha rhythm sources revealed by independent component analysis. In: Ninth international conference on functional mapping of the human brain, 2003, New York, pp 18–22

Golland Y, Golland P, Bentin S, Malach R (2008) Data-driven clustering reveals a fundamental subdivision of the human cortex into two global systems. Neuropsychologia 46:540–553

Gordon EM, Laumann TO, Gilmore AW, Newbold DJ, Greene DJ, Berg JJ, Ortega M, Hoyt-Drazen C, Gratton C, Sun H, Hampton JM, Coalson RS, Nguyen AL, McDermott KB, Shimony JS, Snyder AZ, Schlaggar BL, Petersen SE, Nelson SM, Dosenbach NUF (2017) Precision functional mapping of individual human brains. Neuron 95:791–807.e7

Greicius MD, Krasnow B, Reiss AL, Menon V (2003) Functional connectivity in the resting brain: a network analysis of the default mode hypothesis. Proc Natl Acad Sci U S A 100:253–258

Greicius MD, Srivastava G, Reiss AL, Menon V (2004) Default-mode network activity distinguishes Alzheimer's disease from healthy aging: evidence from functional MRI. Proc Natl Acad Sci U S A 101:4637–4642

Gusnard DA, Raichle ME, Raichle ME (2001) Searching for a baseline: functional imaging and the resting human brain. Nat Rev Neurosci 2:685–694

Hacker CD, Laumann TO, Szrama NP, Baldassarre A, Snyder AZ, Leuthardt EC, Corbetta M (2013) Resting state network estimation in individual subjects. NeuroImage 82:616–633

Hart MG, Price SJ, Suckling J (2017) Functional connectivity networks for preoperative brain mapping in neurosurgery. J Neurosurg 126:1941–1950

Hutchison RM, Gallivan JP, Culham JC, Gati JS, Menon RS, Everling S (2012) Functional connectivity of the frontal eye fields in humans and macaque monkeys investigated with resting-state fMRI. J Neurophysiol 107:2463–2474

Jo HJ, Saad ZS, Simmons WK, Milbury LA, Cox RW (2010) Mapping sources of correlation in resting state FMRI, with artifact detection and removal. NeuroImage 52:571–582

Joel SE, Caffo BS, Van Zijl PC, Pekar JJ (2011) On the relationship between seed-based and ICA-based measures of functional connectivity. Magn Reson Med 66:644–657

Kamran M, Hacker CD, Allen MG, Mitchell TJ, Leuthardt EC, Snyder AZ, Shimony JS (2014) Resting-state blood oxygen level-dependent functional magnetic resonance imaging for presurgical planning. Neuroimaging Clin N Am 24:655–669

Keles GE, Lamborn KR, Berger MS (2001) Low-grade hemispheric gliomas in adults: a critical review of extent of resection as a factor influencing outcome. J Neurosurg 95:735–745

Keles GE, Chang EF, Lamborn KR, Tihan T, Chang CJ, Chang SM, Berger MS (2006) Volumetric extent of resection and residual contrast enhancement on initial surgery as predictors of outcome in adult patients with hemispheric anaplastic astrocytoma. J Neurosurg 105:34–40

Kokkonen SM, Nikkinen J, Remes J, Kantola J, Starck T, Haapea M, Tuominen J, Tervonen O, Kiviniemi V (2009) Preoperative localization of the sensorimotor area using independent component analysis of resting-state fMRI. Magn Reson Imaging 27:733–740

Kundu P, Voon V, Balchandani P, Lombardo MV, Poser BA, Bandettini PA (2017) Multi-echo fMRI: a review of applications in fMRI denoising and analysis of BOLD signals. NeuroImage 154:59–80

Lacroix M, Abi-Said D, Fourney DR, Gokaslan ZL, Shi W, Demonte F, Lang FF, Mccutcheon IE, Hassenbusch SJ, Holland E, Hess K, Michael C, Miller D, Sawaya R (2001) A multivariate analysis of 416 patients with glioblastoma multiforme: prognosis, extent of resection, and survival. J Neurosurg 95:190–198

Larson-Prior LJ, Zempel JM, Nolan TS, Prior FW, Snyder AZ, Raichle ME (2009) Cortical network functional connectivity in the descent to sleep. Proc Natl Acad Sci U S A 106:4489–4494

Laumann TO, Snyder AZ, Mitra A, Gordon EM, Gratton C, Adeyemo B, Gilmore AW, Nelson SM, Berg JJ, Greene DJ, McCarthy JE, Tagliazucchi E, Laufs H, Schlaggar BL, Dosenbach NUF, Petersen SE (2017) On the stability of BOLD fMRI correlations. Cereb Cortex 27:4719–4732

Lecun Y, Boser B, Denker JS, Henderson D, Howard RE, Hubbard W, Jackel LD (1989) Backpropagation applied to handwritten zip code recognition. Neural Comput 1:541–551

Lee MH, Hacker CD, Snyder AZ, Corbetta M, Zhang D, Leuthardt EC, Shimony JS (2012a) Clustering of resting state networks. PLoS One 7:e40370

Lee MH, Smyser CD, Shimony JS (2012b) Resting-state fMRI: a review of methods and clinical applications. AJNR Am J Neuroradiol. https://doi.org/10.3174/ajnr. A3263

Lemee JM, Berro DH, Bernard F, Chinier E, Leiber LM, Menei P, Ter Minassian A (2019) Resting-state functional magnetic resonance imaging versus task-based activity for language mapping and correlation with perioperative cortical mapping. Brain Behav 9:e01362

Lennie P (2003) The cost of cortical computation. Curr Biol 13:493–497

Leuthardt EC, Guzman G, Bandt SK, Hacker C, Vellimana AK, Limbrick D, Milchenko M, Lamontagne P, Speidel B, Roland J, Miller-Thomas M, Snyder AZ, Marcus D, Shimony J, Benzinger TLS (2018) Integration of resting state functional MRI into clinical practice— a large single institution experience. PLoS One 13:e0198349

Liao W, Mantini D, Zhang Z, Pan Z, Ding J, Gong Q, Yang Y, Chen H (2010) Evaluating the effective connectivity of resting state networks using conditional Granger causality. Biol Cybern 102:57–69

Liu H, Buckner RL, Talukdar T, Tanaka N, Madsen JR, Stufflebeam SM (2009) Task-free presurgical mapping using functional magnetic resonance imaging intrinsic activity. J Neurosurg 111:746–754

Lowe MJ, Mock BJ, Sorenson JA (1998) Functional connectivity in single and multislice echoplanar imaging using resting-state fluctuations. NeuroImage 7:119–132

Lu J, Zhang H, Hameed NUF, Zhang J, Yuan S, Qiu T, Shen D, Wu J (2017) An automated method for identifying an independent component analysis-based language-related resting-state network in brain tumor subjects for surgical planning. Sci Rep 7:13769

Luckett P, Lee JJ, Park KY, Dierker D, Daniel AGS, Seitzman BA, Hacker CD, Ances BM, Leuthardt EC, Snyder AZ, Shimony JS (2020) Mapping of the language network with deep learning. Front Neurol 11:819

Lv H, Wang Z, Tong E, Williams LM, Zaharchuk G, Zeineh M, Goldstein-Piekarski AN, Ball TM, Liao C, Wintermark M (2018) Resting-state functional MRI: everything that nonexperts have always wanted to know. AJNR Am J Neuroradiol 39:1390–1399

Macey PM, Macey KE, Kumar R, Harper RM (2004) A method for removal of global effects from fMRI time series. NeuroImage 22:360–366

McGirt MJ, Chaichana KL, Gathinji M, Attenello FJ, Than K, Olivi A, Weingart JD, Brem H, Quinones-Hinojosa AR (2009) Independent association of extent of resection with survival in patients with malignant brain astrocytoma. J Neurosurg 110:156–162

Mhuircheartaigh RN, Rosenorn-Lanng D, Wise R, Jbabdi S, Rogers R, Tracey I (2010) Cortical and subcortical connectivity changes during decreasing levels of consciousness in humans: a functional magnetic resonance imaging study using propofol. J Neurosci 30:9095–9102

Mitchell TH, Hacker CD et al (2013) A novel data driven approach to preoperative mapping of functional cortex using resting state fMRI. Neurosurgery 73:969–982

Mitra A, Snyder AZ, Hacker CD, Pahwa M, Tagliazucchi E, Laufs H, Leuthardt EC, Raichle ME (2016) Human cortical-hippocampal dialogue in wake and slow-wave sleep. Proc Natl Acad Sci U S A 113:E6868–E6876

Murphy K, Birn RM, Handwerker DA, Jones TB, Bandettini PA (2009) The impact of global signal regression on resting state correlations: are anti-correlated networks introduced? NeuroImage 44:893–905

Nasrallah FA, Tay HC, Chuang KH (2013) Detection of functional connectivity in the resting mouse brain. NeuroImage. https://doi.org/10.1016/j. neuroimage.2013.10.025

Ojemann JG, Buckner RL, Corbetta M, Raichle ME (1997) Imaging studies of memory and attention. Neurosurg Clin N Am 8:307–319

Park KY, Lee JJ, Dierker D, Marple LM, Hacker CD, Roland JL, Marcus DS, Milchenko M, Miller-Thomas MM, Benzinger TL, Shimony JS, Snyder AZ, Leuthardt EC (2020) Mapping language function with task-based vs resting-state functional MRI. PLoS One 15:e0236423

Parker Jones O, Voets NL, Adcock JE, Stacey R, Jbabdi S (2017) Resting connectivity predicts task activation in pre-surgical populations. Neuroimage Clin 13:378–385

Pizoli CE, Shah MN, Snyder AZ, Shimony JS, Limbrick DD, Raichle ME, Schlaggar BL, Smyth MD (2011) Resting-state activity in development and maintenance of normal brain function. Proc Natl Acad Sci U S A 108:11638–11643

Posner MIR, Marcus E (1994) Images of mind. Scientific American Library/Scientific American Books, New York

Power JD, Petersen SE (2013) Control-related systems in the human brain. Curr Opin Neurobiol 23:223–228

Power JD, Cohen AL, Nelson SM, Wig GS, Barnes KA, Church JA, Vogel AC, Laumann TO, Miezin FM, Schlaggar BL, Petersen SE (2011) Functional network organization of the human brain. Neuron 72:665–678

Power JD, Barnes KA, Snyder AZ, Schlaggar BL, Petersen SE (2012) Spurious but systematic correlations in functional connectivity MRI networks arise from subject motion. NeuroImage 59:2142–2154

Purdon PL, Weisskoff RM (1998) Effect of temporal autocorrelation due to physiological noise and stimulus paradigm on voxel-level false-positive rates in fMRI. Hum Brain Mapp 6:239–249

Qiu TM, Yan CG, Tang WJ, Wu JS, Zhuang DX, Yao CJ, Lu JF, Zhu FP, Mao Y, Zhou LF (2014) Localizing hand motor area using resting-state fMRI: validated with direct cortical stimulation. Acta Neurochir (Wien) 156:2295–2302

Raichle ME, Mintun MA (2006) Brain work and brain imaging. Annu Rev Neurosci 29:449–476

Rosazza C, Minati L, Ghielmetti F, Mandelli ML, Bruzzone MG (2012) Functional connectivity during resting-state functional MR imaging: study of the correspondence between independent component analysis and region-of-interest-based methods. AJNR Am J Neuroradiol 33:180–187

Rosazza C, Aquino D, D'Incerti L, Cordella R, Andronache A, Zaca D, Bruzzone MG, Tringali G, Minati L (2014) Preoperative mapping of the sensorimotor cortex: comparative assessment of task-based and resting-state FMRI. PLoS One 9:e98860

Rumelhart DE, Hinton GE, Williams RJ (1986) Learning representations by back-propagating errors. Nature 323:533–536

Saad ZS, Gotts SJ, Murphy K, Chen G, Jo HJ, Martin A, Cox RW (2012) Trouble at rest: how correlation patterns and group differences become distorted after global signal regression. Brain Connect 2:25–32

Sadaghiani S, Hesselmann G, Kleinschmidt A (2009) Distributed and antagonistic contributions of ongoing activity fluctuations to auditory stimulus detection. J Neurosci 29:13410–13417

Sair HI, Yahyavi-Firouz-Abadi N, Calhoun VD, Airan RD, Agarwal S, Intrapiromkul J, Choe AS, Gujar SK, Caffo B, Lindquist MA, Pillai JJ (2016) Presurgical brain mapping of the language network in patients with brain tumors using resting-state fMRI: comparison with task fMRI. Hum Brain Mapp 37:913–923

Samann PG, Tully C, Spoormaker VI, Wetter TC, Holsboer F, Wehrle R, Czisch M (2010) Increased sleep pressure reduces resting state functional connectivity. MAGMA 23:375–389

Sanai N, Mirzadeh Z, Berger MS (2008) Functional outcome after language mapping for glioma resection. N Engl J Med 358:18–27

Satterthwaite TD, Wolf DH, Loughead J, Ruparel K, Elliott MA, Hakonarson H, Gur RC, Gur RE (2012) Impact of in-scanner head motion on multiple measures of functional connectivity: relevance for studies of neurodevelopment in youth. NeuroImage 60:623–632

Scholvinck ML, Maier A, Ye FQ, Duyn JH, Leopold DA (2010) Neural basis of global resting-state fMRI activity. Proc Natl Acad Sci U S A 107:10238–10243

Schwarz AJ, Gass N, Sartorius A, Risterucci C, Spedding M, Schenker E, Meyer-Lindenberg A, Weber-Fahr W (2013) Anti-correlated cortical networks of intrinsic connectivity in the rat brain. Brain Connect 3:503–511

Seeley WW, Menon V, Schatzberg AF, Keller J, Glover GH, Kenna H, Reiss AL, Greicius MD (2007) Dissociable intrinsic connectivity networks for salience processing and executive control. J Neurosci 27:2349–2356

Seitzman BA, Snyder AZ, Leuthardt EC, Shimony JS (2019) The state of resting state networks. Top Magn Reson Imaging 28:189–196

Seitzman BA, Gratton C, Marek S, Raut RV, Dosenbach NUF, Schlaggar BL, Petersen SE, Greene DJ (2020) A set of functionally-defined brain regions with improved representation of the subcortex and cerebellum. NeuroImage 206:116290

Shehzad Z, Kelly AM, Reiss PT, Gee DG, Gotimer K, Uddin LQ, Lee SH, Margulies DS, Roy AK, Biswal BB, Petkova E, Castellanos FX, Milham MP (2009) The resting brain: unconstrained yet reliable. Cereb Cortex 19:2209–2229

Shimony JS, Zhang D, Johnston JM, Fox MD, Roy A, Leuthardt EC (2009) Resting-state spontaneous fluctuations in brain activity: a new paradigm for presurgical planning using fMRI. Acad Radiol 16:578–583

Shmuel A, Yacoub E, Chaimow D, Logothetis NK, Ugurbil K (2007) Spatio-temporal point-spread function of fMRI signal in human gray matter at 7 Tesla. NeuroImage 35:539–552

Shulman GL, Fiez JA, Corbetta M, Buckner RL, Miezin FM, Raichle ME, Petersen SE (1997) Common blood flow changes across visual tasks: II. Decreases in cerebral cortex. J Cogn Neurosci 9:648–663

Shulman RG, Rothman DL, Behar KL, Hyder F (2004) Energetic basis of brain activity: implications for neuroimaging. Trends Neurosci 27:489–495

Shulman GL, Pope DL, Astafiev SV, Mcavoy MP, Snyder AZ, Corbetta M (2010) Right hemisphere dominance during spatial selective attention and target detection occurs outside the dorsal frontoparietal network. J Neurosci 30:3640–3651

Smith SM, Fox PT, Miller KL, Glahn DC, Fox PM, Mackay CE, Filippini N, Watkins KE, Toro R, Laird AR, Beckmann CF (2009) Correspondence of the brain's functional architecture during activation and rest. Proc Natl Acad Sci U S A 106:13040–13045

Spitzer M, Kwong KK, Kennedy W, Rosen BR, Belliveau JW (1995) Category-specific brain activation in fMRI during picture naming. Neuroreport 6:2109–2112

Starck T, Remes J, Nikkinen J, Tervonen O, Kiviniemi V (2010) Correction of low-frequency physiological noise from the resting state BOLD fMRI—effect on ICA default mode analysis at 1.5 T. J Neurosci Methods 186:179–185

Thomas CG, Harshman RA, Menon RS (2002) Noise reduction in BOLD-based fMRI using component analysis. NeuroImage 17:1521–1537

Tie Y, Rigolo L, Norton IH, Huang RY, Wu W, Orringer D, et al. Defining language networks from resting-state fMRI for surgical planning—a feasibility study. Hum Brain Mapp. 2014;35(3):1018–30. https://doi.org/10.1002/hbm.22231 PMID: 23288627

Tohka J, Foerde K, Aron AR, Tom SM, Toga AW, Poldrack RA (2008) Automatic independent component labeling for artifact removal in fMRI. NeuroImage 39:1227–1245

Tomasi D, Volkow ND (2012) Resting functional connectivity of language networks: characterization and reproducibility. Mol Psychiatry 17:841–854

Triantafyllou C, Hoge RD, Krueger G, Wiggins CJ, Potthast A, Wiggins GC, Wald LL (2005) Comparison of physiological noise at 1.5 T, 3 T and 7 T and optimization of fMRI acquisition parameters. NeuroImage 26:243–250

Van Den Heuvel M, Mandl R, Hulshoff Pol H (2008) Normalized cut group clustering of resting-state FMRI data. PLoS One 3:e2001

Vincent JL, Snyder AZ, Fox MD, Shannon BJ, Andrews JR, Raichle ME, Buckner RL (2006) Coherent spontaneous activity identifies a hippocampal-parietal memory network. J Neurophysiol 96:3517–3531

Vincent JL, Kahn I, Snyder AZ, Raichle ME, Buckner RL (2008) Evidence for a frontoparietal control system revealed by intrinsic functional connectivity. J Neurophysiol 100:3328–3342

Wise RG, Ide K, Poulin MJ, Tracey I (2004) Resting fluctuations in arterial carbon dioxide induce significant low frequency variations in BOLD signal. NeuroImage 21:1652–1664

Xiong J, Parsons LM, Gao JH, Fox PT (1999) Interregional connectivity to primary motor cortex revealed using MRI resting state images. Hum Brain Mapp 8:151–156

Yahyavi-Firouz-Abadi N, Pillai JJ, Lindquist MA, Calhoun VD, Agarwal S, Airan RD, Caffo B, Gujar SK, Sair HI (2017) Presurgical brain mapping of the ventral somatomotor network in patients with brain tumors using resting-state fMRI. AJNR Am J Neuroradiol 38:1006–1012

Yan CG, Cheung B, Kelly C, Colcombe S, Craddock RC, Di Martino A, Li Q, Zuo XN, Castellanos FX, Milham MP (2013) A comprehensive assessment of regional variation in the impact of head micromovements on functional connectomics. NeuroImage 76:183–201

Yeo BT, Krienen FM, Sepulcre J, Sabuncu MR, Lashkari D, Hollinshead M, Roffman JL, Smoller JW, Zollei L, Polimeni JR, Fischl B, Liu H, Buckner RL (2011) The organization of the human cerebral cortex estimated by intrinsic functional connectivity. J Neurophysiol 106:1125–1165

Zhang D, Raichle ME (2010) Disease and the brain's dark energy. Nat Rev Neurol 6:15–28

Zhang D, Johnston JM, Fox MD, Leuthardt EC, Grubb RL, Chicoine MR, Smyth MD, Snyder AZ, Raichle ME, Shimony JS (2009) Preoperative sensorimotor mapping in brain tumor patients using spontaneous fluctuations in neuronal activity imaged with functional magnetic resonance imaging: initial experience. Neurosurgery 65:226–236

Zuo XN, Kelly C, Adelstein JS, Klein DF, Castellanos FX, Milham MP (2010) Reliable intrinsic connectivity networks: test-retest evaluation using ICA and dual regression approach. NeuroImage 49:2163–2177

Simultaneous EEG-fMRI in Epilepsy

R. Wiest, C. Rummel, and E. Abela

Contents

R. Wiest (✉) · C. Rummel
Support Centre for Advanced Neuroimaging (SCAN),
Institute for Diagnostic and Interventional
Neuroradiology, University Hospital Bern,
Bern, Switzerland
e-mail: roland.wiest@insel.ch;
Christian.Rummel@insel.ch

E. Abela
Department of Basic and Clinical Neuroscience,
Institute of Psychiatry, Psychology and Neuroscience,
King's College London, London, UK

Abstract

Simultaneous recordings of electroencephalogram (EEG) and functional magnetic resonance imaging (fMRI) signals are technically demanding, but offer a unique view onto the spatiotemporal dynamics of large-scale epilepsy-related networks. In this chapter, we present a detailed methodological overview of

© The Author(s), under exclusive license to Springer Nature Switzerland AG 2022
C. Stippich (ed.), *Clinical Functional MRI*, Medical Radiology Diagnostic Imaging,
https://doi.org/10.1007/978-3-030-83343-5_6

simultaneous EEG-fMRI, and provide examples of two clinical applications: (1) identification of syndrome-specific functional correlates in idiopathic generalized epilepsies (IGE) and (2) localization of potentially epileptogenic tissue in patients with pharmacoresistant focal epilepsy syndromes. Studies using EEG-fMRI have shown that there are bilateral areas of deactivation during generalized spike-wave discharges (GSW) in IGE within the thalamus, precuneus, anterior cingulate cortex, and inferior parietal cortex. These results underscore the importance of thalamocortical interactions in GSW generation, as well as the role of the so-called default mode network in sustaining attention and consciousness. In focal epilepsies, EEG-fMRI provides complementary information during the presurgical workup of refractory epilepsy, especially in patients with multifocal or nonlesional epilepsies. Connectivity analysis is used to identify coordinated responses of specific large-scale brain network, whose dynamics are modulated by epilepsy and epilepsy-related treatment. With the recent advent of artificial intelligence technologies, identification of specific EEG fingerprints and their concordance with BOLD responses can be processed and analyzed without human interaction. Overall, simultaneous EEG-fMRI has become an invaluable tool to elucidate the neurophysiology of human epilepsy, and shows promise as a clinical tool for specialized epilepsy centers.

1 Introduction

The simultaneous acquisition of electroencephalography and functional magnetic resonance imaging (simultaneous EEG-fMRI) bridges the gap between neurophysiology and neuroradiology. It extends the application of clinical fMRI from externally driven, task-related protocols to the neurophysiologically driven prediction of hemodynamic responses. This advanced imaging technique was developed during the mid-1990s as a response to one of the most common and difficult problems in clinical neurology: i.e. how to localize the source(s) of epileptic activity in the human brain (Ives et al. 1993; Warach et al. 1996; Seeck et al. 1998; Goldman et al. 2000; Archer et al. 2003b; Laufs 2012). The research agenda was motivated by the need to combine the complementary strengths of the two techniques, i.e., the high temporal resolution of EEG and the high spatial resolution of blood oxygen level-dependent (BOLD) fMRI. Significant progress has been made towards mitigating the weaknesses of the combined approach, e.g., the various EEG artifacts induced by the scanner environment and the analytical difficulties that arise due to the often idiosyncratic hemodynamic responses associated with epileptiform activity. Since its introduction, about 380 papers have been published on simultaneous EEG-fMRI in adult and pediatric epilepsy patients.[1] The technique is applied in many research areas, such as motor imagery (Formaggio et al. 2010), decision-making (Esposito et al. 2009), reward processing (Plichta et al. 2013), spatial attention (Green et al. 2017), and brain oscillations during wakefulness (Goldman et al. 2002; Jann et al. 2009; Mayhew et al. 2013) and sleep (Picchioni et al. 2011; Caporro et al. 2012). It has also spurred a number of methodological developments aiming to integrate multimodal data using advanced signal processing methods (Moosmann et al. 2008; Vulliemoz et al. 2009; Caballero-Gaudes et al. 2013) or generative models of brain function (Daunizeau et al. 2010, 2012). These efforts might lead to insights from which cognitive neuroimaging and neuroscience in general could benefit substantially (Debener et al. 2006). This research has also expanded our understanding of epilepsy as a network disorder, where specific cortical and subcortical networks constitute fundamental elements that contribute to the generation and spread of focal onset seizures throughout

---

[1] Number determined with a PubMed search using "((eeg-fmri) OR (eeg/fmri)) AND epilep*" from 01.01.1993 to 30.06.2020.

the human brain (Spencer 2002; Blumenfeld et al. 2004; Wiest et al. 2013).

Simultaneous EEG-fMRI thus has a direct impact on clinical epileptology, where it serves as an additional diagnostic tool during the preoperative workup of patients being considered for epilepsy surgery, and intense practical and theoretical development is ongoing (Rosenkranz and Lemieux 2010; Gotman and Pittau 2011; Moeller et al. 2013; An et al. 2013, 2015; van Graan et al. 2015; Khoo et al. 2017; Shamshiri et al. 2019). The technique is clinically important since epilepsy is one of the most common neurological conditions worldwide, with a prevalence of 0.5–1% of the global population (~35–70 million patients) and an incidence of around 50 cases per 100,000/year (Sander 2003). Somatic and psychiatric comorbidities are common and lead to an increased risk of premature death (Gaitatzis et al. 2004; Keezer et al. 2016). Indeed, evidence from community-based studies indicates that overall mortality in epilepsy cohorts is 2–3 times higher than in the general population. Causes of death are seizures in young patients with suboptimal pharmacological control (Gaitatzis and Sander 2004; Hitiris et al. 2007; Watila et al. 2018), but also preventable causes such as drowning (Bell et al. 2008) or suicide (Pompili et al. 2006). Randomized controlled trials showed evidence that early surgery for patients with mesial temporal lobe epilepsy (TLE) is superior to medical therapy (Wiebe et al. 2001; Engel Jr et al. 2012). Although long-term outcomes after TLE surgery are fairly well characterized, data on long-term outcomes after extratemporal epilepsy surgery are less consistent with seizure-free rates and range from 27% to 46% (Téllez-Zenteno et al. 2005; de Tisi et al. 2011).

Theoretical concepts used in clinical practice and research divide the epileptic brain into different zones: the seizure-onset zone, the epileptogenic lesion, the epileptogenic zone, the symptomatogenic zone, and the irritative zone (Rosenow and Lüders 2001; Lüders et al. 2006; Zijlmans et al. 2019). The epileptogenic lesion is the cortical region of the brain that, when stimulated, produces spontaneous seizures or auras, whereas the epileptogenic zone is a theoretical

concept defined as the area of cortex that is indispensable for the generation of epileptic seizures. Currently, it cannot be imaged directly and only an outer bound of this zone can be defined retrospectively, if surgery has rendered a patient permanently seizure-free. The symptomatogenic zone is the region of the cortex that produces the initial ictal symptoms or signs. The irritative zone is defined as the area of cortical tissue that generates interictal epileptiform discharges. This zone thus has a functional definition and the interictal epileptiform discharges (IEDs) can be depicted in EEG. It thus forms the basis for investigating the simultaneous hemodynamic response of IEDs that approximately resemble the epileptogenic zone. In patients with cortical dysplasia, widely distributed spike-related BOLD responses were associated with widespread seizure-onset zones and less favorable outcome (Thornton et al. 2011). During surgical evaluation, EEG-fMRI has the potential to improve source localization in complex cases, especially in patients with an unclear focus on EEG (Zijlmans et al. 2007). Other studies have shown that EEG-fMRI correlation patterns are spatially accurate at the level of anatomical brain regions, reflecting an underlying network of IEDs (van Houdt et al. 2013).

In this chapter we provide the reader with a methodological overview of clinical EEG-fMRI, including typical findings in focal and generalized epilepsies, and with a special focus on presurgical applications.

2 Data Acquisition and Analysis

When speaking about simultaneous EEG-fMRI recordings, we distinguish two types of EEG: scalp EEG and intracranial EEG (iEEG). Use of implanted electrodes means that patient safety is a much greater concern for iEEG-fMRI. Despite this, several studies have used iEEG at a field strength of 1.5 T (Vulliemoz et al. 2009; Carmichael et al. 2012; Sharma et al. 2019). Similarly, several attempts to use simultaneous EEG-fMRI at ultrahigh magnetic field strength (i.e., 7 T) have been made (Jorge et al. 2015a, b).

In our review, we concentrate on the more widely applied scalp EEG-fMRI at 1.5 and 3 T. Other authors have published comprehensive reviews on simultaneous EEG-fMRI including technical aspects (Lemieux et al. 1997; Nunez and Silberstein 2000; Gotman et al. 2006; Ritter and Villringer 2006; Cunningham et al. 2008; van Graan et al. 2015).

2.1   The Technology

Three types of magnetic fields are generated in MR scanners:

1. The static and homogeneous magnetic field B0, which aligns the proton spins
2. The gradient fields Gx, Gy, and Gz, which are used to fulfill the resonance condition in one voxel at a time and vary their orientation in space with frequencies in the kHz range
3. The head coil, which produces the radio-frequency electromagnetic B1 field (MHz range) necessary for spin rotation (e.g., 90° pulses, 180° pulses)

The Maxwell's equations (see, e.g., Jackson 1998) demonstrate that the dynamically changing magnetic (MRI) and electric fields (EEG) are inseparably interconnected. This makes simultaneous EEG-fMRI acquisition more ambitious and cumbersome than fMRI or scalp EEG alone. If conductors such as the EEG electrodes and wires are introduced into MR scanners, the changing magnetic fields may induce currents by three different mechanisms (Lemieux et al. 1997):

1. Wire loops may change the loop area perpendicular to the B0 field by deformation or change of orientation.
2. The gradient fields Gx, Gy, and Gz constantly change their spatial orientation relative to the wire loops.
3. The radio-frequency B1 field may induce currents in extended wires (electric field component) and loops (magnetic field component).

Strong induced currents may endanger patients and may cause burns due to focal heating of EEG electrodes and wires. In addition, the interaction between currents and magnetic fields may induce artifacts in both the EEG recordings and the functional and structural MR images. To guarantee patient safety and minimize artifacts of all kinds, special equipment and special data processing algorithms are required. In the following sections, we review the necessary instrumentation and the different types of artifacts occurring in EEG and fMRI data. In each subsection we describe the technical attempts to minimize artifact appearance and data processing algorithms to eliminate residual influences.

2.2   Patient Safety

An early publication by Lemieux et al. (1997) addressed patient safety during simultaneous EEG-fMRI measurements. The authors identified the interaction between the radio-frequency electromagnetic fields produced in the head coil and the EEG wire loops as the primary safety hazard and concluded that "the recording of EEG signals during the acquisition of functional and anatomical images can be performed safely if necessary precautions are taken." They recommended avoiding loops and crossing wires. In addition, serial resistors should be positioned close to the EEG electrodes to limit the currents. The resistor values depend on the instrumentation and must be large enough to limit heating and thus avoid localized burns. Optimal resistor values represent a trade-off between minimization of induced currents and maximization of the EEG signal-to-noise ratio.

2.3   Technical Equipment

The first simultaneous scalp EEG-fMRI recordings were performed on 1.5 T scanners. Today the use of 3 T scanners is standard. Patient safety issues and most artifacts in EEG and MRI data become more frequent with increasing field strength. This suggests that there is an upper limit to the field strengths that can be applied. While there are no special requirements for the MR scanner besides sufficient field strength and the ability to acquire high-resolution structural MRI data and BOLD sequences, this is different for the EEG equipment. For simultaneous EEG-fMRI specialized EEG caps, amplifiers and transmission wires are necessary.

Various MR-compatible EEG caps are commercially available, where the amount of metal in their contacts has been reduced. The rationale is to minimize the danger of focal heating at the contact points of stray electrodes and to reduce scanner artifacts in the EEG traces due to induction. In addition, it minimizes artifacts on MR images caused by local field inhomogeneities. MR-compatible EEG caps avoid wire loops by bundling wires tightly together in straight lines. The montage time may vary considerably between different types of EEG caps. For example, proper montage of the EasyCap (EasyCap GmbH, Inning am Ammersee, Germany) using electrolyte gel may take 30–45 min depending on the patient's hairstyle, whereas the Geodesic EEG system (Electrical Geodesics Inc., Eugene, Oregon, USA) using saline solution can be mounted much faster.

Standard EEG amplifiers may contain larger metal parts, which prevent them from being used in the high magnetic field inside the scanner room. More importantly, to ensure patient safety even during a potential device failure, specialized battery-supplied preamplifiers with galvanic isolation from the power line are needed. Metal transmission wires for EEG signals are kept short since they would otherwise inductively pick up artifacts from the magnetic fields. To minimize this effect, EEG data is transmitted optically to a recording device stationed outside the scanner room via glass fibers.

2.4   Artifacts in EEG Data

EEG recorded inside MR scanners may contain two types of gross artifacts, gradient artifacts and movement artifacts including the ballistocardiogram (see below), which is a special case. Gradient artifacts are caused by the rapidly switching gradient fields Gx, Gy, and Gz and may be 50 times larger in amplitude during scanning than in the background EEG (Gotman et al. 2006). In early applications, they were avoided in large parts of the recording by scanning MR images only in response to visually or computationally identified EEG events ("spike-triggered" or "IED-triggered" EEG-fMRI). For continuous MRI scanning, one can take into account that the timing of the gradient artifacts is precisely known (during acquisition of the BOLD volumes) and that they have a stereotypical shape. This enables us to use a template removal strategy called average artifact subtraction (AAS) (Allen et al. 1998, 2000). To avoid aliasing problems (given the high-frequency components of the scanner artifacts) the EEG data has to be sampled with very high frequency for this purpose (i.e., several kHz in contrast to frequencies of a few hundred Hz, which is ample for ordinary scalp EEG). Currently, two MATLAB toolboxes are available, which allow the combination of different removal algorithms for gradient artifacts: the classic FASTR package (Niazy et al. 2005) which is complemented by FACET (Glaser et al. 2013). Recently, a new EEG cap prototype was introduced. It uses a layer of reference electrodes that pick up the scanner artifacts at almost identical positions, but are electrically isolated from the scalp (Steyrl et al. 2017, 2018). These simultaneously recorded reference signals can be used for online artifact subtraction or adaptive filtering of the EEG. Using the alpha rhythm amplitude ratio between closed and open eyes and the signal-to-noise ratio of visual evoked potentials as metrics, it was shown that a combination of classic AAS and adaptive filtering can reduce scanner (and also pulse artifacts, see below) most effectively.

Movement artifacts in EEG signals are caused by electrode, wire, and patient motion inside the strong magnetic field and are especially relevant when acquiring a long-term recording of EEG-fMRI, for example in sleep studies (Altmann et al. 2016; Bagshaw et al. 2017). To avoid these artifacts we attempt to stabilize the patient's head and to improve patient comfort—especially for EEG-fMRI recordings that take a long time. Foam pads and vacuum cushions are used to fix the head, EEG caps should be elastic, and contacts in occipital regions should be cushioned to avoid pressure marks. As certain movement artifacts (e.g., swallowing, talking, and yawning) may mimic epileptiform EEG activity, it is advisable to use a movement detector so that movement-associated events can be excluded from the analysis. However, these devices require similar precautions to those that apply to the EEG equipment itself. The general advice is to immobilize EEG wires by bundling them closely together (as in most commercially available EEG caps) and fixing the leads to the scanner in straight lines (e.g., by using suitable sandbags).

A special category of movement artifacts is the ballistocardiogram (BCG, sometimes also called a cardioballistogram or pulse artifact). The cardiac cycle induces periodic small amplitude displacements of the head and the EEG electrodes due to scalp arteries pulsating inside the high magnetic field and this may induce electric currents. Since these displacements are time-locked to the heart rate, simultaneous measurement of a high-quality electrocardiogram (ECG) or pulse oximetry makes it possible to remove the BCG by averaging and subtraction techniques similar to those used for gradient artifacts (Allen et al. 1998). Furthermore, it has been demonstrated that the relevant pulse information can also be extracted from the EEG itself and that an ECG might not be needed (Iannotti et al. 2015). In addition, techniques based on principal component analysis (PCA) and independent component analysis (ICA) can be employed (Srivastava et al. 2005). PCA and ICA assume that the BCG is uncorrelated with or statistically independent from brain activation, respectively. Thus the corresponding components can be eliminated, and cleaned EEG signals can be reconstructed.

Another artifact in the EEG signals is caused by the helium pump used for cooling of the superconducting coils that generate the static B0 field. Similar to gradient artifacts and BCG, the timing (and to a lesser extent also the shape) of the artifact is known and could in principle be exploited for artifact reduction. However, a much simpler solution is to switch off the helium pump during short-term EEG-fMRI acquisition. Caution: It must be stressed, however, that neglecting to switch the pump on again after a short time might cause serious damage to the MRI scanner. Therefore, great care is essential when considering this as an option.

One also needs to remove any residual high-frequency artifacts in the EEG signals which are caused by incomplete artifact removal or acquisition of a electromyogram (EMG) rather than neuronal activity. Therefore, as for any scalp EEG, the EEG recorded inside MR scanners should be passed through a low-pass filter with a cutoff frequency of 25 or 30 Hz and can finally be downsampled to a sampling rate of a few hundred Hz before further analysis. Whitham et al. have impressively shown that scalp EEG includes large contributions from EMG at higher frequencies, independent from the application inside the MR scanner (Whitham et al. 2007). If these frequency bands are to be analyzed in scalp EEG, special care is needed to exclude artifact components.

2.5   Artifacts in fMRI Data

EEG artifacts in structural and functional MR images are generally less of an issue in simultaneous EEG-fMRI acquisition than imaging artifacts in EEG. Nevertheless, although minimized in size, currently available MR-compatible EEG equipment contains metal parts (electrodes and wires), which may distort MR images through two effects. First, conducting material may alter the magnetic field locally due to "susceptibility artifacts" and the possibility of eddy current induction. In the worst case, these artifacts can have an electrode-centered radius of 7.5 mm and can thus extend into the cortex (Lemieux et al. 1999). To minimize these effects, special materials with lower magnetic susceptibility can be used (Allen et al. 2000).

Second, high-frequency currents in the EEG leads and electromagnetic radiation emitted from the electronics of the EEG preamplifier may reduce the signal-to-noise level of MR images. Proper magnetic shielding of the amplifier largely reduces this effect.

Similarly to EEG signals, patient movement impairs MR image quality. As already discussed above, movement can effectively be minimized by improving patient comfort. During the preprocessing of fMRI data, the volumes are realigned according to the six estimated rigid-body movement parameters (three translations, three rotations). Despite realignment, the associated parameters (and occasionally also temporal derivatives or time-shifted copies) should be used as nuisance parameters in the data post-processing (Friston et al. 1996). When head movement becomes too large (e.g., more than 1 mm translational displacement or 1-degree rotational displacement), realignment is no longer reliable and the affected volumes or the whole data set might need to be discarded. After movement correction, spatial smoothing using a Gaussian kernel with 6–8 mm full width at half maximum (FWHM) is applied to reduce noise.

2.6   Recording Procedure

Technical equipment for simultaneous EEG-fMRI recording is now available from various manufacturers. MRI scanners with field strengths up to 3 T and standard radio-frequency head coils can be used with multi-slice single-shot T2*-weighted echo planar imaging sequences to record the BOLD fMRI time series. For later co-registration, a high-resolution anatomical T1-weighted sequence should also be acquired.

For EEG, a variety of EEG caps and battery-supplied amplifiers are on the market. Some options are designed to be used with electrode gel or sponges soaked in electrolyte solutions, and come with active or passive shielding. The number of available electrodes ranges from 32 to 256. For efficient removal of pulse and eye movement artifacts, ECG and electro-oculo-gram (EOG) should be recorded in parallel with EEG.

For data acquisition, the patients are positioned in the head coil using standard manufacturer-supplied cushions and earplugs and are asked to stay awake and keep their eyes closed. If necessary, electrode cables are fixed to the cap with bandaging material and sandbags prevent the wires in the scanner from moving during the recording. After off-line visual inspection of the measured EEG, channels with increased impedance and corrupt signals are excluded from further analysis.

2.7   Modeling the Hemodynamic Response

The BOLD signal represents an indirect measurement of neuronal activity. Although its underlying mechanisms are still not fully understood, it is clear that the cerebral blood volume (CBV) and the concentration of deoxygenated hemoglobin both contribute to changes in the BOLD signal; see, e.g., Kim and Ogawa (2012) for a review. The "balloon model" proposed by Buxton et al. (1998) and its variants qualitatively explain the BOLD changes in response to neuronal activation (Buxton et al. 1998). In magnetic fields, oxygenated hemoglobin (HbO) and deoxygenated hemoglobin ("reduced" hemoglobin, HbR) behave differently. HbO molecules do not contain unpaired electrons and are therefore diamagnetic. In contrast, HbR has four unpaired electrons and is thus paramagnetic. In magnetic fields, the strong dipole moment associated with it induces local field inhomogeneities that depend on the HbR concentration. Locally, the proton spin precession will thus dephase faster, leading to shorter transversal relaxation time T2. In T2- and T2*-weighted MR images, the state of hemoglobin oxygenation therefore acts as the body's own contrast agent. Immediately after neurons are activated, the oxygen metabolism and thus the HbR concentration increase locally ("initial dip" for $t < 2$ s). After a short time, the arterioles react by relaxing and widening, and the oxygen demand is overcompensated by increased influx of oxygenated blood. The concentration of HbR decreases, resulting in a localized increase in T2 and thus stronger signal intensities. A positive peak of +2% to +3% signal intensity is reached around 6 s after the stimulus. Approximately 10 s after neuronal activation stops, the signal intensities slightly undershoot due to slower recovery of the CBV than of the cerebral blood flow (CBF) and return to baseline in about 15–20 s. The sequence of initial dip, signal peak, undershoot, and return to baseline is called the hemodynamic response function (HRF).

In the neocortex, the BOLD signal reflects peri-synaptic activity in the form of the local field potential rather than the spiking rate of individual neurons, but dissociations between BOLD, spiking, and local field potential may occur under pathological conditions (Logothetis 2003; Logothetis and Wandell 2004; Ekstrom 2010). For example in patients with epilepsy, a linear relationship between epileptic discharges and hemodynamic responses has been observed in some studies, while others reported contradictory results (Bagshaw et al. 2005; Mirsattari et al. 2006). Similar to many fMRI studies, in simultaneous EEG-fMRI the hemodynamic response of the BOLD signal to neuronal activation is modeled by the canonical HRF (Friston et al. 1998) in the whole brain and linear correlations between a HRF-convolved predictor and each voxel time series are computed within the framework of the general linear model (GLM) (Glover 1999).

Although this procedure is straightforward, it has serious limitations. First, inter- and intraindividual HRF variability is high (Buckner 1998; Aguirre et al. 1998) and stems from multiple sources including nonneural (vascular, breathing) signals, idiosyncratic responses of different brain areas to external stimuli, effects of the experimental session, task demands and cognitive set, as well as influence of aging and medi-

cations (Kannurpatti et al. 2010, 2011). Second, the assumption of linearity, although a useful approximation, does not hold in all situations (Birn et al. 2001; Birn and Bandettini 2005; Wan et al. 2006). It may be violated when several stimuli occur with less than a few seconds' separation as may be the case in epileptogenic tissue and IEDs. Additional analysis may be required to explore the link between IEDs and BOLD signals.

By modifying the HRF in epilepsy patients it has been shown that the BOLD "response" may occur prior to the spike in scalp EEG. Similar observations have been made in animal studies. Acquiring simultaneous electrocorticogram (ECoG) and near-infrared spectroscopy (NIRS)[2] during drug-induced spiking in adult rats has shown that hemodynamic changes may precede the electrophysiological changes even when measured with implanted electrodes (Osharina et al. 2010). One possible explanation is that increased neural activity may already be occurring in a non-synchronized way before it becomes observable in ECoG via the synchronized spike, which may terminate the epileptic discharge, rather than being the main signature itself.

Going beyond model-based assumptions, exploratory data-driven techniques of fMRI analysis, such as ICA or temporal clustering analysis (TCA), are able to capture BOLD signal changes without imposing constraints on the HRF shape (McKeown et al. 1998; Eichele et al. 2009; Calhoun and Adalı 2012).

---

[2]Like BOLD fMRI NIRS is sensitive to hemoglobin oxygenation. However, the mechanism is different. NIRS exploits the different absorption characteristics of oxygenated and deoxygenated hemoglobin. By measuring absorbance at least at two wavelengths in 650 nm $< \lambda < 1000$ nm, separate quantification of the concentration of both chromophores becomes possible. The advantages of NIRS are its comparably low sensitivity to head movements and fast sampling. A major disadvantage is its insensitivity to deeper brain structures.

2.8   Spike-Based Evaluation

The first simultaneous EEG-fMRI recordings in epilepsy patients were made by acquiring manually triggered single BOLD volumes 3 or 4 s after visual recognition of epileptic EEG spikes recorded in the static magnetic B0 field (Warach et al. 1996; Seeck et al. 1998; Krakow et al. 1999). At this delay, the hemodynamic response is assumed to be maximal. A direct comparison with non-spike-reference BOLD volumes allowed spike localization without the need for removal of gradient artifacts from the raw EEG. A disadvantage of this approach is that it requires continuous EEG reading or automated spike detection and is very inefficient when patients have only a few spikes.

In general, the measurability of synchronized neuronal activity by an EEG electrode at a certain distance depends on the orientation of the cortical source dipole to the electrode surface. Only the perpendicular part of the dipole contributes to the EEG signal, implying that scalp EEG is (partially) blind to large parts of the folded cortex. In addition, owing to the low conductance of the skull, in scalp EEG, sources are spread out tangentially and high-frequency signals as well as spikes can be attenuated by a factor of more than 50 with respect to direct measurement on the dura (Nunez and Silberstein 2000). This implies that spikes can easily remain undetected in background EEG, especially after application of all the (still imperfect) artifact removal techniques outlined above. As a result, the spike-triggered approach is overly conservative for two reasons. First, spikes detected on scalp EEG may represent only a fraction of the true epileptic activity. Secondly, the alleged "spike-free" reference epochs may in fact contain epileptic activity that has gone unrecognized.

The Geneva-London team developed a more modern approach to spike-based evaluation of EEG-fMRI (Grouiller et al. 2011). In short, their procedure is as follows. Using the same EEG equipment for long-term scalp monitoring of epilepsy patients during presurgical evaluation as for EEG-fMRI, patient-specific average spike voltage maps can be generated with very good statistics. After preprocessing similar to the procedure outlined above, the correlation coefficient between topographic voltage maps of EEG recorded inside the MR scanner and average spike voltage map is calculated using a moving window approach. The time course of this correlation coefficient is then used as a predictor for the BOLD responses in a GLM. Grouiller et al. showed that this approach significantly improved simultaneous EEG-fMRI data in a group of patients with previously inconclusive results, even when interictal spikes were absent on the in-scanner EEG (Grouiller et al. 2011).

This topography-based approach has been complemented by a template-based approach by Tousseyn et al. (2014). This procedure also starts with EEG recorded outside the scanner and builds a spike template as a multichannel time-amplitude map by spike-locked averaging over many interictal epileptic spikes and band-pass filtering between 1 and 30 Hz. After preprocessing similar to the procedures described above, the spatiotemporal cross-correlation between the EEG recorded inside the scanner and the template is calculated across all channels in a time-windowed manner. When the correlation exceeds a threshold determined from healthy controls, an event is triggered. The event series is finally convolved with the HRF and used as a predictor in a GLM to calculate the BOLD responses.

2.9   ICA-Based Evaluation

A different approach to analyze simultaneous EEG-fMRI data has been developed at our institution (Jann et al. 2008). After EEG preprocessing as outlined above we run an ICA on the channels which are free of permanent artifacts (extended infomax algorithm (Delorme and Makeig 2004)). The primary justification for applying ICA (or PCA)-based techniques for EEG decomposition is to use them to remove artifacts (see above), which can be regarded as statistically independent from neuronal activity. In practice, this technique can also isolate a single component or a small number of components ("factors"), which contain epileptiform activity that coincides with IEDs and separate them from the remainder that does not. ICA separation on EEG recorded during MR scanning proved insufficient but could be considerably improved by including EEG recorded outside the scanner (Jann et al. 2008).

The ICA of these two datasets produces a small set of ICA components that have only a small spectral amplitude outside the scanner but are markedly increased inside the scanner. This is the expected behavior for factors representing scanner-related and BCG artifacts; see above. Factors associated with eye movements are also easily identified and excluded based on their stereotypical signal shape and spatial distribution. The IED-related ICA factors are inspected visually and those showing signatures of epileptiform activity coinciding with IEDs are selected. Additionally the load of these factors onto the individual electrodes (e.g., scalp distribution) is considered and compared with the topographic voltage map during IEDs. Where more than one ICA factor represents epileptiform activity, only the one that most accurately mirrors the IED observed in the EEG is considered for further analysis, corrected, convolved with a double-gamma HRF (Glover 1999), and used as a predictor for the BOLD signal of the fMRI. Voxel-wise correlations between the BOLD signal and the ICA-based predictor are computed using a GLM. The six motion parameters derived from the fMRI preprocessing are used as nuisance parameters in the GLM.

2.10 Evaluation Based on Artificial Intelligence

Over the past decade, artificial intelligence (AI) and machine learning (ML) have increasingly found their way into medical image analysis and neuroimaging. In a review of recent studies using deep learning (DL) in medical image analysis (Litjens et al. 2017), MRI was the most frequently used imaging modality, and the brain the most often imaged organ. The vast majority of tasks were image segmentation and classification, and convolutional neural networks (Lecun et al. 1998) were the most prevalent architectures for image analysis. Regarding resting-state fMRI, classic ML techniques like support vector machines were used to classify epilepsy-related components identified by spatial ICA (Bharath et al. 2019).

Very recently, the application of DL for EEG analysis has also gained momentum (Craik et al. 2019; Rim et al. 2020). Besides detecting seizures and event-related potentials, its main applications are the EEG-based classification of brain functionality, brain disease, emotion, sleep stage, and motion. The detection of focal epileptiform discharges in scalp EEG has been addressed by Tjepkema-Cloostermans et al. (2018) who evaluated several combinations of convolutional and recurrent neural networks. With the best-performing algorithm, they obtained an area under the receiver-operator characteristic curve (AUC) of 0.94 (sensitivity 47.4%, specificity 98.0% and 99.9% in EEGs with focal epileptic discharges and normal EEGs, respectively). Recent studies on DL-based seizure detection have reported high or even very high performance accuracy (Hussein et al. 2019; Yuan et al. 2019).

ML applications to analyze simultaneous EEG-fMRI are still rare and focus on research questions such as revealing specific EEG fingerprints of deep structures like the amygdala in scalp recordings (Meir-Hasson et al. 2014), classification of sleep patterns from resting-state fMRI alone (Altmann et al. 2016), and detection of visual brain activity (Ahmad et al. 2015, 2017). In a study about epilepsy Hao et al. (2018) used deep residual learning (He et al. 2015) to classify EEG recorded inside the MR scanner as containing either one or none of several possible patient-specific spike types. They then generated a GLM predictor similar to the methods described above.

The authors showed that the sensitivity with which a spike in the EEG could be detected was substantially higher than that of the template-based approach described by Tousseyn et al. (2014). Since the false-positive rate was high (about five detections per minute) manual editing was still required to reject the erroneous detections. One advantage of this approach is that it is much less time consuming than manual annotation of the full recording (only about 11% of the dataset needed to be checked). Moreover, Hao et al. were able to show that BOLD responses to manually annotated EEG were reproduced with the semiautomated method on an anatomical level in 73.7% of the cases and on a lobar level in 89.5% of the cases. In some of the discordant cases, the BOLD responses of the semiautomated method were even more plausible than those based on manual annotations. Concordance of BOLD responses with the epileptogenic zone (EZ) defined by intracranial EEG was 76.9%.

2.11 Connectivity-Based Evaluation

A modern view of epilepsy suggests that it is a disorder of large-scale network dynamics (Bernhardt et al. 2015; Gotman 2008; Spencer 2002). Indeed, spike- or ICA-based analyses of EEG-fMRI data commonly reveal multiple brain regions that respond with coordinated BOLD signal increases or decreases to IED (see below). These coordinated responses are often interpreted in terms of networks; that is, if two regions respond similarly, they must be connected to the same large-scale brain network, whose dynamics are modulated and disrupted by IED (Gotman 2008; Pittau et al. 2014; Richardson 2012). In addition to the approaches presented above, EEG-fMRI experiments can also be evaluated using connectivity methods that seek to identify these network modulations more directly (Karl J. Friston 2011). In this context, networks are usually identified in the fMRI part of the data and the EEG part is used to constrain network calcu-

lations in some meaningful way, e.g., by providing time windows of interest to help network interpretation, or dynamic signal features against which network connectivity can be compared.

fMRI data can be screened for two types of brain network connectivity: "functional" or "effective" connectivity (Friston 2011). Functional connectivity (FC) is defined as the "temporal coincidence of spatially distant neurophysiological events" (Friston 1994; Eickhoff and Müller 2015). In other words, two brain areas are functionally connected if their BOLD signals are correlated over time in a statistically significant way. In fMRI, one of the easiest ways to analyze FC is to extract the BOLD signal from one particular region of interest (ROI, also called a "seed"), and correlate that signal with the signals of all the remaining voxels in the brain. Seed regions can be derived from various sources, e.g., neuroanatomical landmarks, template atlases, voxel coordinates reported in previous research papers, or clusters of activation obtained from a previous standard EEG-fMRI analyses. As an example, one of the earliest studies of FC used a seed on the left motor cortex to obtain a map of the sensorimotor network—in essence, a map of brain-wide time-series correlation coefficients (Biswal and Zerrin Yetkin 1995). Notably, these correlations are found in low-frequency BOLD signal fluctuations, typically below 1 Hz. Furthermore, they are susceptible to a plethora of confounders, in particular to noise introduced by participant motion, respiration, and cardiac pulsations (Power et al. 2014; Parkes et al. 2018; Kassinopoulos and Mitsis 2019). Careful preprocessing of data is therefore necessary to obtain valid results. Another robust way to identify functional networks is to do an ICA of the fMRI data (instead of decomposing the EEG, as described in Sect. 2.9) and to then retain independent components that reflect brain networks rather than noise components (Smith et al. 2011). The advantage of this approach is that it is data driven and thus relatively independent of ROI misspecifications or researcher biases. Moreover, it can be extended to "fuse" data modalities, e.g., to find patterns of joint activity across both EEG and fMRI and potentially even genetic and behavioral data (Calhoun and Adalı 2012). It is therefore particularly suited for exploratory analyses of large, multidimensional datasets (Smith et al. 2009; Allen et al. 2011; Elliott et al. 2018). ICA methods have been an indispensable tool to characterize brain networks from resting-state fMRI that can now be considered canonical (Damoiseaux et al. 2006; van den Heuvel and Hulshoff Pol 2010).

Effective connectivity (EC), a newer development, proposes to go even further by investigating causal relationships between brain regions using fMRI (Friston et al. 2003; Marreiros et al. 2008). EC analyses do not use correlations to represent brain networks, but rather employ complex, biologically informed models of how fMRI signals are generated from a network. Different EC models are usually compared using a Bayesian approach, allowing researchers to draw inferences on both model structure and model parameters (driving versus dampening influences). Because the potential space of causal interactions is enormous, precise a priori hypotheses are required, which are instantiated in a few well-defined models, together with careful modeling of group-level effects (Kahan and Foltynie 2013; Zeidman et al. 2019). Overall, EC is conceptually appealing because it offers a promising way to move beyond pure descriptive statements and towards genuine mechanistic insights, which could be exploited for targeted therapeutic interventions (e.g., deep-brain stimulation) (Moran 2015; Papadopoulou et al. 2017). It might also be possible to extend the methods to assess EC over large numbers of regions (Frässle et al. 2017; Razi et al. 2017) and even to integrate models of neuronal microcircuitry with models of BOLD responses—two developments that might be particularly useful for epilepsy research (Wei et al. 2020). However, EC analyses are less straightforward to implement than FC and rest on statistical concepts that need considerable expertise. In addition, whether one can infer causality from fMRI data remains a somewhat controversial question (Mehler and Kording 2018).

3 Clinical Applications

Clinical applications of simultaneous EEG-fMRI in human epilepsy can be broadly divided into two categories. The first one is investigating BOLD correlates of epileptiform EEG signals in clinically well-defined epilepsy syndromes, such as absence epilepsy or mesial temporal lobe epilepsy with hippocampal sclerosis. The aim of this line of investigation is not only to achieve a more complete syndromic description, but also to unravel pathophysiological mechanisms that could lead to a deeper understanding of epileptogenesis and perhaps even to a more refined, evidence-based classification of the epilepsies (Berg et al. 2010). The second application is localizing epileptogenic foci during the preoperative workup of children and adults with pharmacoresistant epilepsies (Salek-Haddadi et al. 2006; De Tiege et al. 2007). Here, the focus is on the localization of the seizure-onset zone, and simultaneous EEG-fMRI has proven especially valuable when no epileptogenic lesion can be detected by conventional MRI protocols (Moeller et al. 2009), or when multifocal seizures are suspected (Zijlmans et al. 2007). We review both types of studies below.

3.1 Simultaneous EEG-fMRI in Genetic Generalized Epilepsy Syndromes

Genetic generalized epilepsies (GGE) comprise a group of heterogeneous syndromes in which a strong genetic component is suspected or has been identified. GGE are common and account for roughly 40% of epilepsy diagnoses. Their hallmark is generalized spike-waves (GSWD) in the EEG; these are synchronous, mostly symmetric, bilateral paroxysmal, short-duration (<200 ms) high-amplitude potentials followed by a slow wave (Seneviratne et al. 2017). They can occur in isolation, but classically appear in short runs with frequencies around 3–4 Hz. Longer series of GSWD impair consciousness for brief periods, leading to the clinical picture of absence seizures. These seizures are further characterized by sudden behavioral arrest, unresponsiveness, staring, and sometimes mild oral automatisms and/or bilateral eye blinks (Holmes et al. 1987; Panayiotopoulos et al. 1992). The co-occurrence of GSWD on EEG and absence seizures define childhood (4–8 years) and juvenile (9–13 years) absence epilepsy (AE). The syndromes represent ~10% of all epilepsies in each age group, are readily amenable to pharmacological treatment, and, in general, have a good prognosis. Other syndromes studied include juvenile myoclonic epilepsy (JME) and benign epilepsy with centro-temporal spikes (BECTS, or Rolandic epilepsy). JME is clinically important in this context, because up to one-third of patients can be refractory to treatment and this type of epilepsy can be accompanied by neurocognitive impairment (Kim et al. 2007; Stevelink et al. 2019).

GGE patients have participated in experimental EEG-fMRI studies which pursued three aims: (1) to identify the (syndrome-specific) networks associated with GSW discharges, (2) to map the neural correlates of attention and vigilance (as surrogates for consciousness), and, more recently, and (3) to validate complex biophysical models of brain connectivity using fMRI, like dynamic causal modeling (DCM). The first goal has been studied more extensively than the other two since the pathophysiology and neuroanatomy of GSWD and absence seizures are surprisingly difficult to understand (Meeren et al. 2005; Crunelli et al. 2020). EEG-fMRI studies have provided crucial evidence that GSWD emerge in cortico-thalamic networks and that frontal and sensorim-otor cortices are key drivers of GSWD dynamics (Tangwiriyasakul et al. 2018).

One of the earliest simultaneous EEG-fMRI studies by Archer et al. investigated cortical and subcortical patterns of BOLD signal change at 1.5 T in five patients (four of whom suffered from childhood AE) who had frequent GSWD during rest (Archer et al. 2003a). Their main finding was a large area of GSWD-related BOLD deactivation in the posterior cingulate cortex (ret-rosplenial cortex) that was highly consistent across patients, supplemented by more variable

regions of BOLD activation in the angular gyrus and around the precentral sulcus bilaterally. Thalamic BOLD activation was seen in only two of the five patients and was not significant at the group level, either because of intrinsic variability of the BOLD response in subcortical structures or because of the low signal-to-noise ratio at low field strengths. Subsequent studies in adults and children with IGE have reliably identified tha-lamic BOLD signal increases, and have confirmed the high degree of inter-individual variability in cortical and subcortical BOLD patterns (Aghakhani et al. 2004; Hamandi et al. 2006; Moeller et al. 2008a, b).

Notably, the set of symmetrical regions that were deactivated during GSWD in GGE, i.e., precuneus, inferior parietal cortex, and ventral medial prefrontal cortex, are core nodes in the now widely known default mode network (DMN). This network is highly active and functionally strongly interconnected during conscious rest (Raichle et al. 2001; Greicius et al. 2003). It probably supports attentional and self-referential processes such as autobiographical memory or envisioning the future (Raichle and Snyder 2007; Buckner et al. 2008). The role of GSWD-related BOLD signal changes within the DMN is still poorly understood, but deviations of DMN activity are commonly seen in neurological disorders, e.g., Alzheimer's disease, multiple sclerosis, and traumatic brain injury (Buckner et al. 2008; Bonnelle et al. 2012; Rocca et al. 2012).

In Figs. 1 and 2 we present typical examples of GSWD-BOLD correlates from our own patient database. Figure 1 shows data from a 44-year-old patient who has had an unclassified GGE since childhood and poor seizure control despite medication. Panel a summarizes the general analysis strategy at our lab (see above for details), where the in-scanner EEG is analyzed using a temporal ICA to derive a predictor of the BOLD response that encodes the continuously fluctuating epileptic activity (Jann et al. 2008). Panel b shows a typical pattern of BOLD signal change, which is linearly correlated with epileptic activity. Widespread cortical deactivations corresponding to the DMN are evident, as well as a very focal

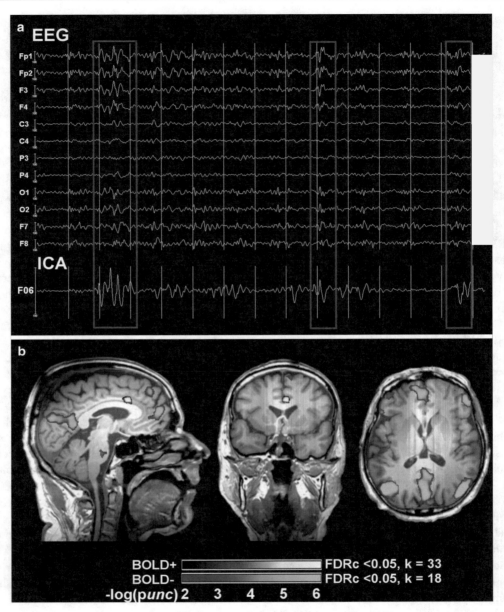

Fig. 1 Example of EEG-fMRI analysis and BOLD correlates of generalized spike-wave discharges (GSWD) in a patient with genetic generalized epilepsy (GGE). Panel (**a**) shows 14 s of artifact-corrected in-scanner electroencephalogram (EEG) and its associated independent component analysis (ICA) factor (F06) that codes for GSWD. Red squares mark three time points (seconds 3, 10, and 14) that contain frontally predominant (EEG electrodes Fp1, Fp2) GSWD. Note the corresponding amplitude oscillations in ICA factor F06. Panel (**b**) shows the statistical parametric maps (SPMs) of functional activations (BOLD+) and deactivations (BOLD−) linearly correlated to F06 (and therefore GSWD), overlaid on an anatomical scan (neurological convention, left in the image is left in the brain). Statistically significant signal increases are seen in the anterior cingulate cortex (warm colors), and widespread decreases in the precuneus, medial prefrontal cortex, inferior parietal, and dorsolateral prefrontal cortices bilaterally (cool colors). SPMs have an uncorrected (unc) peak-level threshold at $p < 0.001$ ($= -\log(2)$) and a corrected false discovery rate cluster-level (FDRc) threshold at $p < 0.05$ (k, critical cluster size)

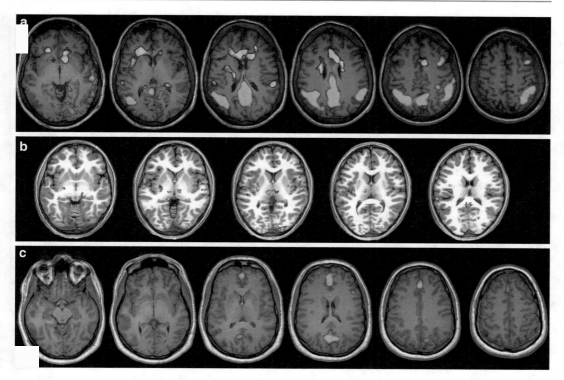

Fig. 2 Examples of the interindividual variability in BOLD correlates of generalized spike-wave discharges in patients with IGE. Hot colors indicate BOLD-signal increase, cool colors show BOLD-signal decrease. All images are in neurological convention (left hemisphere is on the left side of the image). Panel (**a**) 29-year-old patient with generalized seizures. Strong signal increases are seen in the anterior cingulate cortex, and decreases in the pre- cuneus and parietal lobes bilaterally. Panel (**b**) 15-year-old patient with brief visual symptoms followed by generalized seizures. Bilateral BOLD-signal decreases are seen in the thalamus, and unilateral decrease in the right occipital pole. Panel (**c**) 23-year-old patient with generalized seizures. BOLD-signal decreases localize onto the anterior cingulate cortex and precuneus bilaterally

signal increase in the anterior cingulate cortex. As in the study by Archer et al., no thalamic activations are seen in this case. Figure 2 shows a small case series that illustrates the wide interindividual variability of GSWD-related (de)activation patterns.

Besides these observational case series, several controlled experimental studies in patients with absence seizures (AS) have compared GSWD on EEG-fMRI with behavioral changes. These studies focused on the second goal mentioned above, i.e., correlating attentional states with GSWD and their metabolic correlates. AS patients typically show a transient impairment of consciousness that manifests in a sudden cessa-

tion of spontaneous behavior, blank stare, subtle motor automatisms, and reduced attention. Berman et al. investigated these changes in attention in a group of children with AS using simultaneous EEG-fMRI during execution of two tasks, a continuous performance task (CPT), which required sustained attention to letter stimuli, and a simple repetitive motor task. CPT performance dropped significantly more than motor task performance during AS (as recorded with the in-scanner EEG), and this behavioral impairment was associated with the core corticothalamic BOLD network found in the studies mentioned above and illustrated in our examples. This study was the first to establish a link between behavior and simultaneous EEG-fMRI signal, thus indicating that all areas visualized in observational studies with GGE patients (see above) are indeed relevant for the maintenance of attention.

A concomitant study by the same group analyzed the temporal dynamics of the BOLD response to GGE by shifting the HRF from 16 s before the onset of AS to 24 s after it in a large cohort of AE patients ($n = 88$) (Bai et al. 2010). They found bilateral BOLD increases in medial and orbital frontal areas as early as 14 s before AS onset, followed by a late increase in the thalamus (10 s after AS onset) that was paralleled by widespread BOLD decreases in the DMN and bilateral frontoparietal networks, which outlasted the AS by more than 20 s. Moreover, they found that HRF in selected regions (e.g., the thalamus or medial and orbital frontal cortex) was highly variable and did not necessarily conform to a "canonical" HRF. These results suggest that not all events accompanying AS are captured by scalp EEG, and that there might be additional between- and within-subject variability in the neurovascular coupling between electrical and metabolic activity in GGE, which is still poorly understood and cannot be captured with conventional HRF modeling (Bai et al. 2010). Benuzzi et al. analyzed the intersubject variability of BOLD dynamics from 15 s before to 9 s after the GSWD in a mixed group of 15 adolescents and adults with different GGE syndromes (Benuzzi et al. 2012). At the group level, DMN regions (precuneus, bilateral inferior parietal cortex) as well as the bilateral dorsolateral prefrontal cortex showed transient BOLD increases between 12 and 6 s before GSWD, and then an immediate BOLD decrease from GSW start to ~6 s afterwards. The thalamus (together with the cerebellum and anterior cingulate cortex) was most active at GSWD initiation for a short time (roughly 3 s in their analysis). Notably, the individual patterns of the temporal evolution of these changes were highly variable. There were cases of very early or very late decreases in the DMN, short or prolonged increases in the thalamus, and different degrees of overlap between activated and deactivated areas (Benuzzi et al. 2012).

Finally, two studies analyzed the EC within the thalamocortical BOLD-GSW network, i.e., the dynamic couplings and influences of brain regions on each other (Friston 2011). This was accomplished by using dynamic causal modeling (DCM), an advanced biophysical modeling framework that allows (hidden) neural activity to be inferred based on observed BOLD responses (see Sect. 2.11). In one study, Vaudano et al. found that the precuneus has a "permissive" or "gatekeeper" role in GSW generation within the thalamocortical network, which harks back to the idea that a cortical contribution is necessary (Vaudano et al. 2009). Daunizeau et al. took this observation one step further. Using simultaneous EEG-fMRI data from the same study, they showed that spontaneous fMRI signal fluctuations explained frequency modulations of the EEG during GSWD (Daunizeau et al. 2012). This hints at a future area of research, where not only the spatial profiles, but also the temporal dynamics of EEG and fMRI events, are to analyze epileptiform activity.

In summary, simultaneous EEG-fMRI has produced abundant and novel findings on functional correlates in GGE. A common theme is the involvement of thalamocortical functional networks in ictal and interictal GSW and a still incompletely understood intersubject variability in the spatial patterns and temporal dynamics of these networks. This variability is not only due to the different and sometimes heterogeneous populations studied, since it was also found in more tightly defined subgroups, e.g., children with AS (Moeller et al. 2008a; Bai et al. 2010). Therefore, it seems reasonable to assume that it might be biologically meaningful, indicating that GSWD, although relatively stereotypical on scalp EEG, might not reflect a unitary phenomenon but a complex set of brain network interactions. Simultaneous EEG-fMRI may thus serve as a biomarker for different GGE subtypes (even in syndromes that have been thought to be rather homogeneous on clinical grounds).

3.2 Simultaneous EEG-fMRI in the Preoperative Workup of Pharmacoresistant Focal Epilepsies

Simultaneous EEG-fMRI can assist in the preoperative evaluation of patients who have surgically remediable epilepsy syndromes. This is clinically important, as roughly 30% of epilepsy patients have or develop pharmacoresistant disease (Kwan and Brodie 2000), i.e., seizures that cannot be controlled after adequate treatment with two anti-seizure medications (Kwan and Brodie 2001; Kwan et al. 2010). Epilepsy surgery can be highly effective in this group. The first randomized controlled trial on epilepsy surgery was conducted for a carefully selected cohort of adult patients with mesial temporal lobe epilepsy (MTLE). It showed that the number needed to treat (NNT), i.e., how many patients need to receive therapy to obtain one good outcome or prevent a bad one, was two to render one patient free of seizures impairing awareness at 1 year post-surgery, and 3 to render one patient completely seizure-free (Wiebe et al. 2001). In an illustrative example Wiebe (2004) compared these results to carotid endarterectomy, the widely used standard for symptomatic carotid stenosis. For the latter procedure, the NNT is 15 to avoid one disabling ischemic stroke or death in patients with severe stenosis over a follow-up of 2–6 years (Cina et al. 2000). No surgical complications occurred in patients participating in the randomized controlled epilepsy trial, whereas other studies have reported that surgical complications occur in 11% of patients, and that 3% of patients sustain new, permanent neurological deficits (Engel et al. 2003). However, the fact that successful surgery substantially reduces the risk of premature mortality outweighs these risks (Vickrey et al. 1995; Sperling et al. 1999; Bell et al. 2010). A recent study by De Tisi et al. followed 615 adult epilepsy surgery patients over a median follow-up period of 8 years and found a favorable long-term outcome in about 65% of cases. Fifty-one percent of patients were seizure-free immediately after surgery and for a sustained period of time thereafter, and an additional 14% were eventually seizure-free after a complex sequence of remission and relapse (de Tisi et al. 2011). Some 25% can be weaned off medication and can be considered as cured, but 40% of operated epilepsy patients still require anti-seizure drugs (ASD) to stay seizure-free (Téllez-Zenteno et al. 2005). However, large-scale retrospective studies in MTLE patients ($n = 376$, 18 years of follow-up) have shown that even if ASD are continued, roughly 19% of patients in this category can safely switch from poly- to monotherapy, or reduce monotherapy dosage compared to those used preoperatively (Wieser and Häne 2003, 2004). It is likely that owing to seizure freedom and decreased ASD side effects, quality of life will improve significantly in operated patients, even if they suffer from postoperative memory decline (Langfitt et al. 2007). Consequently, patients occupy less healthcare resources and healthcare costs drop in the first 2 years after surgery. Long-term comparisons of medical and surgical costs between operated and non-operated pharmacoresistant epilepsy patients indicate that epilepsy surgery becomes cost effective in as few as 7 or 8 years (King Jr et al. 1997), although this may take as long as 35 years, depending on the type of analysis (Platt and Sperling 2002). Overall, these findings indicate that epilepsy surgery can be highly beneficial. It provides relief from individual suffering, prevents further disability, and reduces healthcare costs to society as a whole (Begley et al. 2000). Pharmacoresistant patients should therefore be identified and offered surgery as early as possible (Kwan and Brodie 2000; Engel Jr et al. 2012). There is still a delay of 18–23 years between development of pharmacoresistance and referral to preoperative evaluation, although recent data suggest that the delay might be slowly shortening (Haneef et al. 2010; Baud et al. 2018).

For epilepsy surgery to be successful, we must precisely identify the tissue to be resected and its spatial relationship to functionally relevant (eloquent) cortex. This requires data from multiple clinical and paraclinical sources, i.e., patient history, seizure semiology, neuropsychological examination, ictal and interictal scalp and/or intracranial EEG, and functional and structural neuroimaging (Rosenow and Lüders 2001). While standard fMRI with motor, sensory, or cognitive paradigms is used to map eloquent cortex (see chapter "Task-Based Presurgical Functional MRI in Patients with Brain Tumors" of this book), simultaneous EEG-fMRI is used as an additional tool to identify the irritative zone (IZ) and thus to restrict the EZ, i.e., "the minimum amount of cortex that must be resected (inactivated or completely disconnected) to produce seizure freedom." As mentioned in the introduction to this chapter, the EZ overlaps with the seizure-onset zone (SOZ) and the IZ that generate seizures and IED, respectively. The IZ can thus serve as a proxy for the SOZ and the EZ for clinical purposes, although the different zones may not be concordant. Every neuroimaging technique used in epileptology has particular strengths and weaknesses when trying to map and disentangle this complex topography. Scalp EEG for instance has a very high temporal resolution, but is relatively insensitive to deep sources of epileptiform activity within the EZ. Positron-emission tomography (PET) and single-photon emission computed tomography (SPECT) require invasive application of radioactive tracers. Structural MRI has a high spatial resolution and can identify even subtle cortical epileptogenic lesions, but these may not overlap with either the IZ or the SOZ. Simultaneous EEG-fMRI is helpful in this regard, as it can show the metabolic correlates of deep-lying IZs (via IED on scalp EEG) and depict the relationship between IED focus and epileptogenic lesion (via co-registration with high-resolution anatomical images). This might be especially important where mapping of the different zones is complicated or equivocal, e.g., in patients with the SOZ outside the temporal lobes, in those with multifocal lesions, and in those in whom no epileptogenic lesion can be identified by standard MRI protocols (Téllez-Zenteno et al. 2005; Jeha et al. 2007; Bien et al. 2009). A few studies have acquired simultaneous EEG-fMRI during the (fortuitous) occurrence of focal seizures (Sierra-Marcos et al. 2013), but in our view safety concerns, movement artifacts,

and unpredictable nature of seizures limit the clinical applicability of this technique.

Several clinical observational studies indicate that local BOLD responses, as mapped with simultaneous EEG-fMRI, co-localize with the SOZ at the lobar level (Fig. 3 shows one example from our institution of how lobe-level localization can be obtained, starting from surface EEG to whole-brain BOLD correlates). Krakow et al. investigated ten patients with focal pharmacoresistant epilepsies (Krakow et al. 1999). BOLD correlates to IED could be found in six of the patients, and in all of them, the BOLD correlate was close to the SW maximum in the EEG. One large study analyzed 63 consecutive patients investigated with frequent IED (Salek-Haddadi et al. 2006). Concordant or approximately concordant BOLD correlates were found in 23 patients (37%), 25 had no IED, and 11 did not show any BOLD correlates, despite the presence of IED. There might have been technical reasons for this low yield since the study was performed at 1.5 T with spike triggering, and higher field strengths (Federico et al. 2005) as well as continuous imaging lead to better results (Al-Asmi et al. 2003). Despite its shortcomings, this study revealed a few interesting results. For instance, there was a pattern of precuneal deactivation in seven patients, reminiscent of the patterns found in GGE (see above). Also, the authors found that, in general, BOLD activations showed better concordance with the presumed spike-wave (SW) focus than BOLD deactivations (the reason for which is still unknown). Finally, they found that most HRF had physiological waveforms, indicating that "standard" modeling approaches might be sufficient for clinical purposes. Kobayashi et al. investigated 35 patients with temporal lobe epilepsy and found concordant responses in 83% of them (Kobayashi et al. 2006). Deactivations were again identified in roughly 50% of cases. Interestingly, these authors found 16 patients with neocortical BOLD correlates of whom 12 had concordant bilateral temporal lobe clusters, indicating that simultaneous EEG-fMRI not only reveals EZ, but can also depict parts of the complete epileptogenic network. In a follow-up study, these authors observed that this network extended not only to bilateral mesial temporal structures, but also to interconnected areas such as the basal ganglia, inferior insula, and lateral temporal gyri (Kobayashi et al. 2009). Notably, contralateral temporal lobe BOLD activity peaked later than the ipsilateral activity. Thus, these results demonstrate that simultaneous EEG-fMRI, despite the low temporal resolution of the latter, might also

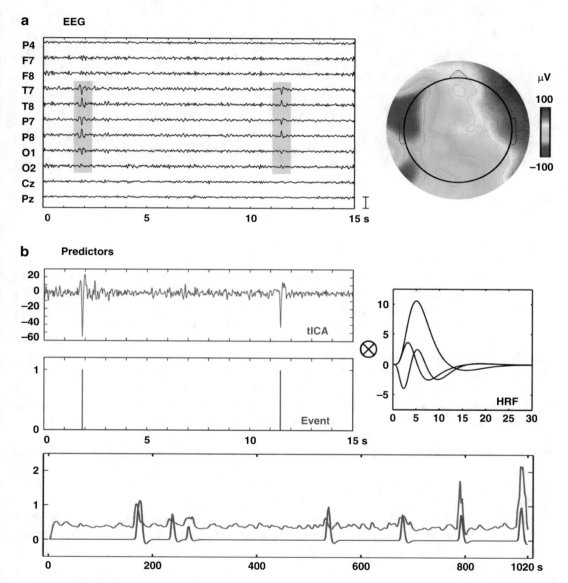

Fig. 3 A standard EEG-fMRI analysis in a patient with left-sided mesial temporal lobe epilepsy. Panel (**a**) shows on the left an artifact-corrected in-scanner EEG trace with two interictal epileptiform discharges (IED, gray areas) and on the right the corresponding scalp topography, with a large negative deflection on the left frontotemporal region. Panel (**b**) displays the steps to obtain predictors for subsequent statistical modeling. IED can be modeled either as a continuous predictor using temporal ICA (red traces, see Fig. 1 and main text for details) or as single events (blue event markers). Convolution with a set of hemodynamic response functions (HRF) leads predictors that are included in a design matrix (panel **c**, left plot) together with multiple confounders that code for physiological and movement-related noise. Statistical analysis across the whole brain revealed in this case distinct clusters of BOLD-signal increase in the left temporal pole and left hippocampus (panel **d**)

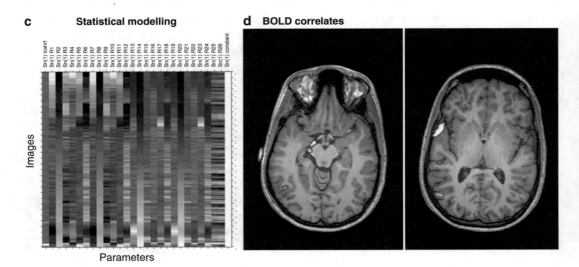

Fig. 3 (continued)

reveal aspects of the temporal dynamics of SW-associated functional networks.

One important question concerning the clinical utility of simultaneous EEG-fMRI is how closely it aligns with two important gold standard measures: results from intracranial EEG and postsurgical outcome (Zhang et al. 2012). This question has been addressed in several retrospective case reports and case series, which suggest overall that EEG-fMRI can be a clinically meaningful aid to the localization of the SOZ. Seeck et al. published one of the first case reports of a patient in whom simultaneous EEG-fMRI activity was concordant with scalp EEG source analysis and electrocorticography (ECoG) (Seeck et al. 1998). In the abovementioned case series by Krakow et al. in which six patients showed BOLD correlates of focal SW, one localization was also confirmed by ECoG (Krakow et al. 1999). Laufs et al. also found excellent concordance of simultaneous EEG-fMRI in one patient with a right frontocentral SOZ (Laufs et al. 2006). Interestingly, this patient did not show clear IED during the combined recording, and a focal abnormality of the EEG (localized delta activity) was used to derive the fMRI regressor. However, mixed results were reported in two studies by Bagshaw et al. (*n* = 4) and Bénar et al. (*n* = 5) (Bagshaw et al. 2004; Bénar et al. 2006). Both

groups validated the findings of simultaneous EEG-fMRI against stereotaxic EEG (sEEG) and found concordant BOLD activations to focal SW in 3/4 and 4/5 patients, respectively, but also discordant BOLD correlates in one patient per study. More recently, Khoo et al. reanalyzed data on 37 patients who had undergone EEG-fMRI and sEEG implantations (Khoo et al. 2017). They found that BOLD responses to IED correctly localized the SOZ in 24 of the patients and that a classifier built on BOLD response statistics could help to identify the most relevant BOLD clusters, i.e., those most likely to correspond to the actual SOZ. Three further studies investigated the overlap between EEG-fMRI responses and postoperative resections in relation to seizure outcomes (Thornton et al. 2010; An et al. 2013; Coan et al. 2016). Although methods for defining the overlap differed, all of these studies showed that concordance between the BOLD response and the resection zone was associated with postoperative seizure freedom, whereas discordant findings were associated with a less favorable outlook, indicating that EEG-fMRI might help in defining surgical targets. This could be particularly important in focal epilepsy patients with frequent IED but discordant findings on standard EEG and MRI. For instance, Ziljmans et al. reviewed 29 patients with simultaneous recordings who had

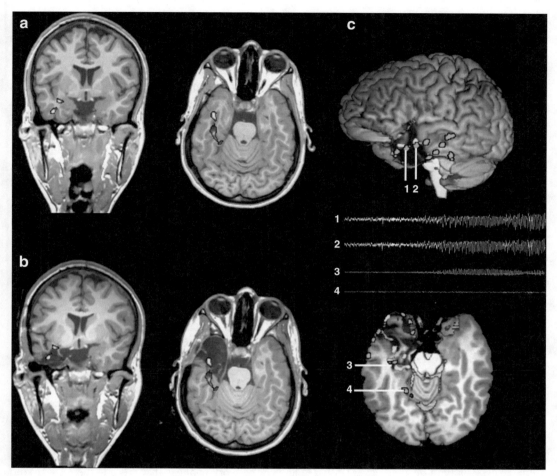

Fig. 4 This figure shows how EEG-fMRI results can relate to intracranial EEG investigations and postsurgical resections in a patient with non-lesional left-sided mesial temporal lobe epilepsy. Panel (**a**) shows a coronal and axial slice of a patient with non-lesional left-sided mesial temporal lobe epilepsy (same patient as in Fig. 1, neurological convention). Color maps indicate clusters of blood oxygen level-dependent (BOLD) signal increases significantly correlated with interictal epileptiform discharges ($p < 0.05$, corrected for multiple comparisons). Panel (**b**) shows the same clusters projected onto a postoperative anatomical MRI. The peak BOLD cluster is included in the resected area. Panel (**c**) shows the correspondence between IED-related BOLD clusters and intracranial EEG signals. The upper image shows a lateral view of the 3D-rendered brain after resection. Green clusters represent intracranial electrode positions, derived from CT-MRI fusion. The lower image shows an axial cut through the upper border of the resection. Traces show the first 10 s of seizure evolution in the temporal pole (electrodes 1 and 2) and the hippocampus (3). Note their proximity to the hemodynamic IED correlates. In contrast, a distant electrode (4) does not show epileptiform activity

not been referred for surgery owing to insufficient certainty in focus localization or multifocality (Zijlmans et al. 2007). In their study, preoperative reevaluation for four patients was considered worthwhile, and two underwent intracranial studies that confirmed EEG-fMRI results. Moeller et al. studied another complex group—patients with non-lesional frontal lobe epilepsy (Moeller et al. 2009). They found BOLD correlates in 8/9 patients. In two patients who had undergone surgery, subtle cortical abnormalities just adjacent to the EEG-fMRI correlates could be identified on histopathology. Figure 4 displays one exemplar case from our own presurgical program, in which EEG-fMRI results, iEEG investigations, and surgical resection showed broad concordance.

While most of the studies reviewed above aimed at finding BOLD correlates that were highly specific for individual patients, another line of research has tried to identify common epileptogenic regions shared among multiple focal epilepsy syndromes. The rationale for this approach is that such common regions could be used as standard therapeutic targets, thus simplifying treatment. Group analyses of EEG-fMRI data did reveal that a region anterior to the amygdala, corresponding to the human piriform cortex, seems to be activated by IED in most focal epilepsy syndromes (Flanagan et al. 2014). The piriform cortex is a brain region with widespread connectivity that was highly seizure-prone in animal experiments (Stripling and Patneau 1990; Löscher and Ebert 1996; Vaughan and Jackson 2014). Interestingly, resection of the piriform cortex has recently been shown to be predictive of a good surgical outcome (Galovic et al. 2019).

In sum, the studies reviewed above testify to the complexity of results that can be obtained with simultaneous EEG-fMRI. This technique clearly has its place in the presurgical workup of patients with focal epilepsy, and seems to be valuable especially in difficult cases (Pittau et al. 2012a; Centeno et al. 2017). However, the fact that mapping epileptogenic tissue with simultaneous EEG-fMRI still mainly depends on the detection of IED is an important limitation: overall, only 50% of patients with refractory epilepsy seem to have sufficient IED during scanning, and again half of the patients with refractory epilepsy will show an identifiable BOLD correlate (Gotman et al. 2004; Salek-Haddadi et al. 2006). Furthermore, the predictive value of IED in localizing the SOZ is not always easy to determine and it seems to depend on the neuroanatomical localization of the EZ and the pathophysiology of the underlying disease. This adds to the complexity already presented by the overlapping zones (or rather networks and network components). For temporal lobe epilepsies, data indicate that IED on scalp EEG does predict the SOZ correctly in ~90% of cases (Blume et al. 2001). However,

for extratemporal sites, e.g., the frontal or parietal lobes, the predictive power of IED is lower, as only ~20% of patients exhibit unilateral, clearly focal IED (Holmes et al. 2000). Thus, techniques that allow mapping of the EZ even without spikes are an important focus of further research on EEG-fMRI (Rodionov et al. 2007; Grouiller et al. 2011). This could lead to a further important goal for simultaneous EEG-fMRI, i.e., guiding the placement of intracranial electrodes in patients with non-lesional or multifocal epilepsies (Zijlmans et al. 2007).

3.3   Connectivity Analyses

Broadly speaking, there are three areas in which connectivity analyses of EEG-fMRI data have provided insightful results: basic mechanisms of GSWD, effects of epileptic discharges (both focal and generalized) on intrinsic connectivity networks, and, finally, refinement of surgical targets. Examples of each of these are provided below.

In terms of GSWD mechanisms, EEG-fMRI studies have shown that GSWD do not emerge suddenly, as their appearance on scalp EEG would suggest, but rather that they are the result of network changes that precede them by around 1 min—a fact that was known from rodent models, but less well recognized in humans (Crunelli et al. 2020). In a recent study, Tangwiriyasakul et al. analyzed phase synchrony in visual, sensorimotor, and frontoparietal networks, using EEG-fMRI data acquired in 43 patients with a total of 95 GSWD events (Tangwiriyasakul et al. 2018). They found that the frontoparietal network showed significantly low synchrony in non-discharge epochs, but increased its intrinsic connectivity steeply before GSWD. They also observed that the motor network was already highly synchronized 1 min before GSWD onset, suggesting some form of pre-ictal network priming. Interestingly, additional significant connections to the sensorimotor network were observed, involving the prefrontal and precuneus regions, as GSWD approached. These findings are in line with previous amplitude-based analyses and suggest that persistently high sensorimotor network synchrony, coupled with transiently low posterior network synchrony, may be a state predisposing to GSWD onset (Bai et al. 2010). Notably, increased sensorimotor connectivity on fMRI has been observed in first-degree relatives of GGE patients, both at rest and during motor tasks (Vollmar et al. 2011). This further supports the idea that increased excitability of motor areas could be a core feature of GGE pathophysiology. How do these network dynamics affect consciousness? To address this question, Guo et al. prospectively investigated a group of 93 pediatric patients using EEG-fMRI and were able to capture more than 1000 AS with GSWD in 39 of them (Guo et al. 2016). They found that rather than being associated with one particular network, impaired consciousness was related to the intensity of signal changes in multiple networks, in this case the DMN, the sensorimotor network, and a frontoparietal attentional network.

The idea that epilepsy can alter multiple existing brain networks has received increasing support from EEG-fMRI studies (Shamshiri et al. 2019). In a study of children with focal epilepsy, Shamshiri et al. found that IED reduced FC in attentional networks, which could explain the cognitive problems seen in this population (Shamshiri et al. 2017). In patients with MTLE, unilateral IED disrupt the connectivity between hippocampus and DMN (Tong et al. 2019). It is noteworthy that connectivity alterations seem to occur not only during focal IED, but even without them (Iannotti et al. 2016). In patients with MTLE, for instance, connectivity in limbic networks, DMN, and attentional networks is reduced prior to IED (Pittau et al. 2012b; Faizo et al. 2014; Burianová et al. 2017). A similar phenomenon was seen in Lennox-Gastaut syndrome, a severe epileptic encephalopathy: interactions between multiple cognitive networks were persistently abnormal after accounting for the effect of IED (Warren et al. 2016). This suggests that connectivity alterations are both a state and trait marker of epilepsy.

Finally, connectivity analyses could help refine surgical targets in patients with focal epi-

lepsy. Negishi et al. found that patients with lateralized FC, as calculated from the maximum of the EEG-fMRI response, had better postsurgical outcome than those with less lateralized networks (Negishi et al. 2011). Similar to the findings with standard analyses, Lee et al. found that concordance of SOZ with local connectivity was associated with a good postsurgical outcome (Lee et al. 2014).

4 Future Directions

Epilepsy is a prototypical dynamic disease that affects a large-scale network and not only a circumscribed area of seizure generation. Normal brain function requires complex interactions between different, highly dynamic neural systems that rely on the integrity of structural and functional networks. Thus, a comprehensive evaluation of a patient with epilepsy requires not only the identification of the EZ, but also an understanding of its functional embedment in and interaction with an epileptic network as well as the potential structural abnormalities (the structural epileptogenic lesion) that predispose to seizure generation. Since the last edition of this textbook, remarkable advances have been made in this area. They include AI technologies which filter artifacts, FC analysis done via DL, and concurrent TMS-EEG-fMRI to monitor causal dependencies of signal propagation through cortico-subcortical networks (Hosseini et al. 2020).

Beyond advances in the application of EEG-fMRI as a diagnostic tool, various complementary structural and functional imaging technologies are currently being tested in clinical environments.

Perfusion imaging has become an important tool for investigating peri-ictal perfusion changes. It is for example used to differentiate ictal stroke mimics from acute ischemic stroke by showing focal areas of increased perfusion on computed tomography or MRI images. Moreover, perfusion imaging can detect abnormalities related to the symptomatogenic zone and to seizure spread. Arterial spin labeling

(ASL) is of particular interest, since it enables quantification of CBF without the need for intravenous gadolinium contrast and can be applied repeatedly during peri-ictal and seizure-free periods (Wiest and Beisteiner 2019). It holds promise for investigating within- and between-subject differences associated with epilepsy-induced state changes and baseline differences in regional CBF. Recent ASL studies have revealed consistent downregulation of CBF in brain areas involved in seizure generation and propagation in the early postictal period as compared to the intraindividual reference CBF during seizure-free periods. Postictal perfusion decrease which overlaps partially or completely with the presumed SOZ has been consistently reported in patients with chronic focal epilepsy (Gaxiola-Valdez et al. 2017). This is in line with electric source imaging data on EEG and hypometabolism of fluorodeoxyglucose-PET (Storti et al. 2014).

Image post-processing of structural MRI is another technique that shows clinical potential in epilepsy. It can assist in the identification of subtle cortical abnormalities related to focal cortical dysplasia, and can automatically segment and parcellate the cortex to derive cortical thickness measures directly from T1-weighted (T1w) MRI. A worldwide study of brain structural changes in patients with epilepsy using quantitative MRI has identified robust structural brain alterations within and across epilepsy syndromes (Whelan et al. 2018). Automated post-processing techniques can help to identify region-wise cortical thickness abnormalities on normal-appearing MRI scans that are labeled as non-lesional epilepsy. Automated surface-based MRI morphometry can nowadays be empowered with AI for automated lesion detection and identification of abnormal structural network patterns across cohorts from different centers and scanners (Jin et al. 2018). New methods using DL technologies allow fast and sensitive data analysis within a fraction of the time required by conventional surface-based morphometric methods and at no cost to the robustness (Rebsamen et al. 2020). Analysis of large-scale gray matter alterations complements EEG-fMRI measurements and can help identify reconfigurations of structural network topology in distinct epilepsy syndromes.

MRI-based methods that detect subtle fluctuations in the electromagnetic fields, and are thus complementary to EEG-fMRI, are currently under investigation (Cassará et al. 2009; Du et al. 2014; Sundaram et al. 2016). Some progress has been made with MRI using the stimulus-induced rotary saturation (SIRS) effect, but interference from the BOLD response still complicates such measurements (Sveinsson et al. 2020). Experimental studies have suggested that MRI could detect oscillating magnetic fields directly using spin locking to investigate contrasts in populations of protons with a Larmor frequency different from that of water. If neuronal signaling during epileptic discharges generates magnetic fields, these interact with the externally applied magnetic field and attenuate local MR signal intensity. Thus, if the Larmor frequency of the MR scanner is adjusted to frequency domains in the high-frequency and ultrahigh-frequency band that match pathological activities recorded in the epileptic brain in vivo, subtle MR signal attenuation can be observed. Neuronal current imaging makes use of changes in ionic currents associated with synaptic and suprathreshold activity of the order of nanoamperes. The first technical report of effects on magnetic field perturbations in a small series of patients that underwent presurgical phase II workup noted a hemispheric concordance in 7/8 patients (Kiefer et al. 2016). Notably, the effects of the spin-lock experiment were absent after successful epilepsy surgery (Engel class I), but remained detectable in patients with a less favorable outcome. While it has not yet made its way into clinical practice, this approach would certainly lead to further insights into human brain functional organization and open a new window for simultaneous recordings of EEG and biological fields with MRI.

5   Conclusions

Simultaneous EEG-fMRI is a methodically challenging technique and it is important to consider certain practical pitfalls. However, the capacity of simultaneous EEG-fMRI to provide detailed three-dimensional whole-brain maps of epileptiform activity is unparalleled, making it an attractive tool for clinical and experimental investigations. Artifact rejection algorithms, statistical analysis techniques, and biophysical models for multimodal data fusion are evolving rapidly as is the range of applications. This is an exciting area of imaging neuroscience that, if properly validated, could have a considerable impact on our understanding and management of epilepsy patients.

References

Aghakhani Y, Bagshaw AP, Bénar CG et al (2004) fMRI activation during spike and wave discharges in idiopathic generalized epilepsy. Brain 127:1127–1144

Aguirre GK, Zarahn E, D'esposito M (1998) The variability of human, BOLD hemodynamic responses. NeuroImage 8:360–369

Ahmad RF, Malik AS, Kamel N, Reza F (2015) Object categories specific brain activity classification with simultaneous EEG-fMRI. Conf Proc IEEE Eng Med Biol Soc 2015:1825–1828

Ahmad RF, Malik AS, Kamel N et al (2017) Visual brain activity patterns classification with simultaneous EEG-fMRI: a multimodal approach. Technol Health Care 25:471–485

Al-Asmi A, Bénar C-G, Gross DW et al (2003) fMRI activation in continuous and spike-triggered EEG-fMRI studies of epileptic spikes. Epilepsia 44:1328–1339

Allen PJ, Polizzi G, Krakow K et al (1998) Identification of EEG events in the MR scanner: the problem of pulse artifact and a method for its subtraction. NeuroImage 8:229–239

Allen PJ, Josephs O, Turner R (2000) A method for removing imaging artifact from continuous EEG recorded during functional MRI. NeuroImage 12:230–239

Allen E, Erhardt E, Damaraju E et al (2011) A baseline for the multivariate comparison of resting-state networks. Front Syst Neurosci 5:2

Altmann A, Schröter MS, Spoormaker VI et al (2016) Validation of non-REM sleep stage decoding from resting state fMRI using linear support vector machines. NeuroImage 125:544–555

An D, Fahoum F, Hall J et al (2013) Electroencephalography/functional magnetic resonance imaging responses help predict surgical outcome in focal epilepsy. Epilepsia 54:2184–2194

An D, Dubeau F, Gotman J (2015) BOLD responses related to focal spikes and widespread bilateral synchronous discharges generated in the frontal lobe. Epilepsia 56:366–374

Archer JS, Abbott DF, Waites AB, Jackson GD (2003a) fMRI "deactivation" of the posterior cingulate during generalized spike and wave. NeuroImage 20:1915–1922

Archer JS, Briellmann RS, Syngeniotis A et al (2003b) Spike-triggered fMRI in reading epilepsy: involvement of left frontal cortex working memory area. Neurology 60:415–421

Bagshaw AP, Aghakhani Y, Bénar C-G et al (2004) EEG-fMRI of focal epileptic spikes: analysis with multiple haemodynamic functions and comparison with gadolinium-enhanced MR angiograms. Hum Brain Mapp 22:179–192

Bagshaw AP, Hawco C, Bénar C-G et al (2005) Analysis of the EEG–fMRI response to prolonged bursts of interictal epileptiform activity. NeuroImage 24:1099–1112

Bagshaw AP, Hale JR, Campos BM et al (2017) Sleep onset uncovers thalamic abnormalities in patients with idiopathic generalised epilepsy. Neuroimage Clin 16:52–57

Bai X, Vestal M, Berman R et al (2010) Dynamic time course of typical childhood absence seizures: EEG, behavior, and functional magnetic resonance imaging. J Neurosci 30:5884–5893

Baud MO, Perneger T, Rácz A et al (2018) European trends in epilepsy surgery. Neurology 91:e96–e106

Begley CE, Famulari M, Annegers JF et al (2000) The cost of epilepsy in the United States: an estimate from population-based clinical and survey data. Epilepsia 41:342–351

Bell GS, Gaitatzis A, Bell CL et al (2008) Drowning in people with epilepsy: how great is the risk? Neurology 71:578–582

Bell GS, Sinha S, de Tisi J et al (2010) Premature mortality in refractory partial epilepsy: does surgical treatment make a difference? J Neurol Neurosurg Psychiatry 81:716–718

Bénar C-G, Grova C, Kobayashi E et al (2006) EEG–fMRI of epileptic spikes: concordance with EEG source localization and intracranial EEG. NeuroImage 30:1161–1170

Benuzzi F, Mirandola L, Pugnaghi M et al (2012) Increased cortical BOLD signal anticipates generalized spike and wave discharges in adolescents and adults with idiopathic generalized epilepsies. Epilepsia 53:622–630

Berg AT, Berkovic SF, Brodie MJ, Buchhalter J, Cross JH, van Emde Boas W, Engel J, French J, Glauser TA, Mathern GW, Moshe SL, Nordli D, Plouin P, Scheffer IE (2010) Revised terminology and concepts for organization of seizures and epilepsies: report of the ILAE Commission on Classification and Terminology, 2005–2009. Epilepsia 51:676–685.

Bernhardt BC, Bonilha L, Gross DW (2015) Network analysis for a network disorder: The emerging role of graph theory in the study of epilepsy. Epilepsy Behav 50: 162–170.

Bharath RD, Panda R, Raj J et al (2019) Machine learning identifies "rsfMRI epilepsy networks" in temporal lobe epilepsy. Eur Radiol 29:3496–3505

Bien CG, Szinay M, Wagner J et al (2009) Characteristics and surgical outcomes of patients with refractory magnetic resonance imaging-negative epilepsies. Arch Neurol 66:1491–1499

Birn RM, Bandettini PA (2005) The effect of stimulus duty cycle and "off" duration on BOLD response linearity. NeuroImage 27:70–82

Birn RM, Saad ZS, Bandettini PA (2001) Spatial heterogeneity of the nonlinear dynamics in the FMRI BOLD response. NeuroImage 14:817–826

Biswal B, Zerrin Yetkin F (1995) Functional connectivity in the motor cortex of resting human brain using echo-planar MRI. Magn Reson Med 34(4):537–541

Blume WT, Holloway GM, Wiebe S (2001) Temporal epileptogenesis: localizing value of scalp and subdural interictal and ictal EEG data. Epilepsia 42:508–514

Blumenfeld H, McNally KA, Vanderhill SD, Paige AL, ChungR, Davis K, Norden AD, Stokking R, Studholme C, Novotny EJ Jr., Zubal IG, Spencer SS, (2004) Positive and negative network correlations in temporal lobe epilepsy. Cereb Cortex 14:892–902.

Bonnelle V, Ham TE, Leech R et al (2012) Salience network integrity predicts default mode network function after traumatic brain injury. Proc Natl Acad Sci U S A 109:4690–4695

Buckner RL (1998) Event-related fMRI and the hemodynamic response. Hum Brain Mapp 6:373–377

Buckner RL, Andrews-Hanna JR, Schacter DL (2008) The brain's default network: anatomy, function, and relevance to disease. Ann N Y Acad Sci 1124:1–38

Burianová H, Faizo NL, Gray M et al (2017) Altered functional connectivity in mesial temporal lobe epilepsy. Epilepsy Res 137:45–52

Buxton RB, Wong EC, Frank LR (1998) Dynamics of blood flow and oxygenation changes during brain activation: the balloon model. Magn Reson Med 39:855–864

Caballero-Gaudes C, Van de Ville D, Grouiller F et al (2013) Mapping interictal epileptic discharges using mutual information between concurrent EEG and fMRI. NeuroImage 68:248–262

Calhoun VD, Adalı T (2012) Multisubject independent component analysis of fMRI: a decade of intrinsic networks, default mode, and neurodiagnostic discovery. IEEE Rev Biomed Eng 5:60–73

Caporro M, Haneef Z, Yeh HJ et al (2012) Functional MRI of sleep spindles and K-complexes. Clin Neurophysiol 123:303–309

Carmichael DW, Vulliemoz S, Rodionov R et al (2012) Simultaneous intracranial EEG–fMRI in humans: protocol considerations and data quality. NeuroImage 63:301–309

Cassará AM, Maraviglia B, Hartwig S et al (2009) Neuronal current detection with low-field magnetic resonance: simulations and methods. Magn Reson Imaging 27:1131–1139

Centeno M, Tierney TM, Perani S (2017) Combined electroencephalography–functional magnetic resonance imaging and electrical source imaging improves localization of pediatric focal epilepsy. Ann Neurol 82(2):278–287

Cina CS, Clase CM, Haynes RB (2000) Carotid endarterectomy for symptomatic carotid stenosis. Cochrane Database Syst Rev 6(6):CD001081

Coan AC, Chaudhary UJ, Grouiller F et al (2016) EEG-fMRI in the presurgical evaluation of temporal lobe epilepsy. J Neurol Neurosurg Psychiatry 87:642–649

Craik A, He Y, Contreras-Vidal JL (2019) Deep learning for electroencephalogram (EEG) classification tasks: a review. J Neural Eng 16:031001

Crunelli V, Lőrincz ML, McCafferty C et al (2020) Clinical and experimental insight into pathophysiology, comorbidity and therapy of absence seizures. Brain. https://doi.org/10.1093/brain/awaa072

Cunningham CJB, Zaamout ME-F, Goodyear B, Federico P (2008) Simultaneous EEG-fMRI in human epilepsy. Can J Neurol Sci 35:420–435

Damoiseaux JS, Rombouts S, Barkhof F et al (2006) Consistent resting-state networks across healthy subjects. Proc Natl Acad Sci 103:13848–13853

Daunizeau J, Vaudano AE, Lemieux L (2010) Bayesian multi-modal model comparison: a case study on the generators of the spike and the wave in generalized spike–wave complexes. NeuroImage 49:656–667

Daunizeau J, Lemieux L, Vaudano AE et al (2012) An electrophysiological validation of stochastic DCM for fMRI. Front Comput Neurosci 6:103

De Tiege X, Laufs H, Boyd SG, Harkness W, Allen PJ, Clark CA, Connelly A, Cross JH (2007) EEGfMRI in children with pharmacoresistant focal epilepsy. Epilepsia 48:385–389.

de Tisi J, Bell GS, Peacock JL et al (2011) The long-term outcome of adult epilepsy surgery, patterns of seizure remission, and relapse: a cohort study. Lancet 378:1388–1395

Debener S, Ullsperger M, Siegel M, Engel AK (2006) Single-trial EEG-fMRI reveals the dynamics of cognitive function. Trends Cogn Sci 10:558–563

Delorme A, Makeig S (2004) EEGLAB: an open source toolbox for analysis of single-trial EEG dynamics including independent component analysis. J Neurosci Methods 134:9–21

Du J, Vegh V, Reutens DC (2014) MRI signal phase oscillates with neuronal activity in cerebral cortex: implications for neuronal current imaging. NeuroImage 94:1–11

Eichele T, Calhoun VD, Debener S (2009) Mining EEG–fMRI using independent component analysis. Int J Psychophysiol 73:53–61

Eickhoff SB, Müller VI (2015) Functional connectivity. In: Toga AW (ed) Brain mapping. Academic, Waltham, pp 187–201

Ekstrom A (2010) How and when the fMRI BOLD signal relates to underlying neural activity: the danger in dissociation. Brain Res Rev 62:233–244

Elliott LT, Sharp K, Alfaro-Almagro F et al (2018) Genome-wide association studies of brain imaging phenotypes in UK Biobank. Nature 562:210–216

Engel J Jr, McDermott MP, Wiebe S et al (2012) Early surgical therapy for drug-resistant temporal lobe epilepsy: a randomized trial. JAMA 307:922–930

Engel J, Wiebe S, French J et al (2003) Practice parameter: temporal lobe and localized neocortical resections for epilepsy: report of the Quality Standards Subcommittee of the American Academy of Neurology, in association with the American Epilepsy Society and the American Association of Neurological Surgeons. Neurology 60:538–547

Esposito F, Mulert C, Goebel R (2009) Combined distributed source and single-trial EEG–fMRI modeling: application to effortful decision making processes. NeuroImage 47:112–121

Faizo NL, Burianová H, Gray M et al (2014) Identification of pre-spike network in patients with mesial temporal lobe epilepsy. Front Neurol 5:222

Federico P, Archer JS, Abbott DF, Jackson GD (2005) Cortical/subcortical BOLD changes associated with epileptic discharges: an EEG-fMRI study at 3 T. Neurology 64:1125–1130

Flanagan D, Badawy RAB, Jackson GD (2014) EEG–fMRI in focal epilepsy: local activation and regional networks. Clin Neurophysiol 125:21–31

Formaggio E, Storti SF, Cerini R et al (2010) Brain oscillatory activity during motor imagery in EEG-fMRI coregistration. Magn Reson Imaging 28:1403–1412

Frässle S, Lomakina EI, Razi A et al (2017) Regression DCM for fMRI. NeuroImage 155:406–421

Friston KJ (1994) Functional and effective connectivity in neuroimaging: a synthesis. Hum Brain Mapp 2(1-2):56–78

Friston KJ (2011) Functional and effective connectivity: a review. Brain Connect 1:13–36

Friston KJ, Williams S, Howard R et al (1996) Movement-related effects in fMRI time-series. Magn Reson Med 35:346–355

Friston KJ, Fletcher P, Josephs O et al (1998) Event-related fMRI: characterizing differential responses. NeuroImage 7:30–40

Friston KJ, Harrison L, Penny W (2003) Dynamic causal modelling. NeuroImage 19:1273–1302

Gaitatzis A, Sander JW (2004) The mortality of epilepsy revisited. Epileptic Disord 6:3–13

Gaitatzis A, Trimble MR, Sander JW (2004) The psychiatric comorbidity of epilepsy. Acta Neurol Scand 110:207–220

Galovic M, Baudracco I, Wright-Goff E et al (2019) Association of piriform cortex resection with surgical outcomes in patients with temporal lobe epilepsy. JAMA Neurol. https://doi.org/10.1001/jamaneurol.2019.0204

Gaxiola-Valdez I, Singh S, Perera T et al (2017) Seizure onset zone localization using postictal hypoperfusion detected by arterial spin labelling MRI. Brain 140:2895–2911

Glaser J, Beisteiner R, Bauer H, Fischmeister F (2013) FACET – a "Flexible Artifact Correction and Evaluation Toolbox" for concurrently recorded EEG/fMRI data. BMC Neurosci 14:138

Glover GH (1999) Deconvolution of impulse response in event-related BOLD fMRI1. NeuroImage 9:416–429

Goldman RI, Stern JM, Engel J Jr, Cohen MS (2000) Acquiring simultaneous EEG and functional MRI. Clin Neurophysiol 111:1974–1980

Goldman RI, Stern JM, Engel J Jr, Cohen MS (2002) Simultaneous EEG and fMRI of the alpha rhythm. Neuroreport 13:2487–2492

Gotman J (2008) Epileptic networks studied with EEG-fMRI. Epilepsia 49:42–51

Gotman J, Pittau F (2011) Combining EEG and fMRI in the study of epileptic discharges. Epilepsia 52(Suppl 4):38–42

Gotman J, Bénar C-G, Dubeau F (2004) Combining EEG and fMRI in epilepsy: methodological challenges and clinical results. J Clin Neurophysiol 21:229–240

Gotman J, Kobayashi E, Bagshaw AP et al (2006) Combining EEG and fMRI: a multimodal tool for epilepsy research. J Magn Reson Imaging 23:906–920

Green JJ, Boehler CN, Roberts KC et al (2017) Cortical and subcortical coordination of visual spatial attention revealed by simultaneous EEG–fMRI recording. J Neurosci 37:7803–7810

Greicius MD, Krasnow B, Reiss AL, Menon V (2003) Functional connectivity in the resting brain: a network analysis of the default mode hypothesis. Proc Natl Acad Sci U S A 100:253–258

Grouiller F, Thornton RC, Groening K et al (2011) With or without spikes: localization of focal epileptic activity by simultaneous electroencephalography and functional magnetic resonance imaging. Brain 134:2867–2886

Guo JN, Kim R, Chen Y et al (2016) Impaired consciousness in patients with absence seizures investigated by functional MRI, EEG, and behavioural measures: a cross-sectional study. Lancet Neurol 15:1336–1345

Hamandi K, Salek-Haddadi A, Laufs H et al (2006) EEG–fMRI of idiopathic and secondarily generalized epilepsies. NeuroImage 31:1700–1710

Haneef Z, Stern J, Dewar S, Engel J Jr (2010) Referral pattern for epilepsy surgery after evidence-based recommendations: a retrospective study. Neurology 75:699–704

Hao Y, Khoo HM, von Ellenrieder N et al (2018) DeepIED: an epileptic discharge detector for EEG-fMRI based on deep learning. Neuroimage Clin 17:962–975

He K, Zhang X, Ren S, Sun J (2015) Deep residual learning for image recognition. arXiv [cs.CV]

Hitiris N, Mohanraj R, Norrie J, Brodie MJ (2007) Mortality in epilepsy. Epilepsy Behav 10:363–376

Holmes GL, McKeever M, Adamson M (1987) Absence seizures in children: clinical and electroencephalographic features. Ann Neurol 21:268–273

Holmes MD, Kutsy RL, Ojemann GA, Wilensky AJ, Ojemann LM (2000) Interictal, unifocal spikes in refractory extratemporal epilepsy predict ictal origin and postsurgical outcome. Clin Neurophysiol 111: 1802–1808.

Hosseini M-P, Tran TX, Pompili D et al (2020) Multimodal data analysis of epileptic EEG and rs-fMRI via deep learning and edge computing. Artif Intell Med 104:101813

Hussein R, Palangi H, Ward RK, Wang ZJ (2019) Optimized deep neural network architecture for robust detection of epileptic seizures using EEG signals. Clin Neurophysiol 130:25–37

Iannotti GR, Pittau F, Michel CM et al (2015) Pulse artifact detection in simultaneous EEG-fMRI recording based on EEG map topography. Brain Topogr 28:21–32

Iannotti GR, Grouiller F, Centeno M et al (2016) Epileptic networks are strongly connected with and without the effects of interictal discharges. Epilepsia 57:1086–1096

Ives JR, Warach S, Schmitt F et al (1993) Monitoring the patient's EEG during echo planar MRI. Electroencephalogr Clin Neurophysiol 87:417–420

Jackson JD (1998) Classical Electrodynamics, 3rd Edition, Wiley

Jann K, Wiest R, Hauf M et al (2008) BOLD correlates of continuously fluctuating epileptic activity isolated by independent component analysis. NeuroImage 42:635–648

Jann K, Dierks T, Boesch C et al (2009) BOLD correlates of EEG alpha phase-locking and the fMRI default mode network. NeuroImage 45:903–916

Jeha LE, Najm I, Bingaman W et al (2007) Surgical outcome and prognostic factors of frontal lobe epilepsy surgery. Brain 130:574–584

Jin B, Krishnan B, Adler S et al (2018) Automated detection of focal cortical dysplasia type II with surface-based magnetic resonance imaging postprocessing and machine learning. Epilepsia 59:982–992

Jorge J, Grouiller F, Gruetter R et al (2015a) Towards high-quality simultaneous EEG-fMRI at 7 T: detection and reduction of EEG artifacts due to head motion. NeuroImage 120:143–153

Jorge J, Grouiller F, Ipek Ö et al (2015b) Simultaneous EEG-fMRI at ultra-high field: artifact prevention and safety assessment. NeuroImage 105:132–144

Kahan J, Foltynie T (2013) Understanding DCM: ten simple rules for the clinician. NeuroImage 83:542–549

Kannurpatti SS, Motes MA, Rypma B, Biswal BB (2010) Neural and vascular variability and the fMRI-BOLD response in normal aging. Magn Reson Imaging 28:466–476

Kannurpatti SS, Motes MA, Rypma B, Biswal BB (2011) Non-neural BOLD variability in block and event-related paradigms. Magn Reson Imaging 29:140–146

Kassinopoulos M, Mitsis GD (2019) Identification of physiological response functions to correct for fluctuations in resting-state fMRI related to heart rate and respiration. NeuroImage 202:116150

Keezer MR, Sisodiya SM, Sander JW (2016) Comorbidities of epilepsy: current concepts and future perspectives. Lancet Neurol 15:106–115

Khoo HM, Hao Y, von Ellenrieder N et al (2017) The hemodynamic response to interictal epileptic discharges localizes the seizure-onset zone. Epilepsia 58:811–823

Kiefer C, Abela E, Schindler K, Wiest R (2016) Focal epilepsy: MR imaging of nonhemodynamic field effects by using a phase-cycled stimulus-induced rotary saturation approach with spin-lock preparation. Radiology 280:237–243

Kim S-G, Ogawa S (2012) Biophysical and physiological origins of blood oxygenation level-dependent fMRI signals. J Cereb Blood Flow Metab 32:1188–1206

Kim S-Y, Hwang Y-H, Lee H-W et al (2007) Cognitive impairment in juvenile myoclonic epilepsy. J Clin Neurol 3:86–92

King JT Jr, Sperling MR, Justice AC, O'Connor MJ (1997) A cost-effectiveness analysis of anterior temporal lobectomy for intractable temporal lobe epilepsy. J Neurosurg 87:20–28

Kobayashi E, Bagshaw AP, Bénar C-G et al (2006) Temporal and extratemporal BOLD responses to temporal lobe interictal spikes. Epilepsia 47:343–354

Kobayashi E, Grova C, Tyvaert L et al (2009) Structures involved at the time of temporal lobe spikes revealed by interindividual group analysis of EEG/fMRI data. Epilepsia 50:2549–2556

Krakow K, Woermann FG, Symms MR et al (1999) EEG-triggered functional MRI of interictal epileptiform activity in patients with partial seizures. Brain 122(Pt 9):1679–1688

Kwan P, Brodie MJ (2000) Early identification of refractory epilepsy. N Engl J Med 342:314–319

Kwan P, Brodie MJ (2001) Effectiveness of first antiepileptic drug. Epilepsia 42:1255–1260

Kwan P, Arzimanoglou A, Berg AT et al (2010) Definition of drug resistant epilepsy: consensus proposal by the ad hoc Task Force of the ILAE Commission on Therapeutic Strategies. Epilepsia 51:1069–1077

Langfitt JT, Westerveld M, Hamberger MJ et al (2007) Worsening of quality of life after epilepsy surgery: effect of seizures and memory decline. Neurology 68:1988–1994

Laufs H (2012) A personalized history of EEG–fMRI integration. NeuroImage 62:1056–1067

Laufs H, Hamandi K, Walker MC et al (2006) EEG–fMRI mapping of asymmetrical delta activity in a patient with refractory epilepsy is concordant with the epileptogenic region determined by intracranial EEG. Magn Reson Imaging 24:367–371

Lecun Y, Bottou L, Bengio Y, Haffner P (1998) Gradient-based learning applied to document recognition. Proc IEEE 86:2278–2324

Lee HW, Arora J, Papademetris X et al (2014) Altered functional connectivity in seizure onset zones revealed by fMRI intrinsic connectivity. Neurology 83:2269–2277

Lemieux L, Allen PJ, Franconi F et al (1997) Recording of EEG during fMRI experiments: patient safety. Magn Reson Med 38:943–952

Lemieux L, Allen PJ, Krakow K, Symms MR, Fish DR (1999) Methodological Issues in EEG-correlated Functional MRI Experiments. Int J Biomagnetism 1:87–95.

Litjens G, Kooi T, Bejnordi BE et al (2017) A survey on deep learning in medical image analysis. Med Image Anal 42:60–88

Logothetis NK (2003) The underpinnings of the BOLD functional magnetic resonance imaging signal. J Neurosci 23:3963–3971

Logothetis NK, Wandell BA (2004) Interpreting the BOLD signal. Annu Rev Physiol 66:735–769

Löscher W, Ebert U (1996) The role of the piriform cortex in kindling. Prog Neurobiol 50:427–481

Lüders HO, Najm I, Nair D et al (2006) The epileptogenic zone: general principles. Epileptic Disord 8(Suppl 2):S1–S9

Marreiros AC, Kiebel SJ, Friston KJ (2008) Dynamic causal modelling for fMRI: a two-state model. NeuroImage 39:269–278

Mayhew SD, Ostwald D, Porcaro C, Bagshaw AP (2013) Spontaneous EEG alpha oscillation interacts with positive and negative BOLD responses in the visual–auditory cortices and default-mode network. NeuroImage 76:362–372

McKeown MJ, Makeig S, Brown GG et al (1998) Analysis of fMRI data by blind separation into independent spatial components. Hum Brain Mapp 6:160–188

Meeren H, van Luijtelaar G, Lopes da Silva F, Coenen A (2005) Evolving concepts on the pathophysiology of absence seizures: the cortical focus theory. Arch Neurol 62:371–376

Mehler DMA, Kording KP (2018) The lure of causal statements: rampant mis-inference of causality in estimated connectivity. arXiv [q-bio.NC]

Meir-Hasson Y, Kinreich S, Podlipsky I et al (2014) An EEG finger-print of fMRI deep regional activation. NeuroImage 102(Pt 1):128–141

Mirsattari SM, Wang Z, Ives JR et al (2006) Linear aspects of transformation from interictal epileptic discharges to BOLD fMRI signals in an animal model of occipital epilepsy. NeuroImage 30:1133–1148

Moeller F, Siebner HR, Wolff S et al (2008a) Changes in activity of striato-thalamo-cortical network precede generalized spike wave discharges. NeuroImage 39:1839–1849

Moeller F, Siebner HR, Wolff S et al (2008b) Simultaneous EEG-fMRI in drug-naive children with newly diagnosed absence epilepsy. Epilepsia 49:1510–1519

Moeller F, Tyvaert L, Nguyen DK et al (2009) EEG-fMRI: adding to standard evaluations of patients with nonlesional frontal lobe epilepsy. Neurology 73:2023–2030

Moeller F, Stephani U, Siniatchkin M (2013) Simultaneous EEG and fMRI recordings (EEG-fMRI) in children with epilepsy. Epilepsia 54:971–982

Moosmann M, Eichele T, Nordby H et al (2008) Joint independent component analysis for simultaneous EEG–fMRI: principle and simulation. Int J Psychophysiol 67:212–221

Moran R (2015) Deep brain stimulation for neurodegenerative disease: a computational blueprint using dynamic causal modeling. Prog Brain Res 222:125–146

Negishi M, Martuzzi R, Novotny EJ et al (2011) Functional MRI connectivity as a predictor of the surgical outcome of epilepsy. Epilepsia 52:1733–1740

Niazy RK, Beckmann CF, Iannetti GD et al (2005) Removal of FMRI environment artifacts from EEG data using optimal basis sets. NeuroImage 28:720–737

Nunez PL, Silberstein RB (2000) On the relationship of synaptic activity to macroscopic measurements: does co-registration of EEG with fMRI make sense? Brain Topogr 13(2):79–96

Osharina V, Ponchel E, Aarabi A et al (2010) Local haemodynamic changes preceding interictal spikes: a simultaneous electrocorticography (ECoG) and near-infrared spectroscopy (NIRS) analysis in rats. NeuroImage 50:600–607

Panayiotopoulos CP, Chroni E, Daskalopoulos C et al (1992) Typical absence seizures in adults: clinical, EEG, video-EEG findings and diagnostic/syndromic considerations. J Neurol Neurosurg Psychiatry 55:1002–1008

Papadopoulou M, Cooray G, Rosch R et al (2017) Dynamic causal modelling of seizure activity in a rat model. NeuroImage 146:518–532

Parkes L, Fulcher B, Yücel M, Fornito A (2018) An evaluation of the efficacy, reliability, and sensitivity of motion correction strategies for resting-state functional MRI. NeuroImage 171:415–436

Picchioni D, Horovitz SG, Fukunaga M et al (2011) Infraslow EEG oscillations organize large-scale cortical–subcortical interactions during sleep: a combined EEG/fMRI study. Brain Res 1374:63–72

Pittau F, Dubeau F, Gotman J (2012a) Contribution of EEG/fMRI to the definition of the epileptic focus. Neurology 78:1479–1487

Pittau F, Mégevand P, Sheybani L, Abela E, Grouiller F, Spinelli L, Michel CM, Seeck M, Vulliemoz S (2014) Mapping epileptic activity: sources or networks for the clinicians? Front Neurol 5:218. https://doi.org/10.3389/fneur.2014.00218. eCollection 2014.

Pittau F, Grova C, Moeller F et al (2012b) Patterns of altered functional connectivity in mesial temporal lobe epilepsy. Epilepsia 53:1013–1023

Platt M, Sperling MR (2002) A comparison of surgical and medical costs for refractory epilepsy. Epilepsia 43(Suppl 4):25–31

Plichta MM, Wolf I, Hohmann S et al (2013) Simultaneous EEG and fMRI reveals a causally connected subcortical-cortical network during reward anticipation. J Neurosci 33:14526–14533

Pompili M, Girardi P, Tatarelli R (2006) Death from suicide versus mortality from epilepsy in the epilepsies: a meta-analysis. Epilepsy Behav 9:641–648

Power JD, Mitra A, Laumann TO et al (2014) Methods to detect, characterize, and remove motion artifact in resting state fMRI. NeuroImage 84:320–341

Raichle ME, Snyder AZ (2007) A default mode of brain function: a brief history of an evolving idea. NeuroImage 37:1083–90; discussion 1097–9

Raichle ME, MacLeod AM, Snyder AZ et al (2001) A default mode of brain function. Proc Natl Acad Sci U S A 98:676–682

Razi A, Seghier ML, Zhou Y et al (2017) Large-scale DCMs for resting-state fMRI. Netw Neurosci 1:222–241

Rebsamen M, Rummel C, Reyes M, Wiest R, McKinley R (2020) Direct cortical thickness estimation using deep learning-based anatomy segmentation and cortex parcellation. Hum Brain Mapp 41(17):4804–4814

Richardson MP (2012) Large scale brain models of epilepsy: dynamics meets connectomics. J Neurol Neurosurg Psychiatry 83:1238–1248.

Rim B, Sung N-J, Min S, Hong M (2020) Deep learning in physiological signal data: a survey. Sensors 20. https://doi.org/10.3390/s20040969

Ritter P, Villringer A (2006) Simultaneous EEG-fMRI. Neurosci Biobehav Rev 30:823–838

Rocca MA, Valsasina P, Martinelli V et al (2012) Large-scale neuronal network dysfunction in relapsing-remitting multiple sclerosis. Neurology 79:1449–1457

Rodionov R, De Martino F, Laufs H, Carmichael DW, Formisano E, Walker M, Duncan JS, Lemieux L, (2007) Independent component analysis of interictal fMRI in focal epilepsy: comparison with general linear model-based EEG-correlated fMRI. Neuroimage 38:488–500.

Rosenkranz K, Lemieux L (2010) Present and future of simultaneous EEG-fMRI. MAGMA 23:309–316

Rosenow F, Lüders H (2001) Presurgical evaluation of epilepsy. Brain 124:1683–1700

Salek-Haddadi A, Diehl B, Hamandi K et al (2006) Hemodynamic correlates of epileptiform discharges: an EEG-fMRI study of 63 patients with focal epilepsy. Brain Res 1088:148–166

Sander JW (2003) The epidemiology of epilepsy revisited. Curr Opin Neurol 16:165–170

Seeck M, Lazeyras F, Michel CM et al (1998) Non-invasive epileptic focus localization using EEG-triggered functional MRI and electromagnetic tomography. Electroencephalogr Clin Neurophysiol 106:508–512

Seneviratne U, Cook MJ, D'Souza WJ (2017) Electroencephalography in the diagnosis of genetic generalized epilepsy syndromes. Front Neurol 8:499

Shamshiri EA, Tierney TM, Centeno M et al (2017) Interictal activity is an important contributor to abnormal intrinsic network connectivity in paediatric focal epilepsy. Hum Brain Mapp 38:221–236

Shamshiri EA, Sheybani L, Vulliemoz S (2019) The role of EEG-fMRI in studying cognitive network alterations in epilepsy. Front Neurol 10:1033

Sharma NK, Pedreira C, Chaudhary UJ et al (2019) BOLD mapping of human epileptic spikes recorded during simultaneous intracranial EEG-fMRI: the impact of automated spike classification. NeuroImage 184:981–992

Sierra-Marcos A, Maestro I, Falcón C et al (2013) Ictal EEG-fMRI in localization of epileptogenic area in patients with refractory neocortical focal epilepsy. Epilepsia 54:1688–1698

Smith SM, Fox PT, Miller KL et al (2009) Correspondence of the brain's functional architecture during activation and rest. Proc Natl Acad Sci U S A 106:13040–13045

Smith SM, Miller KL, Salimi-Khorshidi G et al (2011) Network modelling methods for FMRI. NeuroImage 54:875–891

Spencer SS (2002) Neural networks in human epilepsy: evidence of and implications for treatment. Epilepsia 43:219–227.

Sperling MR, Feldman H, Kinman J et al (1999) Seizure control and mortality in epilepsy. Ann Neurol 46:45–50

Srivastava G, Crottaz-Herbette S, Lau KM, Glover GH, Menon V, (2005) ICA-based procedures for removing ballistocardiogram artifacts from EEG data acquired in the MRI scanner. Neuroimage 24:50–60.

Stevelink R, Koeleman BPC, Sander JW et al (2019) Refractory juvenile myoclonic epilepsy: a meta-analysis of prevalence and risk factors. Eur J Neurol 26:856–864

Steyrl D, Krausz G, Koschutnig K et al (2017) Reference layer adaptive filtering (RLAF) for EEG artifact reduction in simultaneous EEG-fMRI. J Neural Eng 14:026003

Steyrl D, Krausz G, Koschutnig K et al (2018) Online reduction of artifacts in EEG of simultaneous EEG-fMRI using reference layer adaptive filtering (RLAF). Brain Topogr 31:129–149

Storti SF, Boscolo Galazzo I, Del Felice A et al (2014) Combining ESI, ASL and PET for quantitative assessment of drug-resistant focal epilepsy. NeuroImage 102(Pt 1):49–59

Stripling JS, Patneau DK (1990) Seizure mechanisms in the piriform cortex. Adv Behav Biol 37:45–59

Sundaram P, Nummenmaa A, Wells W et al (2016) Direct neural current imaging in an intact cerebellum with magnetic resonance imaging. NeuroImage 132:477–490

Sveinsson B, Koonjoo N, Zhu B et al (2020) Detection of nanotesla AC magnetic fields using steady-state SIRS and ultra-low field MRI. J Neural Eng 17:034001

Tangwiriyasakul C, Perani S, Centeno M et al (2018) Dynamic brain network states in human generalized spike-wave discharges. Brain 141:2981–2994

Téllez-Zenteno JF, Dhar R, Wiebe S (2005) Long-term seizure outcomes following epilepsy surgery: a systematic review and meta-analysis. Brain 128:1188–1198

Thornton R, Laufs H, Rodionov R et al (2010) EEG correlated functional MRI and postoperative outcome in focal epilepsy. J Neurol Neurosurg Psychiatry 81:922–927

Thornton R, Vulliemoz S, Rodionov R (2011) Epileptic networks in focal cortical dysplasia revealed using electroencephalography–functional magnetic resonance imaging. Ann Neurol 70(5):822–837

Tjepkema-Cloostermans MC, de Carvalho RCV, van Putten MJAM (2018) Deep learning for detection of focal epileptiform discharges from scalp EEG recordings. Clin Neurophysiol 129:2191–2196

Tong X, An D, Xiao F et al (2019) Real-time effects of interictal spikes on hippocampus and amygdala functional connectivity in unilateral temporal lobe epilepsy: an EEG-fMRI study. Epilepsia 60: 246–254

Tousseyn S, Dupont P, Robben D et al (2014) A reliable and time-saving semiautomatic spike-template-based analysis of interictal EEG-fMRI. Epilepsia 55:2048–2058

van den Heuvel MP, Hulshoff Pol HE (2010) Exploring the brain network: a review on resting-state fMRI functional connectivity. Eur Neuropsychopharmacol 20:519–534

van Graan LA, Lemieux L, Chaudhary UJ (2015) Methods and utility of EEG-fMRI in epilepsy. Quant Imaging Med Surg 5:300–312

van Houdt PJ, de Munck JC, Leijten FSS et al (2013) EEG-fMRI correlation patterns in the presurgical evaluation of focal epilepsy: a comparison with electrocorticographic data and surgical outcome measures. NeuroImage 75:238–248

Vaudano AE, Laufs H, Kiebel SJ et al (2009) Causal hierarchy within the thalamo-cortical network in spike and wave discharges. PLoS One 4:e6475

Vaughan DN, Jackson GD (2014) The piriform cortex and human focal epilepsy. Front Neurol 5:259

Vickrey BG, Hays RD, Rausch R et al (1995) Outcomes in 248 patients who had diagnostic evaluations for epilepsy surgery. Lancet 346:1445–1449

Vollmar C, O'Muircheartaigh J, Barker GJ, Symms MR, Thompson P, Kumari V, Duncan JS, Janz D, Richardson MP, Koepp MJ (2011) Motor system hyperconnectivity in juvenile myoclonic epilepsy: a cognitive functional magnetic resonance imaging study. Brain 134(Pt 6):1710–9. https://doi.org/10.1093/brain/awr098.

Vulliemoz S, Thornton R, Rodionov R et al (2009) The spatio-temporal mapping of epileptic networks: combination of EEG–fMRI and EEG source imaging. NeuroImage 46:834–843

Wan X, Riera J, Iwata K et al (2006) The neural basis of the hemodynamic response nonlinearity in human primary visual cortex: implications for neurovascular coupling mechanism. NeuroImage 32:616–625

Warach S, Ives JR, Schlaug G et al (1996) EEG-triggered echo-planar functional MRI in epilepsy. Neurology 47:89–93

Warren AEL, Abbott DF, Vaughan DN et al (2016) Abnormal cognitive network interactions in Lennox-Gastaut syndrome: a potential mechanism of epileptic encephalopathy. Epilepsia 57:812–822

Watila MM, Balarabe SA, Ojo O et al (2018) Overall and cause-specific premature mortality in epilepsy: a systematic review. Epilepsy Behav 87:213–225

Wei H, Jafarian A, Zeidman P et al (2020) Bayesian fusion and multimodal DCM for EEG and fMRI. NeuroImage 211:116595

Wiest R, Estermann L, Scheidegger O, Rummel C, Jann K, Seeck M, Schindler K, Hauf M (2013) Widespread grey matter changes and hemodynamic correlates to interictal epileptiform discharges in pharmacoresistant mesial temporal epilepsy. J Neurol 260:1601–1610.

Whelan CD, Altmann A, Botía JA et al (2018) Structural brain abnormalities in the common epilepsies assessed in a worldwide ENIGMA study. Brain 141:391–408

Whitham EM, Pope KJ, Fitzgibbon SP et al (2007) Scalp electrical recording during paralysis: quantitative evidence that EEG frequencies above 20 Hz are contaminated by EMG. Clin Neurophysiol 118:1877–1888

Wiebe S (2004) Effectiveness and safety of epilepsy surgery: what is the evidence? CNS Spectr 9:120–2, 126–32

Wiebe S, Blume WT, Girvin JP et al (2001) A randomized, controlled trial of surgery for temporal-lobe epilepsy. N Engl J Med 345:311–318

Wieser H-G, Häne A (2003) Antiepileptic drug treatment before and after selective amygdalohippocampectomy. Epilepsy Res 55:211–223

Wieser HG, Häne A (2004) Antiepileptic drug treatment in seizure-free mesial temporal lobe epilepsy patients with hippocampal sclerosis following selective amygdalohippocampectomy. Seizure 13:534–536

Wiest R, Beisteiner R (2019) Recent developments in imaging of epilepsy. Curr Opin Neurol 32: 530–538

Yuan Y, Xun G, Jia K, Zhang A (2019) A multi-view deep learning framework for EEG seizure detection. IEEE J Biomed Health Inform 23:83–94

Zeidman P, Jafarian A, Corbin N et al (2019) A guide to group effective connectivity analysis, Part 1: First level analysis with DCM for fMRI. NeuroImage 200:174–190

Zhang J, Liu W, Chen H et al (2012) EEG–fMRI validation studies in comparison with icEEG: a review. Int J Psychophysiol 84:233–239

Zijlmans M, Huiskamp G, Hersevoort M et al (2007) EEG-fMRI in the preoperative work-up for epilepsy surgery. Brain 130:2343–2353

Zijlmans M, Zweiphenning W, van Klink N (2019) Changing concepts in presurgical assessment for epilepsy surgery. Nat Rev Neurol 15:594–606

Diffusion Imaging with MR Tractography for Brain Tumor Surgery

Alberto Bizzi

Contents

A. Bizzi (✉)
Fondazione IRCCS Istituto Neurologico Carlo Besta,
Milan, Italy
e-mail: alberto.bizzi@istituto-besta.it

© The Author(s), under exclusive license to Springer Nature Switzerland AG 2022
C. Stippich (ed.), *Clinical Functional MRI*, Medical Radiology Diagnostic Imaging,
https://doi.org/10.1007/978-3-030-83343-5_7

Abstract

In the last 20 years advances in Neurosurgery, Neuroradiology and Neuro-Oncology have dramatically changed management of brain tumors, especially of gliomas that are seated in eloquent areas and are carrying a higher risk for permanent postoperative neurological deficits.

This chapter aims to provide practical and clinically relevant information with a review of the current literature from glioma biology through MR diffusion basic principles, methodology and clinical application of MR tractography, so that the reader can get a throughout interdisciplinary impression of the state of the art.

In contrast to brain metastases and meningiomas, gliomas extensively infiltrate the extracellular space of the gray and white matter changing the anatomic and functional properties of the brain. MR diffusion imaging has great potentials to contribute to disclose the mechanisms of interaction between gliomas and the host tissue.

Diffusion tensor imaging (DTI) is the most established and validated clinical application of MR tractography and it is increasingly requested by neurosurgeons. More advanced diffusion MR acquisition schemes such as high-angular resolution diffusion imaging (HARDI) and more sophisticated tractography algorithms such as spherical deconvolution (SD) and Q-ball imaging (QBI) have been developed to overcome DTI limitations. The community is beginning to apply the advanced methods in presurgical mapping.

A detailed understanding of the relationship between eloquent white matter fascicles and infiltrating gliomas is mandatory to correctly planning a resection and interpret the functional neurophysiological responses recorded during intraoperative monitoring (IOM) with electromyography (EMG), motor evoked potential (MEP), and direct intraoperative electrical stimulation (IES). It should be emphasized that MR diffusion tractography provides anatomical, not functional information.

The neurosurgical community is increasingly recognizing the value of MR diffusion imaging with tractography in evaluating patients with gliomas. MR tractography is a great educational tool for neurosurgeons and neuroradiologists. Presurgical visualization of eloquent fascicles in the proximity of a mass has been associated with a higher probability of total resection in low and high grade gliomas. Postoperative MR tractography is increasingly used to correlate postoperative deficits with white matter anatomy, and guide rehabilitation strategies.

This chapter presents optimized clinical presurgical HARDI protocols and tractography methods for visualization of the major white matter tracts that are part of the motor, language and visuospatial attention systems. Practical examples of how to interpret MR tractography findings are given, illustrative cases with typical and atypical presurgical findings are presented. Complementary applications with functional MR imaging (fMRI) are highlighted. Finally, the clinical value and limitations of presurgical MR diffusion imaging are discussed.

Abbreviations

AC	Anterior commissure
ADC	Apparent diffusion coefficient
AF	Arcuate fasciculus
AG	Angular gyrus
ALA	5-Aminolevulinic acid
BA	Brodmann area
BOLD	Blood oxygenated level dependent
CC	Corpus callosum
CL	Linear anisotropy coefficient
CP	Planar anisotropy coefficient
CST	Corticospinal tract
DEC	Directionally encoded color
dlPFC	Dorsolateral prefrontal cortex
dODF	Diffusion orientation distribution function
DSI	Diffusion spectrum imaging
DTI	Diffusion tensor imaging
DWI	Diffusion weighted imaging
ECS	Extracellular space
EOR	Extent of resection
EPI	Echo planar imaging
FA	Fractional anisotropy
FAT	Frontal aslant tract
FEF	Frontal eye field
FLAIR	Fluid attenuated inversion recovery
fMRI	Functional magnetic resonance imaging
fODF	Fiber orientation diffusion function
FST	Frontal striatal tract
GBM	Glioblastoma multiforme
HARDI	High-angular resolution diffusion imaging
HGG	High grade glioma
IES	Intraoperative electrical stimulation
IFG	Inferior frontal gyrus
IFOF	Inferior frontal occipital fasciculus
ILF	Inferior longitudinal fasciculus
IOM	Intraoperative monitoring
IPL	Inferior parietal lobule
ITG	Inferior temporal gyrus
LGG	Low grade glioma
M1	Primary motor cortex
MD	Mean diffusivity
MEP	Notor evoked potential
MFG	Medial frontal gyrus
MLF	Medial longitudinal fasciculus
MRI	Magnetic resonance imaging
MTG	Medial temporal gyrus
ND	Neurite density
NODDI	Neurite orientation dispersion and density imaging
ODI	Orientation dispersion index
OR	Optic radiations
PMC	Premotor cortex
PMd	Premotor dorsal
PMv	Premotor ventral
PPC	Posterior parietal cortex
QBI	Q-ball imaging
ROI	Region of interest
S1	Primary somatosensory cortex
SC	Spherical anisotropy coefficient
SCF	Subcallosal fasciculus
SD	Spherical deconvolution
SFG	Superior frontal gyrus
SLF	Superior longitudinal fasciculus
SMA	Supplementary motor area
SMG	Supramarginal gyrus
SPL	Superior parietal lobule
STG	Superior temporal gyrus
T2WI	T2-weighted image
TPFIA	Temporo-parietal fiber intersection area
UF	Uncinate fasciculus
vlPFC	Ventrolateral prefrontal cortex
WHO	World Health Organization
WM	White matter

1 Introduction

In the last 25 years tremendous advancements in Neurosurgery, Neuroradiology and Neuro-Oncology have changed the management of brain tumors. Advancements in Neurosurgery include implementation of microscopic surgery, intraoperative monitoring (IOM) and imaging-guided methods in the operating theater (Keles and Berger 2004). Twenty-five years ago brain tumors infiltrating "eloquent areas" were considered "inoperable" by the majority of neurosurgeons. Implementation of modern surgical techniques has widened the indications for brain tumor surgery to include lesions located in the proximity of the primary motor cortex and of the optic radiations, or infiltrating Broca and Wernicke areas of the language system. The aims of surgery in lower grade gliomas are maximal tumor resection according to "functional margins" and whenever possible to perform "supratotal resection" that extends beyond the areas with MR signal abnormalities. Achievement of these goals significantly increases overall survival by delaying malignant transformation of diffuse gliomas. The aim of surgery in glioblastoma multiforme (GBM) is to remove up to 95% of the enhancing and solid component of the tumor in order to delay recurrence of the tumor. In the last two decades refinement of intraoperative functional mapping methods has resulted in much more reliable identification of functional margins of the motor and language systems.

Advances in Neuroradiology, in particular in the field of functional MR imaging (fMRI) and MR diffusion tensor imaging (DTI) have changed the way surgeons evaluate patients before surgery. Advanced neuroimaging methods can now provide morphological and functional information about the alterations induced by the tumor on the hosting brain. This new information is quite important and relevant, especially when a diffuse infiltrating glioma is growing in an eloquent brain structure. It has been shown that presurgical mapping with fMRI and DTI may improve surgical targeting, guide surgical strategy and intraoperative assessments, reduce intraoperative time (Petrella et al. 2006). It is a fact that neurosurgeons are increasingly requesting fMRI and DTI as part of their routine presurgical evaluation. Functional maps are frequently used to discuss the aims of surgery with the patients and their family, before securing the consent to proceed.

Advances in Neuro-Oncology have been also quite impressive in the last decade. Substantial progresses have been made in the molecular classification of many brain tumors. Large-scale molecular profiling approaches have identified new mutations in gliomas which have allowed subclassification into distinct molecular sub-

groups with characteristic features of age, localization, and outcome (Sturm et al. 2012). Randomized clinical trials have demonstrated that molecular characterization allows identification of subgroups of gliomas that are associated with distinct prognosis and predicted treatment response (Stupp and Hegi 2013). The diagnostic importance of *isocitrate dehydrogenase* (IDH) mutational status in diffuse gliomas was first formally recognized within the updated fourth edition of the WHO Classification of Tumors of the Central nervous System in 2016 (Louis et al. 2016). The incorporation of IDH and other molecular biomarkers into an integrated diagnosis of gliomas provides a more reproducible and clinically meaningful classification of diffuse gliomas in adults (Brat et al. 2020; Eckel-Passow et al. 2015). Thus molecular analyses have become a must of the standard diagnostic workup in all patients with a brain tumor (Thomas et al. 2013). These advances in neuro-oncology emphasize the importance of tumor tissue sampling for molecular studies.

All together the above-mentioned advances have changed treatment strategies for this disease, especially so when the lesion is located in the proximity of eloquent structures. In the early nineties it was quite common to follow a "wait-and-see" strategy or performing a stereotactic needle biopsy, while today radical tumor exeresis has become the standard of care. These advances have paved the way to a *personalized treatment strategy* that is going to influence the outcome of brain tumors in the years to come (Weller et al. 2012).

2 Neuro-Oncology of Gliomas

2.1 Histology and Molecular Markers

Diffusely infiltrative gliomas are by far the most common type of primary brain neoplasms in adults and they are classified by genetics, tumor cell lineage and index of proliferative activity. The historical histopathological classification in astrocytomas and oligodendrogliomas has become less important than the IDH-status. The IDH mutation is the earliest genomic event of tumorigenesis and it is almost always retained during tumor progression. In contrast to IDH-mutant gliomas, IDH-wildtype astrocytic tumors are distinct clinical and genetic entities with more aggressive clinical behavior and they have a poor prognosis (Louis et al. 2016; Brat et al. 2020). The age range of IDH-wildtype (sixth and seventh decades) is higher than that of IDH-mutant gliomas (third and fifth decades).

The term glioblastoma (GBM), corresponding to WHO grade 4, should be reserved for IDH-wildtype diffuse astrocytic gliomas that have genetic and histologic features predictive of a highly aggressive clinical behavior. Among brain neoplasms GBMs have the highest proliferative activity and they may grow very quickly; they usually become symptomatic within a few months. GBMs have a dismal prognosis with a median survival time of 14 months, despite radio and chemotherapy (Stupp et al. 2005).

On the contrary, IDH-mutant gliomas have genetic and histopathologic features predictive of a less aggressive clinical behavior with longer survival times (median 3–5 years) and they occur in younger adults. IDH-mutant gliomas are subdivided into two subgroups: the astrocytic phenotype with co-mutation in *TP53* and *ATRX*, and the oligodendrocytic phenotype with codeletion of 1p/19q chromosomes and *TERT* promoter mutation. These genetic abnormalities are mutually exclusive. *Diffuse astrocytomas* WHO-2 will ultimately progress to WHO-3 (*anaplastic astrocytomas*) and then to WHO-4. *IDH-mutant, codeleted* WHO-2 and WHO-3 *oligodendroglioma* respond well to chemotherapy and they are associated with a relatively longer survival time than IDH-mutant astrocytic tumors (Louis et al. 2007).

2.2 Pattern of Growth and Velocity of Expansion

One important property of gliomas is their skill to infiltrate extensively the extracellular space (ECS) in gray as well as in white matter (WM). Like "guerilla warriors" glioma cells abuse the host "supply" vessels rather than constructing their own for satisfying their oxygen and nutrients requirements (Claes et al. 2007). This property is found in IDH-mutant as well as in IDH-wildtype, implying that the invasive phenotype is acquired early in oncogenesis. Glioma cells have the capability to migrate and modulate the ECS. Glioma cells may follow different patterns of growth that depend on preexisting host tissue elements. This growth pattern has significant prognostic implications and it is a major factor in therapeutic failure. Different glioma subtypes may follow different patterns of infiltration that depend upon the "weapons and tools" used by the invading "guerilla cells" and by the interaction with the environmental factors of the host. Glioma cells of a particular subtype may be extremely successful to infiltrate along myelinated WM tracts (intrafascicular growth), whereas tumor cells of other subtypes may accumulate in the subpial, perivascular, or perineuronal space (Giese and Westphal 1996). Other subtypes preferentially infiltrate the gray matter's neuropil in specific anatomic regions such as the insular cortex or the supplementary motor area in the superior frontal gyrus (SFG) (Duffau and Capelle 2004). The most extreme example of diffuse infiltrative growth is represented by gliomas infiltrating multiple lobes, subcortical nuclei or other anatomic brain regions (Mawrin 2005).

Measuring the spontaneous velocity of diametric expansion is important to predict patient's overall survival. The velocity of diametric expansion is faster in GBMs than in LGG; the latter have a spontaneous velocity in the range of 2–8 mm/year with a mean of 5.8 mm/year (Pallud et al. 2013). While LGG may continue to grow and infiltrate brain tissue at a stable velocity, GBMs grow fast and usually dislocate or destroy adjacent WM fasciculi and gyri (Nimsky et al. 2005). We will see later how these differences in velocity of expansion may have important implications for the interpretation of functional and MR diffusion imaging data.

2.3 Aims of Brain Tumor Surgery

Is surgery still the best treatment option for patients with a new diagnosis of brain tumor, despite the high costs and the relative high morbidity risk? The role of surgery is crucial for determining the diagnosis controlling seizures and planning radio and chemotherapy. The infiltrative nature of diffuse gliomas and their frequent localization in so-called eloquent areas has historically limited the extent of resection (EOR) due to the high risk of causing permanent focal neurological deficits. The controversy about the value of surgery in patients with LGG and HGG has not yet been fully resolved. Stereotactic biopsy is associated with a substantial risk of inaccuracy and sampling error. Currently, indications for biopsy are very limited in gliomas. Furthermore, biopsy has no therapeutic impact. Despite the lack of phase III study, most recent data strongly argue in favor of achieving a maximal resection of the tumor. Accordingly, in the last two decades there has been a paradigm shift from a surgical approach that relied mainly on anatomical landmarks to one based on identification of eloquent brain structures. Observational and retrospective studies have provided indication that radical surgical resection may offer a survival advantage over stereotactic biopsy and subtotal resections. Different considerations apply to surgery in LGG and HGG.

In the past the "wait-and-see" approach in LGG was justified by the lack of prospective randomized controlled clinical trials providing Level I evidence that extensive surgical resection had an impact on the quality of life and overall patients' survival (Laws 2001; Laws et al. 2003). In the majority of clinical studies EOR was not objectively assessed on postoperative MRI scans. Only recently authors have begun to include systematic measurement of residual tumor measured on postoperative MRI scans. Clinical studies have demonstrated that EOR correlates with survival times. LGG patients with resection >90% will have significantly longer overall survival times (Smith et al. 2008). In addition, supratotal resection that extends beyond the areas of signal abnormalities will significantly increase time of progression-free survival (Yordanova et al. 2011).

Until a decade ago in patients with GBM it was an even more open question whether simple debulking was effective or whether the neurosurgeons should strive to achieve maximal cytoreduction. A randomized study demonstrated that elderly GBM patients treated with open craniotomy rather than stereotactic biopsy have longer overall survival times (171 vs. 85 days), but overall benefit of open surgery to patients seemed to be modest, since time of deterioration did not differ between the two treatment groups (Vuorinen et al. 2003). In the past more emphasis has been placed on the role of radio and chemotherapy than on surgery.

The issue of complete resection as a causal, not only prognostic factor for overall survival in patients with GBM has been readdressed in a randomized phase III 5-aminolevulinic acid (ALA) study. This study investigated 5-ALA-induced fluorescence as a tool for improving EOR and provided a very high fraction of patients with postoperative MR imaging data acquired within 72 h. Residual tumor measured in the postoperative MRI scan was defined as tissue with a volume of contrast enhancement greater than 0.175 cm^3. Of the 243 GBM patients included in the ALA study 121 (49%) had incomplete resection and 122 (50.2%) had complete resection: the median overall survival was 11.8 months in the former and 16.9 months in the latter group (Stummer et al. 2008). Long-term survivors (>24 months) were almost exclusively among patients of the complete resection group. It is known that neurosurgeons may be less aggressive during resections in the elderly and when the tumor is near critical areas. It was shown that the difference in survival remained stable and significant when patients were restratified according to age (>60 years) in two groups, corroborating a causal effect of EOR on survival independent of age. The difference in survival among the two groups remained stable also when patients were restratified in two groups of patients with or without tumors in eloquent locations. The EOR not only influences survival, but also the efficacy of adjuvant therapies. The ALA cohort study provided for the first time Level 2b evidence that in GBM as a single factor survival depends on complete resection of the enhancing tumor. This level of evidence is inferior to randomized studies (Level 1) yet superior to case-control studies (Level 3), case series (Level 4), or expert opinions (Level 5).

The same authors (Stummer et al. 2011) reported that extended resections performed using 5-ALA carry a greater risk of temporary impairment of neurological function; patients with a greater risk of developing permanent postoperative deficits were those with preoperative symptoms such as aphasia unresponsive to steroids. Infiltration and destruction of eloquent brain, rather than vasogenic edema, are likely responsible for these preoperative focal neurological deficits. This data emphasizes again the importance of identifying the anatomic boundaries of the lesion with presurgical MR tractography and ultimately the functional limits with subcortical intraoperative electrical stimulation (IES). The importance of EOR as a predictor of overall survival has been shown also in a series of 107 patients with recurrent GBM when gross total (>95% by volume) resection is achieved at recurrence, overall survival is maximized regardless of initial EOR, suggesting that patients with initial subtotal resection may benefit from additional surgery (Bloch et al. 2012).

Detection of functional boundaries during surgery should be achieved with the aid of intraoperative neurophysiology and supported by presurgical fMRI and MR diffusion tractography (Bello et al. 2010). When a temporary deficit is repeatedly elicited with direct subcortical IES in the proximity of the wall of the surgical cavity, the functional limits of the resection are reached and the resection in that part of the tumor should be stopped. Identification of the functional limits is critical especially in gliomas infiltrating the motor system, in particular when the tumor involves the corticospinal tract (CST) (Bello et al. 2014). There is very low possibility of function compensation in the CST network when fast (20 μm thick) fibers are damaged because the function cannot be transferred to a nearby or distant network (Robles et al. 2008). Other critical

networks that if damaged are likely to produce permanent deficits are the inferior frontal-occipital fasciculus (IFOF), the arcuate fasciculus (AF) and the subcallosal fasciculus (SCF) for the language system and the optic radiations (OR) for the visuospatial system. Damage or resection of several other long-range fascicles is likely to induce severe transitory neurological deficits followed by near to complete recovery in the matter of few weeks or months.

Another important parameter to determine is preoperative estimation of the residual tumor volume. Mandonnet et al. computed a probabilistic atlas of glioma residues with preoperative MR imaging data that allowed a preoperative estimation of the expected EOR. The atlas enhances the anatomic regions where tumor cannot be resected. In their series of 65 patients with LGG the success rate of the presurgical classification for partial vs. subtotal resection was 82% (Mandonnet et al. 2007a). The residual volume was underestimated in 9 patients with partial resection, overestimated in 3 patients with subtotal resection. It is remarkable that the regions with the highest probability of residual tumors are essentially located in the WM. Regions with a probability of residual tumor greater than 70% include the CST, the IFOF and the AF. Other regions with high percentage of residual tumor were found in the posterior aspect of the corpus callosum and the anterior perforated substance. The last two anatomic structures are not considered functionally essential, however they are either difficult to access or contain lenticulostriate vessels. This study once again outlines the importance of identifying and safeguarding vital vascular and functional structures during tumor resection.

3 Magnetic Resonance Diffusion Imaging Methods

3.1 Conventional MR Imaging

Magnetic resonance imaging (MRI) is currently the method of choice for detecting brain tumors. MRI is very sensitive to detect alterations in water content that are so common in brain tumors. Water accumulation alters the MR signal on T2- and T1-weighted MR images and it is one of the first macroscopic changes occurring very early in the natural history of the neoplasm. Water accumulation precedes other metabolic and physiologic changes such as elevation of choline, cerebral blood volume (CBV), glucose uptake and protein synthesis that are detected, respectively, by proton MR spectroscopy (H-MRS), perfusion MR imaging and positron emission tomography (PET). MRI accurately defines the size of the mass and its relationship with relevant anatomic landmarks. MRI identifies presence of blood products and/or abnormal vessels within the mass that are important for assessing tumor grade. MRI after intravenous contrast agent injection detects breakdown of the blood–brain barrier, a consistent sign of more aggressive behavior related to the presence of angiogenesis and immature vessels.

However, MRI has several limitations. Like in a guerilla war, visualization of the elusive invasive front may be problematic. MR imaging may significantly underestimate the extent of diffuse infiltrative glioma growth. Infiltrating glioma cells can be found at biopsy beyond the hyperintense area on T2/FLAIR images (Ganslandt et al. 2005). Discrimination of infiltrating tumor from vasogenic edema is often difficult. Radio and chemotherapy-induced changes may mimic tumor progression (pseudoprogression). Thus, evaluation of response to therapy may be problematic due to ambiguous and overlapping MR signal changes in pseudoprogression and recurrent tumor, pseudoresponse and true response.

Finally, one important limitation of conventional MRI at magnetic field strength of 1.5 and 3.0 T is that it is blind to orientation of WM pathways. At ultrahigh field strength (7.0 T and above) only the major WM tracts can be recognized on T2-weighted MR images; in addition susceptibility imaging is a very sensitive method able to detect the orientation of myelinated WM bundles (Duyn 2013; Sati et al. 2013).

3.2 Diffusion Tensor Imaging

MRI with diffusion-weighted sequences measures the effects of tissue microstructure on the random walks of water molecules (Brownian motion) in the brain. When molecules can diffuse equally in all directions diffusion is called *isotropic*, when molecules can diffuse only along a specific direction it is called *anisotropic*. Isotropic diffusion occurs if there are no barriers like in the cerebrospinal fluid or when the barriers are randomly oriented like in the gray matter. Anisotropic diffusion occurs when there are oriented barriers that favor movement of water along rather than across them. In tissues with an orderly oriented microstructure, such as the WM, diffusivity of water varies with orientation since water molecules are likely to encounter different obstacles and barriers according to the direction in which they move (Chenevert et al. 1990; Doran et al. 1990). In WM water diffuses fastest along the principal orientation of the bundles (parallel diffusivity), and slowest along the cross-sectional plane (radial diffusivity). In the WM the degree of anisotropy depends primarily on membrane density, mainly in the form of intact axonal membranes.

In 1994 Basser et al. showed that the classic ellipsoid tensor formalism could be deployed to measure anisotropy in the human body (Basser et al. 1994). The tensor not only describes the magnitude of the water diffusion, but also the degree and the principal directions of anisotropic diffusion. Mathematically the tensor describes the shape of the ellipsoid with three eigenvalues that represent the diffusivities along the three orthogonal axes and three eigenvectors that provide orientation. The three eigenvalues are numbered in decreasing order by magnitude ($\lambda 1 > \lambda 2 > \lambda 3$). DTI is currently the most robust and efficient method to analyze diffusion MR data. DTI has become so popular because it provides several unique insights into tissue microstructure. It quantifies mean diffusivity (MD) and diffusion anisotropy, which are useful indices of WM integrity; with the eigenvector ($\varepsilon 1$)

providing the orientation information that enables for tractography.

Multiple imaging parameters informative about tissue microstructure can be calculated from a single DTI acquisition. Fractional anisotropy (FA) measures the eccentricity of water molecules displacement. Anisotropy is found in other body tissues such as peripheral nerves, kidneys, skeletal and cardiac muscles; however neural bundles show the greatest degree of anisotropy, with parallel diffusion on the order of 2–10 times larger than perpendicular diffusion. In the healthy human brain the intravoxel orientation coherence of WM bundles is probably the most relevant factor affecting FA (Pierpaoli et al. 1996). FA is a scalar value that describes the degree of anisotropy of a diffusion process. FA ranges between zero and one and its values are displayed in gray scale maps. A value of zero means that diffusion is free or equally hindered in all directions ($\lambda 1 = \lambda 2 = \lambda 3$), the ellipsoid reduces to a sphere. A value of one means that diffusion occurs only along one direction and it is hindered or restricted along other directions ($\lambda 1 > 0$; $\lambda 2 = \lambda 3 = 0$); the ellipsoid reduces to a line. This means that the diffusion is confined to that direction alone.

FA is a scalar metric that measures the degree of anisotropy, but does not indicate the shape of the diffusion ellipsoid. Voxels with similar FA value may have different shapes (Alexander et al. 2000). When linear diffusivity prevails ($\lambda 1 \gg \lambda 2 = \lambda 3$) anisotropy has the shape of a cigar, when planar diffusivity prevails ($\lambda 1 = \lambda 2 \gg \lambda 3$) it has the shape of a Frisbee. While both linear and planar anisotropy coefficients (CL and CP) are responsible for increased FA, their relative values indicate the shape of the ellipsoid. CL specifically highlights the region of tubular tensors, whereas CP indicates regions of planar tensors. We will see later how anisotropy shape coefficients at the periphery of a mass may provide relevant information about the modality of growth of the lesion and how they may affect DTI tractography.

MD, parallel ($\lambda 1$), and radial diffusivity (($\lambda 2 + \lambda 3$)/2) provide information about the integrity of WM bundles. These indices have become quite popular and they have been particularly used in the evaluation of neurological diseases such as multiple sclerosis, Alzheimer disease, other dementias, and psychiatric disorders.

The orientation of the largest eigenvalue can be color coded to provide directionally encoded color (DEC) maps. By convention, bundles oriented along the z axis (cranio-caudal) of the MR scanner are displayed in blue, those coursing in the x direction (right to left) in red and those coursing in the y direction (anterior to posterior) in green. DEC maps provide a simple and effective way to visualize orientation information contained in DTI and they clearly show the main projection (blue), commissural (red) and association (green) WM pathways (Pajevic and Pierpaoli 1999). On DEC maps it was possible to identify unambiguously the major projection, commissural and association pathways in the brain of 123 mammalian species (Assaf et al. 2020).

3.3 DTI Metrics and Brain Tumor Microstructure

How do the above parameters relate to changes in tissue microstructure? In imaging protocols for clinical research the spatial resolution of DTI is usually in the range of 2.0 × 2.0 × 2.0 mm. Despite the apparent low spatial resolution, DTI is used as a probe to investigate tissue microstructure and it is sensitive to molecular water displacements on the order of 5–10 µm. There are three main longitudinally oriented structures that could hinder water diffusion perpendicular to neural bundles: (1) microtubules and neurofilaments of the axonal cytoskeleton, (2) the axonal membrane (axolemma), and (3) the myelin sheath surrounding the axons. Additional confounders are fast axonal transport and streaming, and B_0 susceptibility. Multiple studies have shown that there are no major differences in diffusion measurements between myelinated and unmyelinated bundles, thus the axolemma is the primary determinant of anisotropic diffusion of water. Therefore anisotropy should not be considered myelin specific. Notwithstanding, myelin can modulate the degree of anisotropy.

It is more intuitive to correlate changes in parallel and perpendicular diffusivities rather than changes in FA to WM pathological lesions. Injuries with collapse of the axolemma are likely to determine a decrease in parallel diffusivity. Myelin loss and axonal increased permeability to water will likely determine an increase in radial diffusivity, despite integrity of axonal membranes (Beaulieu et al. 1996).

Glioma cells migration and growth cause more complex microstructural changes in the brain tissue. Glioma cells remodel the extracellular matrix by destroying the surrounding tissue through secretion of matrix-degrading enzymes, such as the plasminogen activator and the family of matrix metalloproteinases. In the majority of tumor types widening of the ECS, changes in cellular size, destruction of axonal membranes, and a general disruption of the normal brain architecture are associated with accumulation of water in large amounts. Studies have shown a dramatic increase in the ECS volume of gliomas even during the early infiltration stage (Zamecnik 2005). These microstructural changes lead to higher water diffusivity (i.e., increased MD) and reduction in diffusion anisotropy (i.e., decreased FA), especially in the early avascular stage of growth that is typical of LGG. The above histopathological changes will likely be associated with minimal decrease in axial diffusivity and variable increase in radial diffusivity due to enlargement of the ECS and glioma cell infiltration. Overall the increased amount of water in the ECS appears to be the dominant factor leading to increased MD and decreased FA. However, the enlarged ECS is not filled with water alone. In LGG a dense network of glioma cell processes may hinder diffusion even of small molecules. In GBM the expansion of ECS is associated with the overproduction of aberrant glycoproteins (i.e., tenascin) in the extracellular matrix that not only stabilize the ECS volume, but also serve as a substrate for adhesion and subsequent migration

of the tumor cells through the enlarged ECS. Tumor invasion in WM will likely interrupt thousands of axons thus decreasing tissue anisotropy.

Gliomas have a propensity for microscopic infiltration of WM bundles well beyond their macroscopic borders. Microscopic glioma cells infiltration extends outside of the area of T2-signal hyperintensity and it is typically undetectable by conventional MR imaging. In areas with T2-signal hyperintensity tumor infiltration may be indistinguishable from peritumoral vasogenic edema that has a similar propensity to diffuse along WM bundles. DTI has been the focus of extensive studies that have attempted to answer this relevant clinical question that has important therapy implications. Unfortunately, so far DTI results have been remarkably inconsistent on this topic. The degree of peritumoral edema may be highly variable among tumor types; the degree of glioma cell infiltration along WM bundles also may vary considerably, potentially influenced by multiple factors that are playing a key role in extracellular matrix alteration and in ECS volume expansion such as tumor location, biology and genetics. Early reports suggested that the infiltrating component might be discriminated from tumor-free perilesional vasogenic edema on DEC maps (Field et al. 2004), however this method was not considered reliable. Price et al. advocate using the isotropic (p) and anisotropic (q) components of the diffusion tensor instead of FA to characterize glioma microstructure. The authors demonstrated that it was possible to differentiate areas of solid, high cellular tumor from areas of tumor infiltration on the basis of the anisotropic component q, but not necessarily the latter from areas of perilesional vasogenic edema (Price et al. 2006).

Perhaps the partial failure of the classic DTI parameters (i.e., MD, FA, parallel and radial diffusivities) to reliably characterize the many types of microstructural changes occurring in gliomas should come as no surprise and raise a specificity issue. FA and the other diffusion imaging parameters are sensitive but not enough specific to detect complex microstructural changes. Future research should focus into more advanced multi-compartmental models taking into accounts the many factors involved (Zhang et al. 2012; Papadogiorgaki et al. 2013).

3.4 MR Tractography

DTI fiber tracking or tractography is a natural extension of diffusion ellipsoid imaging (Conturo et al. 1999; Mori et al. 1999; Basser et al. 2000). It is the process of integrating voxel-wise tract orientations into a trajectory that connects remote brain regions. In WM regions (i.e., corpus callosum, CST, and OR) where the fascicles are compact and parallel the diffusion ellipsoid is prolate. The orientation of the principal eigenvector does not change much from one voxel to the next. We can use a mathematical procedure (algorithm) to generate a trajectory connecting consecutive coherently ordered ellipsoids within the brain, a muscle or another fibrous tissue. Starting from a "seed point" voxel trajectories are generated in all directions until "termination" criteria are satisfied. We can choose one seed point and form a tractogram with all streamlines going through that seed point, or delineate two ROIs and generate a tractogram with all streamlines connecting those two brain regions. The algorithm requires two important assumptions that are known as the FA and the angle thresholds. Trajectories cannot extend to voxels with FA values that are close to background noise, because the degree of uncertainty of the ellipsoid orientation would be too high, thus we use a FA threshold >0.15–0.20. Trajectories are interrupted when in consecutive voxels the angle formed by the intersection of their respective principal eigenvectors is smaller than a set angle (i.e., angle threshold <35°–45°), because it is assumed that the majority of WM fascicles do not U-turn. The algorithm aims to generate trajectories through the data field along which diffusion is least hindered. The trajectory or streamline is the basic stone of deterministic

tractography and it cannot be divided into smaller units. It has no direct relationship with any biological structure (axon, bundle, or fascicle) even though it reproduces its macroscopic trajectory in 3D space.

Strategies for generating diffusion tractograms vary greatly among algorithms and they can be broadly classified into local or global, model based or model free, deterministic or probabilistic. Deterministic tractography methods are the most intuitive and they are based upon streamline algorithms where the local tract direction is defined by the major eigenvector of the diffusion tensor as described above (Conturo et al. 1999; Mori et al. 1999). Mathematically a streamline can be represented as a 3D-space curve, as described by Basser et al. (2000). One limitation of the deterministic method is that any errors in calculations of the streamlines will be compounded as the streamline progresses from the seed to the termination point. The accuracy and variance of the tract reconstruction are a function of the algorithm, the signal-to-noise ratio, the diffusion tensor eigenvalues, and the tract length.

Limitations of fiber tracking performed with the streamline approach motivated the development of probabilistic tracking algorithms (Jones 2008). The aim of probabilistic tractography is to develop a full representation of the uncertainty associated with any assumption that might be made. Given a model and the data, probabilistic tractography provides a voxel-based map of high and low confidence (values given in percentage) that the trajectory of least hindrance to diffusion will connect the seed with the target point. From a mathematical point of view, the assumptions and the comparisons that can be made in studies across individual subjects and groups are more complete and flexible with probabilistic than with streamline tractography. Notwithstanding, streamline tractography is easier to implement in clinical practice and its more intuitive approach has contributed to its popularity among neuroanatomists and neuroradiologists.

A DTI tractography atlas for virtual in vivo dissection of the principal human WM tracts using a deterministic approach is very useful and practical for beginners (Catani and Thiebaut de Schotten 2008). The greatest success of fiber tracking is its use for in vivo dissection of major WM fascicles in individual healthy and pathological human brains. Tractography is also of value for segmenting WM pathways and providing quantitative measurements for comparison across subjects or groups.

3.5 Limitations of DTI and MR Tractography

The tensor is the most robust diffusion model, however it has several limitations when it is applied to brain WM. DTI provides two types of new contrasts: diffusion anisotropy and fiber orientation, which carry rich anatomical information about WM complexity. However, when interpreting MR diffusion data it is very important to understand well the inherent limitations of each method: (1) MR diffusion measurements are very sensitive to noise, motion and brain pulsatility, therefore to scanning time; (2) diffusion anisotropy carries information at the microscopic cellular (protein filaments and microtubules, cell membranes, and myelin) and macroscopic (vessels, glial cell networks, and population of bundles with different orientation) level that is averaged over a relative large voxel volume. Partial volume effects may become a problem in WM regions with more than one bundle such as the paraventricular zones, where FA is low and the degree of uncertainty in the estimation of bundle orientation increases. (3) DTI does not measure any specific parameter for the intraaxonal restricted water pool. (4) The calculation of the tensor assumes that fiber structures are homogeneous within a voxel but this assumption is not true when there are two or more fiber populations: one orientation cannot represent accurately the orientations of two fiber populations! Two strategies have been proposed to reduce this problem: increase spatial image resolution by reducing the voxel size or extract information with higher angular resolution from each voxel and abandon the simple tensor model. (5) DTI-based tractography algorithms cannot determine if bundles are crossing or kissing. (6) Diffusion MR cannot differentiate the directionality of axons within bundles. (7) At the spatial resolution currently used in clinical MRI, diffusion cannot track streamlines thru the gray matter, thus it cannot track the trajectories of WM bundles to their cortical terminations.

One of the major limitations of the classic tensor model is that for each voxel it provides only a single fiber orientation: this is a major obstacle for tractography and connectivity studies. Using spherical deconvolution methods with a spatial resolution of $2 \times 2 \times 2$ mm^3 it has been estimated that the proportion of WM voxels containing more than one bundle (crossing fibers) is about 90% (Jeurissen et al. 2013). These findings suggest that the DTI model may be inadequate to measure the complexity of fiber trajectories in the WM.

In voxels with more than one fiber population the orientation measured with classic DTI is the average of the orientations of all bundles present in that voxel. As a result, the shape of the diffusion ellipsoid in voxels with crossing fibers may appear either prolate or oblate. A prolate (stretch out, linear) object has the shape of a spheroid generated by an ellipse rotating about its longer axis with the polar radius much greater than the equatorial radius ($\lambda 1 \gg \lambda 2 = \lambda 3$), while an oblate (flatten, planar) object has the shape of a spheroid generated by rotating an ellipse about its shorter axis with the equatorial radius much greater than the distance between the poles ($\lambda 1 = \lambda 2 \gg \lambda 3$). A geometric analysis of DTI measurements in the human brain using a three-phase tensor shape diagram demonstrated that there is a tensor shape hierarchy between different WM tracts in the order of commissural, deep projection and association WM tracts (Alexander et al. 2000). The CC and the CST show the greatest linear shape, while the AF and the subcortical WM tracts show a significant planar component of their tensor measurements. The causes of planar diffusion in the brain are not perfectly understood. Bundles arranged in sheets could explain planar diffusion (Wedeen et al. 2012); however, a more likely origin is presence of crossing WM tracts within the large voxels typical of the DTI experiment. The linear shape of CC and CST may outline the compacted nature of the bundles in the central segment of those tracts, whereas the planar shape of the AF at the level of the centrum semiovale may reflect that most voxels contain AF and CC crossing fibers.

The shape of the diffusion ellipsoid of the voxels in the proximity of a focal lesion can be affected by mass effect. Especially in voxels near the borders of fast growing gliomas the ellipsoid can become oblate with undefined principal orientation. It is important to evaluate the shape of the ellipsoid when interpreting tractography results in the proximity of a mass, because it might provide a warning sign about false positive results. Oblate voxels are confusing for tractography because the difference between $\lambda 1$ and $\lambda 2$ is minimal and noise will cause the principal eigenvector to have random orientation in the plane: tracking might go either way in oblate voxels.

Detection of WM bundles within a tumor and surrounding areas of vasogenic edema may be also problematic. Intraoperative direct electrical stimulation has detected presence of functioning WM tracts within areas of T2-signal hyperintensity especially so in LGG. It is assumed that a significant number of electrically competent and signal conducting axons are preserved despite infiltration by glioma cells. Tumor infiltration alters MR diffusivity along WM bundles and it may distort their geometry. The increased free water content may artificially decrease FA, thus leading to false negative results if FA decreases below the FA threshold that is commonly used for tractography. It may be responsible for false positive results due to increasing degree of uncertainty in estimating the orientation of the principal eigenvector. DTI studies have shown interruption of streamlines inside the tumor or

areas of vasogenic edema, especially when FA threshold was set at >0.15 (Bastin et al. 2002; Bizzi et al. 2012). This issue raises a sensitivity issue for MR tractography with a relative high rate of false negative results in areas of decreased FA, high diffusivity and T2-hyperintensity that are especially common in LGG. Other authors have validated with IES the tractography findings obtained with FA threshold (>0.10) through regions of tumor infiltration (Bello et al. 2008). An alternative approach is to use advanced diffusion multicompartmental models such as Neurite Orientation Dispersion and Density Imaging (NODDI) method (Zhang et al. 2012) that will be discussed in detail in the next section. NODDI is a practical high-angular resolution diffusion imaging (HARDI) method with two shells for estimating the microstructural complexity of dendrites and axons in vivo on clinical MRI scanners. NODDI allows separation of the restricted intraaxonal compartment from the isotropic and hindered compartments and provides estimates of two parameters that are more specific than FA: neurite density and orientation index.

3.6 Crossing Fibers and the Need for Advanced MR Diffusion Imaging Methods

It is important to understand well the limitations of MR tractography, especially when the method is applied in the interest of neurosurgical patients. Tractography can determine the trajectories of major WM fascicles but it cannot infer in which direction the signal is transmitted along each pathway. It cannot track streamlines to their cortical termination and it may fail at fiber crossing because the DTI model can recover only a single fiber orientation in each voxel. It is a user-dependent method based on a priori anatomic knowledge. It is also important to be aware that tractography does not provide functional information. IES is the only method able to test WM function and generate a subcortical functional map that has proven to maximize tumor resection and minimize hazards.

The ambiguity in determining fiber orientation in a voxel containing more than one fascicle is related to the model applied with DTI, but it is not a limitation of diffusion MRI in general. DTI models the dispersion of water molecules using a Gaussian distribution, thus the assumption is that the scatter pattern during the diffusion time has an ellipsoid shape. Voxels contain hundreds of thousands of axons that are organized in bundles and fascicles that can have a wide range of complex configurations. The fibers within each voxel may be parallel, fanning, bending, and crossing at an acute or perpendicular angle. DTI is accurate to represent parallel fibers, but it cannot distinguish them from fanning and bending fibers, except for a lower FA value. In voxels with crossing fibers at an acute angle the principal orientation measured with DTI is misleading, as the mean fiber orientation that has a prolate shape does not correspond to the direction of any fiber. In voxels with orthogonal crossing fibers DTI fails to identify the two fascicles and its best approximation is an oblate ellipsoid that contains none of the useful directional information.

In the past decade there has been a lot of effort to move beyond DTI and solve the crossing fiber problem. Development of new models and algorithms that exploit more sophisticated imaging acquisition schemes such as HARDI has been addressed (Seunarine and Alexander 2009). The field is very complex and a detailed description of the many advanced methods goes beyond the purpose of this chapter.

Model-based approaches, such as the multi-tensor model, resolve fiber crossing by modeling distinct fiber populations separately. The model-based approaches assume that the voxel contains distinct populations of fibers and that diffusing molecules do not exchange between fiber populations. The multi-tensor model is a generalization of DTI that replaces the Gaussian model with a mixture of Gaussian densities. The "ball and stick" model assumes that water molecules belong to one of two populations: an isotropic component that does not interact with fibers and diffuses freely in the voxel and a restricted component that diffuses inside and immediately around axons (Behrens et al. 2003). The composite hindered and restricted model of diffusion (CHARMED) proposed by Assaf describes the restricted fiber population with a cylinder and the hindered population in extracellular space with an anisotropic Gaussian model (Assaf et al. 2004). The model-based methods do not naturally distinguish fanning and bending configurations from parallel fiber populations.

The aim of non-parametric methods is to estimate from diffusion MRI measurements the fiber orientation diffusion function (fODF) that provides more insight into the underlying fiber configuration. These methods do not rely solely on parametric models of diffusion, but try instead to reconstruct the fODF without placing modeling constraints on its form. Diffusion spectrum imaging (DSI) and Q-ball imaging reconstruct a function called the diffusion orientation distribution function (dODF). Spherical deconvolution (SD) methods recover a more direct estimate of the fODF.

DSI attempts to measure the scatter of diffusion directly and makes no assumptions about tissue microstructure or its shape (Wedeen et al. 2008). The acquisition requirements are the major limitations of DSI: standard protocols require long acquisition times with 500–1000 measurements at the expense of image resolution; stringent hardware with very strong gradients is required in order to apply very short pulses. The acquisition requirements in Q-ball imaging are more manageable than DSI. In its original work Tuch showed that Q-ball can resolve fiber crossing consistently using an acquisition scheme with 252 gradient directions at a $b = 4000$ s/mm^2 (Tuch 2004) although the approximation of the dODF introduces some blurring, which may reduce angular resolution and precision of peak directions.

The SD algorithm has the advantage of relatively short acquisition times, which are close to standard DTI clinical protocols, reduced computational times compared to some of the other methods, and the ability to resolve crossing fibers with a good angular resolution (Dell'Acqua et al. 2010). SD is based on the assumption that the acquired diffusion signals from a single voxel can be modeled as a spherical convolution between the fiber orientation distribution (FOD) and the fiber response function that describes the common signal profile from the WM bundles contained in the voxel (Tournier et al. 2004). A major limitation of SD is its susceptibility to noise, which often results in spurious peaks in the recovered fODF. Acquisition requirements are compatible with clinical protocols: 64 directions with $b = 2000$–3000 s/mm^2 with a total scan time of 16 min. DTI and SD reconstructions can be obtained from the same dataset.

NODDI combines a three-compartmental tissue model with a two-shell HARDI protocol optimized for clinical feasibility. NODDI adopts a tissue model that distinguishes three types of microstructural environment: intracellular (restricted), extracellular space (hindered), and cerebrospinal fluid (isotropic) compartments (Zhang et al. 2012). Each environment affects water diffusion in a unique way and gives rise to a separate normalized MR signal. The intracellular compartment refers to the space bounded by the membrane of neurites and it is modeled as a set of sticks. NODDI provides measurements of several parameters, among which the two most innovative are neurite density and an index of orientation dispersion that defines variation of neurites orientation within each voxel. These parameters have great potential to provide relevant information for brain tumor tissue characterization and may be particularly efficient to track fibers in voxels with an increased amount of water such as those with vasogenic edema and glioma infiltration. Tractography can be performed using the SD algorithm, the NODDI or the DTI model from one HARDI acquisition scheme.

3.7 Clinically Feasible Brain Mapping Imaging Protocols and Pre-processing Requirements

It is mandatory to acquire diffusion data with relatively high spatial and angular resolution in order to perform a state of the art tractography study. High spatial resolution plays in favor of tractography because it reduces the gap in size between voxels and fascicles. High-angular resolution increases the discrimination of crossing fascicles at an acute angle. Unfortunately, improved spatial resolution always comes at the expense of longer acquisition times and lower signal-to-noise ratio. It is important to verify the capability of the MR unit in order to reach a good compromise between spatial resolution, signal-to-noise ratio and total acquisition scan time. In clinical practice the isovolumetric voxel size should be no larger than 1.5 mm when acquiring data with 1.5 T or even better with 3.0 T MR units. One common strategy to improve the angular resolution and the signal-to-noise ratio of the HARDI acquisition scheme is to acquire a dataset with 32 or 64 gradient directions and a b value in the range of 1500–3000 s/mm^2. MR units with strong gradients (high maximum amplitude and fast slew rate) are beneficial to keep the TE to a minimum value. Especially if fMRI is also acquired, scan time inferior to 20 min is recommended in order to keep the total time of the study session within 45 min.

DEC maps are very useful for preliminary interpretation of clinical studies in patients with disease, especially when used by experienced users. Low angular resolution DEC maps can be acquired with DTI acquisitions that use a minimum of 6 gradient directions and b value of 800 s/mm^2; however, the examiner should be aware that performing tractography with a low quality dataset may increase the likelihood of errors.

For NODDI acquisition scheme the following imaging parameters are recommended: two shells (b value of 700 and 2000 s/mm^2) with similar TR and TE, and respectively, 20 and 64 gradient directions will result in a total scan time of about 20 min.

Clinical MRI diffusion studies are performed by acquiring single-shot echo-planar images (EPI) with diffusion sensitizing gradients of different strengths and orientations that are applied for a relative long time in order to achieve the desired b value. EPI read-out is very sensitive to static magnetic field (B_0) inhomogeneity that produces nonlinear geometric distortion primarily along the phase-encoding direction. Susceptibility artifacts are more pronounced at air–tissue interfaces and are most obvious in the orbitofrontal and mesial temporal regions, near the sphenoid sinus and the temporal petrous bone. In addition, patient bulk motion and additional image distortion induced by eddy currents, that do not cancel out when diffusion gradients are applied for a relative long time, cause additional artifacts on DWI. Analysis of diffusion imaging studies requires correction for patient motion and for susceptibility and eddy current artifacts. The many acquired DWIs have to be spatially aligned to avoid systematic errors in the parametric maps computed from misaligned DWI (Rohde et al. 2004). Several software are available for correcting DWI artifacts and confounds (Jenkinson et al. 2012; Leemans et al. 2009; Pierpaoli et al. 2010). Their use for pre-processing of DWI is strongly recommended in order to obtain reliable DTI measurements.

Since March 2012 the American Society of Functional Neuroradiology (ASFNR) has released and updated a document with ASFNR Guidelines for Clinical Application of Diffusion Tensor Imaging that is available on its website (https://www.asfnr.org/clinical-standards).

4 Functional Systems of the Brain and the Connectome

Current view is that the brain is hierarchically organized in terms of anatomical structure and function. The brain is a highly integrated system and for teaching purposes it may be divided into three distinct systems that function as a whole: the sensory, the motor, and the associative systems.

The sensory systems are in charge of processing special somatic sensations coming from the outside world: visual, auditory, tactile, and vestibular systems. Other sensory systems are specialized in processing visceral input: the olfactory, gustatory, and limbic systems. They are organized in primary sensory and unimodal cortical areas that continuously exchange information. Most sensory information is routed to the cerebral cortex via the thalamus. Only olfactory information passes through the olfactory bulb to the olfactory cortex in the uncus, bypassing the thalamus. The sensory systems converge to so-called multimodal areas that are located in the associative cortices of the parietal, temporal, and frontal lobes.

The motor system is responsible for purposeful movement; it plans for action, coordinates and executes the motor programs. The primary motor cortex (M1) plans and executes movements in association with other motor areas including the PMd, PMv, SMA, PPC, and several subcortical brain regions. The PPC plays an important role in generating planned movements by modulating the input received from the three sensory subsystems that localize the body and external objects in space. The PPC modulates planned movements, spatial reasoning, and visuospatial attention. The dlPFC is in charge of executive functions, including working memory, cognitive flexibility, and abstract reasoning. The dlPFC integrates sensory and mnemonic information and the regulation of intellectual function and action. Cognitive flexibility is the ability to switch between thinking about two different concepts and to think about multiple concepts simultaneously.

The associative system integrates current states with past tense states to predict proper responses based on a set of stimuli. The many association areas are located in the prefrontal, parietal, and temporal regions of both cerebral hemispheres; they permit perception and form a cohesive view of the external world. The association areas relate the information to past experiences, before the brain makes a decision and generates a motor response. The association areas are organized as distributed networks, and each network connects areas distributed across widely spaced regions of the cortex.

Network science does quantitative analysis of different aspects of connectivity that are peculiar of a complex system (Sporns 2014). Virtually all complex systems form networks of interacting parts composed of multiple and redundant neural circuits that process and transfer the information either serially or in parallel. A network is made of a group of elementary macro (or micro) components that are closely connected and work as a unit. At the macroscale level nodes and pathways are the basic components of the network. At the microscale level the components are neurons, dendrites, axons, and synapses. Understanding such complex systems will require knowledge of the ways in which these components interact and the emergent properties of their interactions.

The visuospatial, motor, and language systems are of great interest for presurgical mapping because they are in charge of functions that are essential for human life. These systems may share similar elementary components; however, their networks display peculiar different and organized patterns. Each network of a functional system is dedicated to a specific sensory, motor or cognitive modality and it includes several specialized nodes that have different roles in processing information. The *primary sensory cortex* is the brain area containing neurons that receive most of their information directly from the thalamus. The distance from the body sensory receptors at the periphery defines secondary and tertiary cortical sensory areas. These are unimodal and multimodal association areas that play an important role in integration and modulation of the input signals reaching the cortex, and in planning of motor actions. Secondary motor areas located in the SMA and in the PMv and PMd cortices compute programs of movement that are conveyed to the *primary motor cortex*, where are located the cortical pyramidal motor neurons that project directly to the spinal cord.

The organization of functional systems follows several principles. The information conveyed within each network is processed and transformed at every node level. Information may be amplified, attenuated, integrated with information conveyed from other nodes of the same system. There are two main groups of neurons at each stage of the information processing: projecting neurons and local interneurons. The projecting neurons convey the information to the next node stage in the system. Each brain region

may contain nodes of multiple functional systems. Axons leaving the node of a functional system are bundled together in a fascicle that projects to the next node. Bundles belonging to different networks and systems can course temporarily within the same fascicle. Short and long bundles may enter and exit at various locations along the course of a fascicle. All the nodes of the sensory and motor systems have a somatotopic organization that is repeated throughout the network. In this way an orderly neural map of information is retained at each successive level of processing in the brain. Visual, auditory, somatosensory, and motor maps are built at different stages of their respective networks.

Most functional systems are hierarchically organized. In the primary visual cortex an individual neuron may fire only when it receives the signal input from a very specific outside stimulus. Following the same principle multiple neurons in the primary visual cortex converge on individual cells in the association cortical areas. At very advanced stages of information processing, individual cortical neurons are responsive to highly complex information.

In the following sections the functional organization of the three functional systems that are more clinically relevant for presurgical mapping are addressed.

4.1 The Motor System

The task of the motor system is to maintain performance of basic functions such as balance, posture, locomotion, reaching, and communication through speech and gesture by moving body parts, limbs, and eyes. The motor system produces movement by translating neural signals into contractile force in muscles. The agility and dexterity of an athlete or of a piano player reflect the capabilities of his motor system to plan, coordinate, and execute motor programs that have been learnt and practiced many times until they can be executed automatically for the most part.

According to modern theories the motor system acts as a distributed network. The neurons of origin of the network are located in at least five distinct cortical areas of each hemisphere: M1, PMv, PMd, prefrontal, and parietal areas. According to their targets the descending fibers are divided into four groups: the ventromedial and dorsolateral brainstem pathways, the corticobulbar, and the CSTs (Lemon 2008). It is important to emphasize that the CST originates from cortical areas that have different functions: M1, PM, SMA, the cingulate motor area, the primary somatosensory cortex (S1), the posterior parietal cortex, and the parietal operculum. M1 contains the greatest density of neurons giving rise to CST and corticobulbar tract. The human CST consists of about one million axons, of which about 49% originate in M1, 19% in the SMA, 21% in the parietal lobe (S1 and posterior parietal cortex), 7% in the PMd, and 4% PMv (Fig. 1). The axonal projections of the cortical motor neurons converge in the corona radiata, a fan-like array of descending and ascending fibers connecting the cortex with thalamus, basal nuclei,

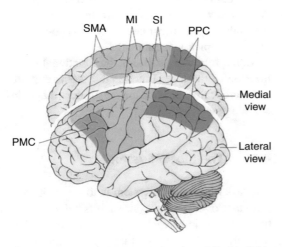

Fig. 1 The corticospinal tract arises from M1, S1, SMA, PMd, and PMv. Approximately 49% of the one million axons arises from M1, 21% from S1. The remaining 30% of the fibers originate from the PMC, the region immediately rostral to the precentral gyrus: 19% arises from SMA, 7% from PMd, and 4% from PMv. The descending axonal projections converge in the corona radiata, then enter the internal capsule maintaining a somatotopic distribution: corticobulbar fibers are located within the genu, corticospinal fiber in the middle third of the posterior limb of the internal capsule with the face-hand-foot represented in the anterior-posterior direction. The PPC does not contribute to the CST but modulates its activity. (Modified from http://what-when-how.com)

and spinal cord. More ventrally the descending tracts enter the internal capsule maintaining a somatotopic distribution: fibers originating from PMv, PMd, and SMA and prefrontal fibers originating from the frontal eye field areas course in the anterior third of the posterior limb, whereas the fibers originating in M1 course in the intermediate third. In the midbrain the fibers of the corticobulbar tract and CST become even more compact and enter the cerebral peduncles. At this level the frontal projections are located medially while tracts originating in the parietal, temporal, and occipital lobes are located more laterally in this order. In the pons the tracts course between the transverse pontine fibers, before beginning to cross to the contralateral side in the decussation of the pyramids at the level of the medulla oblongata. This contingent of the CST continues its course in the lateral columns of the spine. However, about 10% of the fibers of the CST continue their journey to the spine in the ipsilateral anterior columns and will cross side only when they reach their target. The CST terminates widely within the spinal gray matter, presumably reflecting control of nociceptive, somatosensory, reflex, autonomic, and somatic motor functions. These peculiar features explain why a single neuroanatomical pathway can mediate multiple functions (Lemon and Griffiths 2005).

There are striking differences across species in the organization of the descending pathways, and in particular of the CST. Some higher primates have unique direct projections to spinal motor neurons that bypass part of the integrative mechanisms of the spinal cord in order to generate motor output. Tracing studies with retrograde transneuronal transport of rabies virus from single muscles in rhesus monkeys have identified cortico-motoneuronal cells located in the caudal region of M1 that is buried in the central sulcus. This area is the lowest threshold site within M1. These cortico-motoneuronal cells make monosynaptic connections with motoneurons in the spine (Rathelot and Strick 2009). The cortical territories occupied by cortico-motoneuronal cells for different muscles overlap extensively within this region of M1. The findings of these tracing studies are against a focal representation of single muscles in M1. The axons originating in dorsal M1 may have connections with other muscles in addition to the one it was injected with the rabies virus. Thus, the overlap and intermingling among the different populations of neurons may be the neural substrate to create a wide variety of muscle synergies (Rathelot and Strick 2006) and may indeed represent a resource for neuroplasticity. The extent of CST projections from cortico-motoneurons in this newly recognized M1 area correlates with index of dexterity, skilled use of hands and digits across species. Recent studies suggest that the monosynaptic cortico-motoneuronal system is related to voluntary control of relatively independent finger movements. Preservation of the axons originating from M1 monosynaptic neurons is mandatory in order to maintain highly skilled movements in patients with a brain tumor infiltrating the CST or growing in its proximity.

The CST also carries M1 axons that form synapses with interneurons in the spinal cord. This *indirect pathway* is coursing more rostral and it is important for coordinating larger groups of muscles in behaviors such as reaching and walking. The motor information provided by the cortico-motoneuronal system via the CST is significantly modulated by information originated in secondary cortical motor areas. In the macaque it has been shown that electrical stimulation of the PMv could produce powerful stimulation of the M1 outputs to the spine. This neuronal circuit may represent an important parallel route through which a secondary motor area could exert its motor effects (Cerri et al. 2003). In addition, the output of M1 is modulated by neurons located in other motor regions located in the thalamus, basal nuclei, and cerebellum. The activity of these subcortical structures is also very important for the execution of smooth movements.

Mapping of the CST in the operating room is not a trivial procedure. Subcortical direct IES of the CST with the 60 Hz bipolar probe evokes the unnatural and synchronous stimulation of many fascicles and may well exert mixed excitatory and inhibitory effects on target neurons. On the contrary, subcortical direct IES with the monopolar probe is capable to discriminate the different

components of the CST that is so important for brain surgery (Bello et al. 2014).

In summary, in the motor system neuronal information is processed in a variety of discrete networks that are simultaneously active. In the particular case of the CST the signal carrying motor information is conducted along fibers that are originating in different parts of the neuronal network and are converging into the CST that eventually carry them to a common target in the brainstem or in the spinal cord.

For the many different functions it carries, the CST is probably the most complex and important pathway of the entire human brain. For sure it is the most important and eloquent structure that must be safeguarded in brain surgery. Lesions along the CST cause a pyramidal disconnection syndrome with neurological signs that vary according to lesion location and the interval from time of onset. Motor deficits can range from hemiparesis to hemiplegia. Lesions cause a breakdown in fine sensorimotor control of the extremities, implying a deterioration not only in motor function, but also in the capacity to interrogate correctly the sensory feedback from the limb (Lemon and Griffiths 2005). Implicit in modern concepts of a distributed motor network is that neurological signs resulting from lesions to a descending pathway cannot be interpreted any longer as simply being due to the removal of the lesioned pathway. Soon after an acute injury of the CST, activity-dependent, fast neuroplastic changes occur and the clinical outcome must be interpreted as the consequence of compensatory changes of the motor network as a whole, including the response of uninjured fibers.

4.2 The Language System

Language is a native, uniquely human trait that we learn without any formal teaching or training. As humans we use language automatically to communicate, however language is not the only mean we use for communication. People learn to use a highly structured stream of sounds or signs. In contrast, non-human primates and many other animals from bees to whales are able to communicate with sounds and signs, but they are unable to combine words to construct larger utterances. Despite intense training, the ability of binding words to build a linguistic sequence does not exist in other primates. Language emerges spontaneously in all children of the human species and it has a universal design that is based on two components: *words* and *grammar*. A word is an arbitrary association between a sound and a meaning. Grammar has three subsystems: *morphology* defines the rules for combining words and affixes in larger words; *syntax* consists of rules for combining an inventory of words into phrases and sentences; *phonology* consists of rules combining sounds into a consistent pattern that is characteristic of a specific language. In particular, syntax is a specific cognitive system of rules and operations that distinguishes language from other means of communication.

The relationship of specific brain regions with the language system has been more difficult to localize than for the motor and sensory systems. Interest in the structures responsible for the human ability to process speech and language dates back at least to the time of the Greek philosophers. Historically, it was the German neuroanatomist Franz Joseph Gall (1758–1828) who pioneered the study of the localization of mental functions in the brain. Gall suggested that language was located in the left frontal lobe. However, in 1861 the French neurologist Paul Broca began to explore the brain anatomy of language with the invention of the "lesion method." During an autopsy Broca located the stroke lesion in the left inferior frontal gyrus. In 1874 the German Carl Wernicke described the clinical case of a few patients with a deficit in language comprehension. All patients with comprehensive aphasia had lesions in the posterior half of the left superior temporal gyrus. Joseph Jules Dejerine and his wife Augusta made also important contribution to the field of aphasia research. They understood the importance of the association fibers that formed an intricate network that connected the cortical language centers, including Broca and Wernicke areas, and the visual image center in the angular gyrus. The concept of an interconnected *language zone* separated the

Dejerines from the doctrine of the French neurologist Jean-Martin Charcot (1825–1893), who postulated the existence of largely autonomous centers for different language modes (Miraillé 1896).

Knowledge about the neural basis of language processing accelerated 100 years later with the advent of neurophysiology first and more recently of advanced brain imaging methods (Price 2010; Friederici 2011). In the last two decades the classic theory of language localization proposed by Wernicke and Geschwind has been intensely revised thanks to the large amount of imaging data collected with neurophysiology (event-related potential, magnetoencephalography, and IES) and neuroimaging (fMRI and DTI). In the seventies of the twentieth century it was found that neurological patients with Broca aphasia following stroke not only had deficits in language production but they also showed problems in language comprehension when confronted with grammatically complex constructions. Patients with Wernicke aphasia not only had deficits in comprehending the meaning of utterances, but they also had problems in word selection during speech production. These observations led to the theory that Broca's area subserves grammatical processes during both speech production and comprehension. Similarly, the revised language theory suggested that Wernicke's area supports lexical-semantic processes (Caramazza and Zurif 1976). We predict that in the years to come neurosurgical patients will provide a new important source of data, especially now that mapping of brain function before and during removal of a focal brain lesion is recommended according to state of the art medical practice guidelines.

In particular, three important discoveries were made. First, it was confirmed that language is strongly lateralized to the left cerebral hemisphere. This finding was also confirmed with fMRI that showed that language is lateralized to the left in about 96% of right-handed subjects (Pujol et al. 1999). Only 4% of right-handed individuals show a symmetric blood oxygenated level dependent (BOLD) response during a language task. The BOLD response is also lateralized to the left in about 76% of left-handers; it is symmetric in 14% of them, whereas it is lateralized to the right side in the remaining 10%. More recently, the asymmetry of the language network has been demonstrated also with deterministic DTI tractography: the direct AF segment connecting Broca with Wernicke territories is found only on the left side in 62% of right-handed healthy subjects; it is bilateral but left lateralized in 20% and symmetric only in 17.5% of subjects (Catani et al. 2007). The second discovery was that three different aphasic syndromes were associated with damage to three specific brain structures: (1) *Broca aphasia* with damage to pars opercularis of the inferior frontal gyrus; (2) *Wernicke aphasia* with damage to the posterior part of the superior temporal gyrus; (3) *conduction aphasia* with damage to the AF that was thought to be a unidirectional pathway carrying information from Wernicke to Broca area. The third important discovery was that both Wernicke and Broca areas were presumed to interact with heteromodal high-order associative areas in the frontal, parietal, and temporal lobes.

In the first anatomic classic model of language proposed by Wernicke in 1874 there were two cortical centers: Broca area was dedicated to speech production and Wernicke area to auditory comprehension. Wernicke thought that the two centers were indirectly connected by fibers passing through the external capsule and relaying in the insula. It was Dejerine that proposed that the AF was connecting directly the two centers. The classic model was later modified by Geschwind in 1970 who emphasized the importance of a third cortical center located in the angular gyrus (Geschwind 1970).

Recent studies in patients with stroke, head injury, and neurodegenerative diseases (i.e., Alzheimer and frontal temporal dementia) have uncovered other cortical and subcortical regions that belong to the language network. Patients with damage to the left temporal pole (Brodmann area, BA38) may have difficulty to retrieve names of unique places and persons, but can retrieve names of common things. With damage to the mid-portion of the left MTG (BA20 and 21) patients have difficulty to recall both unique and common names, without any associated grammatical and phonemic deficit. Damage to the posterior part of the left inferior temporal gyrus (BA37) instead causes a deficit in recalling words of tools and utensils. The precentral gyrus of the left insula is another language-related area that was not included in the classic models. Patients with stroke lesions in the anterior insula show articulatory planning deficits: a difficulty in pronouncing phonemes in their proper order (Dronkers 1996). Other two areas that were recently considered part the language network are located in the mesial surface of the frontal lobe. The SMA in the left SFG and the left anterior cingulate cortex (BA24) play an important role in the initiation and maintenance of speech. Damage to these areas, especially after surgery is often associated with akinesia and mutism leading patients to fail to communicate by words, gestures, or facial expression. These patients usually recover within a few days (Krainik et al. 2003).

Aphasias are classified in to three major syndromes and few sub syndromes. In *Broca aphasia* the damaged network is involved in both the assembly of phonemes into words and the assembly of words into sentences. The network is thought to be concerned with relational aspects of language, which include the grammatical structure of sentences and the proper use of verbs. The cortical areas damaged in Broca aphasia are frontal BA44, 45, 46, 47, parietal areas BA39 and 40 and the insula. In *Wernicke aphasia* the damaged network is involved in generating speech sounds and in associating the sounds with concepts. Wernicke area is no longer considered the center of auditory comprehension as it was conceived in the Wernicke–Geschwind model (Geschwind 1970). Aphasic patients with lesions in the posterior third of the STG and MTG (BA 22) often shift the order of individual sounds and make frequent phonemic paraphasias. These patients also make semantic paraphasias that are errors in selecting words with substitution of one full word with another that has a meaning relation. In *conduction aphasia* the damaged network is required to assemble phonemes into words and coordinate speech articulation. Patients with conduction aphasia cannot repeat

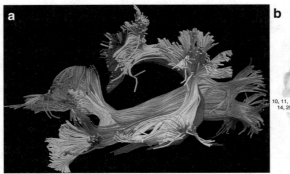
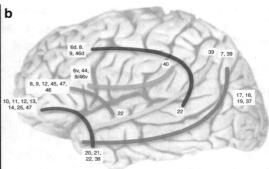

Fig. 2 (**a**) Modern theories about language have recognized that there is a lot of network redundancy in the system. Several models have been proposed, with some differences in connectivity, but all models acknowledge the importance of a dual-stream system with dorsal and ventral networks. The models that are heavily influenced by in humans DTI and post-mortem blunt fiber dissection methods suggest as many as five pathways relevant for language: the direct segment of the AF (red), the posterior segment of the AF (yellow), and the third segment of the SLF-III (green) are part of the dorsal pathway; the inferior fronto-occipital fasciculus (IFOF, orange), UF (cyan), and ILF (magenta) are part of the ventral pathway. The MLF is notably absent in this model. (**b**) Models that are heavily influenced by autoradiographic tract-tracing studies in the macaque monkey suggest as many as six dissociable fiber tracts. The autoradiography data also suggest the existence of a MLF (yellow), but dispute the existence of an IFOF. The extreme capsule (blue), UF (red), MLF and ILF (orange) are part of the ventral pathway connecting the inferior part of the frontal lobe with the temporal, parietal, and occipital lobes. The AF (violet) and SLF-III (green) are part of the dorsal pathway. Numbers refer to the corresponding Brodmann's areas for putative terminations and connections. (Modified from Dick AS et al. - Brain 2012: 135; 3529–3550)

sentences word for word, cannot easily name pictures and objects, they make phonemic paraphasias, but can produce intelligible speech and comprehend simple sentences. Related lesions involve the STG, SMG and AG, the insula and the adjacent WM. Until recently there was not much evidence in the literature that a simple disconnection of the AF alone could cause conduction aphasia, as it was originally suggested by Monakow and later by the Dejerines (Dejerine and Dejerine-Klumpke 1895). Only recently Bizzi and colleagues showed with DTI tractography that preoperative mild conduction aphasia in glioma patients is strictly associated with involvement of the AF (Bizzi et al. 2012).

The large amount of neuroimaging data becoming available is providing new opportunities for testing innovative models of the language network (Fig. 2). In 2004 Hickock and Poeppel outlined a dual-stream model of speech processing with a *dorsal stream* mapping acoustic speech signals to the articulatory subnetworks in the IFG and a *ventral stream* processing signals for comprehension. The model assumed a widely distributed network with a strongly left-lateralized

dorsal pathway and a largely bilateral organized ventral pathway (Hickok and Poeppel 2007). The dorsal stream will connect cortical nodes of the articulatory subnetwork located in the left dominant posterior IFG (pars opercularis and triangularis), ventrolateral premotor cortex, and anterior insula with the sensorimotor interface nodes localized in the posterior STG and AG. The ventral stream will connect a combinatorial subnetwork located in the anterior MTG and inferior temporal sulcus (ITS) with a lexical interface node located in the posterior MTG and ITS and with the articulatory subnetwork already described.

In 2012 Friederici proposed a functional anatomical model of the language network that was focused on different processing steps from auditory perception to comprehension (Friederici 2012). One novelty of this model was that particular attention was dedicated to definition of the structural connections between the cortical nodes of the network. In this model of sentence comprehension several hubs or nodes are connected via the dorsal and ventral pathways. Transformation of sounds in words and phrases occurs within

50–80 ms after acoustic and phonological analysis taking place in the middle portion of the STG. Once the phonological word form is identified, its syntactic and semantic information are retrieved in the anterior STG/STS. This subnetwork operates in the anterior temporal lobe as comprehension moves from phonemes to words and phrases. Lexical-semantic integration occurs in the MTG. Information transfer within this temporal subnetwork is likely provided by short-range bundles within the IFOF.

A second language subnetwork elaborates syntactic and semantic data and requires nodal processors in the anterior (BA47 and 45 for semantic processing) and in the posterior (BA44 for syntactic processing) IFG. Information transfer between the anterior temporal and IFG is assumed to be supported by ventral pathways: semantic information is conveyed via the IFOF connecting the pars orbitalis and triangularis (BA47 and 45) with the temporal and occipital cortices; syntactic information is conveyed via the UF connecting pars opercularis (BA44) with the anterior temporal cortex (Anwander et al. 2007). Patients with lesions involving the ventral language stream have been reported to have semantic and syntactic comprehension deficits (Tyler et al. 2011). A third subnetwork of the model proposed by Friederici is in charge of integrating semantic/syntactic processing at a hierarchical level in order to achieve sentence comprehension. Thus, elaborated information is bidirectional exchanged between the IFG, the posterior MTG (BA22 for semantic processing) and the AG (BA39 for syntactic processing). The connection from the IFG to the AG likely occurs via the direct or indirect route of the AF, whereas it is still under debate whether the connection to the MTG occurs via the ventral (IFOF) or the dorsal (AF) pathway.

The contribution of the dorsal and ventral WM pathways connecting the frontal and temporal speech regions is central to understanding how the cortical areas interact to produce a seamless language system. One emerging concept is that the AF is involved primarily in phonology, articulation, and syntax and the IFOF is mainly implicated in semantics. While authors vary in their claims concerning the extent of functional specialization, all authors argue for some degree of functional differentiation. The authors of a recent study performed in 24 patients with chronic stroke in the left hemisphere suggested that segregation of function for the dorsal and ventral pathways is limited to the phonological and semantic tasks (Rolheiser et al. 2011). On the other hand, morphology and syntax require a synergy between the AF and the IFOF rather than a segregated system. In this DTI study both dorsal and ventral bundles were associated with syntactic performance in both comprehension and production tasks. Comprehending syntax utilizes equally both the AF and IFOF, while syntactic production is predominantly permitted via the AF. By defining the WM architecture as a synergy, the overall determinant of task performance is not dictated by which WM tract is involved, but by how prefrontal and posterior temporal cortical speech regions use and integrate a constant flow of very complex linguistic information.

4.3   The Visuospatial Attention System

What you see is determined by what you attend to. Visuospatial attention is a complex dynamic process that involves filtering relevant information from our spatial environment. We simultaneously attend to and look at objects in a visual scene by means of saccadic eye movements that rapidly bring the fovea onto stimuli of interest. The processing of visual stimuli appearing in the attended spatial location will be enhanced, while stimuli appearing in other parts of the visual field will be suppressed. Visuospatial attention is necessary for selecting and inhibiting visual information over space, because the environment is overloaded with far more perceptual stimuli that our brain can effectively process. Visuospatial attention allows people to select, modulate, and sustain focus on the information that is most relevant to their own behavioral goals. The selected item may enter visual working memory and/or become the target of a movement.

There are multiple forms of attention to external and internal stimuli (Chun et al. 2011). External attention refers to the selection and modulation of sensory information: visual, auditory, olfactory, tactile, and gustatory. Each of these attention systems selects locations in space, or modality-specific output. The visual attention system is by far the most developed in humans while in other animals the auditory or the olfactory attention systems may be in charge of guiding the behavior of the animals in response to environmental stimuli. Internal attention refers to the selection, modulation, and maintenance of internally generated information, such as task rules, responses, long-term memory, or working memory. Visuospatial attention also interacts with other attention processes.

The concept of spatial selective attention refers operationally to the advantage in speed and accuracy of processing for objects lying in attended regions of space as compared to objects located in non-attended regions (Posner 1980). When several events compete for limited processing and comprehending capacity and control of behavior, attention selection may resolve the competition.

fMRI studies in humans have shown that the anatomical structures which are activated during the performance of attention-related functions are located in the parietal and frontal lobes and form multiple functional parietofrontal networks (Corbetta and Shulman 2002). The posterior parietal cortex (PPC) and the frontal eye field/dorsolateral prefrontal cortex are nodes of a dorsal attention network that is active during the orientation period. The temporo-parietal junction and the ventrolateral prefrontal cortex are nodes of a ventral attention network that is active when subjects have to respond to targets presented in unexpected locations. The ventral network is in charge of detecting unexpected but behaviorally relevant events and is responsible for maintaining attention on goals or task demands that are a top-down process. Physiological studies have found that the activity of the frontal and parietal nodes is coordinated during execution of a visual attention task but show distinctive dynamics. In the parietal cortex bottom-up signals appear first and are characterized by an increase of fronto-parietal coherence in the gamma band (25–100 Hz), whereas in the PFC top-down signals emerge first and tend to synchronize in the beta band (12–30 Hz) (Buschman and Miller 2007).

In the monkey brain the activity of neurons dedicated to visuospatial attention has been recorded simultaneously in the parietal and frontal cortices. Axonal tracing studies have shown that parietal and prefrontal neurons are directly and extensively interconnected through a system of fascicles running longitudinally in the centrum semiovale, dorsally to the AF and laterally to the CST. Three distinct parietofrontal long-range segments of the SLF that had been previously described in the rhesus monkey (Petrides and Pandya 1984) have been recently demonstrated also in the human brain using MR tractography with the SD algorithm (Thiebaut de Schotten. 2011a, b).

The dorsal and first segment of the SLF (SLF-I) connects BA5 and 7 in the PPC including the dorsal bank of the intraparietal sulcus with BA8 and 9 in the SFG; the SLF-II connects BA39 and 40 in the inferior parietal lobule (IPL) including the ventral bank of the intraparietal sulcus with BA8 and 9 in the MFG; the ventrally located SLF-III segment connects the AG (BA40) with the BA44, 45 and 47 in the IFG. The SLF-I connects the cortical nodes of the dorsal attention network activated during the voluntary orienting of spatial attention toward visual targets, while the SLF-III overlaps with the ventral network that is activated during the automatic capture of spatial attention by visual targets and damaged in people with visuospatial neglect (Fig. 3). The middle SLF-II segment connects the parietal nodes of the ventral network with the prefrontal nodes of the dorsal network and it may represent a direct communication between the two networks. The SLF-II may act as a modulator for the dorsal network, redirecting goal-directed attention mediated by the SLF-I to events identified as salient by the SLF-III, as suggested by Corbetta in the fMRI study cited above (Corbetta and Shulman 2002).

The parietofrontal network is bilaterally represented with some degree of asymmetry variable among the three segments. By measuring the vol-

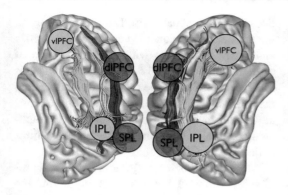

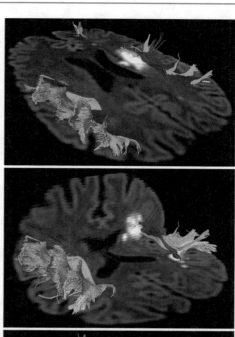

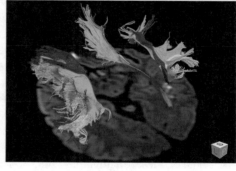

Fig. 3 A schematic representation of the parietofrontal visuospatial attentional networks based on fMRI (Corbetta and Shulman 2002) and MR tractography data (Thiebaut de Schotten et al. 2011a, b). The major cortical nodes are located in the vlPFC and dlPFC, IPL, and SPL. The three segments SLF-I (red), SLF-II (yellow), and SLF-III (green) are believed to connect the parietal and frontal nodes of the dorsal with the ventral attention networks. (Figure as originally published in (Ciaraffa et al. 2012))

umes of the tracts reconstructed with tractography in 20 healthy subjects Thiebaut de Schotten et al. found that the SLF-I is symmetrically represented in the two hemispheres, the SLF-III is right lateralized and the SLF-II shows a trend of right lateralization, but with substantial inter-individual differences that are correlated to behavioral signs of right hemisphere specialization (Thiebaut de Schotten et al. 2011a).

An acute stroke damaging the fronto-parietal network will affect the ability to process visuospatial information and it usually will manifest with neglect. In most of the patients the deficits are transitory and become apparent only with clinical tests that elicit hemispatial neglect. Patients with visual neglect fail to pay attention to objects presented on the side of space contralateral to a brain lesion. While it is undisputed that right lesions provoke more severe and durable signs of neglect than strokes in the left hemisphere, identification of eloquent anatomic structures that, if injured, will cause visual neglect has fostered an intense debate in recent years.

Visual neglect has been associated with right hemisphere lesions in gray matter structures (parietal, frontal, or temporal cortices), in the

Fig. 4 Fifty-five years-old right-handed male presenting with acute onset of severe left visual neglect and left hemiparesis. MR DWI showed small multiple acute ischemic infarcts in the right cerebral WM and no evidence of infarcts in GM. DTI tractography was instrumental to accurately localize one infarct to the SLF-III (green) that is a component of the large-scale networks controlling visuospatial attention. Another infarct was localized in the stem of the AF (AF-direct in red, AF-posterior segment in yellow); the IFOF (orange) and UF (cyan) were not involved. This case report supports the hypothesis that neglect may result from disruption of a distributed attention network (Ciaraffa et al. 2012)

basal nuclei or in the thalami. More recently, visual neglect has been associated with isolated WM injury that was possible to assign to specific fronto-parietal WM tracts with the aid of tractography. In a 55 -years-old man with transient visual neglect tractography was essential to determine that a small acute ischemic WM infarct involved the SLF-III (Fig. 4) (Ciaraffa et al. 2012).

Signs of transient neglect were evoked also in two neurosurgical patients during resection of right hemisphere LGG while they were asked to bisect 20-cm horizontal lines. Patients deviated rightward upon subcortical direct IES of the SMG and of the posterior STG, but made no mistakes when the FEF and the anterior part of the STG were stimulated. However, in one patient it was the stimulation of the SLF-II underneath the IPL that evoked the strongest deviation rightward (Thiebaut de Schotten et al. 2005). The importance of SLF-II damage was replicated with IES in other six neurosurgical patients with right hemisphere gliomas (Vallar et al. 2014) and it is further supported by studies in right hemisphere stroke patients with chronic unilateral neglect, where maximum lesion overlap was along the trajectory of the SLF (Doricchi and Tomaiuolo 2003; Thiebaut de Schotten et al. 2008). The use of a DTI-based atlas of the human brain allowed a detailed analysis of WM lesion involvement in another study in 38 patients with chronic neglect. Results revealed that damage to the SLF-II (and to the SLF-III with lesser significance) was the best predictor of chronic persistence of left visuospatial neglect (Thiebaut de Schotten et al. 2014). Taken together these tractography studies support the importance of parietofrontal disconnection in the pathogenesis of neglect and they outline the important contribution of tractography studies in assigning lesion location to specific WM tracts.

4.4 The Connectome

The human nervous system is an assembly of an average of 86 billion of projecting neurons and local interneurons (Azevedo et al. 2009), wired together by countless, slender axons, and dendrites to form a very dense wiring diagram. Recently this diagram has been renamed "*the connectome.*" This term, like *genome*, implies completeness. A connectome is not made by few or even many connections. It is all the connec-

tions of an individual brain. The connectome of a human being is unique; it has many similarities and many differences with the connectome of other individuals. Unlike the genome, which is relatively fixed from the moment of conception, the connectome changes throughout life. Neurons adjust and rewire their connections by strengthening or weakening them, by creating and eliminating synapses.

More than 100 years ago, Ramon y Cajal predicted that one of the main factors guiding the evolution of the brain was a trade-off between rapid information transfer and the cost of wiring (Ramon y Cajal 1995). The costs of building and running a bigger brain network are metabolically more expensive, but are also quite rigorously controlled to be as low as possible for any given function (Bullmore and Sporns 2012). The results of a recent study with diffusion MRI in 123 species of mammals confirmed that the connectome and the wiring cost are conserved across mammals (Assaf et al. 2020). This conservation principle holds for all mammals, independent of brain size, suggesting a selective evolutionary pressure in favor of efficient connectivity and wiring costs. This conservation principle applies not only to inter- but also to intraspecies variations of the connectome. How is global connectivity maintained despite the large diversity in brain size and shape across mammals? The results of Assaf and colleagues' study found that species with fewer (commissural) interhemispheric connections have more efficient intrahemispheric connectivity. The results suggested that intrahemispheric connectivity compensates for poorer interhemispheric connectivity, maintaining the overall connectivity. The conservation principle may play a role also during ontogeny of the connectome. A recent study showed that patients with agenesis of the corpus callosum have stronger intrahemispheric connections (Owen et al. 2013). Agenesis of the corpus callosum is one of the most common human brain malformations and it can be considered a prototypical human disorder of axon guidance, one in which fibers that would normally have crossed the midline as part of the corpus callosum instead form *Probst bundles*, large white matter tracts that course anterior-posterior parallel to the inter-hemispheric fissure within each cerebral hemisphere.

Neuroanatomical localization is critical to understanding the brain. The Human Connectome Project (HCP) began in 2010 with the goal to develop improved neuroimaging methods and to acquire a data set of unprecedented size and quality for mapping the normal human macroscale connectome. Better maps of the brain's areas and their connections may also improve our ability to understand and treat neurological and psychiatric disorders (Glasser et al. 2016). In the last two decades, comprehensive connectivity maps or connectomes have been generated with functional and diffusion MR imaging data, electroencephalography (EEG) and magneto-electroencephalography (MEG) acquired in healthy human subjects and other organisms. These brain graphs have revealed topological principles of brain network organization. There is now strong evidence that human brain networks have *small-world properties* of high clustering and high global efficiency, a modular community structure and heavy-tailed degree distributions that indicate a number of highly connected nodes or hubs (Achard and Bullmore 2007).

Virtually all systems require the integration of distributed neural activity. Network analysis of human brain systems has consistently identified regions called "hubs" that are critically important for enabling efficient neuronal signaling and communication (Van den Heuvel and Sporns 2013). Hub nodes mediate many of long-range connections between brain modules, and are efficiently interconnected to form a "rich club" (Van den Heuvel and Sporns 2011). The high level of centrality of brain hubs also renders them points of vulnerability that are susceptible to disconnection and dysfunction in brain disorders. It has been shown that in many neurological diseases focal lesions are concentrated in the highly connected hubs of the human connectome (Crossley et al. 2014), also known as the *"anatomical rich club"* (Van den Heuvel and Sporns 2011). Lesions may be concentrated in hubs purely because of their greater topological value. Some diseases might affect brain regions with uniform probability but lead to symptoms when the lesion happened to damage a hub. Regarding presurgical mapping for brain tumor surgery it is important to describe the relationship of the tumor with critical hubs and long-range connections because these are crucial components of eloquent systems.

5 Mapping WM Tracts for Brain Surgery

5.1 Brain Tumor Semeiotic of FA and Directionally Encoded Color Maps

Diffusion imaging with DEC maps and MR tractography is increasingly requested by neurosurgeons because its clinical relevance has been proven. In the motor system DTI has become more popular than functional MRI because it is capable of identifying CST trajectories. MR tractography nicely illustrates the dorsal and ventral language pathways. When a mass dislocates the OR tractography provides necessary information in order to plan the surgical approach to the lesion. DEC maps are immediately available at the console and they can be very practical and useful to determine the relationship of a mass with adjacent tracts. Expert users can identify the course of the main fascicles already on DEC maps. Notwithstanding, it is fiber tracking that best illustrate the trajectory of a tract in 3D and its relationship with the tumor.

On DEC maps and with tractography it is possible to determine whether the main WM tracts are *normal, dislocated, abnormal,* or *interrupted* (Jellison et al. 2004). In the first section we have already pointed out that diffuse infiltrating slow-growing gliomas behave biologically differently from fast expanding GBMs. LGG rarely dislocate WM tracts. LGG infiltrate bundles that remain functional as it was demonstrated by IES. On the contrary HGG, metastases, and meningiomas have the tendency to displace or destroy bundles. Knowledge of this difference in behavior is important preoperatively in order to identify the trajectory of eloquent WM tracts in relationship to the tumor.

It is quite common to observe a tract *dislocated* by a mass becoming more visible on FA and DEC maps because it is compressed and thus more compact with elevated FA. For instance, the CST dislocated by a mass can show paradoxical increased FA value and maintain a blue hue regardless of whether it is shifted (Fig. 5). Gliomas growing in the temporal and occipital lobes are likely to displace the OR in the opposite direction from their point of origin. Presurgical MR tractography will show the trajectory of the OR with exquisite detail and it will be useful to neurosurgeons in planning the point of entry for the corticotomy (Fig. 6). Gliomas infiltrating the perisylvian cortex are likely to displace dorsally the direct segment of the AF. The position of the AF stem or isthmus in the deep temporal occipital WM is easy to recognize and it is a practical landmark on axial DEC maps. The AF stem is color coded in blue and it is frequently dislocated posteriorly by aggressive tumors. Gliomas tend to dislocate the AF stem posteriorly and the frontal arm of the direct AF segment dorsally. A slow-growing tumor growing in the IFG nearby Broca area is likely to dislocate the frontal arm of the direct AF posteriorly without interrupting its major trajectories. Patients with LGG infiltrating Broca area are unlikely to have speech deficits (Plaza et al. 2009). A mass originating in the ventral precentral gyrus may dislocate the AF medially. More aggressive gliomas originating in ventrolateral precentral cortex (BA6) may initially dislocate the AF medially, then as they expand they may interrupt its trajectories causing conduction aphasia (Bizzi et al. 2012).

Intraoperative DTI has been used to show shifting of the CST tract during tumor resection. In a series of 27 patients with glioma the authors used DEC maps to find that dislocation of the CST may occur either inward or outward. The authors underscored that intraoperative updating of the DTI results is important (Nimsky et al. 2005). A WM tract that is compressed by a mass may turn out to be easier to track especially when FA is increased. This phenomenon is likely due to decreased radial diffusivity with minor changes in axial diffusivity. Tracts that are usually more difficult to visualize such as the OR and the contingent of CST fibers projecting to M1 of the face/mouth area may be enhanced when they are compressed by a large mass (Fig. 7).

A WM tract is considered *abnormal* on DEC maps when it is coursing throughout an area of T2-signal hyperintensity, with altered FA and MD but it shows native orientation (color hue). Despite early reports suggesting that DEC maps might separate diffuse infiltrating gliomas from tumor-free vasogenic edema (Jellison et al. 2004), this differentiation is not reliable. The expansion of the ECS deployed by infiltrating glioma cells and the increased water content secondary to vasogenic edema may likely appear with similar and overlapping DTI abnormalities.

LGGs have a predilection to infiltrate associative unimodal and multimodal cortices in the insula, temporal pole, orbitofrontal, and SFG (Duffau and Capelle 2004). Insular gliomas easily infiltrate adjacent IFOF fibers coursing in the ventral floor of the extreme capsule and the UF in the temporal pole. Cancer cells may grow around and move along WM fascicles and infiltrate adjacent frontal and temporal lobes: a swollen temporal stem is a hint that the glioma cells are using the WM tracts as infrastructures to infiltrate additional territory. On axial DEC maps the trajectories of the IFOF in the temporal stem and the extreme capsule is coded in green. Only rarely LGGs may dislocate the IFOF and the UF. On the contrary, GBMs originating in the anterior aspect of the left temporal lobe are more likely to dislocate or interrupt rather than infiltrate the IFOF. MR tractography identifies the trajectories of the IFOF and UF when they are dislocated. Unfortunately, heavy tumor infiltration or vasogenic edema may result in significant MD increase with FA drop. In this scenario MR tractography fails to detect residual bundles because FA decreases below the threshold and the eigenvector may become undetermined. The possibility of false negative findings should be raised in the radiology report to the neurosurgeon. It is important to keep in mind that MR tractography does not provide functional information and that

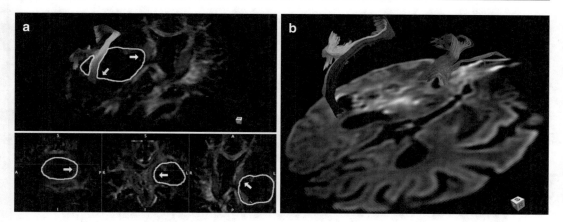

Fig. 5 (**a**) Sixty-five years-old right-handed female with recent onset of severe comprehensive aphasia. MRI showed a large enhancing mass deep seated in the left posterior temporal lobe. DEC maps with tractography showed that the mass dislocated anteriorly and medially the left CST (white arrows) and posteriorly the left AF (yellow arrow). In the upper box MR tractography of the direct segment of the AF with DEC streamlines. In the lower boxes form the left side are sagittal, coronal and axial DEC maps with the margins of the mass outlined. A GBM WHO-IV was removed at surgery. (**b**) DTI tractography of the three segments of the AF (direct in red, anterior in green, posterior in yellow) displayed in 3D over DWI in the axial plane is confirming that the GBM dislocated the AF posteriorly

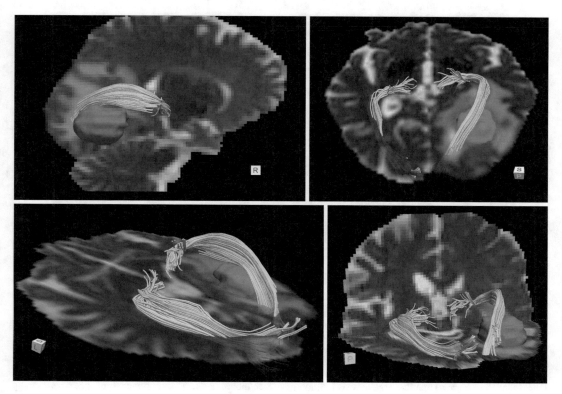

Fig. 6 Seventy-six years-old male with GBM WHO-IV surrounded by abundant perilesional vasogenic edema in the right occipital lobe displacing the OR dorsally. Note the asymmetry with the right OR (light green) displaced dorsally relative to the left OR (yellow) on multiple T2-weighted MR images with overlaid streamline tractography performed with spherical deconvolution. The mass is colored in blue

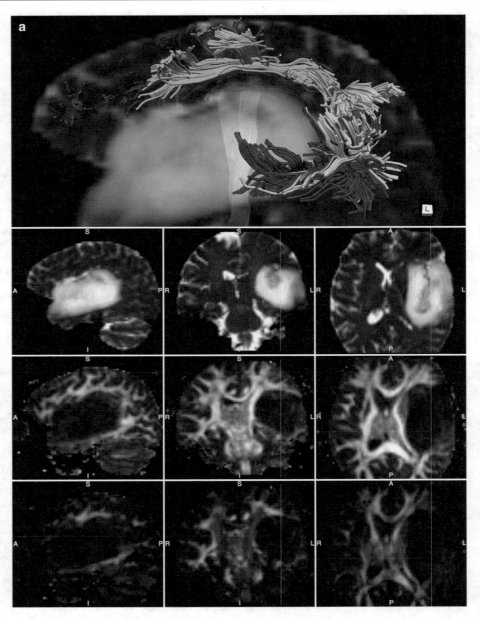

Fig. 7 (**a**) Thirty-six years-old male with astrocytoma WHO-II. The three segments of the left AF (direct segment in red, posterior segment in yellow, and SLF-III in green) and two components of the CST projecting respectively to M1 (yellow) and S1 (cyan) in the area of the face/mouth are displayed over a sagittal T2-weighted MRI (upper row). Note in sagittal, coronal, and axial T2-weighted MRI (second row), FA maps (third row) and DEC maps (bottom row) that the large mass is infiltrating the left insula and the whole temporal lobe and it is displacing the CST medially and the AF dorsally. Presurgical tractography was useful to show that eloquent fascicles (AF and CST) were outside of the mass, thus a complete resection could be attempted after detection of the functional limits with IES mapping. Diffusion data were acquired with HARDI (64 gradient directions, $b = 2000$, $2 \times 2 \times 2$ mm^3) and tractography was performed with spherical deconvolution algorithm. (**b**) Tractograms of the CST and AF are displayed over a coronal T2-weighted MRI (left panel). The severe mass effect paradoxically enhanced detection of the CST fibers projecting to the face/mouth area. This contingent of fibers is usually poorly visualized with normal anatomy due to crossing fibers, even with spherical deconvolution algorithm. Lateral view of the tractograms from below showing CST streamlines crossing the AF (right panel)

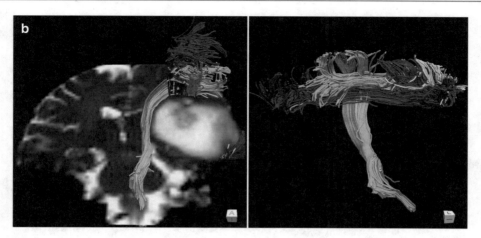

Fig. 7 (continued)

IES is the only method that is reliable in testing WM function and to detecting presence of functional bundles inside a tumor.

A WM tract is considered *interrupted* when the FA value drops below the FA threshold used for tractography and its trajectories are lost in the area of the tumor. From a biophysical perspective, this scenario occurs when diffusion becomes isotropic inside the tumor or the main orientation of anisotropy is not coherent anymore with the native orientation of the tract of interest. A threshold of FA > 0.2 is usually recommended for tractography in healthy tissue; however, it has been shown that lowering the threshold to FA > 0.1 can help to identify residual trajectories inside a tumor (Bello et al. 2008) with the trade-off of raising the chance of false positive results. From a neuro-oncological perspective, interruption of a tract may be due to three conditions: tissue destruction, heavy glioma cell infiltration, or vasogenic edema. In the first condition tractography would provide a true negative result, in the second a result that requires validation with IES or histopathological examination of the surgical specimen, while in the case of vasogenic edema would provide a false negative result. It has been shown that vasogenic edema may be associated with false negative results that should not be confused with bundle destruction (Bizzi et al. 2012; Ducreux et al. 2006). We have already mentioned that the use of advanced diffusion imaging methods that use multicompartmental models such as NODDI (Zhang et al. 2012) has potential to better address this critical issue.

The appearance of a ring of increased anisotropy at the periphery of the mass is another controversial condition that has been described in brain tumors. The cause for high FA values at the interface between the mass and the surrounding brain tissue is not well understood. Few studies have investigated tensor shape indices in the periphery of focal lesions. Significantly higher CL values have been reported near the enhancing ring of GBM rather than of metastasis (Wang et al. 2009). The authors of another study suggested that CL and CP can distinguish true from pseudo WM trajectories inside an abscess cavity (Kumar et al. 2008). CL and CP mean values measured within the abscess cavity were significantly different compared with those of WM tracts; however, FA, MD, and CS values overlapped. High CP with low CL inside an abscess cavity indicates that the shape of the diffusion tensor is predominantly planar, whereas it is linear in WM tracts. These geometrical DTI indices may be used for differentiating true from pseudo WM tracts inside the abscess cavity and in general at the periphery of a tumor. The finding of high FA and CP inside a tumor should be considered non-specific, while high FA and CL may indicate the possibility of residual WM tracts within a glioma. Elevated FA and CL at the periphery of a mass should suggest the proximity

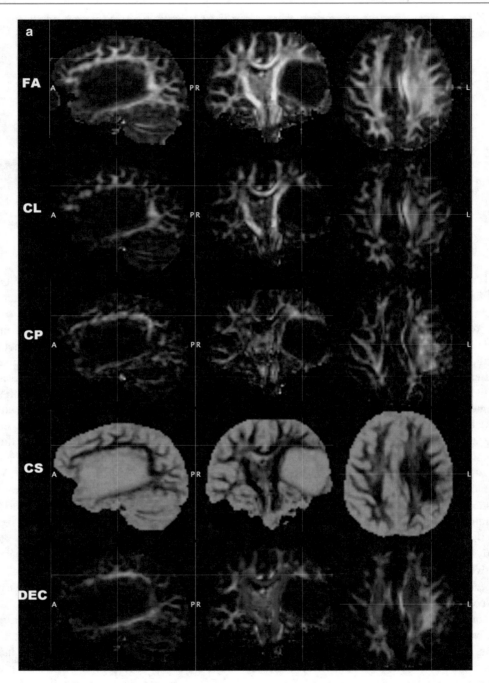

Fig. 8 (a) Parametric maps available from DTI dataset of the same case illustrated in Fig. 7: fractional anisotropy (FA), linear, planar, and spherical anisotropy shape coefficients (CL, CP, CS) and direction encoded color (DEC) maps. A large mass such as this astrocytoma may disrupt the architecture of the WM around it. When CL is high (bright) there is usually one dominant tract such as the CST in the medial boundary of the lesion in this case. When CP is high there may be two crossing fibers such as the AF and the CST in the dorsal boundary. CL and CP maps are often more informative than FA alone. (b) Parametric maps available from NODDI dataset of the same case illustrated in Fig. 7: neurite density (ND) and orientation dispersion index (odi). The very low ND value within the mass is suggesting that unlikely there should be residual fibers within the tumor; odi is elevated within the mass showing a paucity of oriented sticks (fascicles)

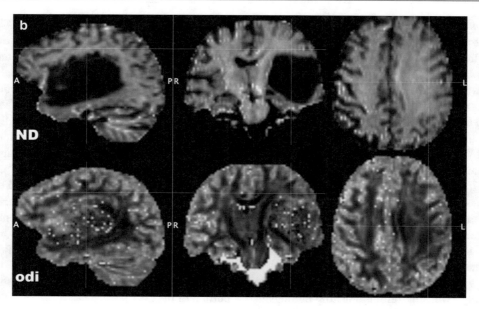

Fig. 8 (continued)

of a compacted WM tract that can be identified with the aid of DEC maps (Fig. 8a). Finding of elevated CP around the periphery of a mass, especially if associated with elevated MD, should raise suspicion for pseudo WM tracts. In this last scenario elevated planar diffusivity might be an epiphenomenon of mass effect at the interface between the tumor and the brain tissue, especially when there is accumulation of water in the ECS (i.e., vasogenic edema). NODDI measures innovative parameters such as neurite density and orientation dispersion index that may also help to characterize tumor infiltration and vasogenic edema within and around a mass (Fig. 8b).

5.2 Mapping Strategies with MR Tractography

The main aims of mapping WM structures in neuro-oncology are (1) presurgical planning; (2) intraoperative guidance during direct subcortical IES and tumor resection; (3) postoperative evaluation after tumor resection.

The advantage of using tractography for presurgical mapping is to show in 3D-space the relationship of the trajectory of the fascicles of interest with a focal lesion and other anatomical landmarks. The neurosurgeon will select the best route to reach the lesion without damaging eloquent tracts, and will choose which tract to test with IES in the operating room. Among neurosurgeons there is consensus that the CST, AF, IFOF, UF, and OR are the most clinically relevant fascicles for presurgical mapping.

The general principle of tractography is to use the orientation information provided by the tensor, the fODF, or the dODF. The most commonly used directional assignment corresponds to the major eigenvector of the diffusion tensor. Starting from one or more "seed" ROI and propagating the trajectories according to the tractography algorithm until the tracts are terminated generates a streamlined tractogram. Specific geometrical and anatomical constraints are used to extract the trajectories that meet specific connection criteria. Geometrical constraints (FA threshold) are used to terminate tracking in voxels with very low FA and undetermined fiber orientation or to avoid unrealistic trajectories with very sharp turns (angle threshold). Rules based on Boolean logic (i.e., true or false) can be applied to select ("IN") or exclude ("OUT") specific streamlines or pathways.

It is tradition since the early days of determin-istic tractography to filter out spurious stream-lines that are known to represent artifacts from a priori knowledge. Spurious tracts represent false positive streamlines that are mainly due to errors to estimate tract orientation with diffusion imag-ing in the presence of crossing, bending, and fan-ning fibers. The number of spurious tracts is variable, it changes with WM fascicles and it depends on the quality and spatial resolution of the HARDI dataset. The number of spurious tracts is usually small in the proximity of a LGG, whereas it may increase significantly in the hemi-sphere ipsilateral to a HGG, especially when the mass is aggressively growing and disarranges WM architecture.

It is important to use a precise and correct ter-minology when describing imaging findings in a radiology report. Diffusion MR tractography pro-vides anatomical (structural) information that has no functional content. *Fasciculus* and *bundle* are anatomic terms: a multitude of axons or fibers form bundles of different diameters; several bun-dles form a fasciculus. The words *streamline* and *trajectory* should be used when describing results in MR tractography studies. The words *pathway* and *stream* are used mainly in functional imaging studies depicting information flow.

5.3   Motor System

5.3.1   Corticospinal Tract

The CST is the most eloquent of all WM struc-tures and damage to the CST leads to permanent motor and speech deficits. Mapping of the CST is requested when a lesion is located in the paracen-tral region, SMA, PMd, PMv, and in the proxim-ity of its course at the level of the thalamus, basal nuclei, or brainstem. The CST carries axons organized in bundles projecting from the M1 (49%), post-central and PPC (21%), SMA-proper (19%), PMd (7%), PMv (4%). IES of the CST is best performed with the high-frequency monopo-lar probe rather than with the low-frequency 60 Hz bipolar probe (Bello et al. 2014). It is man-

datory to identify all components of the CST in order to avoid postoperative motor deficits (Fig. 9). The typical course of the CST and the somatotopic organization of its fascicles is important to know in order to predict potential deficits during removal of a lesion. In M1 the tongue and face areas are located ventrally and laterally to the hand area, the leg and foot are located dorsally and medially in the paracentral lobule. After leaving the cortex the CST curves slightly backwards, then it bends forward before entering the posterior limb of the internal cap-sule. Along this way the somatotopic fibers twist about 90° counter-clockwise so that the tongue and face bundles descend anteriorly and the foot and leg bundles posteriorly. At the level of the internal capsule the hand bundles occupy the mid portion of the CST.

Tracking of the CST should be performed with a two ROIs approach using streamline or probabilistic tractography. Delineation of the seed ROI is usually performed on b_0 (i.e., T2WI) or FA maps in multiple axial slices in the precentral and post-central gyri, posterior third of the SFG (i.e., SMA) and MFG (i.e., PMd and PMv). The ROI should include the subcortical WM since fiber tracking does not reach the corti-cal layers. The ROI in M1 should extend from the mouth to the foot area. Delineation of the target ROI should be done at the level of the pons in the ipsilateral tractus pyramidalis (blue on DEC maps) that is anterior to the pontocerebellar fibers (red on DEC maps) and lemniscus medialis (blue on DEC maps). Some authors prefer to delineate the target ROI in the ipsilateral cerebral peduncle of the midbrain or in the posterior limb of the internal capsule. After connecting the two ROIs the tractogram should be inspected for a priori anatomic consistency.

Spurious streamlines should be removed with "out-ROI" filters with the aim to show the back-bone of a "clean tractogram." Spurious tracts to the contralateral CST are frequently found along the trajectories of the CC and of the pontocere-bellar peduncles. Spurious tracts are due to arti-facts of fiber tracking in voxels with crossing fibers. The number of spurious tracts is variable and depends on the quality and spatial resolution of the HARDI dataset, however some spurious tracts should always be expected in the above regions. Out-ROIs are usually needed in the mid-sagittal plane and in the middle cerebellar peduncles.

Tracking the backbone of the CST from the hand knob area (omega sign) in M1 to the pons is relatively easy. Unfortunately streamline DTI tractography usually fails to reconstruct stream-lines originating in the tongue, face, leg, and foot areas due to the presence of crossing fibers with the CC and the SLF at the level of the centrum semiovale (Mandelli et al. 2014). Implementation of HARDI acquisition scheme with more advanced algorithms such as SD (Dell'Acqua et al. 2013), multi-tensor (Yamada et al. 2007),

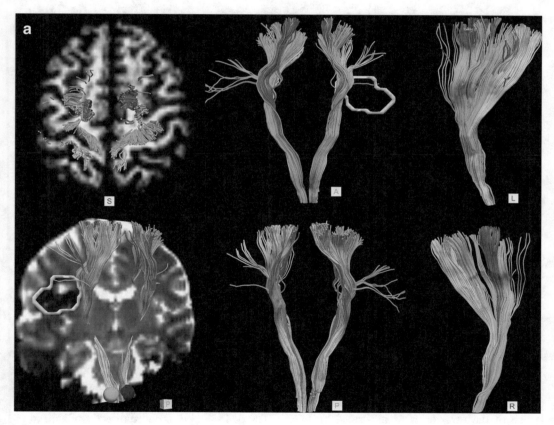

Fig. 9 (a) Thirty-one years-old male with cavernous angioma (white circle) seated in the deep WM below the left SMG. The medial margin of the focal lesion is abutting the left CST. Diffusion data were acquired with HARDI (64 gradient directions, $b = 2000$, $2 \times 2 \times 2$ mm³) and tractography was performed with spherical deconvolution algorithm. Tractography of the CST components originating from M1 (green), SMA (orange), PM dorsal (cyan), and S1 (yellow). The components of both cortico-spinal tracts (CST) are displayed over axial FA map at the level of the central sulcus (upper row, left panel) and coronal T2-weighted MRI (lower row, left panel); anterior and posterior views of both CST in the middle panels; lateral and medial view of the left CST on the right panels. (b) Tractography showing that the components of the left CST projecting to M1 (green) and S1 (yellow) are adjacent to the medial margin of the cavernous angioma. Intraoperative view (left upper corner) showing direct subcortical electrostimulation of the floor of the surgical cavity with the monopolar probe: a current of 8 mA evoked MEP responses of the right hand and leg confirming that the CST was very close to the angioma

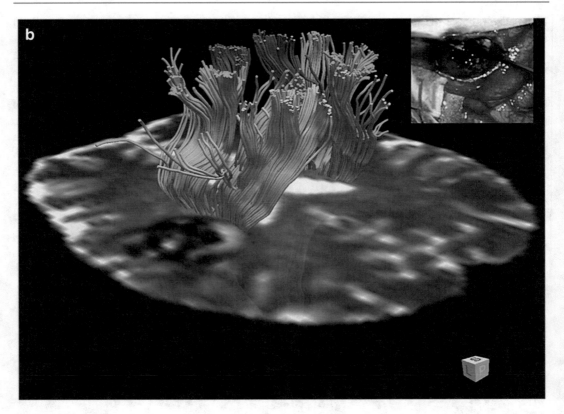

Fig. 9 (continued)

Q-ball, and probabilistic tractography (Bucci et al. 2013) allows depiction of additional trajectories that are originating from the face, tongue, and foot regions of M1.

5.3.2 SMA Connectivity

The SMA is at the center of a rich network of WM connections with motor, language and limbic structures. The connectivity of the SMA is of particular interest for brain tumor surgery since it is one of the favorite areas infiltrated by LGG (Duffau and Capelle 2004). The "SMA syndrome" characterized by transient contralateral akinesia and mutism with a usually complete recovery in 6–12 months can follow surgery in this area. Immediate severe postoperative deficits can be quite stressful for the patient. Knowledge of the connections of the SMA can provide new

insights on the genesis of the SMA syndrome; assessment of the extension of infiltrating tumors can assist the neurosurgeon in predicting the postoperative course of patients.

The SMA is located in the medial posterior third of the SFG and it is functionally and connectively divided into two parts by a virtual line arising from the AC and perpendicular to the AC-PC line. The SMA-proper and pre-SMA play a different role with regard to motor function. The SMA-proper is more directly related to the execution of movement, while the pre-SMA is involved in planning and preparation of higher motor control. Differences in connectivity of the two regions provide an anatomical basis for explaining these functional aspects. The SMA-proper is a component of the CST network and it sends fibers through the corona radiata and the internal capsule to the spinal cord, while the pre-SMA has no direct connection with the cord. The SMA-proper is thought to play a role in the direct execution of movement due to this corticospinal projection. Neuroradiologists should pay particular attention to track also streamlines projecting from the SMA-proper to the spine when mapping the CST.

In a post-mortem dissection and tractography study Vergani et al. identified five main types of connections: (1) short U-fibers in the depth of the precentral sulcus, directly connecting the SMA-proper with M1, especially at the level of the hand region; (2) U-fibers connecting SMA with the cingulate gyrus; (3) an intralobar frontal tract connecting the SMA with pars opercularis BA44 and BA6 (this fascicles has been named by Catani the "frontal aslant tract" (Catani et al. 2012)); (4) fibers connecting the SMA with the striatum; (5) SMA callosal fibers connecting homologous areas (Vergani et al. 2014). Both the SMA-proper and the pre-SMA have direct connections with the head and body of the caudate nucleus. The presence of striatal connections has been demonstrated in a DTI study by Lehericy et al. (2004). This cortico-striatal connection is part of a wider network that reverberates back to the cortex through the thalamus. It is believed that this cortico-basal nuclei-thalamo-cortical network may be implicated in different aspects of motor control, including initiation, sequencing, and modulation of voluntary movements. A predominance of striatal fibers on the left side in right-handed individuals provides evidence for this pathway to play an important role in language.

5.4   Language System

Mapping of the language system is requested when a lesion is located in the perisylvian region of the dominant hemisphere: insula, dorsal aspect of the frontal, temporal, and parietal lobes and in the adjacent WM pathways. Modern theories about language have recognized that there is a lot of network redundancy in the system. The impli-

cations of a dual-stream system with dorsal and ventral networks cannot be overemphasized. The AF is the main component of the dorsal network that is considered critical in syntactic analysis and modulation of acoustic speech signal to the articulatory loop located in the ventrolateral part of the frontal lobe. The IFOF, UF, and inferior longitudinal fasciculus (ILF) are the main fascicles of a ventral perisylvian network that is considered critical for lexical and semantic processing occurring in the anterior temporal lobe. The ventral network is involved in processing sound into meaning and comprehension. However, there are other aspects of language that may rely on a more extended language network with additional fascicles like the middle longitudinal fasciculus (MLF) connecting the STG with the IPL, the frontal aslant tract (FAT), and the subcallosal fascicle connecting language sites with the SMA.

5.4.1   The Dorsal Pathway: Arcuate Fasciculus

The AF is an essential component of the language system connecting regions devoted to formal aspects of language in temporal-parietal areas with regions involved in intentional and social communication in prefrontal areas (Catani and Bambini 2014). According to Catani the AF has three main cortical projections in the ventrolateral prefrontal (Broca), IPL (Geschwind), and posterior third of the temporal (Wernicke) lobe (Catani et al. 2005): (1) a direct (long segment) pathway connecting Broca with Wernicke territories, (2) an anterior segment connecting Broca with the IPL; (3) a posterior segment connecting Geschwind territory with the posterior third of the MTG. The three nodes are used in tractography as seed points to track the trajectories of the three segments that form the AF. Macroscopically the direct segment has two arms that converge in a stem (isthmus) that is located in the deep WM of the posterior temporal lobe. The fronto-parietal arm courses lateral to the corona radiata in the centrum semiovale, then it bends ventrally; the temporal arm of the AF courses along a cranio-caudal axis lateral to other long-range fascicles that are coursing in the deep WM underneath the AG and STG: they are the MLF, IFOF, and OR. The fronto-parietal and temporal arms of the AF-direct converge to form a stem (blue on DEC maps) that is an important landmark for tractography. The anterior and posterior AF segments are lateral to the direct segment; on DEC maps the streamlines of the anterior segment are green, those of the posterior segment are predominantly blue and green.

Tracking of the three segments of the AF should be performed with a two ROIs approach using streamline or probabilistic tractography with delineation of three seed ROIs on sagittal slices in the posterior IFG including BA6 and PMd (Broca territory), posterior third of MTG (Wernicke territory), and IPL (BA39/40, Geschwind territory). DEC and FA maps are quite useful in delineating seed and target ROIs. The ROI in the IPL and in the posterior IFG should include only a small layer of subcortical WM, while ROI delineation in the MTG should include the deep WM and in particular the AF stem.

The three tractograms should be inspected for a priori anatomical consistency after connecting each pair of ROIs. Spurious streamlines should be removed with "out-ROI" filters with the aim to illustrate the backbone of a "clean tractogram." Spurious tracts are often found overlapping with the trajectories of the CC and IFOF, due to fiber-tracking artifacts in voxels with crossing fibers. A statistical significant leftward asymmetry has been reported for the volume and number of streamlines of the direct segment of the AF. Furthermore, left lateralization has been shown in males, while a bilateral distribution has been shown in females. Individuals with more symmetric distribution performed better at remembering words using semantic association. These findings suggest that the degree of lateralization of the long segment of the AF is heterogeneous in the normal population and, paradoxically bilateral representation, not extreme lateraliza-

tion might ultimately be advantageous for specific cognitive functions (Catani et al. 2007). In addition, it was shown in a longitudinal DTI study that the volume of the direct segment of the AF in the right hemisphere is an important predictive factor for recovery of language after stroke in the left dominant hemisphere (Forkel et al. 2014a).

In the past the terms AF and SLF have been used as synonyms, but we agree with Catani that the equivalence of terms is anatomically incorrect despite some overlap between the fascicles. The term SLF should refer to a group of three longitudinal tracts connecting the dorsolateral cortex of the frontal and parietal lobes. The third segment of the SLF (SLF-III) overlaps with the anterior segment of the AF, while SLF-I and SLF-II are not components of the language network. The posterior segment of the AF runs along the cranio-caudal axis and it connects the AG with the posterior third of the MTG. It should not be confused with the MLF that runs longitudinally along the anterior-posterior axis of the SFG.

5.4.2 The Ventral Pathway: IFOF, UF, and ILF

The *IFOF* is a long association fascicle connecting the frontal with the temporal, parietal, and occipital lobes (Catani et al. 2002). The IFOF carries visual information from occipital areas to the temporal lobe and it is likely to play an important role in visual object recognition, and in linking object representation to their lexical labels (Catani and Mesulam 2008). Macroscopically the IFOF has two arms that converge in the temporal stem: the frontal arm projects to the IFG, MFG, dorsolateral prefrontal cortex, orbitofrontal cortex, and frontal pole; the temporo-parieto-occipital arm provides short-range bundles to the anterior temporal and insular cortex, long-range bundles to the posterior STG and MTG, and to the parietal and occipital cortex. Anatomically the IFOF can be subdivided into three segments: frontal, intermediate temporal, and parieto-occipital. Anatomic dissection of 14 post-mortem human cerebral hemispheres using the Klingler method has identified two components of the IFOF: a dorsal component connecting the frontal areas with the superior parietal lobule and posterior portion of the superior and middle occipital gyri and a ventral component connecting the frontal areas with the ventral part of the temporal lobe (fusiform gyrus, temporo-occipital sulcus, and inferior temporal gyrus) and with the inferior occipital gyrus (Martino et al. 2011). IFOF terminations have been demonstrated with post-mortem dissections within the SPL, superior, middle, and inferior occipital gyri (Martino et al. 2010). The ventral fibers of the IFOF partially overlap with the OR projecting into the superior and inferior banks of the calcarine sulcus. Caversazi et al. used Q-ball residual-bootstrap to reconstruct the IFOF using one single ROI delineated in the extreme capsule and thresholds of FA > 0.15 and <60° angle (Caverzasi et al. 2014). The authors were able to duplicate the above reported post-mortem findings. In comparison with classic DTI-based tractograms more extended projections of the anterior arm of the IFOF were found with Q-ball imaging in the lateral and medial orbitofrontal gyri, pars orbitalis and triangularis, rostral portion of the MFG, and even in the SFG. More extended projections of the posterior arm of the IFOF were found to project to the lingula, pericalcarine and lateral occipital cortices, cuneus, and caudal portion of the fusiform gyrus. Trajectories of the dorsal component were found to project to the AG and SPL. The anatomy of the IFOF projections to the occipital lobe was consistent among the 20 healthy subjects with greater than 75% overlap along its entire course.

At the level of the temporal stem the IFOF occupies the posterior and dorsal two-thirds of the stem and the streamlines can easily be distinguished from those of the UF coursing in the anteroventral and lateral part of the stem. As the IFOF exits the temporal stem it runs in the ventral part of both the external and extreme capsules, encasing the inferior part of the claustrum

(Ebeling and von Cramon 1992). The extreme capsule should not be considered a tract but a gross anatomy-defined WM structure. The intermediate segment of the IFOF runs in the roof of the temporal horn, superior and lateral to the OR. Within the posterior temporal region the IFOF trajectories run lateral to the tapetum and medial to the MLF, AF-direct, and posterior segment of the AF.

In the macaque monkey the IFOF is less developed than in humans, as monkeys lack the MTG and their IFOF connects primarily to posterior occipital areas (Forkel et al. 2014b; Schmahmann et al. 2007; Thiebaut de Schotten et al. 2012). In the monkeys the IFOF overlaps to some extent with the extreme capsule and this explains why it has been reported with that name in the literature (Petrides and Pandya 1988; Schmahmann and Pandya 2006). Other authors have adopted the monkey anatomic terminology also for human studies and refer to the extreme capsule as the direct connection between the prefrontal areas and the MTG (Saur et al. 2008, 2010).

Tracking of the IFOF is performed with a two ROIs approach using streamline or probabilistic tractography with delineation of the seed ROI in the temporal stem (green on DEC maps) and the target ROI in the deep WM of the occipital lobe at the level of the calcarine fissure. The seed ROI is delineated in multiple axial slices, whereas the target ROI in one coronal slice is perpendicular to the IFOF trajectories. The tractogram should be inspected for a priori anatomical consistency after connecting the two ROIs. In the human brain the IFOF is an easy tract to reconstruct with tractography because it runs longitudinally in the anterior-posterior direction and it is the dominant tract along most of its course. Spurious streamlines should be removed with "out-ROI" filters. Brain tumors expanding in the temporal or parietal lobe are likely to dislocate its trajectories or even to disrupt its course by increasing the number of spurious streamlines. A statistical significant rightward asymmetry has been reported for the volume and number of streamlines of the IFOF (Thiebaut de Schotten et al. 2011b).

The role of the IFOF in semantic processing is supported by IES mapping studies showing with high reproducibility that stimulation of the fascicle throughout its course from the frontal to the occipital lobe evokes semantic paraphasias (Duffau et al. 2008a). The anterior (frontal) arm of the IFOF should be detected with IES and represents the functional boundary in glioma infiltrating the pars opercularis of the IFG, the PMv or PMd areas of the dominant hemisphere. The intermediate and temporo-occipital segments of the IFOF represent the functional boundary in gliomas infiltrating the insula and the deep temporal lobe.

The *UF* is a hook-shaped bundle connecting the frontal lobe with the anterior temporal lobe. Macroscopically the UF has two arms that converge in the temporal stem: the frontal (dorsal) and the temporal (ventral) arms. From the stem the UF fans out into the frontal and temporal lobes. At the level of the temporal stem and in the proximity of the anteroventral portion of the extreme and external capsules the UF and IFOF look like very compacted bundles with the UF located ventral and anterior to the IFOF. In the frontal lobe the UF bundles project to the lateral and medial orbitofrontal cortex; in the temporal lobe the bundles project to the pole, amygdala, anterior part of the hippocampus, anterior third of STG and MTG (Martino et al. 2011).

The UF is part of the limbic system and it is likely involved in emotion and memory. It also plays a role in lexical retrieval, semantic associations, and specific aspects of naming. In a series of 44 patients who underwent awake surgery for removal of a left frontal or temporal glioma, removal of the UF in 18 patients resulted in long-term deficit of famous face naming, but not of picture naming of objects (Papagno et al. 2010, 2016). Patients were able to retrieve biographical information about people they could not name. Proper name impairment is a post-semantic deficit that requires damage of a functional network

that has several nodes connected by the UF: the orbitofrontal cortex involved in face-encoding, the ventromedial prefrontal cortex involved in the processing of emotions and the temporal pole involved in naming famous faces (Gorno-Tempini et al. 1998).

Tracking of the UF is performed with a two ROIs approach using streamline or probabilistic tractography with delineation of the seed ROI in the temporal stem and the target ROI in the anterior WM of the temporal lobe at the level of the anterior commissure. The seed ROI is delineated in multiple axial slices, whereas the target ROI in one coronal slice is perpendicular to the UF trajectories. The tractogram should be inspected for a priori anatomical consistency after connecting the two ROIs. The UF is an easy tract to reconstruct with tractography despite its bending and fanning trajectory because it does not cross other compact tracts. Spurious streamlines are scarce and they can be removed with "out-ROI" filters. The UF is symmetrical fascicles without significant differences in tract volume between the two hemispheres.

The *ILF* is a ventral associative bundle with long- and short-range fibers connecting the temporal and occipital lobes. The long bundles course medially to the short fibers and connect visual areas to the temporal pole, amygdala, and hippocampus. The ILF trajectories are coursing ventrally and laterally to the IFOF in the deep WM of the temporal and occipital lobes. The streamlines are green on DEC maps, but without tractography they are difficult to distinguish from the other fascicles running in the temporo-parietal fiber intersection area (TPFIA). Short-range fibers of the ILF connect the fusiform gyrus with the posterior part of the inferior occipital gyrus. Long-range fibers run medially to short-range fibers from the anterior temporal lobe to the ventrolateral occipital cortex; they course horizontally along the ventrolateral wall of the temporal and occipital horns with a posterior and lateral orientation. The ILF runs ventrally and laterally to the IFOF and OR for most of its course; the

ILF partially overlaps and crosses the IFOF and OR at the level of the TPFIA.

Tracking of the ILF is performed with a two ROIs approach using streamline or probabilistic tractography with delineation of the seed ROI in the occipital WM and the target ROI in the anterior WM of the temporal lobe at the level of the anterior commissure. Both ROIs are delineated in one coronal slice perpendicular to the ILF trajectories. The tractogram should be inspected for a priori anatomical consistency after connecting the two ROIs. Spurious streamlines can be removed with "out-ROI" filters. The ILF are symmetric fascicles without significant differences in tract volume between the two hemispheres.

The ILF is involved in face and visual object recognition, reading, visual memory, and in linking object representations to their lexical labels (Catani and Mesulam 2008). IES of the ILF systematically impaired reading ability at the level of the posterior surgical area. The ILF is involved in both the direct and indirect transfer of information between extrastriatal visual and anterior temporal areas involved in memory and limbic functions (Mandonnet et al. 2009). Moreover, it has been suggested that the ILF together with the UF provides an indirect pathway between the occipital and frontal language areas supporting semantic and lexical processing. The ILF, MLF, and UF are components of anterior temporal networks involved in selecting verbal labels for objects in a posterior-anterior progression of word comprehension, from generic to specific levels of precision. Overall the anterior temporal network enables mapping sound to meaning (Hickok and Poeppel 2007; Catani and Bambini 2014).

5.4.3 Frontal Aslant Tract and Subcallosal Fasciculus

The FAT is a recently described bilateral frontal intralobar fascicle connecting the anterior part of SMA-proper and the pre-SMA with the pars opercularis (BA44) of the IFG. Some fiber projections reach also the adjacent BA6. The FAT is the only intralobar tract connecting two non-adjacent gyri in the frontal lobe and it has been named "aslant" because of its peculiar oblique orientation in the coronal plane. It has been dissected with streamline tractography using the FACT algorithm (Oishi et al. 2008; Lawes et al. 2008) and with probabilistic tractography (Ford et al. 2010), however it is best visualized with the SD algorithm (Catani et al. 2012). It is one of few (previously unknown) tracts that have been first described with MR tractography (Oishi et al. 2008), then validated with post-mortem dissection studies (Lawes et al. 2008).

A significant leftward asymmetry in track volume in right-handed healthy subjects has been reported (Catani et al. 2012), suggesting a role in language connections. In one of our patients with oligoastrocytoma WHO-II seated in the lobar WM of the left frontal lobe we confirmed the relationship of this tract with language deficits. The presurgical MR tractography study showed that the FAT was adjacent to the medial and ventral margins of the mass, the CST was adjacent to the posterior margin, while the AF was relatively remote from it (Fig. 10). The mass was resected and the patient experienced severe mutism after surgery. Speech initiation deficits lasted longer than expected for a SMA syndrome and approximately 12 months after surgery the patient continued to have delayed reaction time to initiate speech. The postoperative MR tractography study confirmed preservation of the AF and SMA and suggested that the focal neurological deficit was associated with resection of the FAT. The authors of another MR tractography study in 35 patients with primary progressive aphasia showed that fractional anisotropy values of the FAT correlated with deficits in verbal fluency and suggested that this fascicle was part of the speech network (Catani et al. 2013).

Tracking of the FAT is performed with a two ROIs approach using streamline or probabilistic tractography with delineation of the seed ROIs in pars opercularis (BA44) and of the target ROI in the pre-SMA and anterior SMA-proper in multiple axial slices. Placement of spherical ROIs with Trackvis software (http://trackvis.org/) is handily used to explore the frontal region for intralobar streamlines before dissecting the frontal tracts.

The SCF was first described in 1887 by Theodor Meynert who used the term "corona radiata of the caudate nucleus" (Meynert 1887) and later in 1893 by Muratoff (Forkel et al. 2014b). The *SCF* has been described in humans and monkeys. In the monkey Yakovlev and Locke described the SCF as a projection tract connecting the cingulum to the caudate nucleus (Yakovlev and Locke 1961). Moreover, the fronto-striatal fibers also have strong reciprocal connections with BA24 of the cingulate gyrus and the pre-SMA. For this reason the SCF is also named the fronto-striatal tract (FST). In a study of stroke patients using computerized tomography more severe limitation in spontaneous speech was associated with lesions in the most rostral and medial portion of the FST plus the periventricular WM near the body of the lateral

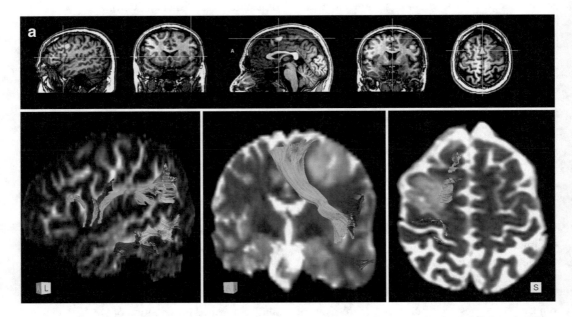

Fig. 10 (**a**) Twenty-nine years-old male with a mass infiltrating the lobar WM and the left MFG. Functional MRI with the verb generation task (upper row, from left to right) is showing BOLD response in left pars opercularis and PMv (sagittal and coronal images), in the pre-SMA and SMA-proper (sagittal image), SMA-proper and PMd (coronal image) and SMA-proper (axial image). Activation areas can be used to assist delineation of ROI for tractography in selected cases. In the left panel of the lower row the projections of the FAT (cyan) in pars opercularis and PMv, projections of the AF-direct (red) in PMv and posterior MTG, projections of the SLF-III (green) in PMv and SMG, projections of the posterior segment of the AF (yellow) in AG and MTG are overlaid on a sagittal FA map. The FAT is the medial and ventral limit of resection of the mass as illustrated in the coronal T2WI (mid panel). The relationship of the mass with the FAT and CST (red-orange scalar) that are, respectively, the medial and posterior margin of the mass is illustrated in the axial T2WI (right panel). (**b**) A left lateral oblique view of the main tracts evaluated in this case is displayed over sagittal and axial FA map. Note how big the FAT is in this case, probably enhanced by interruption of the crossing SLF due to presence of the tumor. Intraoperative monitoring with subcortical IES was not performed in this case and the patient immediately after surgery presented with severe mutism that lasted for a few weeks. Speech initiation deficits lasted longer than expected for a SMA syndrome and approximately 12 months after surgery the patient continued to have delayed reaction time to initiate speech. An oligoastrocitoma WHO-II was removed at surgery. The postoperative tractography study (not shown) confirmed that the severe SMA syndrome was associated with resection of the FAT despite preservation of the AF and SMA. Diffusion data were acquired with HARDI (64 gradient directions, $b = 1000$, $2 \times 2 \times 2$ mm³) and tractography was performed with DTI interpolated streamline algorithm (thresholds FA > 0.15; angle <45°)

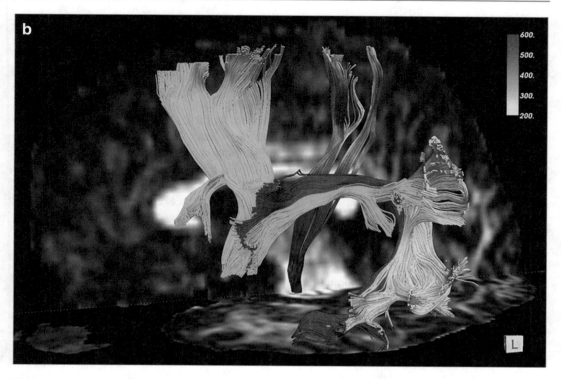

Fig. 10 (continued)

ventricle (Naeser et al. 1989). It is assumed that the FST may play an important role in the development of the intention to act and in the preparation for speech movement, both the initiation and limbic aspects of speech.

The SCF courses within the periventricular zone of the anterior horn of the lateral ventricle, medially to the superior fronto-occipital fasciculus, an association pathway connecting the frontal with the occipital cortex. The two fascicles should be clearly distinguished despite their anatomic proximity in the periventricular zone. To add to the confusion, occasionally the SCF and the superior fronto-occipital fasciculus have been used synonymously in the literature, despite they have clearly different anatomic and physiologic properties.

In a tractography study of 8 healthy subjects Léhericy et al. dissected fronto-strial projections and provided the first demonstration that frontal posterior and anterior premotor areas projections to the striatum are organized in distinct circuits along the caudal-rostral axis (Lehéricy et al. 2004). Fiber tracking of the FST is performed with the two ROI approach: a seed subcortical ROI is delineated in the caudate head and a target ROI in the pre-SMA. The trajectories of the FST ascend around the lateral wall of the frontal horn of the lateral ventricle, and then intermingle with ipsilateral FAT trajectories originating from the pars opercularis before entering into the pre-SMA. Subcortical IES of the FST evokes delayed speech initiation (Vassal et al. 2013).

5.4.4 Which Fascicles Are Eloquent for Speech?

Determination of which brain regions and fascicles are functionally eloquent for language and should be safeguarded during surgery remains an important and debated issue. The aim of IOM is to map the networks underlying different but interactive language processes that will define the functional limits of the resection. Several language tasks are available and selection of which task to administer to the patient depends on the location of the lesion, presurgical imaging mapping and neuropsychological results, handedness, job, and hobbies of the patient (see Table 1).

In gliomas infiltrating the perisylvian region within the dominant hemisphere mapping of the cortical sites on the brain surface begins with identification of the motor strip, PMv, and posterior IFG (Broca area). The PMv (BA6) can be identified asking the patient to count while the neurosurgeon stimulates the surface of the cortex with a low-frequency bipolar probe. When the current depolarizes neurons in the PMv of a patient who is counting or during spontaneous speech, he/she will have a speech arrest (Duffau 2005), even if stimulated in the non-dominant hemisphere (Duffau et al. 2008b). Common and important language tasks are picture naming, reading, comprehension, syntax and language switching from one language to another.

After completing corticotomy, resection of the tumor continues only after all functional limits with eloquent subcortical pathways have been identified and disconnected from the tumor. With gliomas growing in the anterior frontal lobe the FAT and the SCF are found, respectively, laterally and medially. With gliomas growing in the suprasylvian region within the frontal or parietal opercula the SLF-III, AF-direct and CST are encountered in this order. The AF-direct is the deep limit of the resection also in superficial gliomas infiltrating the MTG and STG. The IFOF and OR are the deep limits in gliomas seating deep to the IPL and posterior temporal region. At the level of the ventral temporo-occipital junction the posterior part of the ILF should be identified because it is part of the reading network.

Which of the above fascicles if damaged may relate to permanent language deficits? In a large series of 115 patients with LGG infiltrating language areas Duffau et al. showed that tumor resection by safeguarding functional boundaries avoids permanent postoperative language deficits (Duffau et al. 2008a, b). The AF has been associated with language for a very long time; however, its role together with that of the UF, MLF, and ILF in maintaining the integrity of the network has been questioned by the neurosurgeons. The

AF is a long-range fascicle and a few neurosurgeons suggest that IES of only a focal part of it may evoke phonemic paraphasia. The eloquent part of the AF should be safeguarded, whereas other parts may be removed with the tumor. The eloquent part can only be identified with subcortical direct IES due to a great variability among patients. Stimulation of the AF-direct segment induces transient phonemic paraphasia and repetition errors that are signs of conduction aphasia. Stimulation of the AF can also disrupt syntax (Vidorreta et al. 2011) or a wide network involved in language switching from native to secondary languages, a skill that is important to safeguard in bilingual patients (Bello et al. 2006; Gatignol et al. 2009). Stimulation of the SLF-III induces speech apraxia (Maldonado et al. 2011a) and it may be involved with verbal working memory (Maldonado et al. 2011b), while stimulation of the FAT and SCF induces speech initiation.

We have seen previously how important is direct subcortical IES of the IFOF in preserving semantic processes of language. The IFOF is the medial functional limit in gliomas located in the frontal operculum, insula and temporal lobe of the dominant hemisphere. On the contrary to what applies for the left AF, subcortical IES of the left IFOF throughout its course induces semantic paraphasia (Duffau et al. 2005; Bello et al. 2007).

The UF can be removed without permanent deficits if the IFOF is preserved: in Duffau's large series IES of the left UF did not evoke language deficits (Duffau et al. 2008a, b). However, short and long-lasting deficits in famous face naming in a series of patients with UF resection after removal of left frontal or temporal gliomas have been reported (Papagno et al. 2010, 2016).

In the literature there are conflicting findings about the role of the left ILF in language and semantics. Direct subcortical IES of the left ILF does not particularly impair spoken language generally, especially for picture-naming performances. IES of the left ILF did not induce language errors in 12 patients with LGG in the temporal lobe (Mandonnet et al. 2007b). However, the posterior part of the ILF should be

Table 1 For each System the main fascicles are listed with their cortical terminations. For each fasciculus are indicated the MEP electrode position or the task administered to the patient, the recorded incorrect responses and the neurological deficits occuring when the fasciculus of interest is preserved (transient deficit) or damaged (permanent deficit)

System	Fasciculus	Cortical terminations	IES/task	Response	Preserved	Damaged
Motor	CST	M1, PMv, PMd, SMA	Face, arm, tibialis	MEP or movement disorders (dystonic movement or movement arrest)	Transient motor deficits	Permanent motor deficits
Language	Lt AF	PMd, PMv, MTG	Picture naming	Phonemic paraphasia, anomia	Transient deficits	Conduction aphasia
	Lt IFOF	IFG, OFC, temporal, parietal, occipital	Picture naming	Semantic and verbal paraphasia, anomia	Transient aphasia	Semantic and verbal paraphasia, anomia
	Lt UF	OFC, T-pole	Picture naming, famous face naming	Anomia	Transient deficits	Long-term proper name recall
	Lt ILF	T-pole-occipital and visual word form area	Categorial, reading	Pure anomia, reading disorder	Transient categorial errors	Permanent alexia
	Lt FAT	SMA, BA44	Complex serial articulation	Perseveration, slurring	Speech initiation	Permanent delayed reaction time, deficit of syntax production
	Lt SLF-III	PMd, PMv, SMG and posterior STG	Picture naming, numbering	Number errors, articulatory deficits	Transient deficits	Permanent deficits
Vision	OR	LGN, V1	Alternate picture naming	Missed or "positive" responses (as phosphenes or visual illusion)	Quadrantoanopsia or even hemianopsia	Quadrantoanopsia or even hemianopsia
Visuospatial attention	Rt SLF-II	MFG, AG	Bisection line	Bisection error	Hemispatial neglect	Hemispatial neglect

safeguarded and preserved in gliomas located near the ventral temporo-occipital junction, because the ILF may play a crucial role in reading. In a single glioma patient, direct cortical IES near the visual word form area led to visual paraphasias that were also elicited by subcortical IES of the ILF in the anterior wall of the surgical cavity (Mandonnet et al. 2009). More recently, Duffau and colleagues showed that disruption of the anterior-to-middle segment of the ILF with IES during awake surgery systematically induced pure anomia during a picture-naming task in five patients with LGG in the ITG and posterior temporal lobe, but not in the other six patients with LGG infiltrating the anterior temporal lobe (Herbet et al. 2019). The authors concluded that their results showed that the information conveyed by the ILF is likely rerouted to alternative pathways such as the IFOF when glioma is damaging the anterior temporal cortex. These results also proved that the ILF plays a role in lexical retrieval in normal circumstances. These conclusions are further supported by the case report of a glioma patient who developed a long-lasting anomic aphasia after a presurgically planned interruption of the ILF.

In a series of eight patients with glioma in the left dominant STG subcortical IES of the anterior part of the MLF did not elicited language deficits and the patients did not developed any postoperative permanent language deficit (De Witt Hamer et al. 2011). Thus, the MLF may participate, but is not essential for language processing. Taken together the above studies in patients harboring gliomas seated in the dominant temporal lobe suggest that resections of the UF, ILF, and MLF may cause permanent aphasia in special circumstances when their function cannot be compensated by the IFOF.

Cortical direct IES of the SMA and pre-SMA produces both vocalization and arrest of speech (Penfield and Rasmussen 1950). Patients with lesions of the SMA may present various degrees of speech impairment from a total inability to initiate speech to deficits in phonologic fluency. It has been hypothesized that the SMA through the FAT may facilitate speech initiation. Very recently in a series of 19 patients with WHO-II gliomas infiltrating the SMA, pars opercularis, and/or the caudate nucleus inhibition of speech has been evoked not only by cortical IES of the BA6, pars opercularis or SMA, but also by direct subcortical IES of the left FAT (Kinoshita et al. 2014). Furthermore, the authors found a significant correlation between the severity of postoperative transitory speech initiation deficits and the distance of the FAT from the wall of the resection cavity. In the same study IES of the FST generated negative motor responses suggesting that the FST may be part of the "negative motor network" and may participate in the modulation of motor function including bimanual coordination. Despite the fact that the authors found a relationship between speech initiation postoperative deficits and the left FAT but not the left FST, the average distance between tumor resection and left FST showed a positive correlation with verbal phonemic and semantic fluency scores in the immediate postoperative period and plead in favor of the involvement of the left FST and caudate in speech control. All together these studies emphasize how much valuable is the anatomic information provided by pre- and postoperative tractography studies as a way to integrate IES mapping.

In conclusion, the IFOF, AF-direct, and AF-posterior language fascicles should be identified with presurgical tractography and IES performed in awake patients every time a mass is seated in the perisylvian region of the dominant hemisphere in order to identify the subcortical functional limits of the resection. At present the majority of neurosurgeons performing awake surgery would agree that the IFOF is the most essential of all language-related fascicles, followed by the AF and ILF. Damage to the IFOF is very likely to cause permanent language deficits. A resection very close to the UF, SLF-III, FAT, and SCF is likely to induce transitory speech disorders that may recover in a few weeks or months. We predict that the role of diffusion imaging with tractography in the routine evaluation of pre- and postoperative glioma patients will soon become standard of care in neuro-oncology.

5.5 Visuospatial System: OR

The retinogeniculate fibers originate from neurons in the retina and project to the lateral geniculate nucleus. The OR, also called the geniculostriate fibers, are a large bundle of myelinated fibers that originate from relay neurons in the layers of the lateral geniculate nucleus and project to the ipsilateral primary visual area. The OR are part of the ventral part of the posterior thalamic radiations and can be divided into two main components: the dorsal fibers carrying visual information from the lower quadrants of the contralateral visual hemifield and projecting to the cortex of the cuneus into the superior bank of the calcarine fissure; the ventral fibers carrying visual information from the upper quadrant of the contralateral hemifield and projecting to the cortex of the lingual gyrus into the inferior bank of the calcarine fissure. The dorsal fibers originate from the dorsomedial portion of both lateral geniculate nuclei and arch directly caudally to pass through the retrolenticular limb of the internal capsule before projecting to the cuneus. On the contrary, the ventral fibers originate from the ventrolateral portion of the lateral geniculate nucleus and arch rostral, passing into the WM of the anterior temporal lobes to form a broad U-turn (loop of Meyer) before passing caudally and projecting to the lingula. Damage to the dorsal fibers results in a loss of vision in the contralateral inferior visual field. Damage to the Meyer loop in the anterior temporal lobe or to any other segment of the ventral contingent results in contralateral superior quadrantanopia. Lesions of the OR may result in quadrantanopia or may involve only a portion of a quadrant of the visual field. The closer a lesion is to the primary visual cortex the more congruous the visual field loss of one eye can be superimposed to the other eye. The more anterior a lesion is in the OR, the more

likely it is that the visual deficit will be incongruous in the two eyes.

Tracking of the OR is performed with a two ROIs approach using streamline or probabilistic tractography with delineation of the seed ROI in the lateral geniculate nucleus and of the target ROI in the ipsilateral WM of the occipital lobe at the level of the calcarine fissure. The seed ROI is delineated in the lateral portion of the thalamus in multiple axial slices or using a sphere; the target ROI is delineated in one coronal slice perpendicular to the OR. The OR course together with the IFOF for most of their course (Fig. 6): the dorsal fibers of the OR overlap with the IFOF, as well as the upper two-thirds of the ventral fibers projecting to the inferior bank of the calcarine cortex. Only in the proximity of the more posterior part of the sagittal stratum the OR and IFOF diverge to reach their respective cortical terminations. The tractogram should be inspected for a priori anatomical consistency after connecting the two ROIs. Spurious streamlines can be removed with "out-ROI" filters. The OR are symmetric bundles without significant differences in tract volume between the two hemispheres.

During awake surgery the OR can be identified with IES administering a picture-naming task that displays simultaneously two objects in opposite quadrants. When the surgeon stimulates the dorsal bundles of the OR the patient will fail to name the object in the contralateral inferior hemifield, when he stimulates the ventral bundles the patient will fail to name the object in the contralateral superior hemifield.

5.5.1 Superior Longitudinal Fasciculus

Lesion studies in patients and more recent functional imaging studies in healthy human subjects have provided evidence that visuospatial attention relies on a bilateral fronto-parietal network, with right hemisphere dominance in most, but not all individuals. Synchronous activity of neurons in the frontal and parietal cortices during visual search has been demonstrated using multiple electrodes in monkeys, and scalp EEG in young and elderly human subjects, suggesting that a bilateral fronto-parietal network may play an important role in top-down and bottom-up control mechanisms. Axonal tracing studies in the monkey have demonstrated that frontal and parietal neurons are connected through three separate fascicles coursing longitudinally in the dorsolateral WM of the centrum semiovale (Schmahmann and Pandya 2006). The three segments of the SLF, a major intrahemispheric association fiber pathway that connects the parieto-temporal association areas with the frontal lobe and vice versa, compose the network. In the classical description of Dejerine the AF was also considered part of the SLF; however, studies in monkeys showed that the SLF and AF are two separate entities. The trajectories of three separate segments of the SLF have been demonstrated also in the human brain with post-mortem dissections (Ludwig and Klingler 1956) and more recently with DTI (Makris et al. 2005) and SD (Thiebaut de Schotten et al. 2012) tractography. Overall, the anatomy of the SLF is highly conserved between humans and monkeys.

The *SLF-I* is the most dorsal component and connects the dorsolateral part of the superior parietal lobule and precuneus with the anterior dorsal part of the SFG. The *SLF-II* is the major component of the SLF and it connects the AG and anterior bank of the intraparietal sulcus with the PMd at the junction of the SFG and MFG. Its trajectories are contiguous with the anterior portion of the AF coursing above the Sylvian fissure and insula. The *SLF-III* is the ventral component of the SLF and it connects the IPL (Geschwind territory) with the ventral premotor and prefrontal areas (Broca territory).

Tracking of each of the three segments is performed with a two ROIs approach using streamline or probabilistic tractography. The seed ROI is delineated in a coronal slice at the level of the posterior commissure in the subcortical WM of the SPL and IPL. Three target ROIs are delineated on a coronal slice at the level of the anterior commissure in the dorsal subcortical WM of the superior, middle, and inferior/precentral frontal gyri. An additional ROI should be delineated in the temporal WM to filter out the trajectories of the AF-direct segment that course for some time intermingled with the SLF-II. After connecting the seed ROI in the parietal WM with each target ROI in the frontal WM the tractograms should be inspected for a priori anatomic consistency. Spurious streamlines should be removed with "out-ROI" filters. The SLF-III is an easy tract to reconstruct with DTI tractography in the human brain. Reconstruction of the SLF-I and SLF-II with DTI may be inconsistent because these tracts course along the AF and intersect crossing fibers of the CST and CC. Using the SD algorithm often improves the tracking. A statistical significant rightward asymmetry has been reported for the track volume of the SLF-III; no significant differences were found for the SLF-I and SLF-II (Thiebaut de Schotten et al. 2011a).

Brain tumors expanding in the frontal and parietal lobes may dislocate or interrupt the trajectories of multiple fascicles, including the SLF, FAT, and SCF. The branches of the SLF are only occasionally searched for with IES during surgery, despite the important role they play in the motor and the visuospatial systems. The authors of a recent intraoperative study showed that the SLF-II and the SLF-III together with the AF-direct and the PMv are part of a network involved in motor awareness of voluntary actions (Fornia et al. 2020). Intraoperative IES applied on PMv dramatically altered the patients' motor awareness, making them unconscious of the motor arrest. Another study shed light on a key aspect of cognitive control during the Stroop test: the management of conflicting incoming information to achieve a goal, termed "interference control." The SCF that is connecting the IFG with the striatum was found the key component of cognitive control in the right hemisphere (Puglisi et al. 2019). This latter study suggested that preserving cortico-striatal rather than cortico-cortical connections (i.e., SLF-II, SLF-III, FAT, and IFOF) may be critical for maintaining cognitive control abilities in the surgery of right frontal lobe tumors.

5.6 The Temporo-Parietal Fiber Intersection Area

The TPFIA is a critical neural crossroad with great implications for surgery; it is traversed by seven WM fascicles that connect some of the most eloquent areas in the human brain located in the IPL and posterior temporal lobes. Lesion studies have reported major language deficits such as aphasia (Fridriksson et al. 2010), alexia, agraphia, hemianopia and neglect (Müller-Oehring et al. 2003) in patients with a lesion located in the IPL or in the posterior temporal lobe. In the past clinicians have interpreted neurological deficits of higher cognitive function as a consequence of lesions in associative cortex, neglecting the importance of the WM pathways coursing underneath. Since most focal lesions also affect the subcortical and deep WM, potential damage to adjacent pathways should also be investigated since it may cause a disconnection syndrome (Catani and Ffytche 2005). Recently, unexpectedly high postoperative deficit rates were reported in patients with parietal gliomas. In a series of 119 parietal gliomas Sanai et al. reported a 8.4% permanent language deficit (Sanai et al. 2012), which is fivefold greater compared with the previously reported experience of the UCSF group with gliomas located within language areas (1.6%) (Sanai et al. 2008). The 6.7% rate of permanent visual deficits was also higher than expected in this series. An even higher rate of long-term mild language deficits (42.9%) was reported in a series of 14 consecutive patients with glioma involving the IPL who were operated with cortical and subcortical IES mapping (Maldonado et al. 2011a). This rate is 21-fold greater compared with the 1.7% rate of the overall experience of the same Montpellier group with LGG located within eloquent areas (Duffau et al. 2008a, b). Both studies underscore the importance of the WM pathways coursing underneath the IPL and the posterior temporal lobe that, if damaged, will have consequences far more serious than in other brain cortical and subcortical locations.

Martino et al. elucidated the complex organization and the surgical importance of the TPFIA using post-mortem cortex-sparing fiber dissection and streamline MR tractography (Martino et al. 2013). The TPFIA is seated in the WM underneath the AG, posterior MTG, and ITG and may extend underneath the posterior part of the SMG and STG. The authors described seven long-range WM fascicles passing through the TPFIA. In this section we will discuss the anatomic relationship among the seven tracts and the MLF in detail since the AF, ILF, IFOF, and OR have been already described in other sections.

Starting the virtual or post-mortem dissections from the lateral brain surface at the level of the temporo-parietal junction, the posterior segment of the AF is the most superficial bundle. This fascicle runs vertically and connects the AG with the posterior MTG and ITG. These association fibers had originally been discovered by Wernicke in monkey brains and in the past had been called "Wernicke perpendicular fasciculus." This fascicle is clinically relevant and should be preserved from surgical damage whenever possible. Lesions to the AF-posterior have been associated with preangular alexia without agraphia (Greenblatt 1973). In this peculiar syndrome, patients are unable to read but can still write or text short messages. The closer a lesion is located to the IPL, the more likely it is accompanied by agraphia, whereas the closer a lesion is to the IFG, the more likely it will involve disorders of face or color identification. The anterior aspect of this fascicle may be part of a brain network processing the age of faces (Homola et al. 2012). Bartsch and colleagues have reported four brain tumor patients in which surgical access through the TPFIA has led to alexia without agraphia due to damage of the AF-posterior (Bartsch et al. 2013). Such disconnection syndrome may be transient, but the associated deficit may also persist and turn out to be quite disabling.

Medial and slightly anterior to the posterior segment runs the direct segment of the AF that connects Broca with Wernicke territories. In the TPFIA the bundles of the AF-direct run vertically. Next there is the MLF that is medial to the stem of the AF-direct and lateral to the IFOF.

The *MLF* is a longitudinal fascicle that is coursing with an antero-posterior orientation in the WM of the STG, parallel to the other longitudinal fascicles (SLF and ILF). At the posterior end of the STG the fibers bend dorsally and course in the posterior portion of the corona radiata until they project into the AG. The MLF connects the upper part of the temporal pole and the entire SFG with the AG (Makris and Pandya 2009; Makris et al. 2009). The MLF should not be confused with the posterior segment of the AF, because it is deeper located and it has a longitudinal rather than a vertical orientation. It has been suggested that the MLF has a role in language and attention (Makris and Pandya 2009; Menjot de Champfleur et al. 2013). However, Duffau et al. have evaluated eight patients with glioma infiltrating the STG using IES and have established that damage to the MLF does not cause long-term deficits, thus Duffau concluded that the MLF is not essential for language. No interference with picture naming was observed by IES of the MLF and no new permanent language deficits were detected with the Boston Diagnostic Aphasia Examination after extensive resection of gliomas that included large parts of the MLF. In the same IES study the IFOF was identified in all patients by eliciting semantic paraphasia, thus it can be easily distinguished from the MLF (De Witt Hamer et al. 2011).

The MLF crosses in the upper half of the TPFIA and it is more difficult to reconstruct than the AF with DTI streamline tractography; SD helps to some degree to depict the MLF. The seed ROIs should be delineated on coronal FA/DEC maps in the WM of the anterior part of the SFG at the level of the AC; the target ROIs should be delineated in the WM of the AG at the level of the splenium of the CC (Makris et al. 2009).

In the inferior half of the TPFIA runs the ILF, laterally to the IFOF and ventrally to the MLF. The ILF runs underneath the inferior temporal and lateral occipital gyri and connects the inferior part of the temporal pole with the ITG, the middle and inferior occipital gyri, and the ventral surfaces of the temporal and occipital lobes. Medial to the ILF there is the IFOF, then the OR. Their streamlines are difficult to separate with MR tractography because they are parallel and course together. On axial and coronal DEC maps they appear green along their entire course and they are seated in between two vertically oriented fascicles (blue on color maps): the AF stem on the lateral side, the tapetum on the medial side. The OR fibers are intermingled with those of the IFOF running in the most medial and ventral part of the TPFIA (Fig. 11). The tapetum is the most medial WM structure and consists of

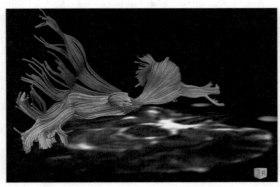
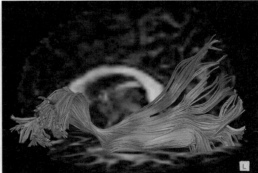

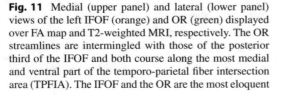

Fig. 11 Medial (upper panel) and lateral (lower panel) views of the left IFOF (orange) and OR (green) displayed over FA map and T2-weighted MRI, respectively. The OR streamlines are intermingled with those of the posterior third of the IFOF and both course along the most medial and ventral part of the temporo-parietal fiber intersection area (TPFIA). The IFOF and the OR are the most eloquent fascicles intersecting in the TPFIA. They course along the lateral wall of the occipital horn of the lateral ventricles and they are difficult to separate with MR tractography. Diffusion data were acquired with HARDI (64 gradient directions, $b = 2000$, $2 \times 2 \times 2$ mm^3) and tractography was performed with DTI interpolated streamline algorithm (thresholds FA > 0.1; angle <35°)

interhemispheric fibers that form the roof and lateral wall of the atrium, temporal, and occipital horns of the lateral ventricles. The tapetum connects both temporal lobes through the posterior part of the corpus callosum.

In summary, the seven tracts can be identified on axial and coronal DEC maps. Three of these tracts have a cranio-caudal orientation and their streamlines are directionally colored in blue; they are the posterior and direct segments of the AF laterally and the tapetum medially. Four tracts with anterior-posterior orientation course in between; the IFOF and the OR course throughout the entire TPFIA, while the MLF and ILF run laterally to the IFOF, respectively, in the upper and lower half of the TPFIA. It is necessary to use MR tractography to distinguish the trajectories of the five antero-posterior oriented tracts.

In the past the transcortical approach through the TPFIA was considered the most direct trajectory from the brain surface to reach a tumor in the posterior hippocampus, temporal, and occipital horns or atrium of the lateral ventricle. Recent postoperative data have shown that the TPFIA is one of the most vulnerable parts of the human brain; therefore knowledge of this important crossroad is now mandatory for surgical planning before a safe resection of deep-seated tumors. When a glioma infiltrating the AG and posterior third of the MTG and ITG extends 2–3 cm into the deep WM it will likely displace, infiltrate, or interrupt the fascicles coursing in the TPFIA. A detailed MR tractography study of the TPFIA should be performed to better understand the relationship between the mass and the seven fascicles. In our practice we have seen several patients with gliomas originating within the TPFIA. We were surprised to note that in a few patients the tumor was causing only mild preoperative neurological deficits. MR tractography was instrumental to explain this unexpected clinical finding. In pauci symptomatic patients the tracts could be reconstructed in their integrity suggesting that the mass was displacing rather than interrupting the tracts. We have seen also rapidly growing gliomas dislocating tracts in the TPFIA (Figs. 12

and 13). Visualization of eloquent tracts in the proximity of a glioma may have a positive predictive value for postoperative outcome, because it suggests that the fascicle is partially spared by the tumor and that an extended resection can be attempted.

It has been shown that MR tractography can reliably reproduce and strengthen the knowledge gathered from intraoperative and post-mortem dissection studies thus having a significant impact on patient management particularly so in cases when the surgical risk should be carefully balanced with the benefits of an extensive resection. Planning a surgical approach anterior or posterior to the TPFIA may preserve the direct and posterior segments of the AF, while in other cases a longitudinal surgical incision may be indicated to safeguard the IFOF, OR, MLF, and ILF that are running in the anterior-posterior orientation (Martino et al. 2013). Moreover, IES should be strongly considered for safe resection of deep-seated tumors, especially in the dominant hemisphere.

5.7 Integration with fMRI

We have seen how tracking of streamlines in the vicinity or within neoplasm is complicated by tumor infiltration, vasogenic edema, mass effect leading to tissue deformation and loss of anatomical landmarks. These changes deform the architecture of the WM and in several cases the use of a priori anatomical approaches for ROI delineation yields unsatisfactory tractography results. Selection of seed and target ROIs based on the results of fMRI has been proposed. Preliminary studies suggested that fMRI-based seed selection may allow for more specific and comprehensive fiber tracking (Schonberg et al. 2006; Smits et al. 2007). The combination and co-registration of clinically feasible fMRI and DTI datasets may help the tractographer to define seed ROIs which are relevant to track the pathway of interest. Schonberg et al. showed that it was feasible and easier to identify the seed and target points, respectively, of the CST and AF with the aid of fMRI maps of finger tapping and speech.

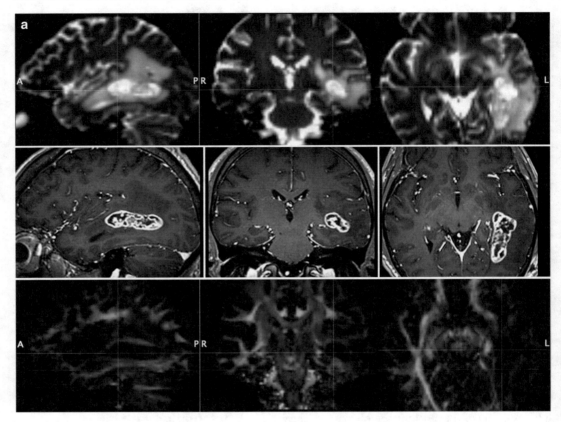

Fig. 12 (a) Fifty years-old male with an enhancing mass seated in the deep left temporo-occipital WM. There is extensive perilesional vasogenic edema that is bright on T2WI, hypointense on T1WI and low on FA maps. A GBM WHO-IV was removed at surgery. DEC maps show decreased hue (FA) and dislocation of several green (associative) tracts in the temporo-parietal fiber intersection area (TPFIA). T2WI upper row, T1WI post-gadolinium middle row, DEC maps lower row. (**b**) Tractography is showing that all fascicles in the TPFIA can be virtually dissected: the mass is dislocating the AF-direct (red) and AF-posterior (yellow) laterally, the IFOF (orange) medially. The AF-direct is the lateral functional boundary, whereas the IFOF is the medial boundary. The functional limits of the resection were confirmed in the operating room with direct subcortical IES. In this case the information provided by tractography is by far superior to that provided by DEC maps. Medial view (left column) showing the relationship of the AF, SLF-III (green), and IFOF with the mass. Anterior view (bottom row, left column) showing the mass splaying the AF-direct from the IFOF. Left lateral view (right column) showing dissection of four of the seven fascicles that form the TPFIA. Diffusion data were acquired with HARDI (64 gradient directions, $b = 2000$, $2 \times 2 \times 2$ mm^3) and tractography was performed with DTI interpolated streamline algorithm (thresholds FA > 0.1; angle <35°)

According to the author's remarks tracking of both fascicles was more accurate than with delineation of a priori anatomical seed points.

The initial enthusiasm about performing tractography in a semi-automated fashion by co-registering and combining the two methods has deflated since the early-published papers. So far, nothing can beat an experienced neuroradiologist in identifying the key anatomic landmarks especially when the anatomy of a network is distorted, displaced, or partially interrupted by a mass. The results of streamline tractography using a priori ROI delineation are quite consistent when using the same acquisition scheme, post-processing, and fiber-tracking routine.

In our practice we routinely acquire fMRI and HARDI during the same study session when we are asked to mapping the language system. We are

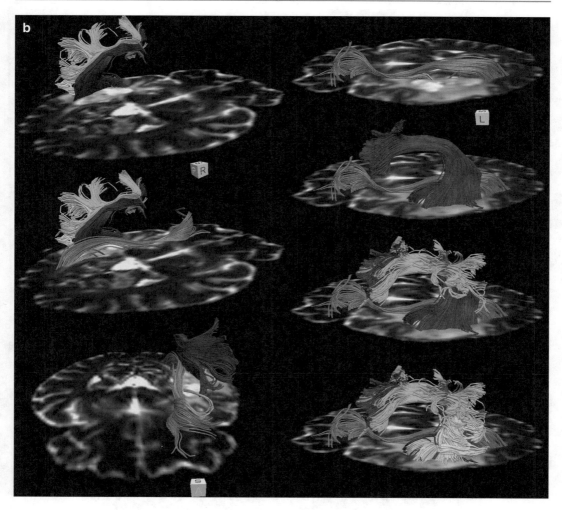

Fig. 12 (continued)

not convinced that combining the two methods in a semi-automatic fashion is worth the effort. fMRI can help identify the seed points of the speech network and to a lesser extent the precentral gyrus when tracking of the CST is requested. We agree with other authors that fMRI is quite helpful to understand the anatomy of sulci and gyri when they are distorted by an infiltrating glioma. When a mass is dislocating the AF or one of its cortical terminations (seed point), the foci of the BOLD response are coherently dislocated (Fig. 14). fMRI is particularly useful to identify the exact anatomy of the IFG and adjacent BA6: despite distortion of the anatomy induced by glioma infiltration a residual cluster of BOLD response is

unequivocally located in the ventral precentral sulcus (neurons of the PMv) between these two key anatomy landmarks (Quiñones-Hinojosa et al. 2003; Bizzi et al. 2012).

5.8 Integration in the Operating Room

Nimsky and colleagues were the first to demonstrate that intraoperative DTI was technically feasible in 38 patients with tumor in the proximity of the CST. DEC maps immediately available in the operating theater showed marked and highly variable shifting of the CST caused by surgical

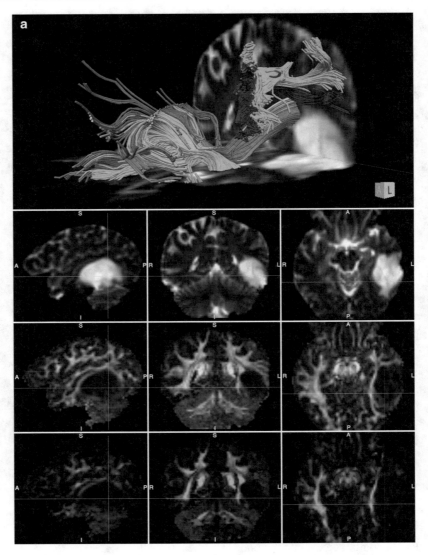

Fig. 13 (**a**) Thirty-one years-old female with a mass expanding in the middle, inferior, and fusiform gyri of the left temporal lobe. Tractography (upper panel) is showing that the main fascicles in the TPFIA can be virtually dissected: the mass is dislocating dorsally the AF-direct (red), medially and superiorly the IFOF (orange) and OR (not shown), medially the ILF (pink). The mass is bright on T2WI (second row) with very low FA (third row). DEC maps (bottom row) are showing that the mass has displayed medially the association tracts but only with tractography it was possible to realize that the IFOF was also displaced dorsally. This information was quite appreciated by the neurosurgeon during presurgical consultation. The functional limits of the resection were confirmed in the operating room with direct subcortical IES. An anaplastic oligodendroglioma WHO-III was removed at surgery. (**b**) Virtual dissection with tractography of the fascicles in the TPFIA. The relationship of five fascicles with the mass (gray) is shown in the upper panel. After "hiding the mass" the medial functional margins of the lesion with the ILF (pink) and IFOF (orange) are illustrated over a FA map in the second panel from above. "Hiding the SLF-III (green)" allows best appreciation of the remarkable dorsal displacement of the temporal arm of the AF-direct (red) in the third panel. "Hiding of the AF-direct" allows appreciation of the ILF and IFOF in the fourth panel. The UF (cyan) is relatively remote from the anterior margin of the lesion. Visualization of eloquent tracts in the proximity of a glioma may have a positive predictive value for postoperative outcome, because it suggests that the fascicle is partially spared by the tumor and that a relatively radical resection can be attempted. Diffusion data were acquired with HARDI (64 gradient directions, $b = 2000$, $2 \times 2 \times 2$ mm^3) and tractography was performed with DTI interpolated streamline algorithm (thresholds FA > 0.1; angle <35°)

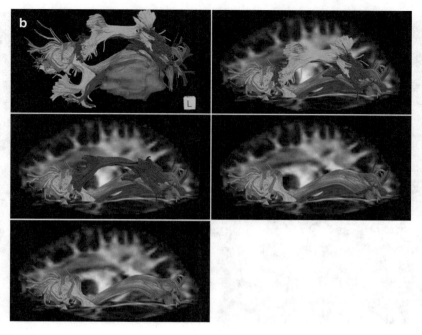

Fig. 13 (continued)

intervention. In the 27 patients who underwent brain tumor resection, CST dislocation ranged from an inward shift of 8 mm to an outward shift of 15 mm (Nimsky et al. 2005).

Another option is fusion of three-dimensional objects of selected tractograms into DICOM post-gadolinium T1WI or T2-FLAIR using a standard neuronavigation system. This method is allowing for intraoperative visualization and localization of the tracts of interest (Nimsky et al. 2007). Display of MR tractograms in the operating room may be useful to determine the relationship of a mass with adjacent fascicles or when the neurosurgeon desires to refresh his anatomical orientation in the operating field, before and after using IES to check the functional limits of a resection on preoperative MRI (Bello et al. 2008).

The long list of important limitations must be well understood and considered when the tractograms are exported to the operating room. Current DTI methods may provide ambiguous results in reconstruction of crossing, kissing, bending, and fanning bundles. MR tractography cannot track the trajectories to their cortical terminations. It is important to be aware that tractography so far is a user-dependent method based on a priori knowledge of the examiner.

The risk of resecting eloquent structures not detected by DTI or HARDI will have to be considered. False negative results may occur especially in areas of T2 signal hyperintensity within a LGG where the trajectories of the tracts appear interrupted due to FA values that are below the recommended 0.10 threshold. The presence of an eloquent tract in the vicinity of the surgical cavity should not be the main reason for stopping the resection prematurely. The finding should be carefully discussed with the surgeon, because an incomplete resection may decrease the impact of surgery on the natural history of the disease. The dangers of using MR tractography in presurgical evaluation of gliomas and intraoperatively has been recently outlined by Duffau (2014). MR tractography does not provide information about the functional status of a fascicle, thus IES should always be used in order to avoid long-term postoperative neurological deficits. IES is the only method able to test WM function in order to create a subcortical functional map that has proven to maximize tumor

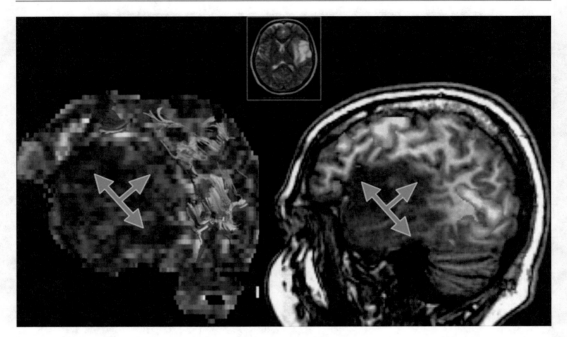

Fig. 14 Forty-one years-old female with a large mass in the left temporal lobe that is hyperintense on T2WI without enhancement after gadolinium injection. Sagittal view of tractography of the left AF (left panel) and fMRI with the verb generation task showing BOLD response in PMv and MTG (right panel). Note that the activation foci on fMRI are coherently dislocated by the mass with the corti-cal terminations of the three segments of the AF. An oligoastrocitoma WHO-II was removed at surgery. The arrows indicate the direction of AF dislocation. Diffusion data were acquired with HARDI (64 gradient directions, $b = 1000$, $2 \times 2 \times 2$ mm³) and tractography was performed with DTI interpolated streamline algorithm (thresholds FA > 0.15; angle <45°)

resection and minimize hazards. The main tasks used with subcortical IES in the operating room with related responses, short and long-term deficits are reported in Table 1 for each of the three functional systems discussed in this chapter.

5.9 Impact in Clinical Practice

Presurgical evaluation of patients with glioma has been so far the most successful application of DTI in clinical practice. Other clinical research applications of MR diffusion imaging are in rehabilitation after stroke, multiple sclerosis, mild traumatic brain injury, and degenerative diseases (Alzheimer disease, amyotrophic lateral sclerosis). However in these diseases DTI is mainly used as a clinical research tool and it is not yet ready for prime time patient management.

MR diffusion imaging is the only non-invasive method allowing in vivo detection of the trajecto-ries of main WM fascicles and it can provide information whether a tract is displaced, infiltrated/edematous, or interrupted by a tumor. The accuracy of MR tractography for detecting motor and speech pathways has been validated with IES, with 82–97% concordance across studies (Bello et al. 2008; Berman et al. 2004; Leclercq et al. 2010; Ohue et al. 2012). DTI provides unique anatomic information, whereas IES provides functional feedback about eloquent subcortical connections that, if not safeguarded, may result in permanent neurological deficits. In many medical centers worldwide DTI is frequently requested as an integral part of the presurgical workup of brain tumor patients and the FA/DEC maps or the tractograms of the relevant fascicles are frequently uploaded to a neuronavigational device in the operating room together with morphological and functional MR images. Tractograms of the CST, OR, AF, and IFOF are the most requested by neurosurgeons.

In a unique prospective randomized controlled (Class I) trial on 238 consecutive glioma patients it has been shown that DTI tractography has an impact on outcome after resection of HGG but not of LGG involving the CST (Wu et al. 2007). The authors reported that gross total resection of HGG was more likely with MR tractography guidance rather than without and that new postoperative motor deficits were less frequent. The study showed clear benefits in increasing EOR, median overall survival and 6-month KPS score and it is key evidence supporting the use of DTI-aided resection of gliomas, despite a few limitations. In a retrospective study on 190 patients with LGG in eloquent areas, the EOR and the difference between the T2WI and T1WI volumes were the strongest independent predictors in improving OS as well as delaying progression-free survival and malignant transformation (Ius et al. 2012). The presurgical difference between T2WI and post-contrast T1WI volumes may discriminate glioma growing mechanism along the WM: when proliferation is the major mechanism of tumor expansion the mass has a regular bulky shape with an equivalent volume on T2WI and post-contrast T1WI; when WM infiltration is the predominant mechanism of growth, the mass has a more irregular and complex shape with digitations along the WM that is better detected on T2WI than T1WI (Skrap et al. 2012). In addition, in the same study two groups of patients who underwent tumor resection with a different intraoperative protocol including subcortical IES with or without overlap of fMRI and diffusion tractography on a neuronavigational device were compared. Patients with fMRI/DTI had a median EOR of 90%, while those without had a median EOR of 77%.

Presurgical estimate of the expected surgical outcome both in terms of EOR and functional outcome is of great interest for patient's counseling and clinical decision making. Information provided by DTI tractography may be extremely useful to identify the candidates that could maximally benefit from surgery. It has been recently shown that DTI could be a useful tool to estimate the chance of performing a total resection in patients with gliomas located near eloquent areas

(Castellano et al. 2012). In a retrospective tractography study performed in 27 patients with HGG and 46 with LGG, detection of intact fascicles was predictive of a higher probability of total resection. On the contrary, detection of infiltrated or displaced fascicles was predictive of a lower probability of total resection, especially for gliomas with a presurgical volume less than 100 cm^3. Infiltration and even displacement of the CST reduced the chance of achieving a total resection. Moreover, IFOF infiltration in the dominant hemisphere was found predictive of incomplete resection. In particular infiltration of the intermediate third of the IFOF was associated with a very low probability of performing a total resection. On the contrary, no significant correlation was found between infiltration of the SLF/AF and EOR. These results can be explained by considering that the anatomical distribution of the SLF/AF is supposed to be larger than the functional distribution identified by IES, thus a large part of the SLF can be safely resected. The TPFIA is likely another critical area where infiltration or dislocation of the fascicles will likely decrease the chances of a complete resection. Taken together these results emphasize that assessment of WM tracts involvement is an essential part of presurgical evaluation of patients with gliomas in the proximity or within eloquent fascicles and the importance of including HARDI with MR tractography in presurgical imaging protocols.

The value of DTI in performing clinical-anatomical correlations has been shown in a prospective preoperative study on 19 patients with gliomas infiltrating the ventrolateral frontal language areas. Anatomical data provided by DTI tractography was used with the lesion method to identify key structures of the language system responsible for speech deficits. Patients with glioma growing in the left PMv were more likely to presenting with presurgical aphasia than those with glioma infiltrating the IFG, including pars opercularis. However, it was tumor extension to infiltrate or interrupt the AF-direct segment that was associated with preoperative speech deficits, in particular with conduction aphasia (Bizzi et al. 2012).

6 Conclusions

Two decades ago the introduction of DTI changed the way neuroscientists look at WM. Since those first pioneer papers MR diffusion has developed into a sophisticated and complex MR multidisciplinary field with the contribution of physicists, biomedical engineers, mathematicians, cognitive neurologists neuroradiologists, and neurosurgeons. With the development of MR tractography the trajectories of multiple WM fascicles can be identified in vivo in the individual subject and their relationship with a focal lesion can be illustrated and used for presurgical brain mapping. It is now recognized that a detailed understanding of the geometric WM changes induced by a tumor is valuable in order to maximize lesion resection, while avoiding permanent postoperative morbidity. This is particularly true in cases of infiltrating gliomas located within eloquent regions of the brain.

Tractography has gained an undisputed educational reputation for teaching WM architecture. Mapping of WM pathways may improve presurgical planning, surgical targeting with neuronavigational devices and it may reduce intraoperative time. Clinical use of advanced MR imaging tools is growing in importance and exams in patients are being increasingly requested by neurosurgeons worldwide. The role of MR tractography in assisting neurosurgeons to correctly plan subcortical IES and interpret the electrophysiological responses in the operating theater is increasingly recognized by the neurosurgical community.

Although advanced diffusion imaging methods are currently available in most MRI scanners, well beyond the framework of clinical research protocols and academic institutions, they are not yet considered "standard of care." The processes that lead to establishing clinical practice are also quite complex, especially at a time when emphasis on economic difficulties affects health care decisions. Functional MRI and DTI are extremely useful methods that can contribute to improve clinical outcome and to reduce complication rates. As all complex methods they work best when all the members of the team acknowledge their limitations and communicate using a common language.

References

Achard S, Bullmore E (2007) Efficiency and cost of economical brain functional networks. PLoS Comput Biol 3(2):e17. https://doi.org/10.1371/journal.pcbi.0030017

Alexander AL, Hasan K, Kindlmann G, Parker DL, Tsuruda JS (2000) A geometric analysis of diffusion tensor measurements of the human brain. Magn Reson Med 44(2):283–291. http://www.ncbi.nlm.nih.gov/pubmed/10918328

Anwander A, Tittgemeyer M, von Cramon DY, Friederici AD, Knosche TR (2007) Connectivity-based parcellation of Broca's area. Cereb Cortex 17(4):816–825. https://doi.org/10.1093/cercor/bhk034

Assaf Y, Freidlin RZ, Rohde GK, Basser PJ (2004) New modeling and experimental framework to characterize hindered and restricted water diffusion in brain white matter. Magn Reson Med 52(5):965–978. https://doi.org/10.1002/mrm.20274

Assaf Y, Bouznach A, Zomet O et al (2020) Conservation of brain connectivity and wiring across the mammalian class. Nat Neurosci 23:805–808. https://doi.org/10.1038/s41593-020-0641-7

Azevedo FA, Carvalho LR, Grinberg LT, Farfel JM, Ferretti RE, Leite RE, Jacob Filho W, Lent R, Herculano-Houzel S (2009) Equal numbers of neuronal and nonneuronal cells make the human brain an isometrically scaled-up primate brain. J Comp Neurol 513(5):532–541. https://doi.org/10.1002/cne.21974

Bartsch AJ, Geletneky K, Jbabdi S (2013) The temporoparietal fiber intersection area and Wernicke perpendicular fasciculus. Neurosurgery 73(2):E381–E382. https://doi.org/10.1227/01.neu.0000430298.25585.1d

Basser PJ, Mattiello J, LeBihan D (1994) MR diffusion tensor spectroscopy and imaging. Biophys J 66(1):259–267. S0006-3495(94)80775-1 [pii]. https://doi.org/10.1016/S0006-3495(94)80775-1

Basser PJ, Pajevic S, Pierpaoli C, Duda J, Aldroubi A (2000) In vivo fiber tractography using DT-MRI data. Magn Reson Med 44(4):625–632. https://doi.org/10.1002/1522-2594(200010)44:4<625::AID-MRM17>3.0.CO;2-O

Bastin ME, Sinha S, Whittle IR, Wardlaw JM (2002) Measurements of water diffusion and T1 values in peritumoural oedematous brain. Neuroreport 13(10):1335–1340. http://www.ncbi.nlm.nih.gov/pubmed/12151798

Beaulieu C, Does MD, Snyder RE, Allen PS (1996) Changes in water diffusion due to Wallerian degeneration in peripheral nerve. Magn Reson Med 36(4):627–631. http://www.ncbi.nlm.nih.gov/pubmed/8892217

Behrens TEJ, Woolrich MW, Jenkinson M, Johansen-Berg H, Nunes RG, Clare S et al (2003) Characterization and propagation of uncertainty in diffusion-weighted MR imaging. Magn Reson Med 50(5):1077–1088. https://doi.org/10.1002/mrm.10609

Bello L, Acerbi F, Giussani C, Baratta P, Taccone P, Songa V et al (2006) Intraoperative language localization in multilingual patients with gliomas. Neurosurgery 59(1):115–125. http://www.ncbi.nlm.nih.gov/entrez/query.fcgi?cmd=Retrieve&db=PubMed&dopt=Citation&list_uids=16823307

Bello L, Gallucci M, Fava M, Carrabba G, Giussani C, Acerbi F et al (2007) Intraoperative subcortical language tract mapping guides surgical removal of gliomas involving speech areas. Neurosurgery 60(1):67–80; discussion 80–82. https://doi.org/10.1227/01.NEU.0000249206.58601.DE

Bello L, Gambini A, Castellano A, Carrabba G, Acerbi F, Fava E et al (2008) Motor and language DTI Fiber Tracking combined with intraoperative subcortical mapping for surgical removal of gliomas. NeuroImage 39(1):369–382. S1053-8119(07)00754-9 [pii]. https://doi.org/10.1016/j.neuroimage.2007.08.031

Bello L, Fava E, Carrabba G, Papagno C, Gaini SM (2010) Present day's standards in microsurgery of low-grade gliomas. Adv Tech Stand Neurosurg 35:113–157. http://www.ncbi.nlm.nih.gov/pubmed/20102113

Bello L, Riva M, Fava E, Ferpozzi V, Castellano A, Raneri F, Pessina F, Bizzi A, Falini A, Cerri G (2014) Tailoring neurophysiological strategies with clinical context enhances resection and safety and expands indications in gliomas involving motor pathways. Neuro-Oncology 16(8):1110–1128. https://doi.org/10.1093/neuonc/not327

Berman JI, Berger MS, Mukherjee P, Henry RG (2004) Diffusion-tensor imaging-guided tracking of fibers of the pyramidal tract combined with intraoperative cortical stimulation mapping in patients with gliomas. J Neurosurg 101(1):66–72. https://doi.org/10.3171/jns.2004.101.1.0066

Bizzi A, Nava S, Ferrè F, Castelli G, Aquino D, Ciaraffa F et al (2012) Aphasia induced by gliomas growing in the ventrolateral frontal region: assessment with diffusion MR tractography, functional MR imaging and neuropsychology. Cortex 48(2):255–272. https://doi.org/10.1016/j.cortex.2011.11.015

Bloch O, Han SJ, Cha S, Sun MZ, Aghi MK, McDermott MW et al (2012) Impact of extent of resection for recurrent glioblastoma on overall survival. J Neurosurg 117(6):1032–1038. https://doi.org/10.3171/2012.9.JNS12504

Brat DJ, Aldape K, Colman H, Figrarella-Branger D, Fuller GN, Giannini C, Holland EC, Jenkins RB, Kleinschmidt-DeMasters B, Komori T, Kros JM, Louis DN, McLean C, Perry A, Reifenberger G, Sarkar C, Stupp R, van den Bent MJ, von Deimling A, Weller M (2020) cIMPACT-NOW update 5: recommended grading criteria and terminologies for IDH-mutant astrocytomas. Acta Neuropathol 139(3):603–608. https://doi.org/10.1007/s00401-020-02127-9. Epub 2020 Jan 29

Bucci M, Mandelli ML, Berman JI, Amirbekian B, Nguyen C, Berger MS, Henry RG (2013) Quantifying diffusion MRI tractography of the corticospinal tract in brain tumors with deterministic and probabilistic methods. NeuroImage Clin 3:361–368. https://doi.org/10.1016/j.nicl.2013.08.008

Bullmore E, Sporns O (2012) The economy of brain network organization. Nat Rev Neurosci 13(5):336–349. https://doi.org/10.1038/nrn3214

Buschman TJ, Miller EK (2007) Top-down versus bottom-up control of attention in the prefrontal and posterior parietal cortices. Science (New York, NY) 315(5820):1860–1862. https://doi.org/10.1126/science.1138071

Cajal SR (1995) Histology of the Nervous System of Man and Vertebrates New York: Oxford Univ. Press

Caramazza A, Zurif EB (1976) Dissociation of algorithmic and heuristic processes in language comprehension: evidence from aphasia. Brain Lang 3(4):572–582. https://doi.org/10.1016/0093-934x(76)90048-1

Castellano A, Bello L, Michelozzi C, Gallucci M, Fava E, Iadanza A et al (2012) Role of diffusion tensor magnetic resonance tractography in predicting the extent of resection in glioma surgery. Neuro-Oncology 14(2):192–202. https://doi.org/10.1093/neuonc/nor188

Catani M, Bambini V (2014) A model for Social Communication And Language Evolution and Development (SCALED). Curr Opin Neurobiol 28C:165–171. https://doi.org/10.1016/j.conb.2014.07.018

Catani M, Ffytche DH (2005) The rises and falls of disconnection syndromes. Brain 128(Pt 10):2224–2239. https://doi.org/10.1093/brain/awh622

Catani M, Mesulam M (2008) The arcuate fasciculus and the disconnection theme in language and aphasia: history and current state. Cortex 44(8):953–961. S0010-9452(08)00111-1 [pii]. https://doi.org/10.1016/j.cortex.2008.04.002

Catani M, Thiebaut de Schotten M (2008) A diffusion tensor imaging tractography atlas for virtual in vivo dissections. Cortex 44(8):1105–1132

Catani M, Howard RJ, Pajevic S, Jones DK (2002) Virtual in vivo interactive dissection of white matter fasciculi in the human brain. NeuroImage 17(1):77–94

Catani M, Jones DK, Ffytche DH (2005) Perisylvian language networks of the human brain. Ann Neurol 57(1):8–16

Catani M, Allin MP, Husain M, Pugliese L, Mesulam MM, Murray RM, Jones DK (2007) Symmetries in human brain language pathways correlate with verbal recall. Proc Natl Acad Sci U S A 104(43):17163–17168

Catani M, Dell'Acqua F, Vergani F, Malik F, Hodge H, Roy P et al (2012) Short frontal lobe connections of the human brain. Cortex 48(2):273–291

Catani M, Mesulam MM, Jakobsen E, Malik F, Martersteck A, Wieneke C et al (2013) A novel frontal pathway underlies verbal fluency in primary progressive aphasia. Brain 136(Pt 8):2619–2628. https://doi.org/10.1093/brain/awt163

Caverzasi E, Papinutto N, Amirbekian B, Berger MS, Henry RG (2014) Q-ball of inferior fronto-occipital fasciculus and beyond. PLoS One 9(6):e100274. https://doi.org/10.1371/journal.pone.0100274

Cerri G, Shimazu H, Maier MA, Lemon RN (2003) Facilitation from ventral premotor cortex of primary motor cortex outputs to macaque hand muscles. J Neurophysiol 90(2):832–842. https://doi.org/10.1152/jn.01026.2002

Chenevert TL, Brunberg JA, Pipe JG (1990) Anisotropic diffusion in human white matter: demonstration with MR techniques in vivo. Radiology 177(2):401–405. https://doi.org/10.1148/radiology.177.2.2217776

Chun MM, Golomb JD, Turk-Browne NB (2011) A taxonomy of external and internal attention. Annu Rev Psychol 62:73–101. https://doi.org/10.1146/annurev.psych.093008.100427

Ciaraffa F, Castelli G, Parati EA, Bartolomeo P, Bizzi A (2012) Visual neglect as a disconnection syndrome? A confirmatory case report. Neurocase. https://doi.org/10.1080/13554794.2012.667130

Claes A, Idema AJ, Wesseling P (2007) Diffuse glioma growth: a guerilla war. Acta Neuropathol 114(5):443–458. https://doi.org/10.1007/s00401-007-0293-7

Conturo TE, Lori NF, Cull TS, Akbudak E, Snyder AZ, Shimony JS et al (1999) Tracking neuronal fiber pathways in the living human brain. Proc Natl Acad Sci U S A 96(18):10422–10427. http://www.ncbi.nlm.nih.gov/entrez/query.fcgi?cmd=Retrieve&db=PubMed&dopt=Citation&list_uids=10468624

Corbetta M, Shulman GL (2002) Control of goal-directed and stimulus-driven attention in the brain. Nat Rev Neurosci 3(3):201–215. https://doi.org/10.1038/nrn755

Crossley NA, Mechelli A, Scott J, Carletti F, Fox PT, McGuire P, Bullmore ET (2014) The hubs of the human connectome are generally implicated in the anatomy of brain disorders. Brain 137(Pt 8):2382–2395. https://doi.org/10.1093/brain/awu132

De Witt Hamer PC, Moritz-Gasser S, Gatignol P, Duffau H (2011) Is the human left middle longitudinal fascicle essential for language? A brain electrostimulation study. Hum Brain Mapp 32(6):962–973. https://doi.org/10.1002/hbm.21082

Dejerine J, Dejerine-Klumpke A (1895) Anatomies des centres nerveux. Rueff et Cie, Paris

Dell'Acqua F, Scifo P, Rizzo G, Catani M, Simmons A, Scotti G, Fazio F (2010) A modified damped Richardson-Lucy algorithm to reduce isotropic background effects in spherical deconvolution. NeuroImage 49(2):1446–1458. https://doi.org/10.1016/j.neuroimage.2009.09.033

Dell'Acqua F, Simmons A, Williams SCR, Catani M (2013) Can spherical deconvolution provide more information than fiber orientations? Hindrance modulated orientational anisotropy, a true-tract specific index to characterize white matter diffusion. Hum Brain Mapp 34(10):2464–2483. https://doi.org/10.1002/hbm.22080

Doran M, Hajnal JV, Van Bruggen N, King MD, Young IR, Bydder GM (1990) Normal and abnormal white matter tracts shown by MR imaging using directional diffusion weighted sequences. J Comput Assist Tomogr 14(6):865–873. http://www.ncbi.nlm.nih.gov/pubmed/2229559

Doricchi F, Tomaiuolo F (2003) The anatomy of neglect without hemianopia: a key role for parietal-frontal disconnection? Neuroreport 14(17):2239–2243. https://doi.org/10.1097/01.wnr.0000091132.75061.64

Dronkers NF (1996) A new brain region for coordinating speech articulation. Nature 384(6605):159–161. https://doi.org/10.1038/384159a0

Ducreux D, Lepeintre J-F, Fillard P, Loureiro C, Tadié M, Lasjaunias P (2006) MR diffusion tensor imaging and fiber tracking in 5 spinal cord astrocytomas. AJNR Am J Neuroradiol 27(1):214–216. http://www.ncbi.nlm.nih.gov/pubmed/16418387

Duffau H (2005) Intraoperative cortico-subcortical stimulations in surgery of low-grade gliomas. Expert Rev Neurother 5(4):473–485. https://doi.org/10.1586/14737175.5.4.473

Duffau H (2014) The dangers of magnetic resonance imaging diffusion tensor tractography in brain surgery. World Neurosurg 81(1):56–58. https://doi.org/10.1016/j.wneu.2013.01.116

Duffau H, Capelle L (2004) Preferential brain locations of low-grade gliomas. Cancer 100(12):2622–2626. https://doi.org/10.1002/cncr.20297

Duffau H, Gatignol P, Mandonnet E, Peruzzi P, Tzourio-Mazoyer N, Capelle L (2005) New insights into the anatomo-functional connectivity of the semantic system: a study using cortico-subcortical electrostimulations. Brain 128(Pt 4):797–810

Duffau H, Gatignol P, Mandonnet E, Capelle L, Taillandier L (2008a) Intraoperative subcortical stimulation mapping of language pathways in a consecutive series of 115 patients with Grade II glioma in the left dominant hemisphere. J Neurosurg 109(September):461–471. https://doi.org/10.3171/JNS/2008/109/9/0461

Duffau H, Leroy M, Gatignol P (2008b) Cortico-subcortical organization of language networks in the right hemisphere: an electrostimulation study in left-handers. Neuropsychologia 46(14):3197–3209. https://doi.org/10.1016/j.neuropsychologia.2008.07.017

Duyn J (2013) MR susceptibility imaging. J Magn Reson 229:198–207. https://doi.org/10.1016/j.jmr.2012.11.013

Ebeling U, von Cramon D (1992) Topography of the uncinate fascicle and adjacent temporal fiber tracts. Acta Neurochir 115(3-4):143–148. http://www.ncbi.nlm.nih.gov/pubmed/1605083

Eckel-Passow JE, Lachance DH, Molinaro AM, Walsh KM, Decker PA, Sicotte H et al (2015) Glioma groups based on 1p/19q, IDH, and TERT promoter mutations in tumors. N Engl J Med 372:2499–2508. https://doi.org/10.1056/NEJMoa1407279

Field AS, Alexander AL, Wu Y-C, Hasan KM, Witwer B, Badie B (2004) Diffusion tensor eigenvector directional color imaging patterns in the evaluation of cerebral white matter tracts altered by tumor. J Magn Reson Imaging 20(4):555–562. https://doi.org/10.1002/jmri.20169

Ford A, McGregor KM, Case K, Crosson B, White KD (2010) Structural connectivity of Broca's area and medial frontal cortex. NeuroImage 52(4):1230–1237. S1053-8119(10)00725-1 [pii]. https://doi.org/10.1016/j.neuroimage.2010.05.018

Forkel SJ, Thiebaut de Schotten M, Dell'Acqua F, Kalra L, Murphy DGM, Williams SCR, Catani M (2014a) Anatomical predictors of aphasia recovery: a tractography study of bilateral perisylvian language networks. Brain 137(Pt 7):2027–2039. https://doi.org/10.1093/brain/awu113

Forkel SJ, Thiebaut de Schotten M, Kawadler JM, Dell'Acqua F, Danek A, Catani M (2014b) The anatomy of fronto-occipital connections from early blunt dissections to contemporary tractography. Cortex 56:73–84. https://doi.org/10.1016/j.cortex.2012.09.005

Fornia L, Puglisi G, Leonetti A, Bello L, Berti A, Cerri G, Garbarini F (2020) Direct electrical stimulation of the premotor cortex shuts down awareness of voluntary actions. Nat Commun 11:705. https://doi.org/10.1038/s41467-020-14517-4

Fridriksson J, Kjartansson O, Morgan PS, Hjaltason H, Magnusdottir S, Bonilha L, Rorden C (2010) Impaired speech repetition and left parietal lobe damage. J Neurosci 30(33):11057–11061. https://doi.org/10.1523/JNEUROSCI.1120-10.2010

Friederici AD (2011) The brain basis of language processing: from structure to function. Physiol Rev 91(4):1357–1392. https://doi.org/10.1152/physrev.00006.2011

Friederici AD (2012) The cortical language circuit: from auditory perception to sentence comprehension. Trends Cogn Sci 16(5):262–268. https://doi.org/10.1016/j.tics.2012.04.001

Ganslandt O, Stadlbauer A, Fahlbusch R, Kamada K, Buslei R, Blumcke I et al (2005) Proton magnetic resonance spectroscopic imaging integrated into image-guided surgery: correlation to standard magnetic resonance imaging and tumor cell density. Neurosurgery 56(2 Suppl):291–298; discussion 291–298. http://www.ncbi.nlm.nih.gov/pubmed/15794826

Gatignol P, Duffau H, Capelle L, Plaza M (2009) Naming performance in two bilinguals with frontal vs. temporal glioma. Neurocase 15(6):466–477. 912523470 [pii]. https://doi.org/10.1080/13554790902950434

Geschwind N (1970) The organization of language and the brain. Science (New York, NY) 170(3961):940–944. http://www.ncbi.nlm.nih.gov/pubmed/5475022

Giese A, Westphal M (1996) Glioma invasion in the central nervous system. Neurosurgery 39(2):235–250; discussion 250–252. http://www.ncbi.nlm.nih.gov/pubmed/8832660

Glasser MF, Smith SM, Marcus DS, Andersson JL, Auerbach EJ, Behrens TE, Coalson TS, Harms MP, Jenkinson M, Moeller S, Robinson EC, Sotiropoulos SN, Xu J, Yacoub E, Ugurbil K, Van Essen DC (2016) The Human Connectome Project's neuroimaging approach. Nat Neurosci 19(9):1175–1187. https://doi.org/10.1038/nn.4361

Gorno-Tempini ML, Price CJ, Josephs O, Vandenberghe R, Cappa SF, Kapur N et al (1998) The neural systems sustaining face and proper-name processing. Brain 121(Pt 11):2103–2118. http://www.ncbi.nlm.nih.gov/pubmed/9827770

Greenblatt SH (1973) Alexia without agraphia or hemianopsia. Anatomical analysis of an autopsied case. Brain 96(2):307–316

Herbet G, Moritz-Gasser S, Lemaitre A-L, Almairac F, Duffau H (2019) Functional compensation of the left inferior longitudinal fasciculus for picture naming. Cogn Neuropsychol 36(3–4):140–157. https://doi.org/10.1080/02643294.2018.1477749

Hickok G, Poeppel D (2007) The cortical organization of speech processing. Nat Rev Neurosci 8(5):393–402. nrn2113 [pii]. https://doi.org/10.1038/nrn2113

Homola GA, Jbabdi S, Beckmann CF, Bartsch AJ (2012) A brain network processing the age of faces. PLoS One 7(11):e49451. https://doi.org/10.1371/journal.pone.0049451

Ius T, Isola M, Budai R, Pauletto G, Tomasino B, Fadiga L, Skrap M (2012) Low-grade glioma surgery in eloquent areas: volumetric analysis of extent of resection and its impact on overall survival. A single-institution experience in 190 patients: clinical article. J Neurosurg 117(6):1039–1052. https://doi.org/10.3171/2012.8.JNS12393

Jellison BJ, Field AS, Medow J, Lazar M, Salamat MS, Alexander AL (2004) Diffusion tensor imaging of cerebral white matter: a pictorial review of physics, fiber tract anatomy, and tumor imaging patterns. AJNR Am J Neuroradiol 25(3):356–369. http://www.ncbi.nlm.nih.gov/entrez/query.fcgi?cmd=Retrieve&db=PubMed&dopt=Citation&list_uids=15037456

Jenkinson M, Beckmann CF, Behrens TEJ, Woolrich MW, Smith SM (2012) FSL. NeuroImage 62(2):782–790. https://doi.org/10.1016/j.neuroimage.2011.09.015

Jeurissen B, Leemans A, Tournier J-D, Jones DK, Sijbers J (2013) Investigating the prevalence of complex fiber configurations in white matter tissue with diffusion magnetic resonance imaging. Hum Brain Mapp 34(11):2747–2766. https://doi.org/10.1002/hbm.22099

Jones DK (2008) Studying connections in the living human brain with diffusion MRI. Cortex 44(8):936–952. S0010-9452(08)00110-X [pii]. https://doi.org/10.1016/j.cortex.2008.05.002

Keles GE, Berger MS (2004) Advances in neurosurgical technique in the current management of brain tumors. Semin Oncol 31(5):659–665. http://www.ncbi.nlm.nih.gov/pubmed/15497119

Kinoshita M, de Champfleur NM, Deverdun J, Moritz-Gasser S, Herbet G, Duffau H (2014) Role of frontostriatal tract and frontal aslant tract in movement and speech: an axonal mapping study. Brain Struct Funct. https://doi.org/10.1007/s00429-014-0863-0

Krainik A, Lehéricy S, Duffau H, Capelle L, Chainay H, Cornu P et al (2003) Postoperative speech disorder after medial frontal surgery: role of the supplementary motor area. Neurology 60(4):587–594. http://www.ncbi.nlm.nih.gov/pubmed/12601097

Kumar M, Gupta RK, Nath K, Rathore RKS, Bayu G, Trivedi R et al (2008) Can we differentiate true white matter fibers from pseudofibers inside a brain abscess cavity using geometrical diffusion tensor imaging metrics? NMR Biomed 21(6):581–588. https://doi.org/10.1002/nbm.1228

Lawes IN, Barrick TR, Murugam V, Spierings N, Evans DR, Song M, Clark CA (2008) Atlas-based segmentation of white matter tracts of the human brain using diffusion tensor tractography and comparison with classical dissection. NeuroImage 39(1):62–79

Laws ER (2001) Resection of low-grade gliomas. J Neurosurg 95(5):731–732. https://doi.org/10.3171/jns.2001.95.5.0731

Laws ER, Parney IF, Huang W, Anderson F, Morris AM, Asher A et al (2003) Survival following surgery and prognostic factors for recently diagnosed malignant glioma: data from the Glioma Outcomes Project. J Neurosurg 99(3):467–473. https://doi.org/10.3171/jns.2003.99.3.0467

Leclercq D, Duffau H, Delmaire C, Capelle L, Gatignol P, Ducros M et al (2010) Comparison of diffusion tensor imaging tractography of language tracts and intraoperative subcortical stimulations. J Neurosurg 112(3):503–511. https://doi.org/10.3171/2009.8.JNS09558

Leemans A, Jeurissen B, Sijbers J, Jones DK (2009) ExploreDTI: a graphical toolbox for processing, analyzing and visualizing diffusion MR data. ISMRM Annu Meeting Proc 17:3537

Lehéricy S, Ducros M, Krainik A, Francois C, Van de Moortele P-F, Ugurbil K, Kim D-S (2004) 3-D diffusion tensor axonal tracking shows distinct SMA and pre-SMA projections to the human striatum. Cereb Cortex 14(12):1302–1309. https://doi.org/10.1093/cercor/bhh091

Lemon RN (2008) Descending pathways in motor control. Annu Rev Neurosci 31:195–218. https://doi.org/10.1146/annurev.neuro.31.060407.125547

Lemon RN, Griffiths J (2005) Comparing the function of the corticospinal system in different species: organizational differences for motor specialization? Muscle Nerve 32(3):261–279. https://doi.org/10.1002/mus.20333

Louis DN, Ohgaki H, Wiestler OD, Cavenee WK et al (2007) WHO classification of tumors of the central nervous system. IARC Press, Lyon, France

Louis DN, Perry A, Reifenberger G, von Deimling A, Figarella-Branger D, Cavenee WK et al (2016) The 2016 World Health Organization Classification of tumors of the central nervous system: a summary. Acta Neuropathol 131:803–820. https://doi.org/10.1007/s00401-016-1545-1

Ludwig E, Klingler J (1956) Atlas cerebri humani. Little, Brown and Company, Boston, MA

Makris N, Pandya DN (2009) The extreme capsule in humans and rethinking of the language circuitry. Brain Struct Funct 213(3):343–358. https://doi.org/10.1007/s00429-008-0199-8

Makris N, Kennedy DN, McInerney S, Sorensen AG, Wang R, Caviness VS, Pandya DN (2005) Segmentation of subcomponents within the superior longitudinal fascicle in humans: a quantitative, in vivo, DT-MRI study.

Cereb Cortex 15(6):854–869. https://doi.org/10.1093/cercor/bhh186

Makris N, Papadimitriou GM, Kaiser JR, Sorg S, Kennedy DN, Pandya DN (2009) Delineation of the middle longitudinal fascicle in humans: a quantitative, in vivo, DT-MRI study. Cereb Cortex 19(4):777–785. bhn124 [pii]. https://doi.org/10.1093/cercor/bhn124

Maldonado IL, Moritz-Gasser S, de Champfleur NM, Bertram L, Moulinié G, Duffau H (2011a) Surgery for gliomas involving the left inferior parietal lobule: new insights into the functional anatomy provided by stimulation mapping in awake patients. J Neurosurg 115(4):770–779. https://doi.org/10.3171/2011.5.JNS112

Maldonado IL, Moritz-Gasser S, Duffau H (2011b) Does the left superior longitudinal fascicle subserve language semantics? A brain electrostimulation study. Brain Struct Funct 216(3):263–274. https://doi.org/10.1007/s00429-011-0309-x

Mandelli ML, Berger MS, Bucci M, Berman JI, Amirbekian B, Henry RG (2014) Quantifying accuracy and precision of diffusion MR tractography of the corticospinal tract in brain tumors. J Neurosurg 121(2):349–358. https://doi.org/10.3171/2014.4.JNS131160

Mandonnet E, Jbabdi S, Taillandier L, Galanaud D, Benali H, Capelle L, Duffau H (2007a) Preoperative estimation of residual volume for WHO grade II glioma resected with intraoperative functional mapping. Neuro-Oncology 9(1):63–69. https://doi.org/10.1215/15228517-2006-015

Mandonnet E, Nouet A, Gatignol P, Capelle L, Duffau H (2007b) Does the left inferior longitudinal fasciculus play a role in language? A brain stimulation study. Brain 130(Pt 3):623–629

Mandonnet E, Gatignol P, Duffau H (2009) Evidence for an occipito-temporal tract underlying visual recognition in picture naming. Clin Neurol Neurosurg 111(7):601–605. https://doi.org/10.1016/j.clineuro.2009.03.007

Martino J, Brogna C, Robles SG, Vergani F, Duffau H (2010) Anatomic dissection of the inferior fronto-occipital fasciculus revisited in the lights of brain stimulation data. Cortex 46(5):691–699. https://doi.org/10.1016/j.cortex.2009.07.015

Martino J, De Witt Hamer PC, Vergani F, Brogna C, de Lucas EM, Vázquez-Barquero A et al (2011) Cortex-sparing fiber dissection: an improved method for the study of white matter anatomy in the human brain. J Anat 219(4):531–541. https://doi.org/10.1111/j.1469-7580.2011.01414.x

Martino J, da Silva-Freitas R, Caballero H, Marco de Lucas E, García-Porrero JA, Vázquez-Barquero A (2013) Fiber dissection and diffusion tensor imaging tractography study of the temporoparietal fiber intersection area. Neurosurgery 72(1 Suppl Operative):87–97; discussion 97–8. https://doi.org/10.1227/NEU.0b013e318274294b

Mawrin C (2005) Molecular genetic alterations in gliomatosis cerebri: what can we learn about the origin and course of the disease? Acta Neuropathol 110(6): 527–536. https://doi.org/10.1007/s00401-005-1083-8

Menjot de Champfleur N, Lima Maldonado I, Moritz-Gasser S, Machi P, Le Bars E, Bonafé A, Duffau H (2013) Middle longitudinal fasciculus delineation within language pathways: a diffusion tensor imaging study in human. Eur J Radiol 82(1):151–157. https://doi.org/10.1016/j.ejrad.2012.05.034

Meynert TH (1887) In: Sachs BT (ed) A clinical treatise on diseases of the fore-brain based upon a study of its structure, functions, and nutrition. G.P. Putman's Sons, New York

Miraillé C (1896) De laphasie sensorielle. G. Steinheil, Paris. http://gallica.bnf.fr/ark:/12148/bpt6k5711953h. Accessed 2 Jan 2021

Mori S, Crain BJ, Chacko VP, van Zijl PC (1999) Three-dimensional tracking of axonal projections in the brain by magnetic resonance imaging. Ann Neurol 45(2):265–269. http://www.ncbi.nlm.nih.gov/entrez/query.fcgi?cmd=Retrieve&db=PubMed&dopt=Citation&list_uids=9989633

Müller-Oehring EM, Kasten E, Poggel DA, Schulte T, Strasburger H, Sabel BA (2003) Neglect and hemianopia superimposed. J Clin Exp Neuropsychol 25(8):1154–1168. https://doi.org/10.1076/jcen.25.8.1154.16727

Naeser MA, Palumbo CL, Helm-Estabrooks N, Stiassny-Eder D, Albert ML (1989) Severe nonfluency in aphasia. Role of the medial subcallosal fasciculus and other white matter pathways in recovery of spontaneous speech. Brain 112(Pt 1):1–38. http://www.ncbi.nlm.nih.gov/pubmed/2917272

Nimsky C, Ganslandt O, Hastreiter P, Wang R, Benner T, Sorensen AG, Fahlbusch R (2005) Intraoperative diffusion-tensor MR imaging: shifting of white matter tracts during neurosurgical procedures—initial experience. Radiology 234(1):218–225

Nimsky C, Ganslandt O, Fahlbusch R (2007) Implementation of fiber tract navigation. Neurosurgery 58(1 Suppl):306–318

Ohue S, Kohno S, Inoue A, Yamashita D, Harada H, Kumon Y et al (2012) Accuracy of diffusion tensor magnetic resonance imaging-based tractography for surgery of gliomas near the pyramidal tract: a significant correlation between subcortical electrical stimulation and postoperative tractography. Neurosurgery 70(2):283–93; discussion 294. https://doi.org/10.1227/NEU.0b013e31823020e6

Oishi K, Zilles K, Amunts K, Faria A, Jiang H, Li X et al (2008) Human brain white matter atlas: identification and assignment of common anatomical structures in superficial white matter. NeuroImage 43(3):447–457

Owen JP, Li YO, Ziv E, Strominger Z, Gold J, Bukhpun P, Wakahiro M, Friedman EJ, Sherr EH, Mukherjee P (2013) The structural connectome of the human brain in agenesis of the corpus callosum. NeuroImage 70:340–355. https://doi.org/10.1016/j.neuroimage.2012.12.031

Pajevic S, Pierpaoli C (1999) Color schemes to represent the orientation of anisotropic tissues from diffusion tensor data: application to white matter fiber tract mapping in the human brain. Magn Reson Med 42(3):526–540. http://www.ncbi.nlm.nih.gov/pubmed/10467297

Pallud J, Blonski M, Mandonnet E, Audureau E, Fontaine D, Sanai N et al (2013) Velocity of tumor spontaneous expansion predicts long-term outcomes for diffuse low-grade gliomas. Neuro-Oncology 15(5):595–606. https://doi.org/10.1093/neuonc/nos331

Papadogiorgaki M, Koliou P, Kotsiakis X, Zervakis ME (2013) Mathematical modelling of spatio-temporal glioma evolution. Theor Biol Med Model 10:47. https://doi.org/10.1186/1742-4682-10-47

Papagno C, Miracapillo C, Casarotti A, Romero Lauro LJ, Castellano A, Falini A et al (2010) What is the role of the uncinate fasciculus? Surgical removal and proper name retrieval. Brain. awq283 [pii]. https://doi.org/10.1093/brain/awq283

Papagno C, Casarotti A, Comi A, Pisoni A, Lucchelli F, Bizzi A, Riva M, Bello L (2016) Long-term proper name anomia after removal of the uncinate fasciculus. Brain Struct Funct 221(1):687–694. https://doi.org/10.1007/s00429-014-0920-8. Epub 2014 Oct 28

Penfield W, Rasmussen T (1950) The cerebral cortex of man: a clinical study of localization of function. Macmillan, New York

Petrella JR, Shah LM, Harris KM, Friedman AH, George TM, Sampson JH et al (2006) Preoperative functional MR imaging localization of language and motor areas: effect on therapeutic decision making in patients with potentially resectable brain tumors. Radiology 240(3):793–802. https://doi.org/10.1148/radiol.2403051153

Petrides M, Pandya DN (1984) Projections to the frontal cortex from the posterior parietal region in the rhesus monkey. J Comp Neurol 228(1):105–116. https://doi.org/10.1002/cne.902280110

Petrides M, Pandya DN (1988) Association fiber pathways to the frontal cortex from the superior temporal region in the rhesus monkey. J Comp Neurol 273:52–66

Pierpaoli C, Jezzard P, Basser PJ, Barnett A, Di Chiro G (1996) Diffusion tensor MR imaging of the human brain. Radiology 201(3):637–648. http://www.ncbi.nlm.nih.gov/entrez/query.fcgi?cmd=Retrieve&db=PubMed&dopt=Citation&list_uids=8939209

Pierpaoli C, Walker L, Irfanoglu MO, Barnett A, Basser P, Chang L-C et al (2010) TORTOISE: an integrated software package for processing of diffusion MRI data. ISMRM Annu Meeting Proc 18:1597

Plaza M, Gatignol P, Leroy M, Duffau H (2009) Speaking without Broca's area after tumor resection. Neurocase 15(4):294–310. 909314371 [pii]. https://doi.org/10.1080/13554790902729473

Posner MI (1980) Orienting of attention. Q J Exp Psychol 32(1):3–25. http://www.ncbi.nlm.nih.gov/pubmed/7367577

Price CJ (2010) The anatomy of language: a review of 100 fMRI studies published in 2009. Ann N Y

Acad Sci 1191:62–88. NYAS5444 [pii]. https://doi.
org/10.1111/j.1749-6632.2010.05444.x

Price SJ, Jena R, Burnet NG, Hutchinson PJ, Dean AF,
Peña A et al (2006) Improved delineation of glioma
margins and regions of infiltration with the use of diffusion tensor imaging: an image-guided biopsy study.
AJNR Am J Neuroradiol 27(9):1969–1974. http://
www.ncbi.nlm.nih.gov/pubmed/17032877

Puglisi G, Howells H, Sciortino T, Leonetti A, Rossi M,
Conti Nibali M, Gabriel Gay L, Fornia L, Bellacicca
A, Viganò L, Simone L, Catani M, Cerri G, Bello L
(2019) Frontal pathways in cognitive control: direct
evidence from intraoperative stimulation and diffusion
tractography. Brain 142(8):2451–2465. https://doi.
org/10.1093/brain/awz178

Pujol J, Deus J, Losilla JM, Capdevila A (1999) Cerebral
lateralization of language in normal left-handed
people studied by functional MRI. Neurology
52(5):1038–1043.   http://www.ncbi.nlm.nih.gov/
pubmed/10102425

Quiñones-Hinojosa A, Ojemann SG, Sanai N, Dillon WP,
Berger MS (2003) Preoperative correlation of intraoperative cortical mapping with magnetic resonance
imaging landmarks to predict localization of the Broca
area. J Neurosurg 99(2):311–318

Rathelot J-A, Strick PL (2006) Muscle representation in
the macaque motor cortex: an anatomical perspective.
Proc Natl Acad Sci U S A 103(21):8257–8262. https://
doi.org/10.1073/pnas.0602933103

Rathelot J-A, Strick PL (2009) Subdivisions of primary
motor cortex based on cortico-motoneuronal cells.
Proc Natl Acad Sci U S A 106(3):918–923. https://doi.
org/10.1073/pnas.0808362106

Robles SG, Gatignol P, Lehéricy S, Duffau H (2008) Long-
term brain plasticity allowing a multistage surgical
approach to World Health Organization Grade II gliomas in eloquent areas. J Neurosurg 109(4):615–624

Rohde GK, Barnett AS, Basser PJ, Marenco S, Pierpaoli
C (2004) Comprehensive approach for correction of motion and distortion in diffusion-weighted
MRI. Magn Reson Med 51(1):103–114. https://doi.
org/10.1002/mrm.10677

Rolheiser T, Stamatakis EA, Tyler LK (2011) Dynamic
processing in the human language system: synergy between the arcuate fascicle and extreme capsule. J Neurosci 31(47):16949–16957. https://doi.
org/10.1523/JNEUROSCI.2725-11.2011

Sanai N, Mirzadeh Z, Berger MS (2008) Functional outcome after language mapping for glioma resection. N
Engl J Med 358:18–27

Sanai N, Martino J, Berger MS (2012) Morbidity profile
following aggressive resection of parietal lobe gliomas. J Neurosurg 116(6):1182–1186. https://doi.org/
10.3171/2012.2.JNS111228

Sati P, van Gelderen P, Silva AC, Reich DS, Merkle H, de
Zwart JA, Duyn JH (2013) Micro-compartment specific
T2* relaxation in the brain. NeuroImage 77:268–278.
https://doi.org/10.1016/j.neuroimage.2013.03.005

Saur D, Kreher BW, Schnell S, Kummerer D, Kellmeyer
P, Vry MS et al (2008) Ventral and dorsal pathways for

language. Proc Natl Acad Sci U S A 105(46):18035–
18040. 0805234105 [pii]. https://doi.org/10.1073/
pnas.0805234105

Saur D, Schelter B, Schnell S, Kratochvil D, Kupper
H, Kellmeyer P et al (2010) Combining functional
and anatomical connectivity reveals brain networks
for auditory language comprehension. NeuroImage
49(4):3187–3197.   S1053-8119(09)01193-8   [pii].
https://doi.org/10.1016/j.neuroimage.2009.11.009

Schmahmann JD, Pandya DN (2006) Fiber pathways of
the brain. Oxford University Press, Oxford

Schmahmann JD, Pandya DN, Wang R, Dai G, D'Arceuil
HE, de Crespigny AJ, Wedeen VJ (2007) Association
fibre pathways of the brain: parallel observations from
diffusion spectrum imaging and autoradiography.
Brain 130(Pt 3):630–653. https://doi.org/10.1093/
brain/awl359

Schonberg T, Pianka P, Hendler T, Pasternak O, Assaf
Y (2006) Characterization of displaced white matter by brain tumors using combined DTI and
fMRI. NeuroImage 30(4):1100–1111. https://doi.
org/10.1016/j.neuroimage.2005.11.015

Seunarine KK, Alexander DC (2009) Multiple fibers:
beyond the diffusion tensor. In: Johansen-Berg H,
Behrens TE (eds) Diffusion MRI: from quantitative measurement to in vivo neuroanatomy. Elsevier,
Oxford, UK, pp 55–72

Skrap M, Mondani M, Tomasino B, Weis L, Budai R,
Pauletto G et al (2012) Surgery of insular nonenhancing gliomas: volumetric analysis of tumoral resection, clinical outcome, and survival in a consecutive
series of 66 cases. Neurosurgery 70(5):1081–1093.;
discussion   1093–1094.   https://doi.org/10.1227/
NEU.0b013e31823f5be5

Smith JS, Chang EF, Lamborn KR, Chang SM, Prados
MD, Cha S et al (2008) Role of extent of resection
in the long-term outcome of low-grade hemispheric
gliomas. J Clin Oncol 26(8):1338–1345. https://doi.
org/10.1200/JCO.2007.13.9337

Smits M, Vernooij MW, Wielopolski PA, Vincent AJPE,
Houston GC, van der Lugt A (2007) Incorporating
functional MR imaging into diffusion tensor tractography in the preoperative assessment of the corticospinal tract in patients with brain tumors. AJNR
Am J Neuroradiol 28(7):1354–1361. https://doi.
org/10.3174/ajnr.A0538

Sporns O (2014) Contributions and challenges for network models in cognitive neuroscience. Nat Neurosci
17(5):652–660. https://doi.org/10.1038/nn.3690

Stummer W, Reulen H-J, Meinel T, Pichlmeier U,
Schumacher W, Tonn J-C et al (2008) Extent of resection and survival in glioblastoma multiforme: identification of and adjustment for bias. Neurosurgery
62(3):564–576.; discussion 564–576. https://doi.
org/10.1227/01.neu.0000317304.31579.17

Stummer W, Tonn J-C, Mehdorn HM, Nestler U, Franz
K, Goetz C et al (2011) Counterbalancing risks and
gains from extended resections in malignant glioma
surgery: a supplemental analysis from the randomized 5-aminolevulinic acid glioma resection study.

Clinical article. J Neurosurg 114(3):613–623. https://doi.org/10.3171/2010.3.JNS097

Stupp R, Hegi ME (2013) Brain cancer in 2012: molecular characterization leads the way. Nat Rev Clin Oncol 10(2):69–70. https://doi.org/10.1038/nrclinonc.2012.240

Stupp R, Mason WP, van den Bent MJ, Weller M, Fisher B, Taphoorn MJB et al (2005) Radiotherapy plus concomitant and adjuvant temozolomide for glioblastoma. N Engl J Med 352(10):987–996. https://doi.org/10.1056/NEJMoa043330

Sturm D, Witt H, Hovestadt V, Khuong-Quang D-A, Jones DTW, Konermann C et al (2012) Hotspot mutations in H3F3A and IDH1 define distinct epigenetic and biological subgroups of glioblastoma. Cancer Cell 22(4):425–437. https://doi.org/10.1016/j.ccr.2012.08.024

Thiebaut de Schotten M, Urbanski M, Duffau H, Volle E, Levy R, Dubois B, Bartolomeo P (2005) Direct evidence for a parietal-frontal pathway subserving spatial awareness in humans. Science 309:2226

Thiebaut de Schotten M, Kinkingnéhun S, Delmaire C, Lehéricy S, Duffau H, Thivard L et al (2008) Visualization of disconnection syndromes in humans. Cortex 44(8):1097–1103. https://doi.org/10.1016/j.cortex.2008.02.003

Thiebaut de Schotten M, Dell'Acqua F, Forkel SJ, Simmons A, Vergani F, Murphy DGM, Catani M (2011a) A lateralized brain network for visuospatial attention. Nat Neurosci 14(10):1245–1246. https://doi.org/10.1038/nn.2905

Thiebaut de Schotten M, Ffytche DH, Bizzi A, Dell'Acqua F, Allin M, Walshe M et al (2011b) Atlasing location, asymmetry and inter-subject variability of white matter tracts in the human brain with MR diffusion tractography. NeuroImage 54(1):49–59. https://doi.org/10.1016/j.neuroimage.2010.07.055

Thiebaut de Schotten M, Dell'Acqua F, Valabregue R, Catani M (2012) Monkey to human comparative anatomy of the frontal lobe association tracts. Cortex 48(1):82–96. https://doi.org/10.1016/j.cortex.2011.10.001

Thiebaut de Schotten M, Tomaiuolo F, Aiello M, Merola S, Silvetti M, Lecce F et al (2014) Damage to white matter pathways in subacute and chronic spatial neglect: a group study and 2 single-case studies with complete virtual "in vivo" tractography dissection. Cereb Cortex 24(3):691–706. https://doi.org/10.1093/cercor/bhs351

Thomas L, Di Stefano AL, Ducray F (2013) Predictive biomarkers in adult gliomas: the present and the future. Curr Opin Oncol 25(6):689–694. https://doi.org/10.1097/CCO.0000000000000002

Tournier J-D, Calamante F, Gadian DG, Connelly A (2004) Direct estimation of the fiber orientation density function from diffusion-weighted MRI data using spherical deconvolution. NeuroImage 23(3):1176–1185. https://doi.org/10.1016/j.neuroimage.2004.07.037

Tuch DS (2004) Q-ball imaging. Magn Reson Med 52(6):1358–1372. https://doi.org/10.1002/mrm.20279

Tyler LK, Marslen-Wilson WD, Randall B, Wright P, Devereux BJ, Zhuang J et al (2011) Left inferior frontal cortex and syntax: function, structure and behaviour in patients with left hemisphere damage. Brain 134(Pt 2):415–431. https://doi.org/10.1093/brain/awq369

Vallar G, Bello L, Bricolo E, Castellano A, Casarotti A, Falini A et al (2014) Cerebral correlates of visuospatial neglect: a direct cerebral stimulation study. Hum Brain Mapp 35(4):1334–1350. https://doi.org/10.1002/hbm.22257

Van den Heuvel MP, Sporns O (2011) Rich-club organization of the human connectome. J Neurosci 31(44):15775–15786. https://doi.org/10.1523/JNEUROSCI.3539-11.2011

Van den Heuvel MP, Sporns O (2013) Network hubs in the human brain. Trends Cogn Sci 17(12):683–696. https://doi.org/10.1016/j.tics.2013.09.012

Vassal F, Schneider F, Sontheimer A, Lemaire J-J, Nuti C (2013) Intraoperative visualisation of language fascicles by diffusion tensor imaging-based tractography in glioma surgery. Acta Neurochir 155(3):437–448. https://doi.org/10.1007/s00701-012-1580-1

Vergani F, Lacerda L, Martino J, Attems J, Morris C, Mitchell P et al (2014) White matter connections of the supplementary motor area in humans. J Neurol Neurosurg Psychiatry. https://doi.org/10.1136/jnnp-2013-307492

Vidorreta JG, Garcia R, Moritz-Gasser S, Duffau H (2011) Double dissociation between syntactic gender and picture naming processing: a brain stimulation mapping study. Hum Brain Mapp 32(3):331–340. https://doi.org/10.1002/hbm.21026

Vuorinen V, Hinkka S, Färkkilä M, Jääskeläinen J (2003) Debulking or biopsy of malignant glioma in elderly people - a randomised study. Acta Neurochir 145(1):5–10. https://doi.org/10.1007/s00701-002-1030-6

Wang S, Kim S, Chawla S, Wolf RL, Zhang W-G, O'Rourke DM et al (2009) Differentiation between glioblastomas and solitary brain metastases using diffusion tensor imaging. NeuroImage 44(3):653–660. https://doi.org/10.1016/j.neuroimage.2008.09.027

Wedeen VJ, Wang RP, Schmahmann JD, Benner T, Tseng WYI, Dai G et al (2008) Diffusion spectrum magnetic resonance imaging (DSI) tractography of crossing fibers. NeuroImage 41(4):1267–1277. https://doi.org/10.1016/j.neuroimage.2008.03.036

Wedeen VJ, Rosene DL, Wang R, Dai G, Mortazavi F, Hagmann P et al (2012) The geometric structure of the brain fiber pathways. Science 335(6076):1628–1634. https://doi.org/10.1126/science.1215280

Weller M, Stupp R, Hegi ME, van den Bent M, Tonn JC, Sanson M et al (2012) Personalized care in neuro-oncology coming of age: why we need MGMT and 1p/19q testing for malignant glioma patients in clinical practice. Neuro-Oncology 14(Suppl 4):iv100–iv108. https://doi.org/10.1093/neuonc/nos206

Wu J-S, Zhou L-F, Tang W-J, Mao Y, Hu J, Song Y-Y et al (2007) Clinical evaluation and follow-up outcome of diffusion tensor imaging-based functional neuronavigation: a prospective, controlled study in patients with gliomas involving pyramidal tracts. Neurosurgery 61(5):935–948.; discussion 948–949. https://doi.org/10.1227/01.neu.0000303189.80049.ab

Yakovlev PI, Locke S (1961) Corticocortical connections of the anterior cingulate gyrus; te cingulum and subcallosal bundle. Trans Am Neurol Assoc 86:252–256. http://www.ncbi.nlm.nih.gov/pubmed/14008718

Yamada K, Sakai K, Hoogenraad FGC, Holthuizen R, Akazawa K, Ito H et al (2007) Multitensor tractography enables better depiction of motor pathways: initial clinical experience using diffusion-weighted MR imaging with standard b-value. AJNR Am J Neuroradiol 28(9):1668–1673. https://doi.org/10.3174/ajnr.A0640

Yordanova YN, Moritz-Gasser S, Duffau H (2011) Awake surgery for WHO Grade II gliomas within "noneloquent" areas in the left dominant hemisphere: toward a "supratotal" resection. Clinical article. J Neurosurg 115(2):232–239. https://doi.org/10.3171/2011.3. JNS101333

Zamecnik J (2005) The extracellular space and matrix of gliomas. Acta Neuropathol 110(5):435–442. https://doi.org/10.1007/s00401-005-1078-5

Zhang H, Schneider T, Wheeler-Kingshott CA, Alexander DC (2012) NODDI: practical in vivo neurite orientation dispersion and density imaging of the human brain. NeuroImage 61(4):1000–1016. https://doi.org/10.1016/j.neuroimage.2012.03.072

Functional Neuronavigation

Volker M. Tronnier and Lennart H. Stieglitz

Contents

V. M. Tronnier (✉)
Department of Neurosurgery, Universitätsklinikum
Schleswig-Holstein, Lübeck, Germany
e-mail: Volker.Tronnier@uksh.de

L. H. Stieglitz
Functional and Stereotactic Neurosurgery Unit,
Department of Neurosurgery, University Hospital
Zurich, Zurich, Switzerland
e-mail: lennart.stieglitz@usz.ch

© The Author(s), under exclusive license to Springer Nature Switzerland AG 2022
C. Stippich (ed.), *Clinical Functional MRI*, Medical Radiology Diagnostic Imaging,
https://doi.org/10.1007/978-3-030-83343-5_8

Abstract

Functional neuronavigation is based on the
visualization of functional images within a
surgical tracking system. This and other developing techniques help the neurosurgeon to tai-
lor surgical procedures in order to increase
diagnostic yield and to preserve brain function
while maximizing the necessary extent of
resection. The final goal is to improve postoperative survival and quality of life. A major
advantage of functional imaging, over other
functional brain mapping techniques, such as
direct cortical stimulation (Electrical Cortical
Stimulation, ECS) is its non-invasiveness.
Furthermore, availability of functional information to the surgeon and patient prior to surgery provides insight not only into a better
evaluation of the procedure's indication, but
also into the planning of a function preserving
operation including the most appropriate surgical access to the respective brain areas. In
order to implement functional neuronavigation into the daily clinical routine, optimized
imaging protocols are indispensable.

regions by detecting indirect effects of neural
activity on local blood volume, flow and oxygen
saturation. Electroencephalography (EEG) and
magnetoencephalography (MEG) allow direct
assessment of the brain's electrophysiology by
displaying the temporal and spatial pattern of the
neuronal populations generating the underlying
neuroelectric and neuromagnetic fields. Positron
Emission Tomography (PET) and Single Photon
Emission Tomography (SPECT) imaging do not
only provide hemodynamic but also metabolic
information, which also holds true for Magnetic
Resonance Spectroscopy (MRS). Subcortical
structures as pyramidal tracts, commissural and
association fibers can nowadays also be integrated in the surgical workflow with
DTI-tractography.

The following chapter will focus on functional
neuronavigation for surgery in eloquent brain
areas. In addition, the importance of functional
imaging in stereotaxy and procedures for pain
and movement disorders will be outlined. Since a
separate chapter (chapter "Simultaneous EEG-
fMRI in Epilepsy") is dedicated to epilepsy surgery, this topic will not be addressed in this
chapter.

1   Introduction

While anatomical MR imaging is widely implemented and has revolutionized surgical decision
making and planning, the emergence of functional neuroimaging techniques localizing brain
activity has significantly expanded the presurgical role of the different imaging modalities. Non-
invasive functional MRI (fMRI) provides the
neurosurgeon with images of activated brain

2   Principles and Technical Aspects of Neuronavigation and Stereotaxy

2.1   Neuronavigation

The development of neuronavigation systems
was a major technical advance in neurosurgery,
especially for small lesions localized in deep or
subcortical regions, where anatomical landmarks

are not available. Such systems facilitate the navigation towards lesions tightly focused avoiding the destruction of eloquent brain areas, in particular when the anatomy is distorted by brain tumors, etc. All navigational systems consist of similar components: The key instrument is a three-dimensional digitizing device (pointer, forceps, ultrasound probe, or other localization device) which enables the surgeon to localize the targets within the physical space (surgical site). This device is linked to a computer where the same targets are displayed on preoperative three-dimensional images. The interface is a reference system, which defines fiducial markers aligning the physical space to the imaging coordinate system. Although morphological information is usually assessed by 3D-T1-weighted MR images with gadolinium for contrast-enhancing lesions or T2-weighted and flair images, respectively, for low-grade gliomas, CT can be used for lesions at the skull base or in the case of maxillofacial, ear-nose-throat and spinal procedures. Different navigational systems are on the market: Arm-based systems with grading scales in usually six joints, providing six degrees of freedom. Based on the known position of the joints by electrogoniometers and the length of the phalanges, the position of a particular instrument connected to the arm can be calculated. The main problem of these arm-based devices is that they are not suitable for fixing the arm in a specific position, which therefore has to be done by the surgeon manually. Therefore, these systems disappeared from the operating theater in favor of wire-connected or wireless pointers.

Optical or acoustic devices based on the principle of satellite navigation are better suitable. These devices work with two or three detecting instruments (IR-cameras, video-or ultrasound systems) with a fixed relationship in space. The distance to active markers (e.g., LEDs) or passive reflectors is calculated via a triangulation method. Obstacles within the line of view, such as the operating microscope can interfere with this type of navigation. One solution is the tracking of the microscope itself, where the focus within the ocular serves as the image-guided "pointer." Computer systems allow the rapid transformation

and correction of new coordinates. Magnetic fields can alternatively serve as detection method, allowing for small attachable references and malleable instruments. Magnetic tracking is often used in patients where surgery without fixation of the skull is required (as in ENT or maxillofacial procedures). However, interference with metallic instruments can lead to inaccuracies (Mascott 2005).

The accuracy of navigational devices depends on the accuracy of the co-registration, e.g., the localization of the patient's individual anatomy on preoperatively acquired images. Determination of registered points in a volume around the suspected lesion is important in order to achieve the highest accuracy in all three planes. For instance, movement of the galea and the skin by head fixation or different patient positioning compared to the supine position inside the scanner creates inaccuracies. Therefore, laser scanning methods detecting the surface of the face with several hundred points increase registration accuracy.

After completion of the registration, each anatomical point can be displayed on a navigational computer. Due to the high amount of data and the need for a rapid image transformation powerful workstations are required for high-end navigational devices.

The use of fMRI or other functional imaging modalities provides additional information, which is helpful for the planning of a tailored tumor resection while minimizing damage to functional areas. Therefore, the integration of functional data with the anatomical information has strongly been endorsed by neurosurgeons and is now possible via so-called functional neuronavigation. The introduction of these frameless intraoperative neuronavigation systems allows the precise co-registration and transfer of fMRI data into the surgical field. Nowadays techniques for displaying sensorimotor, visual, language, and cognitive functions as well as DTI fiber tracking are available as outlined in more detail below.

The sequence of events for functional neuronavigation is as follows:

fMRI should be carried out according to a standardized paradigm protocol (see chapter

"Task-Based Presurgical Functional MRI in Patients with Brain Tumors") at least 1 day prior to neuronavigation-assisted surgery. This ensures sufficient time for the neuroradiologist to analyze the fMRI data, which is still a very labor-intensive task. It also enables the neurosurgeon to critically evaluate the navigational data and plan the surgical approach accordingly. In the same MRI session, a three-dimensional morphological MRI scan is acquired as a reference of co-registration.

The combined functional-anatomical data set is then sent either to the neuronavigation system in the operation room (OR), or to a separate planning station outside the OR for further processing. The boundaries of elements of interest (tumor, vessels, ventricles, etc.) can be outlined and colored in different slices displayed by MRI or CT. The following three-dimensional reconstruction allows a 3-D display of these structures, which facilitates surgical planning. Some commercial neuronavigation software solutions allow automated identification of anatomical structures based on automated volumetric image analysis or on atlas-based segmentation.

At the time of (brain-) surgery, the head is usually fixed in a head holder (Mayfield, Sugita, etc.), to which the registration system (a three to four point star in most optical devices or a magnetic reference) is securely connected. The camera system is adjusted to the surgical field and the surgical microscope. If fiducial markers are used (and no laser scanning method), all defined fiducial markers taped to the patients head have to be identified in the imaging data set for a patient-to-image registration using a rigid body transformation. Alternatively, anatomical landmarks can be defined, and these landmarks can be registered with a pointer using a zoomed image to reach higher accuracy. At least four markers or landmarks are required. However, accuracy correlates with the numbers of registered points. Therefore, in clinical use most often 6–7 fiducial markers are registered. Most modern systems nowadays offer an automated surface matching method, where numerous recognizable points are marked with a laser pointer and detected by three cameras. The computer calculates the best correspondence between the anatomical and imaging data, expressed in RMS (root mean square error) accuracy. Detecting certain well-defined anatomical landmarks (nose tip, e.g., medial or lateral orbita) enables the surgeon to check for the most accurate patient-to-image fusion. The internal root mean square (RMS) of different neuronavigational systems is between 2 and 3.2 mm. The difference between pointer tip and anatomical landmarks is 1.7–2.2 mm, depending on the co-registration method used (see Table 1). This difference has to be added to the well-known difference of 5–10 mm between functional maps and the site of neural activity as determined by direct electrical stimulation (see chapter "Presurgical Functional Localization Possibilities, Limitations, and Validity"). Once the accuracy of the patient to the image registration has been confirmed by the landmark tests, the preplanned contours including the functional voxels are displayed in the surgeons' field of view within the microscope or exoscope.

The additional time required for the use of navigation in the OR is between 15 and 30 min (Wirtz et al. 1998).

The description of the basic principles of neuronavigation and computer-assisted (CAS) or image-guided surgery (IGS) is beyond the scope of this chapter and the reader is asked to refer to other textbooks dealing with this topic (Alexander III and Maciunas 1998; Golby 2015).

2.2 Stereotaxy

Frame-based stereotaxy was the precursor of neuronavigational systems and is based on the concept of overlaying the images' coordinate system onto a coordinate system of the physical space referenced to the stereotactic frame. In order to enhance the diagnostic yield, functional or metabolic imaging is often combined with stereotactic targeting. The main indications are the differentiation between low- and high-grade gliomas and between radionecrosis and recurrent

Table 1 The accuracy of neuronavigation depends mostly on the co-registration method that is used

Accuracy of co-registration techniques	
Anatomical landmarks	Skin fiducials
5.6 mm (Golfinos et al. 1995)	2.5 mm (Watanabe et al. 1987)
3.1 mm (Sipos et al. 1996)	3.0 mm (Laborde et al. 1992)
3.4 mm (Villalobos and Germano 1999)	1–2 mm (Zinreich et al. 1993)
3.2 mm (Wolfsberger et al. 2002)	2.8 mm (Golfinos et al. 1995)
4.0 mm (Woerdeman et al. 2007)	2.3 mm (Sipos et al. 1996)
3.96 mm (Pfisterer et al. 2008)	2.07 mm (Helm and Eckel 1998)
	1.6 mm (Villalobos and Germano 1999)
	4.0 mm (Gumprecht et al. 1999)
	2.9 mm (Wolfsberger et al. 2002)
	2.5 mm (Woerdeman et al. 2007)
	3.49 mm (Pfisterer et al. 2008)
	2.49 mm (Mongen and Willems 2019)
Surface matching (pointer or laser surface matching)	*Bone screws*
4.8 mm (Ryan et al. 1996)	<2 mm (Hassfeld et al. 1997)
1.8–2.8 mm (Raabe et al. 2002)	0.67 mm (Brinker et al. 1998)
4.83 mm (Woerdeman et al. 2007)	2.25 mm (Ammirati et al. 2002)
3.33 mm (Pfisterer et al. 2008)	
5.34 mm (Mongen and Willems 2019)	
2.9 mm (Ballesteros-Zebadúa et al. 2016)	

Sole use of anatomical landmarks allows an acceptable accuracy for orientation purposes. Skin fiducials which can be attached to the patient's skin before volumetric imaging are very easy to use, especially in cases where anatomical landmarks are not in direct "view" of the navigation system's stereoscopic camera. Surface matching and laser surface matching techniques are the most frequently used techniques today. Depending on the distance of the operated brain region from the skin surface used for co-registration, the accuracy may vary between approximately 2 and 5 mm. Accuracies comparable to frame-based stereotaxy below 1 mm mismatch can be achieved by implanting screw markers for point-matching to the bone before cranial CT scan or by use of automated registration methods using intraoperative volumetric imaging

tumor growth. Metabolic imaging procedures with Thallium-SPECT (Hemm et al. 2004; Kuwako et al. 2013), MRS (Son et al. 2001; Raimbault et al. 2014), FDG-PET (Pirotte et al. 2004; Quartuccio et al. 2020) or perfusion-weighted MRI (Maia et al. 2004; Delgado-López et al. 2018) or even CT enable the identification of target areas of higher metabolic activity, such as more aggressive or higher graded tumors. The use of 11-C-methionine, a specific marker for amino-acid transport, as a sensitive indicator of tumor recurrence enables the 11-C-Met-PET to differentiate between radionecrosis and recurrent tumor and renders it useful for stereotactic confirmation (Glaudemans et al. 2013; Kracht et al. 2004; Pirotte et al. 2004). Due to its short half-life (20 min) 11-C-Met-PET is replaced in many

centers by 18-FET-PET, which is equally sensitive although 18-F-FET is not incorporated in proteins (Neuner et al. 2012; Rapp et al. 2013).

2.3 Intraoperative Imaging

Although the development of neuronavigation systems has been a major breakthrough in neurosurgical technique, one serious problem is the so-called brain shift, i.e., tissue movement during tumor resection, by loss of CSF or insertion of brain spatula (Gerard et al. 2017), etc. Despite critical presurgical planning (Kikinis et al. 1996) and modeling of brain shift effects (Miller et al. 2019), there is still a considerable degree of uncertainty concerning the precise match of the surgical site with the images provided by the neuronavigation system. Intraoperative imaging modalities such as intraoperative CT (Okudera et al. 1993), ultrasound (Koivukangas et al. 1993; Unsgaard et al. 2002), or MRI (Black et al. 1997; Nimsky et al. 2000, 2001; Roberts et al. 1999; Tronnier et al. 1997) are important measures to overcome the problems with brain shift. Since several years also functional data were implemented into intraoperative imaging (Mikuni et al. 2007; Moche et al. 2001; Nimsky et al. 2004; Rasmussen et al. 2007; Risholm et al. 2011; Stadlbauer et al. 2004) as well as updated during surgery (Gering and Weber 1998; Kuhnt et al. 2011; Lu et al. 2013).

3 Aims and Indications for Functional Neuronavigation

Combining neuronavigation with functional data, usually acquired by fMRI or MEG, helps to minimize postoperative neurological deficits and at the same time allows maximal removal of pathological tissue. Consequently, the application of functional neuronavigation results in a better selection of surgical candidates, a safer resection with reduced morbidity, and finally shortens hospital stays and therefore minimizes hospital costs. The advantage of fMRI over other functional imaging techniques is that MRI is already used for the navigation itself in most cases due to the high contrast between normal and pathological brain tissue. Therefore, morphological three-dimensional MRI can be easily matched with fMRI data yielding an overlay of functional areas onto anatomical images (Fig. 1). There is no need for additional instrumentation or for the matching of different image formats. Being non-invasive, it can be performed repeatedly hereby providing information on postoperative reorganization or neuroplasticity (Fandino et al. 1999; Jiao et al. 2020).

Historically, neurosurgeons have mapped cortical functions invasively by direct cortical stimulation either intraoperatively or preoperatively using implanted subdural grids. However, these

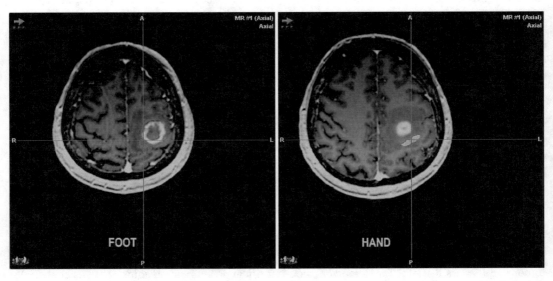

Fig. 1 Overlay of functional activation maps with morphological images (contrast enhanced T1 weighted 3D-data set) visualizing the critical spatial relationship between the left precentral high-grade glioma and the primary motor foot (orange cluster) and hand (yellow cluster) representations. Transverse sections. (Images: courtesy of C. Stippich, MD)

methods have severe limitations in terms of pre-surgical planning and direct intraoperative evaluation of function and are nowadays only used for the confirmation or validation of functional imaging data or intraoperatively when the anatomy has changed due to the procedure. The same applies nowadays for subcortical diffusion tensor imaging of white matter tracts compared to subcortical stimulation (see later).

fMRI imaging studies of motor, somatosensory, and language function as part of the presurgical evaluation process are considered very helpful and are used to define the patient's individual risk for a decline in neurological function. This enables most patients to decide between a more aggressive (gross total) and conservative (subtotal or extended biopsy) resection. Finally, this information is used to choose the "cortical entry" of lowest risk and to plan the surgical approach avoiding functional "no entry" areas in all cases. fMRI is confirmed intraoperatively with surgical inspection, intraoperative neuronavigation and, in selected cases, with cortical or subcortical stimulation or evoked potentials. Optimized preoperative protocols were developed by Stippich et al. (1999, 2000, 2003) and performed together with a 3D T1-weighted MR sequence used for neuronavigation. These protocols demonstrated robust stability for presurgical localization over a long time span (Tyndall et al. 2017). Limitations are a reduced patient compliance, motion artifacts, uncontrolled movements during the resting phase or co-movements of other parts of the body, or a paresis due to tumor growth. Minor inaccuracies can be eliminated by correction algorithms. In rare cases, however, the data acquisition has to be repeated.

Implementation of fMRI information in navigation systems is straight-forward for the surgeon when the functional information is already integrated and displayed in the data volume normally read into these systems. When the anatomical and functional information is acquired in the same session, no additional registration of fMRI data is necessary, hereby reducing the amount of registration errors.

A major drawback is the fact that fMRI is still very labor-intensive, requiring a group of MRI specialists for patient training, acquisition of MRI and fMRI data, and the post-processing of the data which requires several hours. Meanwhile there are novel technical and software solutions available that substantially facilitate the applicability of presurgical fMRI. Also real-time fMRI packages (see later) help to solve some of the technical challenges (Moeller et al. 2004).

The importance and usefulness of navigation in neurosurgical cases have been evaluated in 200 neurosurgical cases (Wirtz et al. 1998, 2000) with regard to the planning of the surgical approach, the determination of functional areas, the detection of lesion and its boundaries, and finally the radicality of glioma resection.

For the planning of the operative approach the following beneficial percentages have been given by six neurosurgeons: 90% for the use of neuronavigation, 80% for the definition of the anatomy and functional areas, 90% for lesion detection, 75% for the assessment of the tumor boundaries, and 65% for resection accuracy.

In another study (Winkler et al. 2005) the additional use of functional MRI has been considered especially helpful for glioma surgery enabling an extended amount of resection and a reduction of postoperative morbidity as compared to landmark oriented resection alone. This has been confirmed in a larger meta-analysis recently (Caras et al. 2020). Less impressive were the results for metastases or meningiomas.

A study involving higher magnetic field strengths (3–7 T) has conclusively shown an increase in spatial resolution and signal to noise ratio (Chen and Ugurbil 1999; Roessler et al. 2005; Thulborn 1999). The future use of nanoparticles as contrast media will possibly demonstrate larger lesions, which can be identified and encircled with the navigation tool. Both developments will have further implications for functionally presurgical evaluation with regard to lesion delineation, preservation of neurological function, and selection of the best therapeutical options (Cheng et al. 2014; Wegscheid et al. 2014).

4 Applications of Functional Neuronavigation

4.1 Motor and Sensory Systems

Integration of functional data for sensorimotor function into the neuronavigational system is of substantial benefit for patients with perirolandic tumors, in terms of preoperative risk assessment, surgical access, and trajectory planning (Fig. 2) (Wengenroth et al. 2011). For example, a patient admitted with a hemiparesis due to a focal central lesion with surrounding edema is first treated with corticosteroids (e.g., 16 mg dexamethasone) in order to evaluate whether the neurological symptoms ameliorate with reduction of the

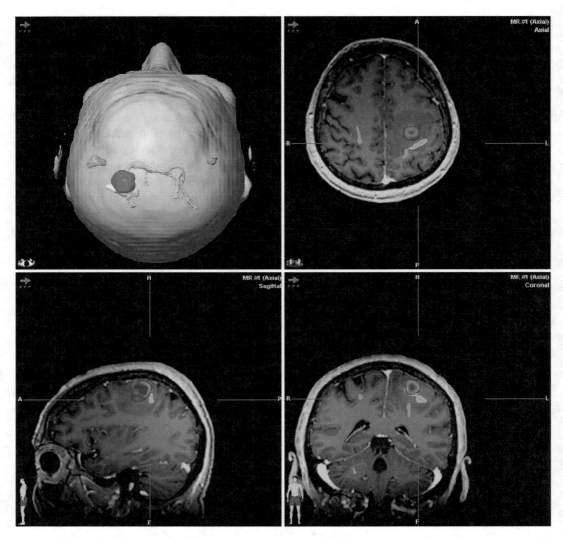

Fig. 2 Integration of BOLD-fMRI somatotopic mapping of the primary motor cortex and of Diffusion Tensor Imaging (DTI) tractography of the pyramidal tract for functional neuronavigation in a patient with a left precentral glioblastoma (same patient in Fig. 1). Segmented tumor (pink), foot and tongue representations (orange clusters), hand representation (yellow cluster), pyramidal tract (green lines). The neurosurgeon is provided with detailed information about the spatial relationship between envisaged site of surgery, functional cortex and fiber tracts, facilitating the planning and the performance of function preserving resection. Conventional surgical view (top left: left–left, right–right). Transverse, sagittal and coronal views, radiological imaging convention (right–left, left–right). (Images: courtesy of C. Stippich, MD)

mass effect. Persisting paresis strongly indicates tumor involvement in the precentral gyrus or subcortical fiber tracts, which can be confirmed by morphological MRI and diffusion tensor imaging (DTI, see below). In this case, a functional task (e.g., finger tapping) cannot typically be performed contralaterally to the lesion due to the impaired neurological function. However, some information can be obtained from an ipsilateral task eliciting bilateral brain responses (Stippich et al. 2003, 2007; Stoeckel et al. 2010; Tozakidou et al. 2013). Thus, voluntary movements of the unimpaired hand can display the ipsilateral precentral gyrus and premotor area, which—together with postcentral activation induced by contralateral passive somatosensory stimulation—can serve as functional landmarks of the affected motor cortex (see Sect. 4.6). In patients with distinct motor deficiencies, a more robust approach is required with tasks like opening and closing a fist to establish signal changes with fMRI (Fig. 3). Also resting-state fMRI is increasingly used to investigate patients with impaired motor function, bypassing such patient-specific problems (Mannfolk et al. 2011; Mitchell et al. 2013).

Thus, functional imaging allows the display of sensorimotor activation in relation to rolandic brain tumors (Bittar et al. 2000; Fandino et al. 1999; Gallen et al. 1994; Jannin et al. 2002), and its validity has been confirmed by direct electrocortical stimulation during surgery (Leherici et al. 2000; Yousry et al. 1995; Meier et al. 2013). However, effects of neuroplastic changes and reorganization also need to be considered (Fandino et al. 1999), and certain limitations with regard to the variability in the venous drainage and regional hemodynamic responses according to the pathology have to be taken into account.

Finally, DTI can be employed as a further imaging adjunct to track subcortical fibers through the corona radiata, the internal capsule, and the crura cerebri (Coenen et al. 2003; Krings et al. 2001; Le Bihan 2003; Zhu et al. 2012; Seidel et al. 2020) (see chapters "Diffusion Imaging with MR Tractography for Brain Tumor Surgery", "Presurgical Functional Localization Possibilities, Limitations, and Validity", and "Multimodal Functional Neuroimaging"). However this technique is limited, when tracts pass through the tumor or surrounding edema. In such situations correlations between DTI data

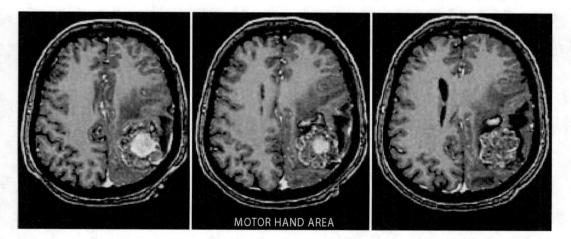

MOTOR HAND AREA

Fig. 3 Hemiparetic patient with a left rolandic metastasis from adenocarcinoma. BOLD-fMRI was performed using hand opening and closure (fist) as motor task. Primary sensorimotor fMRI activation indicated tumor growth into the central region via the postcentral gyrus. A parietal approach was chosen to resect the lesion from a posterior direction. Transverse sections with an overlay of functional activation maps on a T1-weighted contrast enhanced 3D-data set readily prepared for DICOM export to neuronavigation

and electrophysiological information from sub-cortical stimulation identifying fiber tracts (Duffau et al. 2002, 2003; Keles and Berger 2004) still need to be performed. In any case the integration of DTI and fMRI into a neuronaviga-tion system is a major step towards a safer surgi-cal planning and achievement of more extensive cortical and subcortical tumor resection, espe-cially when these data can be updated intraopera-tively (D'Andrea et al. 2017; Kamada et al. 2003; Wu et al. 2007).

4.2 Language

Classical functional neuroanatomy locates the motor output of language to the left inferior fron-tal gyrus (Broca's area, BA 44, 45) and the per-ception of language to the left posterior temporal lobe (Wernicke's area, BA 22). Before the advent of fMRI, language-related functional mapping for neurosurgical planning relied solely on two invasive procedures, the Wada test (intracarotid amytal injection) and intraoperative direct corti-cal stimulation. Language mapping is especially important in patients with lesions in and around the language-dominant hemisphere as well as in epilepsy surgery where it determines the extent of resection. The distance of resection from lan-guage sites, as determined by cortical stimula-tion, is the most important variable predicting recovery from postoperative speech disturbances. Thus, an accurate localization of all essential lan-guage areas is critical for the speed of recovery as well as the avoidance of postoperative neurologi-cal deficits.

For neurosurgical purposes it was first impor-tant to demonstrate whether fMRI could replace the Wada test or not (Massot-Tarrús 2019; see also chapter "Diffusion Imaging with MR Tractography for Brain Tumor Surgery"). In general, there is an excellent correlation between the findings of the Wada test and fMRI for lan-guage lateralization (Binder et al. 1996; Rutten et al. 2002), especially in patients with epilepsy (Benson et al. 1999; Woermann et al. 2003). fMRI studies were also correlated with direct electrical cortical stimulation and a good corre-lation was found, depending on the language task (Benson et al. 1999; FitzGerald et al. 1997; Signorelli et al. 2003). Based on the preoperative findings in functional imaging, the decision will be made, whether a biopsy, a subtotal resection, or a maximal resection using awake craniotomy will be carried out in brain tumor patients (Fig. 4). Different paradigms have been tried to determine the lateralization of expressive and receptive language areas (Partovi et al. 2012; Zacà et al. 2012), especially in patients with brain tumors or epilepsy. Meanwhile a consen-sus recommendation is published (Black et al. 2017). Also in cases with functional deficits nowadays, resting-state fMRI can be used to demonstrate language neuronal networks (Tie et al. 2014).

4.3 Visual Cortex

Up to one-third of the cerebral cortex is involved in vision. This reflects the importance of vision in everyday life. Visual information is transferred from the retina to the lateral geniculate nucleus and finally to the visual cortex following a well-known retinotopic organization. Originally, this information was obtained from PET imaging studies (Fox et al. 1986, 1987) and later con-firmed by fMRI (Belliveau et al. 1991, 1992). Since it is important to select an optimal stimula-tion frequency for visual paradigms (Fox and Raichle 1984; Kwong et al. 1992), stimulation was originally performed with LED goggles. Nowadays, computer-simulated patterns are commercially available. Tumors afflicting the visual cortex around the calcarine fissure or the optic radiation can produce changes in functional imaging tasks. Particularly in high-grade gliomas involving the occipital lobe or tumors situated in the posterior temporal horn, such as intraventric-ular meningeomas or plexus papillomas, critical planning regarding the extent of resection or the surgical access is necessary to avoid disruption of the optic radiation (Fig. 5). Despite the wide-spread use of functional mapping in surgery, the identification of visual structures is rarely reported with fMRI (Hirsch et al. 2000; Roux

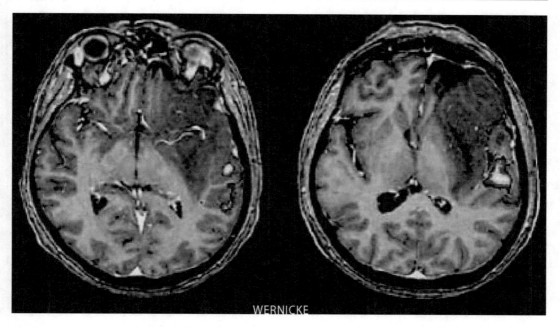

Fig. 4 Functional localization of the Wernicke language area in relation to a left fronto-temporal low-grade glioma involving the basal ganglia and insula. Word listening (auditory stimulation) was used to elicit BOLD-activation. Transverse sections with an overlay of functional activation maps on a T1-weighted contrast enhanced 3D-data set

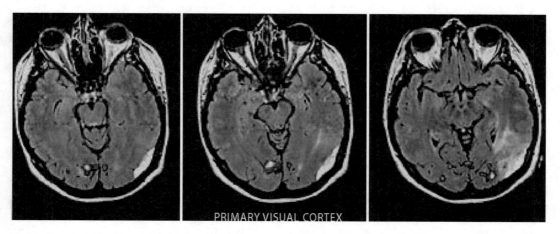

Fig. 5 Functional localization of the primary visual cortex in relation to a left parieto-occipital meningioma with signal alterations (perifocal edema) in the left optic radiation. Transverse sections with an overlay of functional activation maps on a T2-weighted fluid attenuated inversion recovery MR sequence (FLAIR)

et al. 2001a; Schulder et al. 1999; Li et al. 2013), MEG (Nakasato and Yoshimoto 2000) or PET (Fried et al. 1995). More often DTI is nowadays applied to identify the optic radiation in temporal lobe surgery for tumors or epilepsy (Taoka et al. 2008; Winston et al. 2011; James et al. 2015; Faust and Vajcoczy 2016). In addition, the first reports of electrical subcortical stimulation of the optical pathways (Gras-Combe et al. 2012) have been published. A combination of fMRI and DTI displaying visual cortical areas as well as the optic radiation would be desirable to minimize the postoperative risk of visual field defects, which can tremendously affect the quality of life.

4.4 Auditory Cortex

Functional activation of the auditory cortex has rarely been used for neurosurgical procedures or neuronavigation (Hale 2018). It is well known that a tonotopic organization of blood flow responses to different tonal frequencies exists. Sound stimulation activates the primary auditory cortex in the contralateral hemisphere, whereas speech causes bilateral activation (Binder et al. 1994; Lauter et al. 1985). Based on new hypotheses about the origins or consequences of tinnitus, causing neuroplastic changes in the auditory cortex (Langguth et al. 2003; Mahlke and Wallhauser-Franke 2004; Mühlnickel et al. 1998), a case report described the effects of chronic auditory cortex stimulation implanted with the help of auditory-fMRI neuronavigation (DeRidder et al. 2004). Auditory-fMRI was superimposed on morphological 3D-MRI and displayed together in a neuronavigation system, which was used to place an epidural paddle electrode. After successful test stimulation, an impulse generator was implanted with excellent results after 10 months.

4.5 Pain

There are numerous studies dealing with the activation of different cortical and subcortical brain areas evoked by mechanical or thermal noxious stimuli. In addition, therapeutic effects of surgical and non-surgical measures have been studied. fMRI is used for neuronavigation in cases with central or peripheral neuropathic pain and therapeutic motor cortex stimulation (Pirotte et al. 2005; Rasche and Tronnier 2016; Roux et al. 2001b; Sol et al. 2001). Depending on the localization of the painful area and the patients' ability to perform the required tasks a mapping of the motor cortex is performed. The fMRI data are integrated into a neuronavigation system and displayed in the operating room together with the

morphological MRI images. In cases of missing limbs or in plegic patients virtual movements can be trained or the opposite healthy motor cortex is projected onto the affected site, although in these latter cases neuroplastic distortions have to be taken into consideration. Via a burr hole approach an epidural lead electrode can then be placed over the somatotopic representation corresponding to the painful body area (Figs. 6 and 7). One challenge is that the functional areas might differ from the morphological data due to neuroplastic changes. This is known from several studies on neuroplasticity in pain (Flor 2003; Karl et al. 2004). However, a valid correlation between direct cortical stimulation and fMRI with a mean distance of 3.8 mm has been found in the majority of cases (Pirotte et al. 2005). DTI is used to detect the integrity of corticothalamic tracts as presurgical assessment for motor cortex stimulation in central post-stroke pain (Goto et al. 2008). Furthermore, DTI has meanwhile been integrated into functional surgery as well. Apart from indications in neuropsychiatric diseases (Bathia et al. 2012; Coenen et al. 2011; Tohyama et al. 2020) it is also used for the stimulation of fiber tracts in chronic pain (Hunsche et al. 2013; Coenen et al. 2015).

4.6 Psychological Function, Memory

Functional imaging has revolutionized our understanding in different neuropsychiatric diseases. Task-related and resting-state fMRI have revealed the neural circuits and functional connectivity in untreated and treated patients as compared to controls (Cheng et al. 2013; Jung et al. 2013). Additionally, morphometric and MR-spectroscopy is used to highlight treatment effects (Athmaca 2013; Zurowski et al. 2012). Presurgical fMRI reveals lateralization variants and is especially used to predict memory deficits in patients undergoing epilepsy surgery (Mandonnet et al. 2020; Buck and Sidhu 2020). Morphological, functional metabolic, and volumetric data point to several brain regions that are important to the etiology and maintenance of

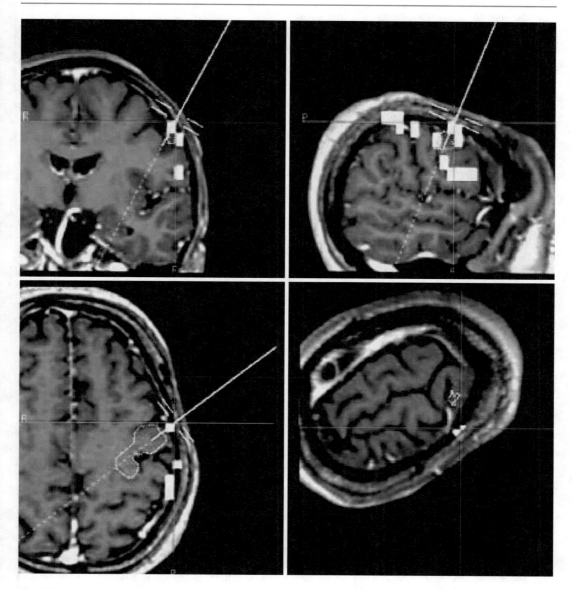

Fig. 6 Functional neuronavigation used for computer-assisted placement of an epidural motor cortex stimulation lead in treatment of chronic pain. The fused images display anatomical and functional information as well as the planned electrode placement site (yellow circular lines) along with the navigation device (pointer instrument, blue line). Coronal (top left), sagittal (top right), and transverse views (bottom left), "navigation view" (bottom right). White clusters indicate primary sensorimotor BOLD-activation after DICOM export

obsessive compulsive disorder (OCD). However, these imaging techniques have not been used for individual deep brain stimulation targeting although first attempts are well on the way (Gutman et al. 2009). Another interesting topic is the possibility to predict memory changes or deficits after surgical procedures (Henke et al. 2003).

This is most important in patients undergoing epilepsy surgery, especially temporal lobectomy (Powell et al. 2004; Rabin et al. 2004). The implementation of activation patterns in the medial temporal lobe (for episodic-like or "event"-memory) or temporal cortex (for semantic-like or "fact" memory) into a

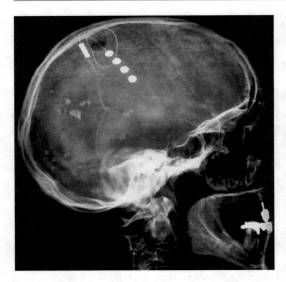

Fig. 7 Lateral X-ray plain film showing the localization of a paddle electrode implanted via a burr hole

neuronavigation system will decrease the probability of postoperative memory deficits. This also holds true for frontal lesions, where the patients, different from temporal amnesia, exhibit impairments in memory of temporal events (order, source, or context). The (pre-) frontal cortex is responsible for the active retrieval of memory and encoding while the temporal cortex is mainly responsible for memory storage and automatic retrieval (Miyashita 2004). Therefore in the future specifically designed event-related fMRI paradigms will help to predict the risk of certain types of postoperative memory deficits. Also the use of preoperative non-invasive neurostimulation techniques in combination with fMRI (so-called concurrent TMS-fMRI), and the integration of these data in a neuronavigation system will be a territory of future research (Bestmann and Feredoes 2013; Blankenburg et al. 2010; Zaehle et al. 2010)

4.7   Resting-State fMRI

There has been an increasing number of studies using resting-state fMRI to characterize abnormal brain connectivity in patients with different neurological and psychiatric disorders (Horwitz

et al. 2013). The technology is based on the brain oxygen level dependency (BOLD) principle just as paradigm- or task-based fMRI, but does not require the patient's cooperation (Lv et al. 2018). However, it has not been proven that these functional (neuroplastic) changes can be correlated with anatomical structural changes relevant for the planning of surgical approaches. Although measuring spontaneous activity and generating resting-state correlation maps similar to functional maps from activation tasks, imaging of these networks is technically very labor-intense and underlies several conditions as the selection of the "seed regions" in order to identify reference networks from examination and statistical analysis of large groups of individuals. A recent study integrated resting-state data into surgical decision making in a restricted number of patients with epilepsy. The authors described an advantage in identifying areas responsible for speech arrest but they did not look for paraphasic errors, which are also important for the functional outcome (Mitchell et al. 2013). For more details on resting-state fMRI we refer the reader to chapter "Presurgical Resting-State fMRI".

4.8   Diffusion Tensor Imaging (DTI)

While fMRI may be used to highlight cortical structures, DTI is used to map white matter structures and specific fiber connections (Fig. 8). It is based on the preferential diffusion of water along white matter tracts within the CNS and allows the neurosurgeon to delineate a lesion with respect to subcortical projection fibers. DTI data can be incorporated into navigational data sets to facilitate more radical tissue resections as well as a reduced risk of postoperative new neurological deficits (Elhawary et al. 2011; Wu et al. 2007). Deterministic tractography algorithms have been integrated in most commercially available navigation systems, are easy to use, and can be applied without the requirement for support by a specialist. While these features helped a great deal making DTI useable for surgical approaches, they are also the main target for controversy (Jones 2010; Jones et al. 2013; Thomas et al.

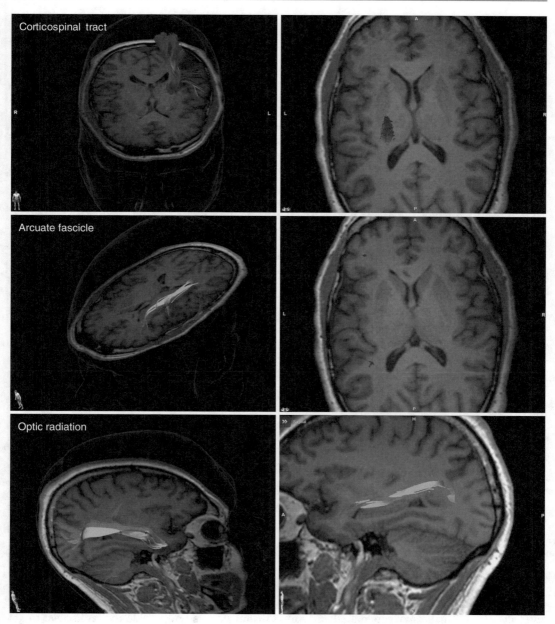

Fig. 8 Three fiber systems with high relevance for surgical approaches. The underlying imaging is a DTI sequence with 30 motion probing gradients scanned on a 3 T Siemens Magnetom. The tractography was performed using Brainlab Elements. Top: The corticospinal tract is critical for limb movement and locomotion. For tractography, usually two regions of interest are selected, the brainstem and the precentral gyrus. Middle: The arcuate fascicle of the dominant hemisphere connects sensory and motor speech areas with each other as well as with further brain regions. Mostly, Broca's area (opercular portion of inferior frontal gyrus) and Wernicke's area (posterior third of superior temporal gyrus) are used as seed volumes. Bottom: The optic radiation connects the lateral geniculate body with the visual cortex in the occipital lobe. The fibers run anteriorly towards the temporal lobe, take a sharp turn, and run backwards towards the occipital lobe on the roof of the lateral ventricle's temporal horn and trigone. Because of the tight bend close to the temporal pole, this portion, the Meyer's loop, is very difficult to visualize and is often not included in the tractography result

2014). DTI imaging is susceptible to MR artifacts such geometric aberrations or in the vicinity of metal, bone, or air. This fact as well as the usually limited spatial resolution of the acquired data is not obvious to the user after overlying the data with high-resolution structural MRI datasets. Furthermore, deterministic tractography algorithms have weaknesses if fibers cross within a single voxel (leading to a seemingly low focal anisotropy, FA), in the case of tight turns of fibers (such as the Meyer's loop) and regarding thin fiber tracts, which only have a limited influence on the overall FA within the passed voxels. These weaknesses and the high dependency on the selected seed volumes for tracking may lead to unreliable tractography results and unfavorable decision making by inexperienced users. Despite the easy application of DTI today, surgery still requires the surgeon to have thorough anatomical and technical knowledge (Pujol et al. 2015).

Probabilistic tractography algorithms are less likely to propagate errors from one voxel to the next than deterministic algorithms, but generate multiple possible trajectories between two seed volumes. By estimation and visualization of their individual likelihood, many of the above mentioned weaknesses of tractography may be overcome (Jeurissen et al. 2019). Many different algorithms have been developed and there is far less standardization among probabilistic tractography than for deterministic ones. Furthermore, a higher degree of expertise is required on the user side along with a need for computation power and time. Consequently, probabilistic tractography only has a minor impact on surgery today.

Because also the white matter undergoes anatomical changes due to brain shift, the intraoperative update of neuronavigational data with high-field MRI is a promising tool for image-guided surgery. The gold-standard for the detection of subcortical fibers remains intraoperative subcortical stimulation. Correlational studies estimate that the white matter tracts determined via DTI are in a vicinity of 8 mm of the stimulated areas (a range from 0 to 15 mm was described by Maesawa et al. 2010, Prabhu et al. 2011, Seidel et al. 2020, Zolal et al. 2012). Therefore, a combination of DTI integrated neu-

ronavigation with subcortical stimulation is considered the most effective way for a safe resection within subcortical areas.

Another new approach for intraoperative decision making or preoperative planning is the use of navigated transcranial stimulation (nTMS) for neuronavigation. NTMS is currently examined for its applicability and reliability for the delineation of cortical and subcortical projection areas, which have to be spared during surgical resection of brain lesions (Krieg et al. 2012, 2013). The information obtained with nTMS has been compared with direct cortical stimulation, preoperative fMRI, and fiber tracking (Frey et al. 2012). Although nTMS has advantages over fMRI because it does not rely on patients' compliance, it depends on several parameters (resting motor threshold, intraoperative brain shift) and the value of its use in the daily clinical routine has yet to be determined (Rosenstock et al. 2020; Sollmann et al. 2020) .

4.9 Implementation of Functional Imaging Data into Intraoperative Imaging

The benefits of integrating functional imaging data into a neuronavigation system have been described above. In contrast to MEG, fMRI is more widely distributed and is therefore nowadays used on a clinical routine basis. fMRI however, depending on the technique and the special requirements, still needs an intense and time-consuming processing phase before the data can be merged into a neuronavigational system. Real-time fMRI packages provided by MR scanner manufacturers now enable the radiologist to get immediate post-imaging results for more "simple" activation tasks. In an earlier study (Moeller et al. 2004) two different routine clinical 1.5-T scanners were used (Magnetom Vision, Siemens and Intera, Philips) for a motor paradigm (finger tapping). The integrated software performed an automatic motion correction and cluster filtering displaying the activated brain area during each scan. An overlay with the 3D T1-weighted data set could be performed semiautomatically.

Integrating these software packages into high-field MR scanners situated in the operating room allows direct intraoperative functional imaging (Nimsky et al. 2004). The extent of resection of brain tumors or lesions in epilepsy surgery can nowadays be further tailored according to the functional information obtained from intraoperative fMRI.

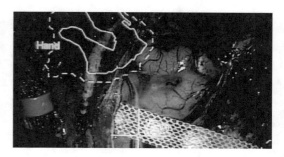

Fig. 9 Operative site showing the correlation of intraoperative cortical stimulation and fMRI localization

4.10 Implementation of Functional Imaging Data into Intraoperative Mapping

The delineation of cortical structures can be performed intraoperatively either via direct visualization, anatomical correlation to a navigational device or neurophysiological methods. In case of a large craniotomy the surgeon is able to identify anatomical landmarks on the exposed cortex and to determine various gyri. The localization of eloquent areas by direct inspection of the brain's surface is very limited as there are no reliable landmarks except for the motor hand area of the precentral gyrus. Especially in cognitive functions, localization of the recruited brain areas is highly variable precluding any reliable prediction in individual patients. In patients with distorted anatomy or limited surgical exposure, neuronavigational devices or neurophysiological techniques help the surgeon to reliably determine the boundaries of eloquent brain regions. Especially in perirolandic tumors, neurophysiological methods facilitate the delineation of the motor or sensory cortex. Direct electrical stimulation elicits movements in muscle groups corresponding to the homunculus. However intraoperatively, electrical cortical stimulation can be hampered by agents, such as relaxants, causing a neuromuscular blockade or by the depth of anesthesia. On the other hand, motor responses are also elicited by stimulation of premotor and even sensory areas. Sensory responses to electrical stimulation of the median or the tibial nerve can delineate the sensory cortex. The combination of somatosensory evoked potentials (SEPs) and cortical stimulation has already been described in the late 1970s (Woolsey et al. 1979) and was later refined by the

use of the phase reversal to differentiate between the motor and sensory cortex (Cedzich et al. 1996; Romstöck et al. 2002) in brain tumor surgery. Nowadays these techniques are used for the validation of functional imaging data by displaying the distance between cortical activation and neurophysiological response and finally by correlating the data with the clinical outcome or neurological function (Cosgrove et al. 1996; Kober et al. 2001; Krishnan et al. 2004; Puce et al. 1995; Schiffbauer et al. 2003) (Fig. 9). Functional imaging has the advantage of being able to depict activation deep in a sulcus, which is not easily accessible for direct stimulation. For further data regarding the validity of functional imaging data see chapter "Presurgical Functional Localization Possibilities, Limitations, and Validity". A combination of both techniques is also used in functional surgery, e.g., in motor cortex stimulation for chronic pain states or tinnitus (Sol et al. 2001; Tronnier et al. 1996).

To prevent damage to the subcortical fiber tracts during resection of eloquent cortical and subcortical lesions, low-threshold monopolar motor-mapping using train-of-5 stimuli for the identification of a motor threshold and estimation of the distance to the respective motor-fibers may be considered gold-standard today (Seidel et al. 2012). The combination with visualization and overlaying of the microscopic or exoscopic image with preoperatively identified subcortical structures in an augmented-reality environment may further improve safety in subcortical tumor resection. In contrast to continuous monopolar motor-mapping, brain shift effects have to be taken into account.

Interesting developments are operations using a real-time atlas-based neuronavigation which adapts to intraoperative changes, such as brain shift, and applies them to all morphological and functional images (Vabulas et al. 2014).

4.11   Cost-Effectiveness

There are no direct cost analyses of functional imaging in presurgical evaluation. However, it is well demonstrated that neuronavigation is able to lower the duration of the hospital stay (Paleologos et al. 2000) hereby significantly reducing the incoming expenses. A study reported the costs of the Wada test to be 3.7 times higher as compared to fMRI (Medina et al. 2004). Increasing the amount of preoperative (functional) imaging will certainly increase the costs produced by manpower and hardware. However the improved postoperative quality of life is difficult to balance by money. At least in benign lesions or epilepsy surgery it seems obvious that less invasive procedures will reduce postoperative morbidity and therefore lower the financial burden (Eljamel and Mahboob 2016).

5   Perspectives

5.1   Single-Rack Solution

The creation of a single-rack information system for the surgeon consisting of a collection of data for functional imaging (MEG, fMRI, DTI, and Perfusion-MRI), navigation, and electrophysiological monitoring with online information to support the surgeon's intraoperative decisions is an important goal (Cartucho et al. 2020). A special focus should be put on the imaging and electrophysiological localization of subcortical pathways. This integrated "functional" neuronavigational approach should be beneficial in surgical planning and pre- and intraoperative decision making, providing online information to facilitate surgical resection and decrease postoperative morbidity by protecting eloquent cortical and subcortical areas. Up to now the surgeon has to

work with different information systems and thus has to integrate all this information during surgery separately when appropriate. An integrated multimodal navigation system taking over all these tasks would reduce the time of surgery, allows a safer resection of brain tumors and presumably ultimately improves the patients' outcome.

Several topics have to be addressed to create such a system:

– The integration of more complex resting-state fMRI data to allow prediction of neuropsychological changes in brain tumor surgery.
– The correlation of fusion inaccuracies based on the fact that up to now only a few anatomic landmarks are used for the merging of data.
– The correction of distortions of the different techniques (reduction of distortion by new imaging techniques; correction of remaining distortion by data processing) and their fusion.
– Automated export of electrophysiological data into a navigation system.
– The automatic recognition of electrode or grid configurations by the navigational system and their display on the monitor or microscope (see below) for the operating surgeon.

The development of so-called Smart (cyber-) Operating Theatres in a few centers around the world tries to solve these problems and combine the comprehension of diagnostic information with a connection to the different therapeutic medical devices via communicating interfaces.

5.2   Overlay of Functional Imaging Data in the Operation Microscope or Exoscope

It would be desirable to overlay the operation site with the operation microscope or exoscope with all available imaging data in order not only to delineate the tumor volume but also functional cortical and subcortical sites. Interruptions or distractions caused by switching the focus between the monitor and the microscope repeatedly are disturbing and time consuming. Using the methods of augmented reality can realize a more efficient use of the different planning data. This could be achieved by superimposing heads-up-displays upon the microscopic view or by a respective planning of the data in the microscopic view (Tronnier et al. 2000; Alfonso-Garcia et al. 2019; Carl et al. 2020). Dedicated micro-optical overlay modules are already designed for inserting and overlaying three-dimensional data within the operating microscope (Aschke et al. 2003; Makela et al. 2001). Further refinements to enhance the surgeon's three-dimensional perception and a fast integration of these data are required to make intraoperative imaging data implementable.

Special tracking methods or computational models which compensate for intraoperative brain shift have to be developed. Tracking points could be vessel branches, other anatomical landmarks, or implanted markers (e.g., LEDs). Additional information provided by intraoperative imaging such as ultrasound should be integrated into the surgical workflow by automated actualization and integration of these imaging data into the microscopic view. This will require different import filters and a merging of different data formats.

5.3 Imaging the Basal Ganglia

First trials examining the basal ganglia with functional somatotopic mapping (Maillard et al. 2000) have been performed. If it were possible to demonstrate the somatotopy of the hand, foot, or face areas in distinct basal ganglia nuclei, such as the internal pallidum or the subthalamic nucleus, these data could be used for surgical planning of the target and trajectories in stereotactic functional procedures such as pallidotomies or deep brain stimulation (DBS). Unfortunately, despite major advances in MRI technology and nearly exclusive use of high-field strengths (1.5 and 3 T), reliable differentiation of the different thalamic nuclei is still not possible. Due to the increased use of DBS for neuropsychiatric disorders, functional imaging such as DTI or tractography is more often required as a preoperative

imaging method (Coenen et al. 2011; Gutman et al. 2009; Owen et al. 2007) as well as to study the postoperative effect of DBS on neuronal circuits (Albaugh and Shih 2014; Rozanski et al. 2014). An alternative to indirect segmentation of the thalamus using DTI is the elastic adaptation of atlas data on the individual three-dimensional anatomy (Su et al. 2019; Chakravarty et al. 2008; Ranjan et al. 2019).

Interestingly, despite these techniques for safer orientation within the basal ganglia, a substantial portion of thalamotomies, pallidotomies, and DBS procedures is still performed based on indirect atlas-based targeting. The reason might be, that the results, especially in awake procedures, are mostly very good (Dallapiazza et al. 2019) and the need for improvement is relatively low.

5.4 Neuroplasticity

Although it is known that over- or under use of a specific function will create cortical neuroplasticity, either by enhanced afferent normal or pathological activity (musicians, writer's cramp), decreased afferent activity (blind individuals, patients with amputation) or disproportion of agonist/antagonist function (focal dystonia), pathological changes of the cortex (stroke, brain tumor, brain surgery) also demonstrate the brain's capacity for plastic changes (Fujii and Nakada 2003). This has serious implications for the different forms of therapy (Lotze et al. 1999; Wu and Kaass 1999; You et al. 2005). To the best of our knowledge, no longitudinal study has been performed looking for immediate postoperative changes in fMRI and long-term changes after surgical resection and neurological recovery. This will be one of the most interesting applications of resting-state and activation task fMRI pre- and postoperatively in the future.

5.5 Imaging the Spinal Cord

Functional imaging of the spinal cord is still in development. Movement artifacts of the cord itself, CSF flow, its small cross diameter, and inhomogeneities caused by the surrounding bone and cartilage make the interpretation of the images difficult. The detection of changes of function by pathological lesions is far from being technically solved (Giove et al. 2004; Stroman et al. 2005). DTI techniques are recently used to examine microstructural changes in degenerative disease (as cervical myeolopathy), infection (multiple sclerosis), and pain (Shabani et al. 2020; Ropele and Fazekas 2019; Zhang et al. 2020).

5.6 Molecular Imaging

A variety of imaging technologies are being investigated as tools for studying gene expression in living subjects, especially after gene therapy. The application of such tools for presurgical planning in humans is desired though it still seems like a long way to implement them and overcome technical difficulties. SPECT and PET are the most mature of the current imaging technologies with high sensitivity and good access to scanners. MRI is also currently used for molecular imaging of different pathologies including brain tumors in rodents in order to evaluate gene therapy protocols (Moffat et al. 2003; Rehemtulla et al. 2002; Varma et al. 2013). PTPmu labeled nanoparticles were successfully used to label pediatric and adult glioblastomas in stereotactic surgical procedures (Covarrubias et al. 2020). It can be expected that in the near future personalized treatment concepts based on application of fluorescent nanoparticles for intraoperative MRI will become available and possibly improve treatment outcome in glioma surgery (Šamec et al. 2020).

6 Summary

Functional imaging can provide information on the localization of essential functional cortex and subcortical pathways preoperatively. It enables the surgeon to assess the surgical risk, to take therapeutic decisions, and to advise the patient

carefully about the estimated risks and benefits of the procedure. Functional imaging enables the surgeon to make his resection plan by estimating the position and relationship of the abnormal and the important functional tissue that should be preserved. In addition, functional imaging allows function-guided resection rather than the resection relying only on morphology which neuro-navigation alone can offer. Limiting factors are the interference with tumor mass and/or surrounding edema compromising local blood flow and the possible presence of preoperative neurological deficits preventing the performance of functional tasks during imaging. To date, the resection borders cannot be determined reliably based on fMRI data. However first reports in a very limited number of patients have suggested that resection of tumor at a distance of at least 10 mm may be safe and may cause no decline in neurological function (Roessler et al. 2005). On the other hand, resection in an area less than 5 mm away from functional cortex will most likely result—at least temporarily—in neurological deficits. To overcome the problem of intraoperative brain shift, a correlation with direct electrical stimulation for motor cortex, as well as SEPs for visual, auditory, and sensory cortex can be applied (Cirillo et al. 2019; Sanvito et al. 2020). Finally, the use of intraoperative high-field MR scanners will provide insight into the evaluation of some functions intraoperatively. Eventually, intraoperative mapping of speech and other higher cognitive functions still requires awake craniotomy.

References

Albaugh DL, Shih Y-YI (2014) Neural circuit modulation during deep brain stimulation at the subthalamic nucleus for Parkinson's disease: what have we learned from neuroimaging studies. Brain Connect 4(1):1–14

Alexander E III, Maciunas RJ (1998) Advanced neurosurgical navigation. Thieme, Stuttgart

Alfonso-Garcia A, Bec J, Weaver SS et al (2019) Real-time augmented reality for delineation of surgical margins during neurosurgery using autofluorescence lifetime contrast. J Biophotonics 13:e2019001008

Ammirati M, Gross JD, Ammirati G, Dugan S (2002) Comparison of registration accuracy of skin- and bone-implanted fiducials for frameless stereotaxis of the brain: a prospective study. Skull Base 12(3):125–130

Aschke M, Wirtz CR, Raczkowsky J et al (2003) Augmented reality in operating microscopes for neurosurgical interventions. Proc IEEE:652–655

Athmaca M (2013) The effect of psychopharmacologic and therapeutic approaches on neuro-imaging in obsessive compulsive disorder. Curr Neuropharmacol 11:109–113

Ballesteros-Zebadúa P, García-Garduño OA, Galván de la Cruz OO, Arellano-Reynoso A, Lárraga-Gutiérrez JM, Celis MA (2016) Assessment of an image guided neurosurgery system using a head phantom. Br J Neurosurg 30(6):606–610

Bathia KD, Henderson L, Ramsey-Stewart G et al (2012) Diffusion tensor imaging to aid subgenual cingulum target selection for deep brain stimulation in depression. Stereotact Funct Neurosurg 90:225–232

Belliveau JW, Kennedy DN, McKinstry RC et al (1991) Functional mapping of the human visual cortex by magnetic resonance imaging. Science 254:716–719

Belliveau JW, Kwong KK, Kennedy DN et al (1992) Magnetic resonance imaging mapping for brain function. Human visual cortex. Investig Radiol 27:S59–S65

Benson RR, FitzGerald DB, LeSueur LL et al (1999) Language dominance determined by whole brain functional MRI in patients with brain lesions. Neurology 52:798–809

Bestmann S, Feredoes E (2013) Combined neurostimulation and neuroimaging in cognitive neuroscience: past present and future. Ann N Y Acad Sci 1296:11–30

Binder JR, Rao SM, Hammeke TA et al (1994) Functional magnetic resonance imaging of human auditory cortex. Ann Neurol 35:662–672

Binder JR, Swanson SJ, Hammeke TA et al (1996) Determination of language dominance using functional MRI: a comparison with the Wada test. Neurology 46:978–984

Bittar RG, Olivier A, Sadikot AF et al (2000) Cortical and somatosensory representation: effect of cerebral lesions. J Neurosurg 92:242–248

Black PM, Moriarty TM, Alexander EA III et al (1997) The development and implementation of intraoperative magnetic resonance imaging and its neurosurgical applications. Neurosurgery 41:831–845

Black DF et al (2017) American Society of Functional Neuroradiology-recommended fMRI paradigm algorithms for presurgical language assessment. AJNR Am J Neuroradiol 38:65–73

Blankenburg F, Ruff CC, Bestmann S et al (2010) Studying the role of the parietal cortex in visuospatial attention with concurrent TMS-fMRI. Cereb Cortex 20:2711

Brinker T, Arango G, Kaminsky J, Samii A, Thomas U, Vokapic P, Samii M (1998) An experimental approach to image guided skull base surgery employing a microscope-based neuronavigation system. Acta Neurochir 140(9):883–889

Buck S, Sidhu MK (2020) A guide to designing a memory fMRI paradigm for pre-surgical evaluation in temporal lobe epilepsy. Front Neurol 10:1354. https://doi.org/10.3389/fneur.2019.01354. eCollection 2019

Caras A et al (2020) Usefulness and impact of intraoperative imaging for glioma resection on patient outcome and extent of resection: a systematic review and meta-analysis. World Neurosurg 134:98–110

Carl B, Bopp M, Saß B et al (2020) Spine surgery supported by augmented reality. Glob Spine J 10:415–455

Cartucho J, Shapira D, Ashrafian H et al (2020) Multimodal mixed reality visualisation for intraoperative surgical guidance. Int J Comput Assist Radiol Surg 15:819–826

Cedzich C, Taniguchi M, Schaefer S et al (1996) Somatosensory evoked potential phase reversal and direct motor cortex stimulation during surgery in and around the central region. Neurosurgery 38:962–970

Chakravarty MM et al (2008) Towards a validation of atlas warping techniques. Med Image Anal 12(6):713–726

Chen W, Ugurbil K (1999) High spatial resolution functional magnetic resonance imaging at very high magnetic field. Top Magn Reson Imaging 10:63–78

Cheng Y, Xu J, Nie B (2013) Abnormal resting-state activities and functional connectivities of the anterior and posterior cortexes in medication-naive patients with obsessive-compulsive disorders. PLoS One 8:e67478

Cheng Y, Morshed RA, Auffinger B et al (2014) Multifunctional nanoparticle for brain tumor imaging and therapy. Adv Drug Deliv Res 66:42–57

Cirillo S, Caulo M, Pieri V, Falini A, Castellano A (2019) Role of functional imaging techniques to assess motor and language cortical plasticity in glioma patients: a systematic review. Neural Plast 2019:4056436

Coenen VA, Krings T, Axer H et al (2003) Intraoperative three-dimensional visualization of the pyramidal tract in a neuronavigation system (PTV) reliably predicts true position of principal pathways. Surg Neurol 60:381–390

Coenen VA, Mädler B, Schiffbauer H et al (2011) Individual fiber anatomy of the subthalamic region revealed with diffusion tensor imaging: a concept to identify the deep brain stimulation target for tremor suppression. Neurosurgery 68:1069–1075

Coenen V, Kieselbach K, Mader I et al (2015) Diffusion tensor magnetic resonance imaging (DTI) tractography-guided deep brain stimulation in neuropathic pain. Acta Neurochir 157:739–741

Cosgrove GR, Buchbinder BR, Jiang H (1996) Functional magnetic resonance imaging for intracranial neuronavigation. Neurosurg Clin N Am 7:313–322

Covarrubias G et al (2020) PTPmu-targeted nanoparticles label invasive pediatric and adult glioblastoma. Nanomedicine 28:102216

D'Andrea G et al (2017) Functional magnetic resonance imaging (fMRI), pre-intraoperative tractography in neurosurgery: the experience of Sant' Andrea Rome University Hospital. Acta Neurochir Suppl 124:241–250

Dallapiazza RF et al (2019) Outcomes from stereotactic surgery for essential tremor. J Neurol Neurosurg Psychiatry 90(4):474–482

Delgado-López PD, Riñones-Mena E, Corrales-García EM (2018) Treatment-related changes in glioblastoma: a review on the controversies in response assessment criteria and the concepts of true progression, pseudoprogression, pseudoresponse and radionecrosis. Clin Transl Oncol 20:939–953

DeRidder D, De Mulder G, Walsh V et al (2004) Magnetic and electrical stimulation of the auditory cortex for intractable tinnitus. Case report. J Neurosurg 100:560–564

Duffau H, Capelle L, Sichez N et al (2002) Intraoperative mapping of the subcortical language pathways using direct stimulations. An anatomo-functional study. Brain 125:199–214

Duffau H, Capelle L, Denvil D et al (2003) Usefulness of intraoperative electrical subcortical mapping during surgery for low-grade gliomas located within eloquent brain regions: functional results in a series of 103 patients. J Neurosurg 98:764–768

Elhawary H, Liu H, Patel P et al (2011) Intraoperative real-time querying of white matter tracts during frameless stereotactic neuronavigation. Neurosurgery 68:506–516

Eljamel MS, Mahboob SO (2016) The effectiveness and cost-effectiveness of intraoperative imaging in high-grade glioma resection; a comparative review of intraoperative ALA, fluorescein, ultrasound and MRI. Photodiagn Photodyn Ther 16:35–43

Fandino J, Kollias S, Wieser HG et al (1999) Intraoperative validation of functional magnetic resonance imaging and cortical reorganization patterns in patients with brain tumors involving the motor cortex. J Neurosurg 91:238–250

Faust K, Vajcoczy P (2016) Distinct displacements of the optic radiation based on tumor location revealed using preoperative diffusion tensor imaging. J Neurosurg 124:1343–1352

Fitzgerald DB, Cosgrove GR, Ronner S et al (1997) Location of language in the cortex: a comparison between functional MR imaging and electrocortical stimulation. AJNR Am J Neuroradiol 18:1529–1539

Flor H (2003) Remapping somatosensory cortex after injury. Adv Neurol 93:195–204

Fox PT, Raichle ME (1984) Stimulus rate dependence of regional cerebral blood flow in human striate cortex, demonstrated by positron emission tomography. J Neurophysiol 51:1109–1120

Fox PT, Mintum MA, Raichle ME et al (1986) Mapping human visual cortex with positron emission tomography. Nature 323:806–809

Fox PT, Miezin FM, Allman JM et al (1987) Retinotopic organization of human visual cortex mapped with positron-emission tomography. J Neurosci 7:913–922

Frey D, Strack V, Wiener E et al (2012) A new approach for corticospinal tract reconstruction based on navigated transcranial stimulation and standardized fractional anisotrophy values. NeuroImage 62:1600–1609

Fried I, Nenov V, Ojemann SG et al (1995) Functional MR and PET imaging of rolandic and visual cortices for neurosurgical planning. J Neurosurg 83:854–861

Fujii Y, Nakada T (2003) Cortical reorganization in patient with subcortical hemiparesis: neural mechanisms of functional recovery and prognostic implication. J Neurosurg 98:64–73

Gallen CC, Bucholz RD, Sobel DF (1994) Intracranial neurosurgery guided by functional imaging. Surg Neurol 42:523–530

Gerard IJ, MartaKersten-Oertel M, Petrecca K et al (2017) Brain shift in neuronavigation of brain tumors: a review. Med Image Anal 35:403–420

Gering DT, Weber DM (1998) Intraoperative, real-time, functional MRI. J Magn Reson Imaging 8:254–257

Giove F, Gareffa G, Giuletti G et al (2004) Issues about the fMRI of the human spinal cord. Magn Reson Imaging 22:1505–1516

Glaudemans AWJM, Enting RH, Heesters MAAM et al (2013) Value of 11C-methionine PET in imaging brain tumours and metastases. Eur J Nucl Med Mol Imaging 40:615–635

Golby A (2015) Image-guided neurosurgery, 1st edn. Academic Press, Elsevier, London

Golfinos JG, Fitzpatrick BC, Smith LR, Spetzler RF (1995) Clinical use of a frameless stereotactic arm: results of 325 cases. J Neurosurg 83(2):197–205

Goto T, Saitoh Y, Hashimoto N, Hirata M, Kishima H, Oshino S, Tani N, Hosomi K, Kakigi R, Yoshimine T. Diffusion tensor fiber tracking in patients with central post-stroke pain; correlation with efficacy of repetitive transcranial magnetic stimulation. Pain. 2008;140:509–518

Gras-Combe G, Moritz-Gasser S, Herbet G et al (2012) Intraoperative subcortical electrical mapping of optic radiation in awake surgery for gliomas in visual pathways. J Neurosurg 117:466–473

Gumprecht HK, Widenka DC, Lumenta CB (1999) BrainLab VectorVision Neuronavigation System: technology and clinical experiences in 131 cases. Neurosurgery 44(1):97–104

Gutman DA, Holtzheimer PE, Behrens TE (2009) A tractography analysis of deep brain stimulation white matter targets for depression. Biol Psychiatry 65:276–282

Hale MD (2018) A novel functional magnetic resonance imaging paradigm for the preoperative assessment of auditory perception in a musician undergoing temporal lobe surgery. World Neurosurg 111:63–67

Hassfeld S, Muehling J, Wirtz CR, Knauth M, Lutze T, Schulz HJ (1997) Intraoperative guidance in maxillofacial and craniofacial surgery. Proc Inst Mech Eng H 211(4):277–283

Helm PA, Eckel TS (1998) Accuracy of registration methods in frameless stereotaxis. Comput Aided Surg 3(2):51–56

Hemm S, Vaissiere N, Zanca M et al (2004) Thallium SPECT-based stereotactic targeting brain tumor biopsies. A technical note. Stereotact Funct Neurosurg 82:70–76

Henke K, Treyer V, Weber B et al (2003) Functional neuroimaging studies predicts individual memory outcome after amygdalohippocampectomy. Neuroreport 14:1197–1202

Hirsch J, Ruge MI, Kim KHS et al (2000) An integrated functional magnetic resonance imaging procedure for preoperative mapping of cortical areas associated with tactile, motor, language and visual functions. Neurosurgery 47:711–722

Horwitz B, Hwang C, Alstott J (2013) Interpreting the effects of altered brain anatomical connectivity on fMRI functional connectivity: a role for computational neural modeling. Front Human Neurosci 7:649

Hunsche S, Sauner D, Runge MJR et al (2013) Tractography-guided stimulation of somatosensory fibers for thalamic pain relief. Stereotact Funct Neurosurg 91:328–334

James JS, Radhakrishnan A, Thomas B, Madhusoodanan M, Kesavadas C, Abraham M, Menon R, Rathore C, Vilanilam G (2015) Diffusion tensor imaging tractography of Meyer's loop in planning resective surgery for drug-resistant temporal lobe epilepsy. Epilepsy Res 110:95–104

Jannin P, Morandi X, Fleig OJ et al (2002) Integration of sulcal and functional information for multimodal neuronavigation. J Neurosurg 96:713–723

Jeurissen B et al (2019) Diffusion MRI fiber tractography of the brain. NMR Biomed 32(4):e3785

Jiao Y et al (2020) Plasticity in language cortex and white matter tracts after resection of dominant inferior parietal lobule arteriovenous malformations: a combined fMRI and DTI study. J Neurosurg 20:1–8. https://doi.org/10.3171/2019.12.JNS191987. Online ahead of print

Jones DK (2010) Challenges and limitations of quantifying brain connectivity in vivo with diffusion MRI. Imaging Med 2(3):341–355

Jones DK, Knösche TR, Turner R (2013) White matter integrity, fiber count, and other fallacies: the do's and don'ts of diffusion MRI. NeuroImage 73:239–254

Jung WH, Kang DH, Kim E et al (2013) Abnormal corticostriatal-limbic functional connectivity in obsessive compulsive disorder during reward processing and resting-state. Neuroimage Clin 3:27–38

Kamada K, Houkin K, Takeuchi F et al (2003) Visualization of the eloquent motor system by integration of MEG, functional, and anisotropic diffusion-weighted MRI in functional neuronavigation. Surg Neurol 59:353–362

Karl A, Mühlnickel W, Kurth R et al (2004) Neuroelectric source imaging of steady-state movement-related cortical potentials in human upper extremity amputees with and without phantom limb pain. Pain 110:90–102

Keles GE, Berger MS (2004) Advances in neurosurgical technique in the current management of brain tumors. Semin Oncol 31:659–665

Kikinis R, Gleason PL, Moriarty TM et al (1996) Computer-assisted interactive three-dimensional planning for neurosurgical procedures. Neurosurgery 38:640–651

Kober H, Nimsky C, Moeller M et al (2001) Correlation of sensorimotor activation with functional magnetic resonance imaging and magnetoencephalography in presurgical functional imaging: a spatial analysis. NeuroImage 14:1214–1228

Koivukangas J, Louhisalmi Y, Alakuijala J et al (1993) Ultrasound-controlled neuronavigator-guided brain surgery. J Neurosurg 79:36–42

Kracht LW, Miletic H, Busch S et al (2004) Delineation of brain tumor extent with (11C)L methionine positron emission tomography: local comparison with stereotactic histopathology. Clin Cancer Res 10:7163–7170

Krieg S, Shiban E, Buchmann N et al (2012) Utility of presurgical navigated transcranial magnetic brain stimulation for the resection of tumors in eloquent motor areas. J Neurosurg 116:994–1001

Krieg SM, Shiban E, Buchmann N et al (2013) Presurgical navigated transcranial magnetic brain stimulation for recurrent gliomas in motor eloquent areas. Clin Neurophysiol 124:522–527

Krings T, Reinges MH, Thiex R et al (2001) Function and diffusion-weighted magnetic resonance images of space-occupying lesions affecting the motor system: imaging the motor cortex and pyramidal tracts. J Neurosurg 95:816–824

Krishnan R, Raabe A, Hattingen E et al (2004) Functional magnetic resonance imaging-integrated neuronavigation: correlation between lesion-to-motor cortex distance and outcome. Neurosurgery 55:904–915

Kuhnt D et al (2011) Quantification of glioma removal by intraoperative high-field magnetic resonance imaging: an update. Neurosurgery 69:852–862

Kuwako T, Mizumura S, Murakami R et al (2013) Voxel-based analysis of (2013) Tl SPECT for grading and diagnostic accuracy of gliomas: comparison with ROI analysis. Ann Nucl Med 27:493–501

Kwong KK, Belliveau JW, Chesler DA et al (1992) Dynamic magnetic resonance imaging of human brain activity during primary sensory stimulation. Proc Natl Acad Sci U S A 89:5675–5679

Laborde G, Gilsbach J, Harders A, Klimek L, Moesges R, Krybus W (1992) Computer assisted localizer for planning of surgery and intra-operative orientation. Acta Neurochir 119(1–4):166–170

Langguth B, Eichhammer P, Wiegand R et al (2003) Neuro-navigated rTMS in a patient with chronic tinnitus. Effects of 4 weeks treatment. Neuroreport 23:977–980

Lauter JL, Herscowitch P, Formby C et al (1985) Tonotopic organization in human auditory cortex revealed by positron emission tomography. Hear Res 20:199–205

Le Bihan D (2003) Looking into the functional architecture of the brain with diffusion MRI. Nat Rev Neurosci 4:469–480

Leherici S, Duffeau H, Cornu P et al (2000) Correspondence between functional magnetic resonance imaging somatotopy and individual brain anatomy of the central region: comparison with intraoperative stimulation in patients with brain tumors. J Neurosurg 92:589–598

Li W, Wait SD, Oqq RJ et al (2013) Functional magnetic resonance imaging of the visual cortex performed in children under sedation to assist in presurgical planning. J Neurosurg Pediatr 11:543–546

Lotze M, Grodd W, Birbaumer N et al (1999) Does use of a myoelectric prosthesis prevent cortical reorganization and phantom limb pain. Nat Neurosci 2:501–502

Lu JF et al (2013) "Awake" intraoperative functional MRI (ai-fMRI) for mapping the eloquent cortex: is it possible in awake craniotomy? Neuroimage Clin 2:132–147H

Lv Z, Wang E, Tong LM, Williams G, Zaharchuk M, Zeineh AN, Goldstein-Piekarski TM, Ball CL, Wintermark M (2018) Resting-state functional MRI: everything that nonexperts have always wanted to know. Am J Neuroradiol 39(8):1390–1399

Maesawa S, Fuji M, Nakahara N et al (2010) Intraoperative tractography and motor evoked potential (MEP) monitoring in surgery for gliomas around the corticospinal tract. World Neurosurg 74:153–161

Mahlke C, Wallhauser-Franke E (2004) Evidence for tinnitus-related plasticity in the auditory and limbic system, demonstrated by arg3.1 and c–fos immunocytochemistry. Hear Res 195:17–34

Maia AC, Malheiros SM, da Rocha AJ et al (2004) Stereotactic biopsy guidance in adults with supratentorial nonenhancing gliomas: role of perfusion-weighted magnetic resonanced imaging. J Neurosurg 101:970–976

Maillard L, Ishii K, Bushara K et al (2000) Mapping the basal ganglia. FMRI evidence for somatotopic representation of face, hand and foot. Neurology 55:377–383

Makela JP, Kirveskari E, Seppa M et al (2001) Three-dimensional integration of brain anatomy and functions to facilitate intraoperative navigation around the sensorimotor strip. Hum Brain Mapp 12:180–192

Mandonnet E, Mellerio C, Barberis M et al (2020) When right is on the left (and vice versa): a case series of glioma patients with reversed lateralization of cognitive functions. J Neurol Surg A Cent Eur Neurosurg 81:138–146

Mannfolk P et al (2011) Can resting-state functional MRI serve as a complement to task-based mapping of sensorimotor function? A test-retest reliability study in healthy volunteers. J Magn Reson Imaging 34:511–517

Mascott CR (2005) Comparison of magnetic tracking and optical tracking by simultaneous use of two independent frameless stereotactic systems. Neurosurgery 57(ONS Suppl 3):295–301

Massot-Tarrús A (2019) Comparing the Wada test and functional MRI for the presurgical evaluation of memory in temporal lobe epilepsy. Curr Neurol Neurosci Rep 19(6):31. https://doi.org/10.1007/s11910-019-0945-8

Medina LS, Aguirre E, Bernal B et al (2004) Functional MR imaging versus Wada test for evaluation of language lateralization: cost analysis. Radiology 230:49–54

Meier MP, Ilmberger J, Fesl G et al (2013) Validation of functional motor and language MRI with direct cortical stimulation. Acta Neurochir 155:675–683

Mikuni N, Okada T, Enatsu R et al (2007) Clinical impact of integrated functional neuronavigation and subcortical stimulation to preserve motor function during resection of brain tumors. J Neurosurg 106:593–598

Miller K, Joldes GR, Bourantas G et al (2019) Biomechanical modeling and computer simulation of the brain during neurosurgery. Int J Numer Method Biomed Eng 35:e3250

Mitchell TJ, Hacker CD, Breshears JD (2013) A novel data-driven approach to preoperative mapping of functional cortex using resting-state functional magnetic resonance imaging. Neurosurgery 73:969–983

Miyashita Y (2004) Cognitive memory: cellular and network machineries and their top-down control. Science 306:435–440

Moche M, Busse H, Dannenberg C et al (2001) Fusion von MRT-, fMRT-und intraoperativen MRT-Daten. Radiologe 41:993–1000

Moeller M, Freund M, Greiner C et al (2004) Real-time fMRI: a tool for the routine presurgical localisation of the motor cortex. Eur Radiol 15:292–295

Moffat BA, Reddy GR, McKonville P et al (2003) A novel polyacrylamide magnetic nanoparticle contrast agent for molecular imaging using MRI. Mol Imaging 2:324–332

Mongen MA, Willems PWA (2019) Current accuracy of surface matching compared to adhesive markers in patient-to-image registration. Acta Neurochir 191(5):865–870

Mühlnickel W, Elbert T, Taub E et al (1998) Reorganization of auditory cortex in tinnitus. Proc Natl Acad Sci U S A 95:10340–10343

Nakasato N, Yoshimoto T (2000) Somatosensory, auditory and visual evoked magnetic fields in patients with brain diseases. J Clin Neurophysiol 17:20–22

Neuner I, Kaffanke JB, Langen K-J et al (2012) Multimodal imaging utilising integrated MR-PET for human brain tumor assessment. Eur Radiol 22:2568–2580

Nimsky C, Ganslandt O, Cerny S et al (2000) Quantification of, visualization of, and compensation for brain shift using intraoperative magnetic resonance imaging. Neurosurgery 47:1070–1079

Nimsky C, Ganslandt O, Kober H et al (2001) Intraoperative magnetic resonance imaging combined with neuronavigation: a new concept. Neurosurgery 48:1082–1091

Nimsky C, Ganslandt O, Fahlbusch R (2004) Functional neuronavigation and intraoperative MRI. Adv Tech Stand Neurosurg 29:229–263

Okudera H, Takemae T, Kobayashi K (1993) Intraoperative computer tomographic scanning during transsphenoidal surgery. Neurosurgery 32:1041–1043

Owen SL, Heath J, Kringelbach ML et al (2007) Preoperative DTI and probabilistic tractography in an amputee with deep brain stimulation for lower limb stump pain. Br J Neurosurg 21:485–490

Paleologos TS, Wadley JP, Kitchen ND et al (2000) Clinical utility and cost-effectiveness of interactive image-guided craniotomy: clinical comparison between conventional and image-guided meningioma surgery. Neurosurgery 47:40–47

Partovi S, Jacobi B, Rapps N et al (2012) Clinical standardized fMRI reveals altered language lateralization in patients with brain tumor. AJNR Am J Neuroradiol 33:2151–2157

Pfisterer WK, Papadopoulos S, Drumm DA, Smith K, Preul MC (2008) Fiducial versus nonfiducial neuronavigation registration assessment and considerations of accuracy. Neurosurgery 62(3 suppl 1):201–207

Pirotte B, Goldman S, Massager N et al (2004) Combined use of 18F-fluorodeoxyglucose and 11C-methionine in 45 positron emission tomography guided stereotactic brain biopsies. J Neurosurg 101:476–483

Pirotte B, Voordecker P, Neugroschl C et al (2005) Combination of functional magnetic resonance imaging-guided neuronavigation and intraoperative cortical brain mapping improves targeting of motor cortex stimulation in neuropathic pain. Neurosurgery 56(ONS Suppl):344–359

Powell HWR, Koepp MJ, Richardson MP et al (2004) The application of functional MRI of memory in temporal lobe epilepsy: a clinical review. Epilepsia 45:855–863

Prabhu SS, Gasco J, Tummala S et al (2011) Intraoperative magnetic resonance imaging-guided tractography with integrated monopolar subcortical functional mapping for resection of brain tumors. J Neurosurg 114:719–726

Puce A, Constable RT, Luby ML et al (1995) Functional magnetic resonance imaging of sensory and motor cortex: comparison with electrophysiological localization. J Neurosurg 83:262–270

Pujol S et al (2015) The DTI challenge: toward standardized evaluation of diffusion tensor imaging tractography for neurosurgery. J Neuroimaging 25(6):875–882

Quartuccio N, Laudicella R, Vento A et al (2020) The additional value of 18 F-FDG PET and MRI in patients with glioma: a review of the literature from 2015 to 2020. Diagnostics 10:357. https://doi.org/10.3390/diagnostics10060357

Raabe A, Krishnan R, Wolff R, Hermann E, Zimmermann M, Seiffert V (2002) Laser surface scanning for patient registration in intracranial image-guided surgery. Neurosurgery 50(4):797–801

Rabin ML, Narayan VM, Kimberg DY et al (2004) Functional MRI predicts post surgical memory following temporal lobectomy. Brain 127:2286–2298

Raimbault A, Cazals X, Lauvin M-A et al (2014) Radionecrosis of malignant glioma and cerebral metastasis: a diagnostic challenge in MRI. Diagn Interv Imaging 95:985–1000

Ranjan M et al (2019) Tractography-based targeting of the ventral intermediate nucleus: accuracy and clinical utility in MRgFUS thalamotomy. J Neurosurg 27:1–8

Rapp M, Foeth FW, Felberg J et al (2013) Clinical value of O-(2-[18F]-fluoroethyl)-L-tyrosine positron emission tomography in patients with low grade glioma. Neurosurg Focus 34(2):E13

Rasche D, Tronnier VM (2016) Clinical significance of invasive motor cortex stimulation for trigeminal facial neuropathic pain syndromes. Neurosurgery 79:655–666

Rasmussen IA, Lindseth F, Rygh OM et al (2007) Functional neuronavigation combined with intraoperative 3D ultrasound: initial experiences during surgical resections close to eloquent brain areas and future directions in automatic brain shift compensation of preoperative data. Acta Neurochir 149:365–378

Rehemtulla A, Hall DE, Stegman LD et al (2002) Molecular imaging of gene expression and efficacy following adenoviral-mediated brain tumour gene therapy. Mol Imaging 1:43–55

Risholm P, Golby AJ, Wells W III et al (2011) Multimodal image registration for preoperative planning and image-guided neurosurgical procedures. Neurosurg Clin N Am 22:197–206

Roberts DW, Miga MI, Hartov A et al (1999) Intraoperatively updated neuroimaging using brain modeling sparse data. Neurosurgery 45:1199–1206

Roessler K, Donat M, R Lanzenberger R et al (2005) Evaluation of preoperative high magnetic field motor functional MRI (3 Tesla) in glioma patients by navigated electrocortical stimulation and postoperative outcome. J Neurol Neurosurg Psychiatry 76:1152–1157

Romstöck J, Fahlbusch R, Ganslandt O et al (2002) Localisation of the sensorimotor cortex during surgery for brain tumours: feasibility and waveform patterns of somatosensory evoked potentials. J Neurol Neurosurg Psychiatry 72:221–229

Ropele S, Fazekas F (2019) Quantification of cortical damage in multiple sclerosis using DTI remains a challenge. Brain 142:1848–1850

Rosenstock T, Picht T, Schneider H et al (2020) Pediatric navigated transcranial magnetic stimulation motor and language mapping combined with diffusion tensor imaging tractography: clinical experience. J Neurosurg Pediatr 24:1–11. https://doi.org/10.3171/2020.4.PEDS20174. Online ahead of print

Roux FE, Ibarrola D, Lotterie JA et al (2001a) Perimetric visual field and functional MRI correlation: implications for image-guided surgery in occipital brain tumors. J Neurol Neurosurg Psychiatry 71:505–514

Roux FE, Ibarrola D, Tremoulet M et al (2001b) Methodological and technical issues for integrating functional magnetic resonance imaging data in a neuronavigational system. Neurosurgery 49:1145–1157

Rozanski VE, Vollmar C, Cunha JP et al (2014) Connectivity patterns of pallidal DBS electrodes in focal dystonia: a diffusion tensor tractography study. NeuroImage 84:435–442

Rutten GJ, Ramsey NF, van Rijen PC et al (2002) FMRI-determined language lateralization in patients with unilateral or mixed language dominance according to the Wada test. NeuroImage 17:447–460

Ryan MJ, Erickson RK, Levin DN, Pelizzari CA, Macdonald RL, Dohrmann GJ (1996) Frameless stereotaxy with real-time tracking of patient head movement and retrospective patient-image registration. J Neurosurg 85(2):287–292

Šamec N et al (2020) Nanomedicine and immunotherapy: a step further towards precision medicine for glioblastoma. Molecules 25(3):490

Sanvito F, Caverzasi E, Riva M, Jordan KM, Blasi V, Scifo P, Iadanza A, Crespi SA, Cirillo S, Casarotti A, Leonetti A, Puglisi G, Grimaldi M, Bello L, Gorno-Tempini ML, Henry RG, Falini A, Castellano A (2020) fMRI-targeted high-angular resolution diffusion MR tractography to identify functional language tracts in healthy controls and glioma patients. Front Neurosci 14:225

Schiffbauer H, Berger MS, Ferrari P et al (2003) Preoperative magnetic source imaging for brain tumor surgery: a quantitative comparison with intraoperative sensory and motor mapping. Neurosurg Focus 15:E7

Schulder M, Holodny A, Liu WC et al (1999) Functional magnetic resonance image-guided surgery of tumors in or near the primary visual cortex. Stereotact Funct Neurosurg 73:31–36

Seidel K et al (2012) Low-threshold monopolar motor mapping for resection of primary motor cortex tumors. Neurosurgery 71(1 Suppl Operative):104–114. discussion 114–115

Seidel K et al (2020) Continuous dynamic mapping to identify the corticospinal tract in motor eloquent brain tumors: an update. J Neurol Surg A Cent Eur Neurosurg 81:105–110

Shabani S, Kaushal M, Budde MD, Wang MC, Kurpad SN (2020) Diffusion tensor imaging in cervical spondylotic myelopathy: a review. J Neurosurg Spine 28:1–8

Signorelli F, Guyotat J, Schneider F et al (2003) Technical refinements for validating functional MRI-based neuronavigation data by electrical stimulation during cortical language mapping. Minim Invasive Neurosurg 46:265–268

Sipos EP, Tebo SA, Zinreich SJ, Long DM, Brem H (1996) In vivo accuracy testing and clinical experience with the ISG Viewing Wand. Neurosurgery 39(1):194–202

Sol JC, Casaux J, Roux FE et al (2001) Chronic motor cortex stimulation for phantom limb pain: correlations between pain relief and functional imaging. Stereotact Funct Neurosurg 77:172–176

Sollmann N, Zhang H, Fratini A et al (2020) Risk assessment by presurgical tractography using navigated TMS maps in patients with highly motor- or language-eloquent brain tumors. Cancers 12(5):1264. https://doi.org/10.3390/cancers12051264

Son BC, Kim MC, Choi BG et al (2001) Proton magnetic resonance chemical shift imaging (1H CSI)-directed stereotactic biopsy. Acta Neurochir 143:45–49

Stadlbauer A, Moser E, Gruber S et al (2004) Integration of biochemical images of a tumor into frameless stereotaxy achieved using a magnetic resonance imaging/magnetic resonance spectroscopy hybrid data set. J Neurosurg 101:287–294

Stippich C, Hofmann R, Kapfer D et al (1999) Somatotopic mapping of the human primary somatosensory cortex by fully automated tactile stimulation using functional MRI. Neurosci Lett 277:25–28

Stippich C, Kapfer D, Hempel E et al (2000) Robust localization of the contralateral precentral gyrus in hemiparetic patients using the unimpaired ipsilateral hand. Neurosci Lett 285:155–159

Stippich C, Kress B, Ochmann H et al (2003) Preoperative functional magnetic resonance imaging (fMRI) in patients with rolandic brain tumors: indication, investigation strategy, possibilities and limitations of clinical application. Fortschr Roentgenstr 175:1042–1050

Stippich C, Rapps N, Dreyhaupt J et al (2007) Localizing and lateralizing language in patients with brain tumors: feasibility of routine preoperative functional MR imaging in 81 consecutive patients. Radiology 243:828–836

Stoeckel MC, Binkofski F (2010) The role of ipsilateral primary motor cortex in movement control and recovery from brain damage. Exp Neurol 221:13–17

Stroman PW, Kornelsen J, Lawrence J (2005) An improved method for spinal functional MRI with large volume coverage of the spinal cord. J Magn Reson Imaging 21:520–526

Su JH et al (2019) Thalamus Optimized Multi Atlas Segmentation (THOMAS): fast, fully automated segmentation of thalamic nuclei from structural MRI. NeuroImage 194:272–282

Taoka T, Sakamoto M, Nagakawa H et al (2008) Diffusion tensor tractography of the Meyer loop in cases of temporal lobe resection for temporal lobe epilepsy. Correlation between postoperative visual field defect and anterior limit of Meyer loop on tractography. AJNR Am J Neuroradiol 29:1329–1334

Thomas C, Ye FQ, Irfanoglu MO et al (2014) Anatomical accuracy of brain connections derived from diffusion MRI tractography is inherently limited. Proc Natl Acad Sci U S A 111(46):16574–16579

Thulborn KR (1999) Clinical rationale for very-high-field (3.0 Tesla). Functional magnetic resonance imaging. Top Magn Reson Imaging 10:37–50

Tie Y, Rigolo L, Norton IH et al (2014) Defining language networks from resting-state fMRI for surgical planning – a feasibility study. Hum Brain Mapp 35(3):1018–1030

Tohyama S, Walker MR, Sammartino F et al (2020) The utility of diffusion tensor imaging in neuromodulation: moving beyond conventional Magnetic Resonance Imaging. Neuromodulation 23:427–435

Tozakidou M, Wenz H, Reinhardt J et al (2013) Primary motor cortex activation and lateralization in patients with tumors of the central region. Neuroimage Clin 2:221–228

Tronnier VM, Wirtz CR, Knauth M et al (1996) Intraoperative computer-assisted neuronavigation in functional neurosurgery. Stereotact Funct Neurosurg 66:65–68

Tronnier VM, Wirtz CR, Knauth M et al (1997) Intraoperative diagnostic and interventional magnetic resonance imaging in neurosurgery. Neurosurgery 40:891–902

Tronnier V, Staubert A, Bonsanto MM et al (2000) Virtuelle Realität in der Neurochirurgie. Radiologe 40:211–217

Tyndall AJ et al (2017) Presurgical motor, somatosensory and language fMRI: technical feasibility and limitations in 491 patients over 13 years. Eur J Radiol 27:267–278

Unsgaard G, Gronningsaeter A, Ommedahl S et al (2002) Brain operations guided by real-time two-dimensional ultrasound: new possibilities as a result of improved image quality. Neurosurgery 51:402–412

Vabulas M, Kumar VA, Hamilton JD et al (2014) Real-time atlas-based stereotactic neuronavigation. Neurosurgery 74(1):128–134

Varma NR, Barton KN, Janic B, Shankar A, Iskander A, Ali MM, Arbab AS (2013) Monitoring adenoviral based gene delivery in rat glioma by molecular imaging. World J Clin Oncol 4(4): 91–101

Villalobos H, Germano IM (1999) Clinical evaluation of multimodality registration in frameless stereotaxy. Comput Aided Surg 4(1):45–49

Watanabe E, Watanabe T, Manaka S, Mayanagi Y, Takakura K (1987) Three-dimensional digitizer (neuronavigator): new equipment for computed tomography-guided stereotactic surgery. Surg Neurol 27:543–547

Wegscheid ML, Morshed RA, Cheng Y et al (2014) The art of attraction: application of multifunctional magnetic nanomaterials for malignant glioma. Expert Opin Drug Deliv 11:957–975

Wengenroth M, Blatow M, Guenther J et al (2011) Diagnostic benefits of presurgical fMRI in patients with brain tumours in the primary sensorimotor cortex. Eur Radiol 21:1517–1525

Winkler D, Strauss G, Lindner D et al (2005) The importance of functional magnetic resonance imaging in neurosurgical treatment of tumors in the central region. Clin Neuroradiol 15:182–189

Winston GP, Yogarajah M, Symms MR (2011) Diffusion tensor imaging tractography to visualize the relationship of the optic radiation to epileptogenic lesion prior to neurosurgery. Epilepsia 52:1430–1438

Wirtz CR, Knauth M, Hassfeld S et al (1998) Neuronavigation – first experience with three commercially available systems. Zentralbl Neurochir 59:14–22

Wirtz CR, Albert FK, Schwaderer M et al (2000) The benefit of neuronavigation for neurosurgery analyzed by its input on glioblastoma surgery. Neurol Res 22:354–360

Woerdeman PA, Willems PWA, Noordmans HJ, Tulleken CAF, Berkelbach van der Sprenkel JW (2007) Application accuracy in frameless image-guided neurosurgery: a comparison study of three patient-to-image registration methods. J Neurosurg 106(6):1012–1016

Woermann FG, Jokeit H, Luerding R et al (2003) Language lateralization by Wada test and fMR in 100 patients with epilepsy. Neurology 61:699–701

Wolfsberger S, Rössler K, Regatschnig R, Ungersböck K (2002) Anatomical landmarks for image registration in frameless stereotactic neuronavigation. Neurosurg Rev 25(1–2):68–72

Woolsey CN, Erickson TC, Gilson WE (1979) Localization in somatic sensory and motor areas of human cerebral cortex as determined by direct recording of evoked responses and electrical stimulation. J Neurosurg 51:476–506

Wu CWH, Kaass JH (1999) Reorganization in primary motor cortex of primates with long-standing therapeutic amputations. J Neurosci 19:7679–7697

Wu JS, Zhou LF, Tang WJ et al (2007) Clinical evaluation and follow-up outcome of diffusion tensor imaging-based neuronavigation: a prospective, controlled study in patients with gliomas involving pyramidal tracts. Neurosurgery 61:935–948

You SH, Jang SH, Kim YH et al (2005) Virtual-reality-induced cortical reorganization and associated locomotor recovery in chronic stroke: an experimenter-blinded study. Stroke 36:1166–1171

Yousry TA, Schmid U, Jassoy AG et al (1995) Topography of the cortical motor hand area: prospective study with functional MR imaging and direct motor mapping at surgery. Radiology 195:23–29

Zacà D, Nickerson JP, Deib G et al (2012) Effectiveness of four different clinical fMRI paradigms for preoperative regional determination of language lateralization in patients with brain tumors. Neuroradiology 54:1015–1025

Zaehle T, Rach S, Herrmann CS (2010) Transcranial alternating current stimulation enhances individual alpha activity in human EEG. PLoS One 5:e13766

Zhang Y, Vakhtin AA, Jennings JS, Massaband P, Wintermark M, Craig PL, Ashford JW, Clark JD, Fürst AJ (2020) Diffusion tensor tractography of brainstem fibers and its application in pain. PLoS One 15(2):e0213952

Zhu FP, Wu JS, Song YY et al (2012) Clinical application of motor pathway mapping using diffusion tensor imaging tractography and intraoperative direct subcortical stimulation in cerebral glioma surgery: a prospective cohort study. Neurosurgery 71:1170–1184

Zinreich SJ, Tebo SA, Long DM, Brem H, Mattox DE, Loury ME, van der Kolk CA, Koch WM, Kennedy DW, Bryan RN (1993) Frameless stereotaxic integration of CT imaging data: accuracy and initial applications. Radiology 188(3):735–742

Zolal A, Hejcl A, Vachata P et al (2012) The use of diffusion tensor images of the corticospinal tract in intrinsic brain tumor surgery: a comparison with direct subcortical stimulation. Neurosurgery 71:331–340

Zurowski B, Kordon A, Weber-Fahr W (2012) Relevance of orbito-frontal neurochemistry for the outcome of cognitive-behavioural therapy in patients with obsessive compulsive disorder. Eur Arch Psychiatry Clin Neurosci 262:617–624

Presurgical Functional Localization Possibilities, Limitations, and Validity

Lydia Chougar, Delphine Leclercq, Pierre-François Van de Moortele, and Stéphane Lehéricy

Contents

L. Chougar (✉) · S. Lehéricy
Centre de NeuroImagerie de Recherche—CENIR,
Institut du Cerveau et de la Moelle—ICM, Sorbonne
Universités, UPMC Univ Paris 06, UMR S 1127,
CNRS UMR 7225, Paris, France

Department of Neuroradiology, Groupe Hospitalier
Pitié-Salpêtrière, Université Pierre et Marie
Curie—Paris 6, 47-83, Boulevard de l'Hôpital,
Paris, France
e-mail: stephane.lehericy@psl.aphp.fr

D. Leclercq
Department of Neuroradiology, Groupe Hospitalier
Pitié-Salpêtrière, Université Pierre et Marie
Curie—Paris 6, 47-83, Boulevard de l'Hôpital,
Paris, France

P.-F. Van de Moortele
Center for Magnetic Resonance Research, University
of Minnesota, Minneapolis, MN, USA
e-mail: vande094@umn.edu

Abstract

Presurgical mapping using functional neuroimaging techniques—and particularly fMRI—is now commonly used in clinical practice and not just for research applications. Presurgical functional neuroimaging with its contributions *to surgical planning and to the prediction of postoperative outcome is now well established.*

Validation studies of functional imaging techniques have shown the potential of fMRI to *localize motor* areas and to *lateralize and localize language and memory functions.* However, particularly for cognitive brain functions, the imaging results strongly depend

© The Author(s), under exclusive license to Springer Nature Switzerland AG 2022
C. Stippich (ed.), *Clinical Functional MRI*, Medical Radiology Diagnostic Imaging,
https://doi.org/10.1007/978-3-030-83343-5_9

on the methodology and require optimal clinical standard procedures. Currently, functional neuroimaging is considered *complementary to direct electrical stimulation (DES)* providing *additional information*, such as information on the entire functional network and on the contralateral hemisphere, which is not accessible to DES. Until now, fMRI cannot fully replace DES. In contrast, for language functions, and more recently, for memory functions, fMRI has supplanted the *intracarotid amobarbital procedure (IAP) or Wada test*. *Diffusion tensor imaging (DTI) fiber tracking*, which determines anatomical relationship between the tumor and adjacent fiber tracks, also plays a major role for presurgical mapping.

1 Possibilities and Limitations of Functional Brain Mapping

In presurgical functional mapping, determining the accuracy of functional maps is essential, the presurgical localization of eloquent areas at risk allowing to avoid postoperative deficits. Among the available and established functional imaging methods, functional MRI (fMRI) is the most widely used. FMRI can be easily performed using clinical MRI scanners. Within the same scanning session, high-resolution three-dimensional (3D) images of the brain and functional images with or without contrast injection are acquired (depending on the brain tumor entity), providing accurate anatomic detail about the lesion. The following paragraphs will focus on the possibilities and limitations of blood-oxygen-level-dependent (BOLD) contrast fMRI.

1.1 Spatial Localization of BOLD Signal

Because fMRI maps are based on secondary metabolic and hemodynamic events that follow neuronal activity and not on the electrical activity itself, it remains unclear what the exact spatial specificity of fMRI is, despite proven congruence of fMRI localization and neuronal activation (Logothetis and Wandell 2004). Moreover, the physiological phenomenon underlying BOLD contrast is not yet fully understood. For details, see chapter "Revealing Brain Activity and White Matter Structure Using Functional and Diffusion-Weighted Magnetic Resonance Imaging."

1.1.1 Spatial Specificity of Deoxyhemoglobin-Based (BOLD fMRI) Methods

Experimental multiple-site single-unit recordings and fMRI studies on the same animal have suggested that the spatial specificity of T_2^* BOLD contrast might be in the range of 4–5 mm for single-condition maps, i.e., the task compared with the rest condition (Ugurbil et al. 2003). This may be adequate for presurgical brain mapping currently performed in the human brain with an image resolution of 3–5 mm, but a much better resolution can be achieved under certain circumstances (Harel et al. 2006).

The explanation for this low resolution is that deoxyhemoglobin changes which are initiated at the point of increased neuronal activity do not remain stationary and propagate into large *draining* vessels. Thus, deoxyhemoglobin changes incorrectly appear as *activation* away from the actual site of neuronal activity. Therefore, increased contribution of small vessels (capillaries) versus large *draining* vessels is a critical issue for improving the spatial resolution of BOLD contrast images. The respective contribution of small versus large vessels depends on several factors, including the field strength and the type of MR-sequence used for BOLD-imaging.

1.1.2 The Type of Sequence: Spin Echo (T_2) Versus Gradient Echo (T_2^*) BOLD fMRI

1.1.2.1 The Intra- and Extravascular Components of BOLD Signal

The most commonly used fMRI approach was introduced in 1992 and is based on T_2^* (i.e., gradient echo) BOLD contrast, which visualizes regional alterations in deoxyhemoglobin accompanying changes in neuronal activity (Heeger et al. 2002; Logothetis and Wandell 2004).

BOLD contrast originates from the intravoxel magnetic field inhomogeneity induced by paramagnetic deoxyhemoglobin inside the red blood cells, which in turn are compartmentalized within the blood vessels. Magnetic susceptibility differences between the deoxyhemoglobin-containing compartments and the surrounding space generate magnetic field gradients across and near the boundaries of these compartments. Consequently, BOLD contrast has thus an intravascular and extravascular contribution (Fig. 1).

The intravascular T2-BOLD effect is associated with the magnetic field gradient generated outside the red blood cells and inside the vessels.

The field gradients around the red blood cells are very small compared to diffusion distances around and across the membranes of these cells (Fig. 1). Therefore, the effect is dynamically averaged and is detectable as a T_2 effect. When regional deoxyhemoglobin content increases, the T_2 of blood decreases (Thulborn et al. 1982). This intravascular effect is present in large as well as in small vessels.

The extravascular BOLD effect is associated with the magnetic field gradient generated outside the boundaries of the blood vessels. This gradient is due to the difference in magnetic susceptibility induced by deoxyhemoglobin between the vessels and the surrounding diamagnetic tissue. For small vessels such as capillaries, water diffusion during image acquisition (typically 50–100 ms for echo planar images (EPI)) dynamically averages the magnetic field gradient and

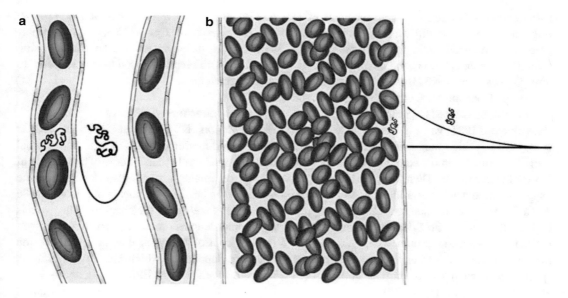

Fig. 1 The extravascular BOLD effect is associated with the magnetic field gradient generated outside the boundaries of the blood vessels, which is due to the difference in magnetic susceptibility induced by deoxyhemoglobin between the vessel and the surrounding diamagnetic tissue (after Hoppel et al. 1993). The black curves outside the vessels represent the field gradient produced by the blood, which is inside the vessels. (**a**) For small vessels such as capillaries, the field gradients around the vessels are large compared to diffusion distances; therefore, the extravascular BOLD is a T2 effect as water diffusion

dynamically averages in the magnetic field gradient. (**b**) For large vessels, the field gradients around the vessels are small compared to diffusion distances. The signal loss in the voxel is the result of a static averaging; therefore, the extravascular BOLD is a T2* effect. In (**a**, **b**), the intravascular BOLD effect is associated with the magnetic field gradient generated outside the red blood cells inside the vessels. Similarly to the extravascular BOLD effect around capillaries, the intravascular BOLD is detectable as a T2 effect results in a T_2 effect, similarly to the intravascular BOLD effect. For large vessels, dynamic averaging is not possible anymore. In contrast, static averaging will result in a signal loss within the voxel. A water molecule located in the vicinity of the blood vessel will see a static magnetic field, which will vary with the proximity to the vessel (Fig. 1). As this magnetic field varies across the voxel, the signal of the entire voxel will be dephased, resulting in a T_2^* effect.

1.1.2.2   Specificity of Spin Echo (T_2) Versus Gradient Echo (T_2^*) BOLD

As detailed above, the T2-BOLD response arises from intra- and extravascular effects originating from small and large vessels. The intravascular contribution originates from both large and small vessels, whereas the extravascular part is dominated by small vessel contributions (Boxerman et al. 1995). Thus, the spin echo (SE) BOLD fMRI response is due to apparent changes in T_2 originating from the diffusion of water in the presence of magnetic field gradients generated in the extravascular space around the microvasculature (Ogawa et al. 1993; Boxerman et al. 1995), as well as from the exchange of water into and out of red blood cells within the blood itself (Pawlik et al. 1981; van Zijl et al. 1998; Ugurbil et al. 1999). At high magnetic fields, blood has a short T_2, shorter than the echo times that are used in fMRI experiments. Therefore, the blood is not expected to contribute significantly to the measured BOLD signal changes. Consequently, at high field strength, the SE BOLD mainly originates from the extravascular space around the microvasculature and hence provides greater specificity to changes in neuronal activity (Lee et al. 1999; Duong et al. 2003; Ugurbil et al. 2003; Yacoub et al. 2003).

1.1.2.3   Field Dependence of BOLD Signal

Both the signal-to-noise ratio (SNR) and spatial resolution of BOLD fMRI increase with the main magnetic field strength. Higher magnetic fields will also *preferentially attenuate the macrovascular contribution* (Ugurbil et al. 2003).

The BOLD response is expected to behave differently with increasing magnetic fields in small versus large blood vessels (Ogawa et al. 1993). The BOLD signal increases quadratically with the magnetic field strength for capillaries and linearly for larger vessels (Ogawa et al. 1993). Therefore, in addition to increasing the fMRI signal, higher magnetic fields will specifically enhance the signal from parenchymal capillary tissue. In contrast, BOLD signal originating from large vessels will be overrepresented at lower magnetic field strengths (Ciobanu et al. 2015; Ladd et al. 2018).

1.2   fMRI Artifacts and Limitations

In clinical fMRI, we need to consider several types of artifacts and methodological limitations, the most important of which we discuss below. *For details, see chapter "Clinical BOLD fMRI and DTI: Artifacts, Tips and Tricks."* It is important to note that even validation studies using established reference procedures are prone to such interferences.

1.2.1   Movement Artifacts

Head motion is a critical issue in BOLD fMRI. Head motion consists of rigid body global deformations and translations. The effect of motion on image artifacts also depends on the extent of the head's movements in relation to the size of the voxels used for imaging. When voxels have side lengths smaller than a millimeter, motion control becomes crucial. Head motion does not depend on which part of the brain is imaged. In single-shot EPI, each image is virtually devoid of motion artifacts since the acquisition time is very short (<100 ms). However, head motion may occur between successive images within fMRI series. Most fMRI studies are currently performed with a spatial resolution of 3–4 mm (in-plane voxel size) and a slice thickness of 4–5 mm (e.g., matrix: 64 × 64, field of view = 24 cm). Head motion artifacts predominantly affect tissue interfaces with large changes

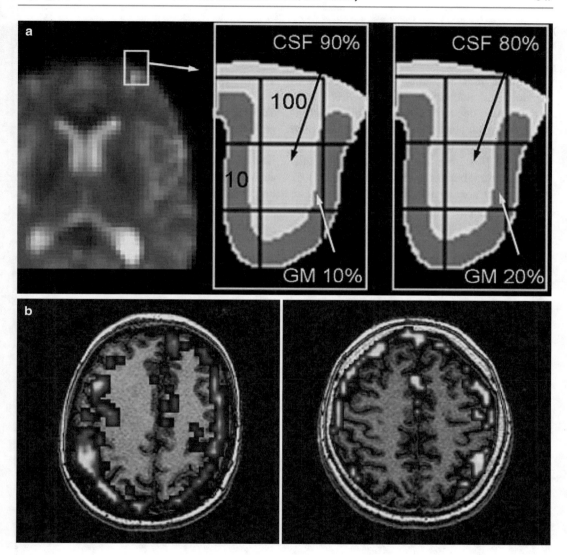

Fig. 2 Head motion artifact. A movement of one tenth of a voxel (300–400 μm) may result in signal changes similar or even larger than the physiological signal increase due to task performance, and, unfortunately, the motion correction software cannot distinguish between the two signals. Artifacts most severely affect tissue interfaces. An example is provided in (**a**). The picture shows the frontal sulcus. In the left diagram, the 4 mm voxel of interest (middle) contains 90% cerebrospinal fluid (CSF, signal = 100 arbitrary units) and 10% gray matter (GM, signal = 10) resulting in an average signal of 91 (left diagram). A 0.4 mm motion (one tenth of the voxel size) will result in an average signal intensity of 82 (80% CSF and 20% GM, right diagram). (**b**) Typical head motion artifacts in two different subjects

in signal intensity (Fig. 2). A movement of one tenth of a voxel (300–400 μm) may lead to similar or larger signal changes than the physiological signal increase due to the task performance (Fig. 2). One can reduce these artifacts by care-

fully setting up the subject in the magnet (padding foams). External devices, such as a bite bar setup, can further minimize head motion but are rarely used in clinical practice. Carefully explaining the task to the subject may also reduce head motion. Furthermore, nowadays, motion correction is implemented in all fMRI preprocessing software.

Cardiac and respiratory motion results in physiological fluctuations of the BOLD signal. Brain motion due to cardiac pulsation is negligible in the motor cortex but becomes significant in the upper brain stem and diencephalon (Enzmann and Pelc 1992). Brain motion has a small amplitude (0.16 mm) but can represent as much as 30% of the voxel size at ultrahigh spatial resolution (0.5 mm in plane). EPI images are particularly sensitive to changes in resonance frequency which can arise from respiration and are more significant at high magnetic field strengths (Van de Moortele et al. 2002). Noise generated from respiration-induced phase and frequency fluctuations and from cardiac-induced fluctuations can be corrected using different algorithms (Pfeuffer

et al. 2002), some of them based on physiological recordings (Hu et al. 1995).

1.2.2 Magnetic Susceptibility Artifacts

These artifacts are due to differences in the magnetic susceptibility of bone, air, and brain structures. These susceptibility differences generate field gradients which result in an inhomogeneous static magnetic field. The consequences are signal loss and distortion in EPI images. These artifacts are particularly predominant in regions containing air and bone, such as sinuses and inner ear structures. They are prevalent in calcified structures and after brain hemorrhage because of metallic particle deposition, such as in vascular malformations (Fig. 3). They are also frequently observed following brain surgery because of the presence of metallic particles deposited during surgery.

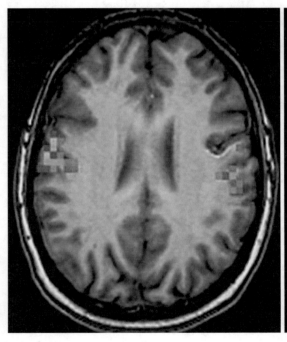 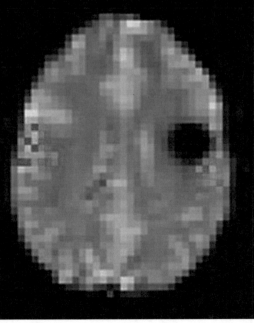

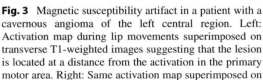

Fig. 3 Magnetic susceptibility artifact in a patient with a cavernous angioma of the left central region. Left: Activation map during lip movements superimposed on transverse T1-weighted images suggesting that the lesion is located at a distance from the activation in the primary motor area. Right: Same activation map superimposed on a transverse EPI T2* image showing the lesion surrounded by a large area of signal drop due to T2* shortening susceptibility artifact. Although no activation is visible inside the area of signal drop, it is not possible to conclude that the functional area does not extend inside this area

Magnetic susceptibility artifacts increase with field strength. Their impact can be reduced by using higher bandwidths, shorter TE, thinner slices, and better shimming procedures in order to improve static magnetic field homogeneity.

1.2.3 BOLD Response Alterations Induced by the Lesion

Neurovascular coupling that underlies BOLD contrast can be altered in normal aging and in vascular diseases and can thus affect the BOLD signal (Pineiro et al. 2002; D'Esposito et al. 2003; Hamzei et al. 2003). This is particularly important in BOLD fMRI studies in patients with brain tumors because the abnormal vasculature is an essential feature of tumor growth (Folkman et al. 1989). Decreased activation has been reported on the side of the tumor predominantly in high-grade glioma (Holodny et al. 1999, 2000). It has been suggested that negative BOLD responses correlate with decreased neuronal activity (Shmuel et al. 2006) or neuronal inhibition in epilepsy (Kobayashi et al. 2005), but the different factors contributing to decreased BOLD activation in patients with brain tumors are not fully understood. They may also include a loss of autoregulation in the tumor vasculature and venous or pressure effects (Holodny et al. 1999, 2000). Several studies have suggested that the regional cerebral blood volume (rCBV) measured by perfusion MRI is altered in gliomas (Ludemann et al. 2001; Cha et al. 2003; Law et al. 2004) and that fMRI activation decreases in the vicinity of brain tumors (Holodny et al. 2000; Fujiwara et al. 2004; Hou et al. 2006; Jiang et al. 2010). Studies which used DES as a reference have shown that glioma grade influences the diagnostic performance of presurgical fMRI for motor and language mapping: in WHO grade II and III gliomas they found higher sensitivity and lower specificity than in glioblastoma multiforme (Bizzi et al. 2008; Castellano et al. 2017). Similarly, tumor type influenced fMRI activation in the ipsilateral primary motor cortex which was significantly reduced in glioblastoma (Fraga de Abreu et al. 2016; Castellano et al. 2017).

In patients with brain arteriovenous malformations (AVMs), flow abnormalities may interfere with fMRI detection of language-related areas (Lehericy et al. 2002). Wada tests and/or postembolization fMRI have shown that severe flow abnormalities contribute to abnormal language lateralization and impair the detection of the BOLD signal (Lehericy et al. 2002). Neurovascular coupling can be altered in several ways in patients with brain AVMs. Hypotension or the presence of a so-called steal phenomenon may negatively influence the normal functions in areas adjacent to the lesion (Barnett et al. 1987; Fogarty-Mack et al. 1996). Changes in cerebral blood flow (Barnett et al. 1987; Young et al. 1990), perfusion pressure (Hassler and Steinmetz 1987; Fogarty-Mack et al. 1996), oxygen metabolism (Fink 1992), autoregulation processes, and vasoreactivity (Barnett et al. 1987; Hassler and Steinmetz 1987; Young et al. 1994; Fogarty-Mack et al. 1996), all of which have been reported in areas adjacent to AVMs, may alter the BOLD signal intensity and its detection.

1.2.4 Effect of Subject Task Performance and Statistical Threshold

For a given task, the magnitude of the BOLD signal variation depends on the subject' task performance. For example, activation of the primary motor cortex increases with movement frequency, amplitude, and force (Waldvogel et al. 1999). Similarly, activation in language areas will become more important as the number of words produced increases during a verbal fluency task. Therefore, monitoring the subject performance during the task is important for correct data interpretation.

The statistical threshold used for activation maps determines the displayed size of the cluster of active voxels. A low threshold means high sensitivity but poor specificity and comes with the risk of false-positive activations. Conversely, a high threshold will increase specificity, on the cost of sensitivity, and of increasing the risk of false negatives (Fig. 4).

1.2.5 Alternatives to Task-Based fMRI

Task-based fMRI comes with a few limitations. Preoperative task-based fMRI requires subject

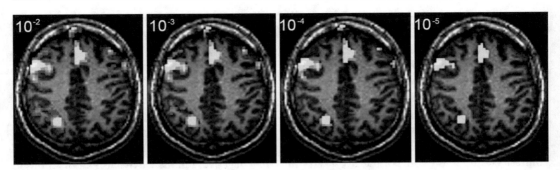

Fig. 4 Variation in brain activations detected with statistical thresholds ranging from $p < 0.01$ (left) to $p < 0.00001$ (right). A low threshold may increase the number of nonessential areas (false positives) and the size of the critical areas, whereas a high threshold may exclude eloquent areas from reaching statistical significance (false negatives)

cooperation, and, therefore, is not feasible in patients with neurological deficits, or impaired consciousness or in young children. Choosing the appropriate task is another important factor for the reliable activation of eloquent brain areas. These difficulties can be overcome by several approaches, e.g., by passive movement for motor mapping (Ogg et al. 2009). More recent approaches rely on functional connectivity techniques. Functional connectivity refers to the temporal correlation between various fMRI signals in spatially unconnected regions. It can be studied by measuring coherent signal fluctuations in BOLD fMRI time series in the resting brain (Biswal et al. 1995). For instance, resting-state functional imaging studies have revealed covarying fluctuations in distributed brain networks.

Previous studies have shown that brain tumors induce a loss of functional connectivity (Bartolomei et al. 2006; Guggisberg et al. 2008). This decreased resting-state functional connectivity in the tumor area has been shown to be strongly associated with the absence of eloquent cortex in DES experiments (Martino et al. 2011). In addition, resection of areas with reduced connectivity bears a low risk of postoperative deficits (Guggisberg et al. 2008). Resting-state fMRI could also efficiently detect the motor and language network when compared with DES (Mitchell et al. 2013). A recent study in brain tumors has shown that sensorimotor and language resting-state networks were identifiable

within 1 min of scan time with high concordance between DES, task-based fMRI and resting-state fMRI (within 5–10 mm Euclidean distance in the motor cortex, Broca's, and Wernicke's areas) (Vakamudi et al. 2019).

In the future, resting-state fMRI may be used as a surrogate for task-based fMRI when task performance is limited, e.g., in patients with poor cooperation or impaired consciousness (Castellano et al. 2017). For more details see chapter "Presurgical Resting-State fMRI."

2 Validation of Presurgical Mapping Using Established Reference Procedures

2.1 Direct Electrical Stimulations

Currently, invasive electrophysiological investigations remain the reference procedure (*gold standard*) for brain surgery, in particular for tumors located near or within eloquent cortical and/or subcortical structures (Keles and Berger 2004; Duffau et al. 2005). Direct electrical stimulation (DES) allows mapping large numbers of motor, somatosensory, and cognitive functions. DES also permits the study of anatomo-functional connectivity by directly stimulating white matter tracts (Duffau et al. 2002, 2003b; Keles et al. 2004). Therefore, DES is viewed as an accurate and reliable technique to localize cortical and subcortical regions at surgical risk regarding brain function. Consequently, a reproducible functional disturbance induced by DES will indicate where to stop with the resection, both for cortical and subcortical structures. Tumor removal is hence performed around functional boundaries to optimize the accuracy of tumor removal and to minimize the risk of postoperative functional deficits.

However, DES has some limitations. It only allows loco-regional and not whole brain mapping. Further, it is a time-consuming and invasive procedure, and the number of tasks that can be performed during surgery is limited. *Therefore, DES should be combined with other metabolic and functional imaging methods.*

2.1.1 Basic Principles

Electrical stimulation increases membrane excitability via an initial phase of passive modification of the local membrane potential (MP) at the level of the cathode (the negative electrode). The inner side of the membrane becomes progressively less negative than the outer side (the membrane becomes inversely hyperpolarized with regard to the anode). The intensity of this phenomenon depends on the stimulation parameters and on the characteristics of the membrane (Jayakar 1993). Stimulation of the membrane is easier at the initial segment of axons in myelinated fibers and in fibers of greater diameter (Ranck Jr 1975). If the MP reaches the depolarization threshold, voltage-dependent ion channels will open and Na^+ ions will enter into the neuron. This Na^+ entry will invert the MP between +20 mV and +30 mV. A secondary outflow of K^+ ions, associated with an inhibition of the inward flux of Na^+ ions, brings the MP back to its resting state. This rapid sequence of MP fluctuations—the action potential—is always the same, regardless of the stimulation parameters (law of *all or nothing*).

2.1.2 Risks Associated with DES

Direct electrical stimulations can damage the brain. Tissue damage can result from numerous causes. Accumulation of negative charges at the cathode or of metal ions at the anode can damage the brain (Agnew and McCreery 1987).

Biphasic impulses in DES can prevent this because the second stimulus inverses the effects of the first one. Excessive heat produced by hydrolysis induces vacuolization and chromatolysis (Doty and Barlett 1981). An intracellular current leakage from the anode to the cathode through the cytoplasm can damage the mitochondria and the endoplasmic reticulum (Pudenz et al. 1977). Repetitively and synchronously stimulated neurons can alter neuronal homeostasis (Fertziger and Ranck Jr 1970; Agnew and McCreery 1987). These risks are directly linked to the charge density. Animal studies have shown that no lesions occur when the charge does not exceed 55 µC/cm^2/phase (Gordon et al. 1990). Stimulations can also generate seizures. The frequency of seizures is estimated at 5–20% (Sartorius and Berger 1998). Monitoring the stimulation with electrocorticography helps detecting *after discharge* in patients (corresponding to discharge occurring after the stimulation has ceased) (Lesser et al. 1984), except for children who have nonmyelinated fibers (Jayakar et al. 1992). The recording electrodes should ideally be located in the immediate proximity of each stimulation location and therefore should *follow* the stimulation electrode. They should also have a small diameter to allow stimulation of the cortex.

Finally, any conductive substance such as cerebrospinal fluid or blood can distribute the current beyond the target tissue, thus increasing the risk of false negatives of DES. Any stimulated structure must therefore be kept dry.

2.1.3 Practical Stimulation Methods

The optimal stimulation parameters (best benefit/risk ratio) have been extensively studied (Nathan et al. 1993; Duffau 2004). They can differ significantly depending on the degree of cerebral maturation and fiber myelination (Jayakar et al. 1992), as well as anesthetic drugs and pathological processes (tumor, epilepsy, postictal status) (Jayakar 1993).

Bipolar stimulation is usually performed using a probe with two tips which are 5 mm apart (Fig. 5) and using the following parameters: rectangular impulses, biphasic current at 50 Hz

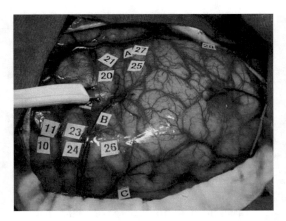

Fig. 5 Intraoperative view showing bipolar stimulation of a patient using a probe with two tips which are 5 mm apart. During surgery, the probe is placed on the cortical surface of the patient. Stimulation sites are labeled using small tags

Motor functions can be mapped in patients who are awake or under general anesthesia, by inducing involuntary motor responses. Awake patients have to stay generally passive during stimulation. Rarely, when looking for *negative motor areas* in the premotor cortex (Luders et al. 1995), the patient is asked to make regular movements which are then altered during the stimulation. Changes in movement parameters are recorded (slowdown, decrease in precision or amplitude, interruption). Under general anesthesia, small movements can be overlooked. This is a frequent problem for neck movements because the intubation cannula often prevents muscular contractions from being perceived. Concomitant intraoperative electromyographic recording and motor evoked potentials improve the detection (Yingling et al. 1999). However, these measures require additional effort. They require additional equipment, the presence of an electrophysiologist in the operating room, and electrodes on the entire hemibody contralateral to the stimulation side if the lesion is in the vicinity of the corona radiata and/or the internal capsule (Duffau et al. 2003a). Sensory functions are mapped intraoperatively by patient-reported dysesthesia (responses are therefore subjective).

For cognitive function, language (spontaneous speech, naming, comprehension, etc.), calculation, memory, reading, or writing are evaluated in awake patients by generating transient disturbances (Ojemann et al. 1989; Duffau et al. 2002). Selecting the most appropriate tests is critical here. Eloquent sites can be detected only if the *proper* function has been tested. This is why sensitive tasks are used rather than specific ones.

Language mapping usually includes a counting test followed by an object-naming task. The counting test detects articulatory dysfunctions including slowing down, dysarthria, anarthria, complete speech arrest, more or less associated with facial movements and/or hoarseness and/or automatic swallowing. During the object-naming task, various symptoms such as articulatory disorders, pure anomia, phonemic or semantic paraphrasias, or even perseverations, are induced. These tasks are short (less than 4 s duration) and therefore compatible with surgical requirements

(Lesser et al. 1987) or 60 Hz (Ojemann et al. 1989; Berger 1995), and intensities of 1–18 mA. Under local anesthesia, current intensities of less than 6–8 mA with an impulse duration of 0.3 ms (Lesser et al. 1987) to 1 ms (Ojemann et al. 1989; Berger 1995) are standard parameters. Typically, the stimulation intensity is progressively increased from 4 mA (under general anesthesia) or 1 mA (under local anesthesia), by increments of 1 mA in order to find the optimal threshold generating responses without causing seizures.

In children, the response rates are lower than in adults (less than 20% <5 years or even 0% <1 year) because of the immaturity of fibers (higher chronaxie in nonmyelinized fibers). Therefore, a progressively and alternately sequential increase of impulse intensity and duration has been proposed (Jayakar et al. 1992).

2.1.4 Neuropsychological Evaluation

Defining the *eloquent* cortical areas using DES requires appropriate tasks and an accurate recording of the clinical response to determine whether stimulation of the site interferes with function. For this purpose, speech therapists or psychologists are present in the operation room in order to interpret DES-induced dysfunctions (Duffau et al. 2002).

under local anesthesia. Depending on the localization of the lesion, a third more specific task is also performed. This task is chosen in each patient based on the individual cortical language organization, as evaluated preoperatively by a neuropsychological assessment and by functional neuroimaging. Tasks include verb generation, tasks in foreign languages for bilingual individuals, memory, calculation, repetition, reading, or even comprehension tasks for patients with posterior temporoparietal lesions (Gatignol et al. 2004).

2.1.5 Co-registration with Functional Imaging Data

Several methods have been used to compare DES with functional imaging data. Initially, simple visual comparisons were obtained between intraoperative views of DES and fMRI data (Jack Jr et al. 1994; Yousry et al. 1995). Co-registration has also been performed by comparing pictures of DES positive sites with the preoperative 3D rendering of the brain (Pujol et al. 1996; Lehericy et al. 2000b) (Fig. 6). However, these methods are not quantitative. 3D rendering displays brain activation as viewed transparently from the surface of the brain. Therefore, the display includes activation that is located in the depth of the sulci and gyri. More recently, co-registration has been obtained using stereotactic neuronavigation procedures (Lehericy et al. 2000b; Krings et al. 2001b; Krishnan et al. 2004). This technique allows a 3D multiplanar comparison of the DES positive sites with functional data, as well as measurements of distances and overlap.

2.1.6 Limitations of Functional and DES Comparison

DES and functional imaging methods provide fundamentally different types of data. DES interferes directly and only locally with neuronal function, thus blocking the ability of the patient to perform a task. Therefore, it is assumed that DES allows identification of critical language areas only. In contrast, functional imaging methods provide activation maps obtained during performance of motor, language, or cognitive tasks in primary and secondary functional areas.

Consequently, imaging techniques do usually not only include the primary target area, but also activity in nonessential areas that are associated with task performance, but could potentially be resected without permanent functional deficit. As mentioned above, functional maps and areas are visualized based on a statistical threshold. Therefore, a low threshold may increase both the number of nonessential areas and the size of the critical areas, whereas a stringent threshold may not allow critical areas to reach statistical significance. Craniotomy and debulking may induce deformation, which impairs image registration (Hill et al. 2000; Krings et al. 2001b). Finally, tasks performed during neurofunctional imaging and intraoperative procedures are not identical because of the different setups in the MR-scanner or OR, respectively (Lurito et al. 2000). These limitations need to be kept in mind when comparing the different techniques.

2.2 Intracarotid Amobarbital Procedure (IAP) or Wada Test

The intracarotid amobarbital procedure (IAP), or Wada test, was first reported as a means to identify the hemisphere of language dominance in patients with epilepsy in the 1950s (Wada and Rasmussen 1960). IAP was then modified to also measure memory function in patients undergoing surgery for epilepsy (Milner et al. 1962). The role of IAP is to assess language and amnesic risks by ensuring that the hemisphere contralateral to the operated one is able to subserve language and memory functions. Thus, IAP helps to predict and prevent postoperative language and memory deficits and to give an estimate of linguistic and neuropsychological outcome (Sperling et al. 1994; Loring et al. 1995).

2.2.1 Methods

IAP is performed in an angiography suite in the presence of a neurology and neuroscience team (Rausch et al. 1993; Akanuma et al. 2003). The patient is positioned on the angiography table. EEG monitoring is performed. After local skin anesthesia and femoral artery access, a diagnostic

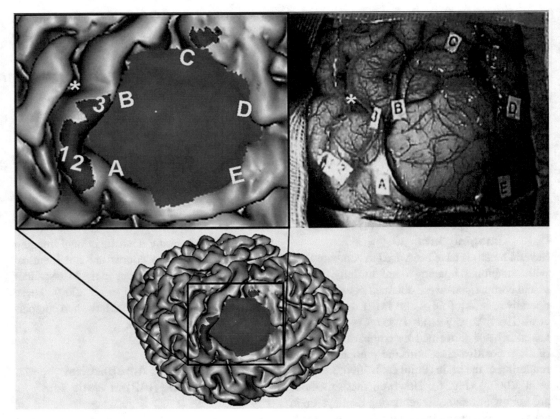

Fig. 6 Concordance of fMRI and intraoperative cortical stimulation. Upper left: Surface rendering of the cortex in a patient with a left premotor low-grade glioma (enlarged view of the figure in the lower row). The tumor is represented in blue. Activation during performance of right-hand movement is shown in red. Upper right: Intraoperative view of the same patient (same orientation). The letters outline the tumor margins. The numbers indicate the stimulation sites that elicited hand movements. Note the good correspondence between the fMRI activation map and direct electrical stimulations

catheter is placed selectively in the internal carotid arteries (ICA) under fluoroscopic guidance. Then amobarbital is injected in the ICA for each side separately. Therefore, the IAP induces a temporary inactivation of the cortex supplied by the anterior and middle cerebral arteries in the hemisphere ipsilateral to the injection. Rarely, both hemispheres are tested on two consecutive days. During the 10–15 min of the procedure, patients receive a battery of language and memory tasks following amobarbital injection (Jones-Gotman 1987). Language tasks usually include speech production (serial speech, naming), speech reception (simple motor commands, token test), and other speech tasks, such as reading aloud and spelling. Tasks are scored so that a lateralization index (LI) can be calculated for each task. The LI can be expressed as the difference between the scores during left injection minus the scores during right injection of amobarbital, divided by the maximum possible score.

2.2.2   Risks and Limitations of the Wada Test

The IAP has several disadvantages (Simkins-Bullock 2000). Its risks include those of intracarotid catheterization. Following cerebral angiography, the ischemic event rate has been estimated to be between 0.3% and 1.8% (0.07–0.3% permanent) (Dion et al. 1987; Cloft et al.

1999). Test–retest reliability and external validation cannot be performed. IAP evaluation is performed within a short period of time (approximately 3–10 min). Anesthesia can induce behavioral effects (e.g., aphasia, attention deficits, neglect, and somnolence). Amobarbital injected via the ICA will inactivate the amygdala and the anterior hippocampus but never or rarely the posterior two-thirds of the hippocampus (Jack Jr et al. 1989; Hong et al. 2000b). This represents a critical concern for the validity of memory assessment. Moreover, in some patients, mesial temporal perfusion can be unaffected during IAP (de Silva et al. 1999). In addition, IAP also inactivates the rest of the hemisphere ipsilateral to the injection and in some patients also the contralateral hemisphere (Hong et al. 2000b). To overcome these limitations, selective IAP via an injection in the posterior cerebral artery has therefore been proposed to test for memory function (Jack Jr et al. 1989). The risk of morbidity of this procedure is much greater than via direct ICA injection, and thus it is not widely used (Jack Jr et al. 1989). For language functions, the IAP provides information on the hemispheric language dominance but not on the anatomical location of language areas and their relation to the lesion. Lastly, the total direct costs of the Wada test have been estimated to be 3.7 times that of fMRI (Medina et al. 2004).

2.2.3 Validation of the Wada Test

IAP has been validated in several ways. Recording of intrahippocampal activity using depth electrodes has shown that the EEG background activity can be significantly suppressed in the posterior hippocampal regions even in the absence of amobarbital perfusion in these areas (Kurthen et al. 1999). Using HMPAO-SPECT, hypoperfusion in the territories of the anterior and middle cerebral arteries was observed during IAP (de Silva et al. 1999). Hypoperfusion in medial temporal structures was noticed in the great majority of these patients (de Silva et al. 1999). Further, in the epileptogenic hemisphere, the degree of hippocampal damage correlated with the impairment in Wada memory performance (Sass et al. 1991; O'Rourke et al. 1993; Davies et al. 1996).

In a few patients with unilateral temporal lobe epilepsy, IAP may also paradoxically lateralize memory function. In these patients, IAP showed poorer memory performance in the non-epileptogenic hemisphere (Davies et al. 1996; Rouleau et al. 1997; Detre et al. 1998; Spencer et al. 2000). Paradoxical IAP memory lateralization (i.e., ipsilateral to the seizure focus) was still concordant with fMRI lateralization scores in two patients with temporal lobe epilepsy (Detre et al. 1998). Spencer et al. (2000) suggested that in patients with medial temporal lobe epilepsy not well lateralized by noninvasive evaluation and in patients with neocortical or mesial frontal epilepsy, IAP may provide incorrect localization which ultimately alters surgical management (Spencer et al. 2000). This paradoxical lateralization has rarely been reported using FDG-PET (Sperling et al. 1995; Nagarajan et al. 1996). In such cases, combined FDG-PET with IAP studies did not report memory impairment contralateral to the hypometabolic zone (Salanova et al. 1992).

3 Important Results of Validation Studies in Brain Tumors and Epilepsies, Overview, and Current State

3.1 Motor Function

3.1.1 Functional Mapping

Validation of more recent functional noninvasive methods, such as fMRI, magnetoencephalography (MEG), and transcranial magnetic stimulation (TMS), can be performed by comparison with earlier techniques such as PET. Nevertheless, DES remains the current reference procedure, and therefore comparison of functional noninvasive methods with DES is the best validation method.

Functional mapping of motor areas can be performed either to localize the central area or to locate motor areas at risk of functional deficits. Therefore, there are two different levels of validation.

The first level is to determine whether functional imaging methods can accurately *localize the central sulcus.* In the normal brain, the hand area and therefore the central sulcus can be accurately localized using anatomical landmarks only (Yousry et al. 1997) (Fig. 7). In patients with brain tumors, however, mass effect frequently distorts normal cortical anatomy and can make localization of the central area difficult by using anatomical landmarks alone (Lehericy et al. 2000b). In such cases, preoperative functional localization is of special interest. See also chapter "Task-Based Presurgical Functional MRI in Patients with Brain Tumors."

3.1.1.1 fMRI vs. DES

Compared to DES, fMRI was very reliable in localizing the motor cortex, with complete or almost complete agreement using visual comparison with 3D MRI (Jack Jr et al. 1994; Yousry

et al. 1995; Pujol et al. 1996, 1998; Roux et al. 1999) (Fig. 6) or preoperative ultrasonography (Fandino et al. 1999), co-registration of preoperative pictures with 3D rendering of the brain (Puce et al. 1995; Lehericy et al. 2000b), or neuronavigation procedures (Hirsch et al. 2000; Lehericy et al. 2000b). Early studies in 28 patients with surgical brain lesions reported that 100% of positive MR activation sites were within 20 mm of DES positive sites and that 87% of correlations were within 10 mm of DES (Yetkin et al. 1997). Another study in 8 patients with brain tumors reported a good correlation between fMRI activation and DES sites, with all fMRI activations related to positive DES responses (Roux et al. 1999). In patients with intra-axial lesions, overlapping results were obtained in 25–63% (<1 cm) and neighboring zones in 29–75% (<2 cm), while

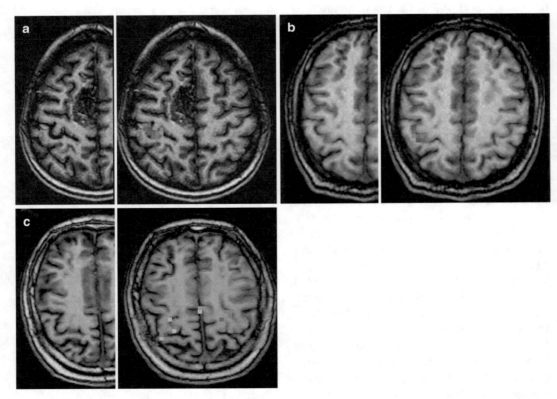

Fig. 7 Typical variations of anatomy of the hand area. Movements of the left hand in three different subjects. Activated pixels are overlaid onto anatomical T1-weighted images in the right hemisphere. (**a**) Typical omega-shaped hand area (patient with a right medial frontal arteriovenous malformation). (**b**) Epsilon-shaped hand knob. (**c**) More complex aspect of the hand area (three-digit aspect)

contradictory results were observed (Krings et al. 2001b; Reinges et al. 2004). Results were less good in patients with extra-axial lesions, with contradictory results in 42% (activation in a different gyrus or >2 cm from DES site) (Reinges et al. 2004). Other more studies reported an agreement between fMRI and DES regarding localization in 92% (Lehericy et al. 2000b), 92.3% (Spena et al. 2010), 83.7% (Gonzalez-Darder et al. 2010), and 77% of subjects (Bartos et al. 2009). The choice of statistical thresholds to display activation maps is also an important factor to take into account as the optimal threshold varies between subjects (Chang et al. 2010).

3.1.1.2 fMRI vs. TMS

Compared to TMS, fMRI peaks produced no motor evoked potential (MEP) when located more than 2 cm away from TMS sites (Krings et al. 1997b).

The next level is to determine whether functional imaging data can accurately *localize motor areas* and to assess how reliable this information is to assess where to stop with the surgical resection in order to prevent functional deficits.

3.1.1.3 fMRI vs. PET

fMRI produced very similar results as PET (Bittar et al. 1999a). The average distance between fMRI and PET activation peaks was 7.9 ± 4.8 mm, with 96% of the peaks being located on either the same or adjacent sulci or gyri. Overlapping voxels activated by each modality occurred in 92% of the studies.

Agreement between PET and fMRI functional localization was 95.6% for intra-axial lesions and spatially concordant as determined by intracranial stimulation (Bittar et al. 1999b). PET results overlapped with DES in 60–92% (<1 cm) and in neighboring zones in 29–75% (<2 cm) (Krings et al. 2001b; Reinges et al. 2004). The mean localization difference between fMRI and PET was 8.1 ± 4.6 mm (range, 2–18 mm) (Reinges et al. 2004). Another study reported that the evaluation of PET findings by cortical stimulation had a 94% sensitivity and a 95% specificity for the identification of motor-associated brain areas (Schreckenberger et al. 2001). PET results for

extra-axial lesions were even superior to those obtained with fMRI with 75% overlapping and 25% neighboring activation, showing no contradictory results (Reinges et al. 2004).

3.1.1.4 TMS vs. DES/fMRI

TMS combined with neuronavigation has also been used for presurgical motor mapping (Picht et al. 2011; Coburger et al. 2013; Krieg et al. 2013) evaluated by comparison to fMRI and DES. TMS sites were close (within 5 mm) to DES positive sites (Picht et al. 2011). Compared to DES, TMS responses fell within 1 cm of the electrical cortical stimulation sites (Krings et al. 1997a; Forster et al. 2011).

TMS sites further than 2 cm away from fMRI peaks produced no motor evoked potentials (MEPs) (Krings et al. 1997b, 2001b), while the mean distance between the fMRI and TMS activation peaks was below 1.5 cm (Krings et al. 2001a; Forster et al. 2011). Further, TMS was able to locate the motor cortex when fMRI failed (Coburger et al. 2013).

3.1.1.5 fMRI vs. MSI

Magnetic source imaging (MSI) using somatosensory stimulation has also been evaluated in patients with brain tumors (Schiffbauer et al. 2002). In one study, the distance between two corresponding points determined using MSI and DES was 12.5 ± 1.3 mm for somatosensory–somatosensory and 19 ± 1.3 mm for somatosensory–motor comparisons. Intraoperative sites at which DES evoked the same patient response exhibited a spatial variation of 10.7 ± 0.7 mm (Schiffbauer et al. 2002).

Overall, these studies suggest that the localization accuracy among the different functional methods is similar. Earlier studies have suggested that in patients with a minimum distance of 2 cm between tumor and activation site, no deficits in motor function are expected after surgery (Mueller et al. 1996; Yetkin et al. 1997). Other studies have suggested that even a shorter distance of <1 cm (lesion to function site) can be achieved (Krishnan et al. 2004; Bartos et al. 2009). Therefore, fMRI methods are considered a useful adjunct to DES.

The value of functional imaging techniques for the accurate localization of functionally important areas at risk for postoperative deficits can also be assessed empirically by a comparison to the postoperative outcome. In this regard, fMRI has proven to be very accurate for the prediction of occurrence of motor and language deficits after medial frontal lobe surgery (Krainik et al. 2001, 2003; Wood et al. 2011). Furthermore, it has been shown that the fMRI results for the presurgical localization of motor and sensory areas as well as language areas are consistent across different MR-scanners at 1.5 and 3.0 T (Tyndall et al. 2017).

It should be kept in mind that fMRI results should be interpreted cautiously as they highly depend on several factors, such as the quality of the examination (movement artifacts), data processing (smoothing), statistical thresholds, and ultimately the experience of the reader. Lastly, functional brain mapping techniques alone cannot assess subcortical white matter tracts. Therefore, combined fMRI and DTI fiber tracking methods have the potential to provide a more complete presurgical mapping than any other functional technique by its own.

3.1.2 DTI Fiber Tracking of the Corticospinal Tract

Compared to the already described functional imaging techniques, fewer validation studies have been published for DTI fiber tracking. Previous studies have shown the reconstruction of well-known fiber tracts, including the corticospinal, long association (Roux et al. 1999; Mori et al. 2002), and brainstem fiber tracts (Stieltjes et al. 2001). Results of fiber tracking have also been correlated with postmortem animal studies in formalin-fixed hearts in rabbits (Holmes et al. 2000) and in the skeletal muscle of rats in vivo (Damon et al. 2002). In vivo DTI has been compared to ex vivo DTI and also to the uptake of wheat germ agglutinin-horseradish peroxidase (WGA-HRP)-stained histological sections in the macaque monkey (Dauguet et al. 2007). A good correspondence has been reported between DTI fiber tracts originating in the left somatosensory cortex and the histological reference. In humans,

tractography results have been compared with the expected known anatomy, dissections, or DES (Lawes and Clark 2010).

Validation studies of DTI fiber tracking have been performed using subcortical DES in patients with brain lesions. Two studies from the same group used cortical positive DES as seeding points for fiber tracking (Berman et al. 2004; Henry et al. 2004). Tracts originating from DES sites eliciting movement of the face matched somatotopically correct the known connections of the primary motor area of the face. For the corticospinal tract, a good agreement was reported in 92–95% between DTI reconstructed tracts and positive functional subcortical DES sites (Coenen et al. 2003; Kamada et al. 2005; Bello et al. 2008, 2010; Ohue et al. 2012; Zhu et al. 2012). The mean distance range between the stimulated sites and the corticospinal tract was 6–14 mm (Bozzao et al. 2010; Gonzalez-Darder et al. 2010; Prabhu et al. 2011; Zhu et al. 2012; Vassal et al. 2013). These distances depended on the intensity used for stimulation (Kamada et al. 2009). Using a 1.5 T intraoperative MRI, a 86% agreement between DTI-based tractography and DES was found, with a linear correlation between the distance to the corticospinal tract and the intensity of DES. In the false-positive cases, the location of the corticospinal tract using tractography was not confirmed by DES, which might be due to tumor infiltration. Indeed, tumor infiltration and gliosis might alter the tissue conductivity and result in negative DES (Javadi et al. 2017). DTI tractography may underestimate the presence of functional fibers in the border of the lesions (Spena et al. 2010). Finally, the topography of the tract, i.e., inside or at the boundary of the tumor, has been confirmed by DES (Bello et al. 2008, 2010).

Conventional diffusion tensor imaging models and tractography techniques are often suboptimal in areas of fiber crossing or fanning. For the corticospinal tract, these techniques are often unable to show the superior medial and lateral portions of the tract. Improved diffusion modeling using high angular resolution diffusion imaging (HARDI) allows a better reconstruction of these parts showing a good agreement with cortical and subcortical DES (Berman et al. 2008; Berman 2009; Bucci et al. 2013).

Therefore, even though the current data are encouraging, further improvement in tractography techniques and more comparisons between DTI and DES in larger series of patients are required.

3.2 Language Function

Regarding language, functional imaging can determine language dominance and localize the various language areas. For the validation of functional imaging techniques for the hemispheric language dominance, the IAP is used as a reference. In contrast, DES serves as a reference for the validation of the localization of different language areas (corticography).

3.2.1 Hemispheric Dominance for Language

FMRI has shown a high concordance (>90%) with IAP for the degree of asymmetric activation between brain hemispheres during language tasks indicating language dominance (Desmond et al. 1995; Binder et al. 1996; Bahn et al. 1997; Hertz-Pannier et al. 1997; Benson et al. 1999; Lehericy et al. 2000a; Carpentier et al. 2001; Gaillard et al. 2002; Rutten et al. 2002b; Sabbah et al. 2003; Woermann et al. 2003). A meta-analysis including 22 studies with 504 patients showed that fMRI correctly classified 94% of patients with typical language lateralization with the Wada test, indicating that fMRI is a reliable triage test for language (Bauer et al. 2014). For patients with a clear left lateralization result on fMRI, further language testing with the Wada test is unnecessary. For patients in whom fMRI fails to show clear left-lateralization, further testing would be warranted (Bauer et al. 2014; Kundu et al. 2019). A good correlation has been observed using productive tasks, such as word or verb generation, and semantic decision tasks, whereas no correlation has been observed for receptive tasks (Lehericy et al. 2000a) (Fig. 8).

Overall, language fMRI studies largely agree on a 10% failure rate to lateralize language as compared to the IAP (Desmond et al. 1995; Binder et al. 1996; Bahn et al. 1997; Hertz-Pannier et al. 1997; Benson et al. 1999; Lehericy et al. 2000a; Carpentier et al. 2001; Gaillard et al. 2002; Rutten et al. 2002b; Sabbah et al. 2003; Woermann et al. 2003). A false categorization using fMRI was more frequent in patients with left temporal lobe epilepsy (Woermann et al. 2003).

The use of well-controlled paradigms with the recording of a patient's performance (such as semantic decision making or picture naming) apparently does not provide better results than more simple paradigms without the control of the patient's performance (such as a silent generation task with a low-level reference condition). The same may also apply to quantitative post-processing (counting the number of activated voxels to calculate the laterality indices) versus visual examination of fMRI maps (Woermann et al. 2003).

3.2.2 Localization of Language Areas

Fewer studies have been performed for quantitative comparison between language functional imaging data and DES. DES was consistent with the MEG-based localization in 13 patients during a visual and auditory word-recognition task (Simos et al. 1999). Using a verb generation task

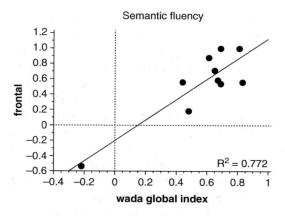

Fig. 8 Correlation between fMRI and Wada results. Pearson linear regression between the Wada and fMRI laterality indices in the frontal lobes in a semantic fluency task obtained in ten patients with temporal lobe epilepsy. (From Lehericy et al. (2000a) with permission)

in eight patients with glioma, via PET-activated areas, showed a 73% sensitivity and 81% specificity to predict aphasic disturbance during intraoperative stimulation (Herholz et al. 1997). In seven patients with intractable epilepsy, cortical regions that showed increased rCBF (PET) during both visual and auditory naming tasks were located in the same regions as subdural electrodes disrupting language during electrical stimulation (Bookheimer et al. 1997). In contrast, cortical regions underlying electrodes that did not disrupt language did also not show any consistent rCBF changes during PET activation (Bookheimer et al. 1997).

In three patients with primary tumors, regions involved in receptive language function identified by fMRI and DES were similar but not identical (Lurito et al. 2000). In 11 patients with surgical brain lesions, the sensitivity/specificity of a set of five different language tasks ranged from 81%/53% for areas that touched DES positive sites to 92%/0% for areas separated by 2 cm (FitzGerald et al. 1997). Using a combination of three different fMRI tasks, the sensitivity of fMRI was 100% in seven of eight patients with temporal lobe epilepsy (<6.4 mm of the DES site). In the remaining patient, the sensitivity was only 38% (Rutten et al. 2002a). Overall, these data yielded a specificity of 61% (Rutten et al. 2002a). Compared to DES, the sensitivity and specificity of language tasks were 22% and 97% for a naming task and 36% and 98% for a verb generation task, respectively (Roux et al. 2003). A better correlation (sensitivity, 59%; specificity, 97%) was achieved by combining the two fMRI tasks (Roux et al. 2003). A more recent study reported a correlation between fMRI and DES in only 42.8% (Spena et al. 2010). In a meta-analysis of nine studies which compared preoperative fMRI and DES for language mapping, the sensitivity and specificity of fMRI in comparison with DES as a gold standard ranged from 59% to 100% and from 0% to 97%, respectively (Giussani et al. 2011). The variety of methods used in these studies contributed to this large range of values. The correspondence between

fMRI and DES mapping depended heavily on the statistical threshold used for fMRI data evaluation and varied between patients, tasks, and studies (FitzGerald et al. 1997; Rutten et al. 2002a; Roux et al. 2003; Giussani et al. 2011). Individual language tasks were not as sensitive as a set of language tasks (Fig. 9). In patients with gliomas, the sensitivity and specificity of fMRI combining three language tasks (letter word generation, category word generation, semantic association) as compared with DES, were 37.1% (95% confidence interval [CI] 20.7–57.2) and 83.4% (95% CI 77.1–88.3), respectively (Kuchcinski et al. 2015). Astrocytoma subtype, tumor rCBV less than 1.5 and a distance to tumor greater than 1 cm were independently associated with fMRI false-positive occurrence (Kuchcinski et al. 2015).

Therefore, fMRI results for language mapping largely depend on the quality of the equipment, the type of tasks, the expertise of the analysis and its interpretation (Giussani et al. 2011; Garrett et al. 2012), as well as tumor grade and perfusion characteristics (Kuchcinski et al. 2015).

3.2.3 DTI Fiber Tracking of Language Tracts

Only few comparisons between DTI fiber tracking of language tracts and DES have been performed in patients with brain lesions (Fig. 10). DTI fiber tracking has been used to delineate the pathways between functional regions (Henry et al. 2004). Tracts from stimulated sites in the inferior frontal cortex resulting in face motor, speech arrest, and anomia have been generated from the DTI data. Connections were found between speech arrest, face motor, and anomia sites and the SMA proper and cerebral peduncle (Henry et al. 2004). Fiber tracking has been performed in brain tumor patients and normal controls to study the connection between the frontal and parietotemporal lobes through the arcuate fascicle (Henry et al. 2004). Tracts connecting the inferior frontal gyrus to the supramarginal gyrus, the posterior superior temporal gyrus, and the middle temporal gyrus were closely located to the

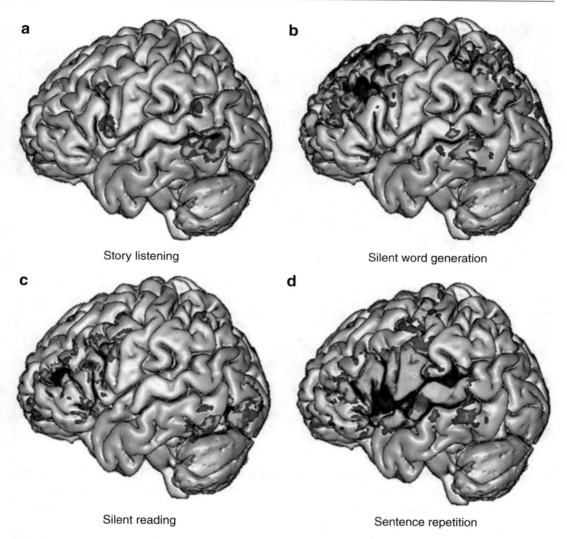

Fig. 9 Activation pattern of four language tasks. Left: Receptive tasks. (**a**) Story listening task compared to the listening to the same story played backward. Activation is mainly located in posterior temporal areas. (**b**) Silent reading compared to fixation. Activation is located in the inferotemporal cortical areas and Broca's area. Right: Productive tasks. (**c**) Silent word generation task com-pared to rest. Activation predominates in the dorsolateral frontal areas and inferior parietal areas, including the angular gyrus. (**d**) Sentence repetition aloud compared to rest. Activation includes frontal (Broca's area and the lower part of the primary sensorimotor area in the face region) and temporal areas (including the primary auditory cortex)

intraoperative cortical stimulation speech arrest sites (Henry et al. 2004). More recent studies combining DES and tractography for language tracts have shown that DES positive subcortical sites correspond with DTI fiber tracts in 81–97% (Bello et al. 2008; Leclercq et al. 2010).

3.3 Memory Functions

Mesial temporal sclerosis or hippocampal sclerosis is the most common cause of intractable temporal lobe epilepsy, the treatment of which is temporal lobectomy or selective

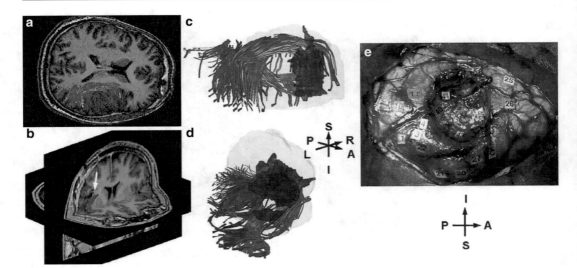

Fig. 10 Relationship between DTI fiber tracking and pre-operative electrical stimulations in a patient with a low-grade glioma of the left insula. Electrical stimulations performed during surgery in the depth of the resection cavity resulted in speech arrest. (**a**) DTI fiber tract reconstruction of the arcuate fasciculus (transverse section; the fiber tract is represented in blue as if viewed from above). (**b**) Oblique 3D reconstruction of the arcuate fasciculus in blue showing the close proximity between the deep part of the resection cavity and the fiber tract (arrow). (**c**, **d**) 3D reconstructions of the fiber tract (blue), the tumor (light green), and the surgical resection site (red) showing the close proximity between the deep part of the surgical resection and the fiber tract (**c** superior view as in **a**; **d** oblique 3D reconstruction, same view as in **b**). Note that the resection cavity touches the fiber tract in agreement with DES findings. (**e**) Surgical view showing positive DES sites for motor responses (1–4 and 40), somatosensory responses (10–11), and speech responses (paraphrasias: 25–26 and 41–43). Sites positive for language were obtained in the depth of the resection cavity (41–43). *Abbreviations*: *A* anterior, *I* inferior, *L* left, *P* posterior, *R* right, *S* superior

amygdalohippocampectomy. As mesial temporal lobes are key structures for memory functions, their resection can result in verbal and non-verbal memory impairment depending on language lateralization. Connectivity with temporal and extratemporal language areas in the speech-dominant hemisphere, usually the left, makes the ipsilateral hippocampus relatively specialized in verbal memory tasks. Conversely, connectivity between posterior cortical regions and the non-dominant hemisphere, usually the right, involves the ipsilateral hippocampus in visuospatial memory functions (Massot-Tarrús et al. 2019). After temporal lobe resection involving the speech-dominant hemisphere, verbal memory decline is well documented (Lee et al. 2002) in comparison with visual memory loss in the nondominant hemisphere (Lee et al. 2002; Witt et al. 2015; Schmid et al. 2018). In a systematic review, risk of verbal memory decline after left-sided tempo-

ral lobe surgery was estimated at 44% (vs. 20% after right-sided surgery). For visual memory, no difference with regard to side of surgery was seen (21% after left-sided surgery vs. 23% after right-sided surgery) (Sherman et al. 2011; Schmid et al. 2018).

The Wada test has been widely used to determine the hemispheric dominance of verbal memory in order to predict postoperative verbal memory performance (Schmid et al. 2018; Massot-Tarrús et al. 2019). However, unlike language lateralization assessment, memory lateralization and its predictive value for postoperative decline are less valid if based on the Wada test. As detailed above, the posterior two-thirds of the hippocampus and the parahippocampal cortex are not explored by the Wada test since their vascularization is supplied by the posterior cerebral artery. Furthermore, aphasia may have a major impact on verbal memory testing during cortical anesthesia of the speech-dominant hemisphere. A superselective Wada test with injection of amobarbital into the posterior cerebral artery or anterior choroidal artery may overcome these limitations and allow memory testing while preserving language functions but has higher risk of complications. On the other hand, the action of amobarbital being limited in 3–5 min, an exhaustive and reliable evaluation of memory functions under anesthesia conditions is difficult. To address these issues, non-invasive procedures including PET, fMRI, and MEG have been applied to presurgical evaluation of language and memory functions (Schmid et al. 2018; Massot-Tarrús et al. 2019).

A good correlation has been demonstrated between PET and IAP results. Patients with mesial temporal lobe epilepsy showed an ^{18}F-fluorodeoxyglucose (FDG) PET hypometabolism in the hemisphere ipsilateral to the lesion, functional deficits on the IAP, or both, as well as verbal memory and word fluency impairment (Rausch et al. 1994; Arnold et al. 1996; Salanova et al. 2001). IAP hemispheric memory performance and hippocampal glucose metabolism showed a positive correlation with the frequency of seizures and a negative correlation with the duration of epilepsy (Jokeit et al. 1999). The results of FDG-PET were predictive for an impaired IAP memory performance (Salanova et al. 2001). Memory impairment contralateral to PET hypometabolism in the temporal lobe has never been seen (Salanova et al. 2001). Finally, in patients with temporal lobe epilepsy, the FDG-PET asymmetry index in the mesial temporal lobe correlated with the IAP asymmetry index for memory performance (Hong et al. 2000a).

Functional MRI studies have shown consistent activation of medial temporal structures during memory tasks in normal subjects (Small et al. 1999; Dupont et al. 2000, 2010; Zeineh et al. 2003). In patients with epilepsy, several studies have evaluated the lateralization value of fMRI activation for memory functions (Detre et al. 1998; Dupont et al. 2001, 2010; Jokeit et al. 2001; Golby et al. 2002; Rabin et al. 2004; Janszky et al. 2005; Richardson et al. 2006; Binder et al. 2010). The preoperative fMRI asym-

metry index of memory function correlated with the changes between pre- and postsurgical measures for memory retention (Rabin et al. 2004; Janszky et al. 2005). Asymmetry ratios in the medial temporal lobe also significantly correlated with memory lateralization by IAP testing (Detre et al. 1998; Golby et al. 2002; Rabin et al. 2004). In ten right-handed patients with hippocampal sclerosis, fMRI provided the strongest independent predictor of memory outcome after surgery (Richardson et al. 2004). At the individual subject level, fMRI data had a high positive predictive value for memory decline (Richardson et al. 2004). Overall, preoperative fMRI can predict postoperative verbal memory alterations and improve the accuracy of the prediction of these deficits in patients with temporal lobe epilepsy (Binder 2011). Thus, fMRI has proven to be efficient for the preoperative evaluation and prediction of memory functions following surgery and has gradually replaced the Wada test (Schmid et al. 2018; Massot-Tarrús et al. 2019).

4 Conclusion

Despite its limitations, fMRI is now increasingly used as a clinical noninvasive tool to locate eloquent brain areas, lateralize language and memory functions, and predict postoperative outcome. Care should be taken to control and reduce artifacts stemming from different sources, including motion, magnetic susceptibility, and alterations in BOLD contrast. DTI tractography is used in addition to fMRI to evaluate white matter fiber tracts in surgical candidates with brain lesions. Motor mapping has been largely validated by using DES. Language lateralization using fMRI has replaced the Wada test in most centers. Localization of language areas using fMRI mainly depends on the choice of tasks, activation thresholds, and subject's performance and is less well validated than DES. FMRI has also supplanted the Wada test for memory lateralization and the prediction of memory impairment after temporal lobectomy for temporal lobe epilepsy. Overall, preoperative mapping with fMRI can be considered a useful adjunct to DES.

References

Agnew WF, McCreery DB (1987) Considerations for safety in the use of extracranial stimulation for motor evoked potentials. Neurosurgery 20:143–147

Akanuma N, Koutroumanidis M, Adachi N, Alarcon G, Binnie CD (2003) Presurgical assessment of memory-related brain structures: the Wada test and functional neuroimaging. Seizure 12:346–358

Arnold S, Schlaug G, Niemann H, Ebner A, Luders H, Witte OW, Seitz RJ (1996) Topography of interictal glucose hypometabolism in unilateral mesiotemporal epilepsy. Neurology 46:1422–1430

Bahn MM, Lin W, Silbergeld DL, Miller JW, Kuppusamy K, Cook RJ, Hammer G, Wetzel R, Cross D III (1997) Localization of language cortices by functional MR imaging compared with intracarotid amobarbital hemispheric sedation. AJR Am J Roentgenol 169: 575–579

Barnett GH, Little JR, Ebrahim ZY, Jones SC, Friel HT (1987) Cerebral circulation during arteriovenous malformation operation. Neurosurgery 20: 836–842

Bartolomei F, Bosma I, Klein M, Baayen JC, Reijneveld JC, Postma TJ, Heimans JJ, van Dijk BW, de Munck JC, de Jongh A, Cover KS, Stam CJ (2006) How do brain tumors alter functional connectivity? A magnetoencephalography study. Ann Neurol 59:128–138

Bartos R, Jech R, Vymazal J, Petrovicky P, Vachata P, Hejcl A, Zolal A, Sames M (2009) Validity of primary motor area localization with fMRI versus electric cortical stimulation: a comparative study. Acta Neurochir 151:1071–1080

Bauer PR, Reitsma JB, Houweling BM et al (2014) Can fMRI safely replace the Wada test for preoperative assessment of language lateralisation? A meta-analysis and systematic review. J Neurol Neurosurg Psychiatry 85:581–588

Bello L, Gambini A, Castellano A, Carrabba G, Acerbi F, Fava E, Giussani C, Cadioli M, Blasi V, Casarotti A, Papagno C, Gupta AK, Gaini S, Scotti G, Falini A (2008) Motor and language DTI fiber tracking combined with intraoperative subcortical mapping for surgical removal of gliomas. NeuroImage 39:369–382

Bello L, Castellano A, Fava E, Casaceli G, Riva M, Scotti G, Gaini SM, Falini A (2010) Intraoperative use of diffusion tensor imaging fiber tractography and subcortical mapping for resection of gliomas: technical considerations. Neurosurg Focus 28:E6

Benson RR, FitzGerald DB, LeSueur LL, Kennedy DN, Kwong KK, Buchbinder BR, Davis TL, Weisskoff RM, Talavage TM, Logan WJ, Cosgrove GR, Belliveau JW, Rosen BR (1999) Language dominance determined by whole brain functional MRI in patients with brain lesions. Neurology 52:798–809

Berger MS (1995) Functional mapping-guided resection of low-grade gliomas. Clin Neurosurg 42:437–452

Berman J (2009) Diffusion MR tractography as a tool for surgical planning. Magn Reson Imaging Clin N Am 17:205–214

Berman JI, Berger MS, Mukherjee P, Henry RG (2004) Diffusion-tensor imaging-guided tracking of fibers of the pyramidal tract combined with intraoperative cortical stimulation mapping in patients with gliomas. J Neurosurg 101:66–72

Berman JI, Chung S, Mukherjee P, Hess CP, Han ET, Henry RG (2008) Probabilistic streamline q-ball tractography using the residual bootstrap. NeuroImage 39:215–222

Binder JR (2011) Functional MRI is a valid noninvasive alternative to Wada testing. Epilepsy Behav 20:214–222

Binder JR, Swanson SJ, Hammeke TA, Morris GL, Mueller WM, Fischer M, Benbadis S, Frost JA, Rao SM, Haughton VM (1996) Determination of language dominance using functional MRI: a comparison with the Wada test. Neurology 46:978–984

Binder JR, Swanson SJ, Sabsevitz DS, Hammeke TA, Raghavan M, Mueller WM (2010) A comparison of two fMRI methods for predicting verbal memory decline after left temporal lobectomy: language lateralization versus hippocampal activation asymmetry. Epilepsia 51:618–626

Biswal B, Yetkin FZ, Haughton VM, Hyde JS (1995) Functional connectivity in the motor cortex of resting human brain using echo-planar MRI. Magn Reson Med 34:537–541

Bittar RG, Olivier A, Sadikot AF, Andermann F, Pike GB, Reutens DC (1999a) Presurgical motor and somatosensory cortex mapping with functional magnetic resonance imaging and positron emission tomography. J Neurosurg 91:915–921

Bittar RG, Olivier A, Sadikot AF, Andermann F, Comeau RM, Cyr M, Peters TM, Reutens DC (1999b) Localization of somatosensory function by using positron emission tomography scanning: a comparison with intraoperative cortical stimulation. J Neurosurg 90:478–483

Bizzi A, Blasi V, Falini A et al (2008) Presurgical functional MR imaging of language and motor functions: validation with intraoperative electrocortical mapping. Radiology 248:579–589

Bookheimer SY, Zeffiro TA, Blaxton T, Malow BA, Gaillard WD, Sato S, Kufta C, Fedio P, Theodore WH (1997) A direct comparison of PET activation and electrocortical stimulation mapping for language localization. Neurology 48:1056–1065

Boxerman JL, Hamberg LM, Rosen BR, Weisskoff RM (1995) MR contrast due to intravascular magnetic susceptibility perturbations. Magn Reson Med 34:555–566

Bozzao A, Romano A, Angelini A, D'Andrea G, Calabria LF, Coppola V, Mastronardi L, Fantozzi LM, Ferrante L (2010) Identification of the pyramidal tract by neuronavigation based on intraoperative magnetic resonance tractography: correlation with subcortical stimulation. Eur Radiol 20:2475–2481

Bucci M, Mandelli ML, Berman JI, Amirbekian B, Nguyen C, Berger MS, Henry RG (2013) Quantifying diffusion MRI tractography of the corticospinal tract in brain tumors with deterministic and probabilistic methods. Neuroimage Clin 3:361–368

Carpentier A, Pugh KR, Westerveld M, Studholme C, Skrinjar O, Thompson JL, Spencer DD, Constable RT (2001) Functional MRI of language processing: dependence on input modality and temporal lobe epilepsy. Epilepsia 42:1241–1254

Castellano A, Cirillo S, Bello L et al (2017) Functional MRI for surgery of gliomas. Curr Treat Options Neurol 19:34

Cha S, Johnson G, Wadghiri YZ, Jin O, Babb J, Zagzag D, Turnbull DH (2003) Dynamic, contrast-enhanced perfusion MRI in mouse gliomas: correlation with histopathology. Magn Reson Med 49:848–855

Chang CY, Peck KK, Brennan NM, Hou BL, Gutin PH, Holodny AI (2010) Functional MRI in the presurgical evaluation of patients with brain tumors: characterization of the statistical threshold. Stereotact Funct Neurosurg 88:35–41

Ciobanu L, Solomon E, Pyatigorskaya N et al (2015) fMRI contrast at high and ultrahigh magnetic fields: insight from complementary methods. NeuroImage 113:37–43

Cloft HJ, Joseph GJ, Dion JE (1999) Risk of cerebral angiography in patients with subarachnoid hemorrhage, cerebral aneurysm, and arteriovenous malformation: a meta-analysis. Stroke 30:317–320

Coburger J, Musahl C, Henkes H, Horvath-Rizea D, Bittl M, Weissbach C, Hopf N (2013) Comparison of navigated transcranial magnetic stimulation and functional magnetic resonance imaging for preoperative mapping in rolandic tumor surgery. Neurosurg Rev 36:65–75; discussion 75–66

Coenen VA, Krings T, Axer H, Weidemann J, Kranzlein H, Hans FJ, Thron A, Gilsbach JM, Rohde V (2003) Intraoperative three-dimensional visualization of the pyramidal tract in a neuronavigation system (PTV) reliably predicts true position of principal motor pathways. Surg Neurol 60:381–390; discussion 390

D'Esposito M, Deouell LY, Gazzaley A (2003) Alterations in the BOLD fMRI signal with ageing and disease: a challenge for neuroimaging. Nat Rev Neurosci 4:863–872

Damon BM, Ding Z, Anderson AW, Freyer AS, Gore JC (2002) Validation of diffusion tensor MRI-based muscle fiber tracking. Magn Reson Med 48:97–104

Dauguet J, Peled S, Berezovskii V, Delzescaux T, Warfield SK, Born R, Westin CF (2007) Comparison of fiber tracts derived from in-vivo DTI tractography with 3D histological neural tract tracer reconstruction on a macaque brain. NeuroImage 37:530–538

Davies KG, Hermann BP, Foley KT (1996) Relation between intracarotid amobarbital memory asymmetry

scores and hippocampal sclerosis in patients undergoing anterior temporal lobe resections. Epilepsia 37:522–525

de Silva R, Duncan R, Patterson J, Gillham R, Hadley D (1999) Regional cerebral perfusion and amytal distribution during the Wada test. J Nucl Med 40:747–752

Desmond JE, Sum JM, Wagner AD, Demb JB, Shear PK, Glover GH, Gabrieli JD, Morrell MJ (1995) Functional MRI measurement of language lateralization in Wada-tested patients. Brain 118(Pt 6):1411–1419

Detre JA, Maccotta L, King D, Alsop DC, Glosser G, D'Esposito M, Zarahn E, Aguirre GK, French JA (1998) Functional MRI lateralization of memory in temporal lobe epilepsy. Neurology 50:926–932

Dion JE, Gates PC, Fox AJ, Barnett HJ, Blom RJ (1987) Clinical events following neuroangiography: a prospective study. Stroke 18:997–1004

Doty RW, Barlett JR (1981) Stimulation of the brain via metallic electrodes. In: Paterson MM, Kesner RP (eds) Electrical stimulation research methods. Academic, New York, pp 71–103

Duffau H (2004) Intraoperative functional mapping using direct electrical stimulations. Methodological considerations. Neurochirurgie 50:474–483

Duffau H, Capelle L, Sichez N, Denvil D, Lopes M, Sichez JP, Bitar A, Fohanno D (2002) Intraoperative mapping of the subcortical language pathways using direct stimulations. An anatomo-functional study. Brain 125:199–214

Duffau H, Capelle L, Denvil D, Gatignol P, Sichez N, Lopes M, Sichez JP, Van Effenterre R (2003a) The role of dominant premotor cortex in language: a study using intraoperative functional mapping in awake patients. NeuroImage 20:1903–1914

Duffau H, Capelle L, Denvil D, Sichez N, Gatignol P, Taillandier L, Lopes M, Mitchell MC, Roche S, Muller JC, Bitar A, Sichez JP, van Effenterre R (2003b) Usefulness of intraoperative electrical subcortical mapping during surgery for low-grade gliomas located within eloquent brain regions: functional results in a consecutive series of 103 patients. J Neurosurg 98:764–778

Duffau H, Lopes M, Arthuis F, Bitar A, Sichez JP, Van Effenterre R, Capelle L (2005) Contribution of intraoperative electrical stimulations in surgery of low grade gliomas: a comparative study between two series without (1985–96) and with (1996–2003) functional mapping in the same institution. J Neurol Neurosurg Psychiatry 76:845–851

Duong TQ, Yacoub E, Adriany G, Hu X, Ugurbil K, Kim SG (2003) Microvascular BOLD contribution at 4 and 7 T in the human brain: gradient-echo and spin-echo fMRI with suppression of blood effects. Magn Reson Med 49:1019–1027

Dupont S, Van de Moortele PF, Samson S, Hasboun D, Poline JB, Adam C, Lehericy S, Le Bihan D, Samson Y, Baulac M (2000) Episodic memory in left temporal lobe epilepsy: a functional MRI study. Brain 123(Pt 8):1722–1732

Dupont S, Samson Y, Van de Moortele PF, Samson S, Poline JB, Adam C, Lehericy S, Le Bihan D, Baulac M (2001) Delayed verbal memory retrieval: a functional MRI study in epileptic patients with structural lesions of the left medial temporal lobe. NeuroImage 14:995–1003

Dupont S, Duron E, Samson S, Denos M, Volle E, Delmaire C, Navarro V, Chiras J, Lehericy S, Samson Y, Baulac M (2010) Functional MR imaging or Wada test: which is the better predictor of individual postoperative memory outcome? Radiology 255:128–134

Enzmann DR, Pelc NJ (1992) Brain motion: measurement with phase-contrast MR imaging. Radiology 185:653–660

Fandino J, Kollias SS, Wieser HG, Valavanis A, Yonekawa Y (1999) Intraoperative validation of functional magnetic resonance imaging and cortical reorganization patterns in patients with brain tumors involving the primary motor cortex. J Neurosurg 91:238–250

Fertziger AP, Ranck JB Jr (1970) Potassium accumulation in interstitial space during epileptiform seizures. Exp Neurol 26:571–585

Fink GR (1992) Effects of cerebral angiomas on perifocal and remote tissue: a multivariate positron emission tomography study. Stroke 23:1099–1105

FitzGerald DB, Cosgrove GR, Ronner S, Jiang H, Buchbinder BR, Belliveau JW, Rosen BR, Benson RR (1997) Location of language in the cortex: a comparison between functional MR imaging and electrocortical stimulation. AJNR Am J Neuroradiol 18:1529–1539

Fogarty-Mack P, Pile-Spellman J, Hacein-Bey L, Ostapkovich N, Joshi S, Vulliemoz Y, Young WL (1996) Superselective intraarterial papaverine administration: effect on regional cerebral blood flow in patients with arteriovenous malformations. J Neurosurg 85:395–402

Folkman J, Watson K, Ingber D, Hanahan D (1989) Induction of angiogenesis during the transition from hyperplasia to neoplasia. Nature 339:58–61

Forster MT, Hattingen E, Senft C, Gasser T, Seifert V, Szelenyi A (2011) Navigated transcranial magnetic stimulation and functional magnetic resonance imaging: advanced adjuncts in preoperative planning for central region tumors. Neurosurgery 68:1317–1324; discussion 1324–1315

Fraga de Abreu VH, Peck KK, Petrovich-Brennan NM et al (2016) Brain tumors: the influence of tumor type and routine MR imaging characteristics at BOLD functional MR imaging in the primary motor gyrus. Radiology 281:876–883

Fujiwara N, Sakatani K, Katayama Y, Murata Y, Hoshino T, Fukaya C, Yamamoto T (2004) Evoked-cerebral blood oxygenation changes in false-negative activations in BOLD contrast functional MRI of patients with brain tumors. NeuroImage 21:1464–1471

Gaillard WD, Balsamo L, Xu B, Grandin CB, Braniecki SH, Papero PH, Weinstein S, Conry J, Pearl PL, Sachs B, Sato S, Jabbari B, Vezina LG, Frattali C, Theodore WH (2002) Language dominance in partial epilepsy patients identified with an fMRI reading task. Neurology 59:256–265

Garrett MC, Pouratian N, Liau LM (2012) Use of language mapping to aid in resection of gliomas in eloquent brain regions. Neurosurg Clin N Am 23:497–506

Gatignol P, Capelle L, Le Bihan R, Duffau H (2004) Double dissociation between picture naming and comprehension: an electrostimulation study. Neuroreport 15:191–195

Giussani C, Roux FE, Ojemann J, Sganzerla EP, Pirillo D, Papagno C (2011) Is preoperative functional magnetic resonance imaging reliable for language areas mapping in brain tumor surgery? Review of language functional magnetic resonance imaging and direct cortical stimulation correlation studies. Neurosurgery 66:113–120

Golby AJ, Poldrack RA, Illes J, Chen D, Desmond JE, Gabrieli JD (2002) Memory lateralization in medial temporal lobe epilepsy assessed by functional MRI. Epilepsia 43:855–863

Gonzalez-Darder JM, Gonzalez-Lopez P, Talamantes F, Quilis V, Cortes V, Garcia-March G, Roldan P (2010) Multimodal navigation in the functional microsurgical resection of intrinsic brain tumors located in eloquent motor areas: role of tractography. Neurosurg Focus 28:E5

Gordon B, Lesser RP, Rance NE, Hart J Jr, Webber R, Uematsu S, Fisher RS (1990) Parameters for direct cortical electrical stimulation in the human: histopathologic confirmation. Electroencephalogr Clin Neurophysiol 75:371–377

Guggisberg AG, Honma SM, Findlay AM, Dalal SS, Kirsch HE, Berger MS, Nagarajan SS (2008) Mapping functional connectivity in patients with brain lesions. Ann Neurol 63:193–203

Hamzei F, Knab R, Weiller C, Rother J (2003) The influence of extra- and intracranial artery disease on the BOLD signal in FMRI. NeuroImage 20:1393–1399

Harel N, Lin J, Moeller S, Ugurbil K, Yacoub E (2006) Combined imaging-histological study of cortical laminar specificity of fMRI signals. NeuroImage 29:879–887

Hassler W, Steinmetz H (1987) Cerebral hemodynamics in angioma patients: an intraoperative study. J Neurosurg 67:822–831

Heeger DJ, Huk AC, Geisler WS, Albrecht DG (2002) What does fMRI tell us about neuronal activity? Nat Rev Neurosci 3:142–151

Henry RG, Berman JI, Nagarajan SS, Mukherjee P, Berger MS (2004) Subcortical pathways serving cortical language sites: initial experience with diffusion tensor imaging fiber tracking combined with intraoperative language mapping. NeuroImage 21:616–622

Herholz K, Reulen HJ, von Stockhausen HM, Thiel A, Ilmberger J, Kessler J, Eisner W, Yousry TA, Heiss WD (1997) Preoperative activation and intraoperative stimulation of language-related areas in patients with glioma. Neurosurgery 41:1253–1260; discussion 1260–1252

Hertz-Pannier L, Gaillard WD, Mott SH, Cuenod CA, Bookheimer SY, Weinstein S, Conry J, Papero PH, Schiff SJ, Le Bihan D, Theodore WH (1997) Noninvasive assessment of language dominance in children and adolescents with functional MRI: a preliminary study. Neurology 48: 1003–1012

Hill DL, Smith AD, Simmons A, Maurer CR Jr, Cox TC, Elwes R, Brammer M, Hawkes DJ, Polkey CE (2000) Sources of error in comparing functional magnetic resonance imaging and invasive electrophysiological recordings. J Neurosurg 93:214–223

Hirsch J, Ruge MI, Kim KH, Correa DD, Victor JD, Relkin NR, Labar DR, Krol G, Bilsky MH, Souweidane MM, DeAngelis LM, Gutin PH (2000) An integrated functional magnetic resonance imaging procedure for preoperative mapping of cortical areas associated with tactile, motor, language, and visual functions. Neurosurgery 47:711–721; discussion 721–722

Holmes AA, Scollan DF, Winslow RL (2000) Direct histological validation of diffusion tensor MRI in formaldehyde-fixed myocardium. Magn Reson Med 44:157–161

Holodny AI, Schulder M, Liu WC, Maldjian JA, Kalnin AJ (1999) Decreased BOLD functional MR activation of the motor and sensory cortices adjacent to a glioblastoma multiforme: implications for image-guided neurosurgery. AJNR Am J Neuroradiol 20:609–612

Holodny AI, Schulder M, Liu WC, Wolko J, Maldjian JA, Kalnin AJ (2000) The effect of brain tumors on BOLD functional MR imaging activation in the adjacent motor cortex: implications for image-guided neurosurgery. AJNR Am J Neuroradiol 21:1415–1422

Hong SB, Roh SY, Kim SE, Seo DW (2000a) Correlation of temporal lobe glucose metabolism with the Wada memory test. Epilepsia 41:1554–1559

Hong SB, Kim KW, Seo DW, Kim SE, Na DG, Byun HS (2000b) Contralateral EEG slowing and amobarbital distribution in Wada test: an intracarotid SPECT study. Epilepsia 41:207–212

Hoppel BE, Weisskoff RM, Thulborn KR, Moore JB, Kwong KK, Rosen BR (1993) Measurement of regional blood oxygenation and cerebral hemodynamics. Magn Reson Med 30:715–723

Hou BL, Bradbury M, Peck KK, Petrovich NM, Gutin PH, Holodny AI (2006) Effect of brain tumor neovasculature defined by rCBV on BOLD fMRI activation volume in the primary motor cortex. NeuroImage 32:489–497

Hu X, Le TH, Parrish T, Erhard P (1995) Retrospective estimation and correction of physiological fluctuation in functional MRI. Magn Reson Med 34:201–212

Jack CR Jr, Nichols DA, Sharbrough FW, Marsh WR, Petersen RC, Hinkeldey NS, Ivnik RJ, Cascino GD, Ilstrup DM (1989) Selective posterior cerebral artery injection of amytal: new method of preoperative memory testing. Mayo Clin Proc 64:965–975

Jack CR Jr, Thompson RM, Butts RK, Sharbrough FW, Kelly PJ, Hanson DP, Riederer SJ, Ehman RL, Hangiandreou NJ, Cascino GD (1994) Sensory motor cortex: correlation of presurgical mapping with functional MR imaging and invasive cortical mapping. Radiology 190:85–92

Janszky J, Jokeit H, Kontopoulou K, Mertens M, Ebner A, Pohlmann-Eden B, Woermann FG (2005) Functional MRI predicts memory performance after right mesiotemporal epilepsy surgery. Epilepsia 46:244–250

Javadi SA, Nabavi A, Giordano M et al (2017) Evaluation of diffusion tensor imaging-based tractography of the corticospinal tract: a correlative study with intraoperative magnetic resonance imaging and direct electrical subcortical stimulation. Neurosurgery 80:287–299

Jayakar P (1993) Physiological principles of electrical stimulation. Adv Neurol 63:17–27

Jayakar P, Alvarez LA, Duchowny MS, Resnick TJ (1992) A safe and effective paradigm to functionally map the cortex in childhood. J Clin Neurophysiol 9:288–293

Jiang Z, Krainik A, David O, Salon C, Tropres I, Hoffmann D, Pannetier N, Barbier EL, Bombin ER, Warnking J, Pasteris C, Chabardes S, Berger F, Grand S, Segebarth C, Gay E, Le Bas JF (2010) Impaired fMRI activation in patients with primary brain tumors. NeuroImage 52:538–548

Jokeit H, Ebner A, Arnold S, Schuller M, Antke C, Huang Y, Steinmetz H, Seitz RJ, Witte OW (1999) Bilateral reductions of hippocampal volume, glucose metabolism, and Wada hemispheric memory performance are related to the duration of mesial temporal lobe epilepsy. J Neurol 246:926–933

Jokeit H, Okujava M, Woermann FG (2001) Memory fMRI lateralizes temporal lobe epilepsy. Neurology 57:1786–1793

Jones-Gotman M (1987) Psychological evaluation-testing of hippocampal function. In: Engel J (ed) Surgical treatment of the epilepsies. Raven, New York, pp 203–211

Kamada K, Todo T, Masutani Y, Aoki S, Ino K, Takano T, Kirino T, Kawahara N, Morita A (2005) Combined use of tractography-integrated functional neuronavigation and direct fiber stimulation. J Neurosurg 102:664–672

Kamada K, Todo T, Ota T, Ino K, Masutani Y, Aoki S, Takeuchi F, Kawai K, Saito N (2009) The motor-evoked potential threshold evaluated by tractography and electrical stimulation. J Neurosurg 111:785–795

Keles GE, Berger MS (2004) Advances in neurosurgical technique in the current management of brain tumors. Semin Oncol 31:659–665

Keles GE, Lundin DA, Lamborn KR, Chang EF, Ojemann G, Berger MS (2004) Intraoperative subcortical stimulation mapping for hemispherical perirolandic gliomas located within or adjacent to the descending motor pathways: evaluation of morbidity and assessment of functional outcome in 294 patients. J Neurosurg 100:369–375

Kobayashi E, Bagshaw AP, Jansen A, Andermann F, Andermann E, Gotman J, Dubeau F (2005) Intrinsic epileptogenicity in polymicrogyric cortex suggested by EEG-fMRI BOLD responses. Neurology 64:1263–1266

Krainik A, Lehericy S, Duffau H, Vlaicu M, Poupon F, Capelle L, Cornu P, Clemenceau S, Sahel M, Valery CA, Boch AL, Mangin JF, Bihan DL, Marsault C (2001) Role of the supplementary motor area in motor deficit following medial frontal lobe surgery. Neurology 57:871–878

Krainik A, Lehericy S, Duffau H, Capelle L, Chainay H, Cornu P, Cohen L, Boch AL, Mangin JF, Le Bihan D, Marsault C (2003) Postoperative speech disorder after medial frontal surgery: role of the supplementary motor area. Neurology 60:587–594

Krieg SM, Shiban E, Buchmann N, Meyer B, Ringel F (2013) Presurgical navigated transcranial magnetic brain stimulation for recurrent gliomas in motor eloquent areas. Clin Neurophysiol 124:522–527

Krings T, Buchbinder BR, Butler WE, Chiappa KH, Jiang HJ, Rosen BR, Cosgrove GR (1997a) Stereotactic transcranial magnetic stimulation: correlation with direct electrical cortical stimulation. Neurosurgery 41:1319–1325; discussion 1325–1316

Krings T, Buchbinder BR, Butler WE, Chiappa KH, Jiang HJ, Cosgrove GR, Rosen BR (1997b) Functional magnetic resonance imaging and transcranial magnetic stimulation: complementary approaches in the evaluation of cortical motor function. Neurology 48:1406–1416

Krings T, Foltys H, Reinges MH, Kemeny S, Rohde V, Spetzger U, Gilsbach JM, Thron A (2001a) Navigated transcranial magnetic stimulation for presurgical planning—correlation with functional MRI. Minim Invasive Neurosurg 44:234–239

Krings T, Schreckenberger M, Rohde V, Foltys H, Spetzger U, Sabri O, Reinges MH, Kemeny S, Meyer PT, Moller-Hartmann W, Korinth M, Gilsbach JM, Buell U, Thron A (2001b) Metabolic and electrophysiological validation of functional MRI. J Neurol Neurosurg Psychiatry 71:762–771

Krishnan R, Raabe A, Hattingen E, Szelenyi A, Yahya H, Hermann E, Zimmermann M, Seifert V (2004) Functional magnetic resonance imaging-integrated neuronavigation: correlation between lesion-to-motor cortex distance and outcome. Neurosurgery 55:904–914; discussion 914–915

Kuchcinski G, Mellerio C, Pallud J et al (2015) Three-tesla functional MR language mapping: comparison with direct cortical stimulation in gliomas. Neurology 84:560–568

Kundu B, Rolston JD, Grandhi R (2019) Mapping language dominance through the lens of the Wada test. Neurosurg Focus 47:E5

Ladd ME, Bachert P, Meyerspeer M et al (2018) Pros and cons of ultra-high-field MRI/MRS for human application. Prog Nucl Magn Reson Spectrosc 109:1–50

Law M, Kazmi K, Wetzel S, Wang E, Iacob C, Zagzag D, Golfinos JG, Johnson G (2004) Dynamic susceptibility contrast-enhanced perfusion and conventional MR imaging findings for adult patients with cerebral primitive neuroectodermal tumors. AJNR Am J Neuroradiol 25:997–1005

Lawes INC, Clark CA (2010) Anatomical validation of DTI and tractography. In: Jones DK (ed) Diffusion MRI. Theory, methods and applications. Oxford University Press, New York, pp 439–447

Leclercq D, Duffau H, Delmaire C, Capelle L, Gatignol P, Ducros M, Chiras J, Lehericy S (2010) Comparison of diffusion tensor imaging tractography of language tracts and intraoperative subcortical stimulations. J Neurosurg 112:503–511

Lee SP, Silva AC, Ugurbil K, Kim SG (1999) Diffusion-weighted spin-echo fMRI at 9.4 T: microvascular/tissue contribution to BOLD signal changes. Magn Reson Med 42:919–928

Lee TMC, Yip JTH, Jones-Gotman M (2002) Memory deficits after resection from left or right anterior temporal lobe in humans: a meta-analytic review. Epilepsia 43:283–291

Lehericy S, Cohen L, Bazin B, Samson S, Giacomini E, Rougetet R, Hertz-Pannier L, Le Bihan D, Marsault C, Baulac M (2000a) Functional MR evaluation of temporal and frontal language dominance compared with the Wada test. Neurology 54:1625–1633

Lehericy S, Duffau H, Cornu P, Capelle L, Pidoux B, Carpentier A, Auliac S, Clemenceau S, Sichez JP, Bitar A, Valery CA, Van Effenterre R, Faillot T, Srour A, Fohanno D, Philippon J, Le Bihan D, Marsault C (2000b) Correspondence between functional magnetic resonance imaging somatotopy and individual brain anatomy of the central region: comparison with intraoperative stimulation in patients with brain tumors. J Neurosurg 92:589–598

Lehericy S, Biondi A, Sourour N, Vlaicu M, du Montcel ST, Cohen L, Vivas E, Capelle L, Faillot T, Casasco A, Le Bihan D, Marsault C (2002) Arteriovenous brain malformations: is functional MR imaging reliable for studying language reorganization in patients? Initial observations. Radiology 223:672–682

Lesser RP, Luders H, Klem G, Dinner DS, Morris HH, Hahn J (1984) Cortical afterdischarge and functional response thresholds: results of extraoperative testing. Epilepsia 25:615–621

Lesser RP, Luders H, Klem G, Dinner DS, Morris HH, Hahn JF, Wyllie E (1987) Extraoperative cortical functional localization in patients with epilepsy. J Clin Neurophysiol 4:27–53

Logothetis NK, Wandell BA (2004) Interpreting the BOLD signal. Annu Rev Physiol 66:735–769

Loring DW, Meador KJ, Lee GP, King DW, Nichols ME, Park YD, Murro AM, Gallagher BB, Smith JR (1995) Wada memory asymmetries predict verbal memory decline after anterior temporal lobectomy. Neurology 45:1329–1333

Ludemann L, Grieger W, Wurm R, Budzisch M, Hamm B, Zimmer C (2001) Comparison of dynamic contrast-enhanced MRI with WHO tumor grading for gliomas. Eur Radiol 11:1231–1241

Luders HO, Dinner DS, Morris HH, Wyllie E, Comair YG (1995) Cortical electrical stimulation in humans. The negative motor areas. Adv Neurol 67:115–129

Lurito JT, Lowe MJ, Sartorius C, Mathews VP (2000) Comparison of fMRI and intraoperative direct cortical stimulation in localization of receptive language areas. J Comput Assist Tomogr 24:99–105

Martino J, Honma SM, Findlay AM, Guggisberg AG, Owen JP, Kirsch HE, Berger MS, Nagarajan SS (2011) Resting functional connectivity in patients with brain tumors in eloquent areas. Ann Neurol 69:521–532

Massot-Tarrús A, White K, Mirsattari SM (2019) Comparing the Wada test and functional MRI for the presurgical evaluation of memory in temporal lobe epilepsy. Curr Neurol Neurosci Rep 19:31

Medina LS, Aguirre E, Bernal B, Altman NR (2004) Functional MR imaging versus Wada test for evaluation of language lateralization: cost analysis. Radiology 230:49–54

Milner B, Branch C, Rasmussen T (1962) Study of short-term memory after intracarotid injection of sodium amytal. Trans Am Neurol Assoc 87:224–226

Mitchell TJ, Hacker CD, Breshears JD, Szrama NP, Sharma M, Bundy DT, Pahwa M, Corbetta M, Snyder AZ, Shimony JS, Leuthardt EC (2013) A novel data-driven approach to preoperative mapping of functional cortex using resting-state functional magnetic resonance imaging. Neurosurgery 73:969–983

Mori S, Kaufmann WE, Davatzikos C, Stieltjes B, Amodei L, Fredericksen K, Pearlson GD, Melhem ER, Solaiyappan M, Raymond GV, Moser HW, van Zijl PC (2002) Imaging cortical association tracts in the human brain using diffusion-tensor-based axonal tracking. Magn Reson Med 47:215–223

Mueller WM, Yetkin FZ, Hammeke TA, Morris GL III, Swanson SJ, Reichert K, Cox R, Haughton VM (1996) Functional magnetic resonance imaging mapping of the motor cortex in patients with cerebral tumors. Neurosurgery 39:515–520; discussion 520–521

Nagarajan L, Schaul N, Eidelberg D, Dhawan V, Fraser R, Labar DR (1996) Contralateral temporal hypometabolism on positron emission tomography in temporal lobe epilepsy. Acta Neurol Scand 93:81–84

Nathan SS, Lesser RP, Gordon B, Thakor NV (1993) Electrical stimulation of the human cerebral cortex. Theoretical approach. In: Devinsky O, Beric A, Dogali M (eds) Electrical and magnetic stimulation of the brain and spinal cord. Raven, New York

O'Rourke DM, Saykin AJ, Gilhool JJ, Harley R, O'Connor MJ, Sperling MR (1993) Unilateral hemispheric memory and hippocampal neuronal density in temporal lobe epilepsy. Neurosurgery 32:574–580; discussion 580–581

Ogawa S, Menon RS, Tank DW, Kim SG, Merkle H, Ellermann JM, Ugurbil K (1993) Functional brain mapping by blood oxygenation level-dependent contrast magnetic resonance imaging. A comparison of signal characteristics with a biophysical model. Biophys J 64:803–812

Ogg RJ, Laningham FH, Clarke D, Einhaus S, Zou P, Tobias ME, Boop FA (2009) Passive range of motion functional magnetic resonance imaging localizing sensorimotor cortex in sedated children. J Neurosurg 4:317–322

Ohue S, Kohno S, Inoue A, Yamashita D, Harada H, Kumon Y, Kikuchi K, Miki H, Ohnishi T (2012) Accuracy of diffusion tensor magnetic resonance imaging-based tractography for surgery of gliomas near the pyramidal tract: a significant correlation between subcortical electrical stimulation and postoperative tractography. Neurosurgery 70:283–293; discussion 294

Ojemann G, Ojemann J, Lettich E, Berger M (1989) Cortical language localization in left, dominant hemisphere. An electrical stimulation mapping investigation in 117 patients. J Neurosurg 71:316–326

Pawlik G, Rackl A, Bing RJ (1981) Quantitative capillary topography and blood flow in the cerebral cortex of cats: an in vivo microscopic study. Brain Res 208:35–58

Pfeuffer J, Van de Moortele PF, Ugurbil K, Hu X, Glover GH (2002) Correction of physiologically induced global off-resonance effects in dynamic echo-planar and spiral functional imaging. Magn Reson Med 47:344–353

Picht T, Schmidt S, Brandt S, Frey D, Hannula H, Neuvonen T, Karhu J, Vajkoczy P, Suess O (2011) Preoperative functional mapping for rolandic brain tumor surgery: comparison of navigated transcranial magnetic stimulation to direct cortical stimulation. Neurosurgery 69:581–588; discussion 588

Pineiro R, Pendlebury S, Johansen-Berg H, Matthews PM (2002) Altered hemodynamic responses in patients after subcortical stroke measured by functional MRI. Stroke 33:103–109

Prabhu SS, Gasco J, Tummala S, Weinberg JS, Rao G (2011) Intraoperative magnetic resonance imaging-guided tractography with integrated monopolar subcortical functional mapping for resection of brain tumors. Clinical article. J Neurosurg 114:719–726

Puce A, Constable RT, Luby ML, McCarthy G, Nobre AC, Spencer DD, Gore JC, Allison T (1995) Functional magnetic resonance imaging of sensory and motor cortex: comparison with electrophysiological localization. J Neurosurg 83:262–270

Pudenz RH, Agnew WF, Yuen TG, Bullara LA, Jacques S, Shelden CH (1977) Adverse effects of electrical energy applied to the nervous system. Appl Neurophysiol 40:72–87

Pujol J, Conesa G, Deus J, Vendrell P, Isamat F, Zannoli G, Marti-Vilalta JL, Capdevila A (1996) Presurgical identification of the primary sensorimotor cortex by functional magnetic resonance imaging. J Neurosurg 84:7–13

Pujol J, Conesa G, Deus J, Lopez-Obarrio L, Isamat F, Capdevila A (1998) Clinical application of functional magnetic resonance imaging in presurgical identification of the central sulcus. J Neurosurg 88:863–869

Rabin ML, Narayan VM, Kimberg DY, Casasanto DJ, Glosser G, Tracy JI, French JA, Sperling MR, Detre JA (2004) Functional MRI predicts post-surgical memory following temporal lobectomy. Brain 127:2286–2298

Ranck JB Jr (1975) Which elements are excited in electrical stimulation of mammalian central nervous system: a review. Brain Res 98:417–440

Rausch R, Silfvenius H, Wieser HG, Dodrill CB, Meader KJ, Jones-Gotman M (1993) Interarterial amobarbital procedures. In: Engel JJ (ed) Surgical treatment of the epilepsies. Raven, New York, pp 341–357

Rausch R, Henry TR, Ary CM, Engel J Jr, Mazziotta J (1994) Asymmetric interictal glucose hypometabolism and cognitive performance in epileptic patients. Arch Neurol 51:139–144

Reinges MH, Krings T, Meyer PT, Schreckenberger M, Rohde V, Weidemann J, Sabri O, Mulders EJ, Buell U, Thron A, Gilsbach JM (2004) Preoperative mapping of cortical motor function: prospective comparison of functional magnetic resonance imaging and [15O]-H2O-positron emission tomography in the same co-ordinate system. Nucl Med Commun 25:987–997

Richardson MP, Strange BA, Thompson PJ, Baxendale SA, Duncan JS, Dolan RJ (2004) Pre-operative verbal memory fMRI predicts post-operative memory decline after left temporal lobe resection. Brain 127:2419–2426

Richardson MP, Strange BA, Duncan JS, Dolan RJ (2006) Memory fMRI in left hippocampal sclerosis: optimizing the approach to predicting postsurgical memory. Neurology 66:699–705

Rouleau I, Robidoux J, Labrecque R, Denault C (1997) Effect of focus lateralization on memory assessment during the intracarotid amobarbital procedure. Brain Cogn 33:224–241

Roux FE, Boulanouar K, Ranjeva JP, Tremoulet M, Henry P, Manelfe C, Sabatier J, Berry I (1999) Usefulness of motor functional MRI correlated to cortical mapping in Rolandic low-grade astrocytomas. Acta Neurochir 141:71–79

Roux FE, Boulanouar K, Lotterie JA, Mejdoubi M, LeSage JP, Berry I (2003) Language functional magnetic resonance imaging in preoperative assessment of language areas: correlation with direct cortical stimulation. Neurosurgery 52:1335–1345; discussion 1345–1347

Rutten GJ, Ramsey NF, van Rijen PC, Noordmans HJ, van Veelen CW (2002a) Development of a functional magnetic resonance imaging protocol for intraoperative localization of critical temporoparietal language areas. Ann Neurol 51:350–360

Rutten GJ, Ramsey NF, van Rijen PC, Alpherts WC, van Veelen CW (2002b) FMRI-determined language lateralization in patients with unilateral or mixed language dominance according to the Wada test. NeuroImage 17:447–460

Sabbah P, Chassoux F, Leveque C, Landre E, Baudoin-Chial S, Devaux B, Mann M, Godon-Hardy S, Nioche C, Ait-Ameur A, Sarrazin JL, Chodkiewicz JP, Cordoliani YS (2003) Functional MR imaging in assessment of language dominance in epileptic patients. NeuroImage 18:460–467

Salanova V, Morris HH III, Rehm P, Wyllie E, Dinner DS, Luders H, Gilmore-Pollak W (1992) Comparison of the intracarotid amobarbital procedure and interictal cerebral 18-fluorodeoxyglucose positron emission tomography scans in refractory temporal lobe epilepsy. Epilepsia 33:635–638

Salanova V, Markand O, Worth R (2001) Focal functional deficits in temporal lobe epilepsy on PET scans and the intracarotid amobarbital procedure: comparison of patients with unitemporal epilepsy with those requiring intracranial recordings. Epilepsia 42:198–203

Sartorius CJ, Berger MS (1998) Rapid termination of intraoperative stimulation-evoked seizures with application of cold Ringer's lactate to the cortex. Technical note. J Neurosurg 88:349–351

Sass KJ, Lencz T, Westerveld M, Novelly RA, Spencer DD, Kim JH (1991) The neural substrate of memory impairment demonstrated by the intracarotid amobarbital procedure. Arch Neurol 48:48–52

Schiffbauer H, Berger MS, Ferrari P, Freudenstein D, Rowley HA, Roberts TP (2002) Preoperative magnetic source imaging for brain tumor surgery: a quantitative comparison with intraoperative sensory and motor mapping. J Neurosurg 97:1333–1342

Schmid E, Thomschewski A, Taylor A et al (2018) Diagnostic accuracy of functional magnetic resonance imaging, Wada test, magnetoencephalography, and functional transcranial Doppler sonography for memory and language outcome after epilepsy surgery: a systematic review. Epilepsia 59:2305–2317

Schreckenberger M, Spetzger U, Sabri O, Meyer PT, Zeggel T, Zimny M, Gilsbach J, Buell U (2001) Localisation of motor areas in brain tumour patients: a comparison of preoperative [18F]FDG-PET and intraoperative cortical electrostimulation. Eur J Nucl Med 28:1394–1403

Sherman EM, Wiebe S, Fay-McClymont TB et al (2011) Neuropsychological outcomes after epilepsy surgery: systematic review and pooled estimates. Centre for Reviews and Dissemination, UK

Shmuel A, Augath M, Oeltermann A, Logothetis NK (2006) Negative functional MRI response correlates with decreases in neuronal activity in monkey visual area V1. Nat Neurosci 9:569–577

Simkins-Bullock J (2000) Beyond speech lateralization: a review of the variability, reliability, and validity of the intracarotid amobarbital procedure and its nonlanguage uses in epilepsy surgery candidates. Neuropsychol Rev 10:41–74

Simos PG, Papanicolaou AC, Breier JI, Wheless JW, Constantinou JE, Gormley WB, Maggio WW (1999) Localization of language-specific cortex by using magnetic source imaging and electrical stimulation mapping. J Neurosurg 91:787–796

Small SA, Perera GM, DeLaPaz R, Mayeux R, Stern Y (1999) Differential regional dysfunction of the hippocampal formation among elderly with memory decline and Alzheimer's disease. Ann Neurol 45:466–472

Spena G, Nava A, Cassini F, Pepoli A, Bruno M, D'Agata F, Cauda F, Sacco K, Duca S, Barletta L, Versari P (2010) Preoperative and intraoperative brain mapping for the resection of eloquent-area tumors. A prospective analysis of methodology, correlation, and usefulness based on clinical outcomes. Acta Neurochir 152:1835–1846

Spencer DC, Morrell MJ, Risinger MW (2000) The role of the intracarotid amobarbital procedure in evaluation of patients for epilepsy surgery. Epilepsia 41:320–325

Sperling MR, Saykin AJ, Glosser G, Moran M, French JA, Brooks M, O'Connor MJ (1994) Predictors of outcome after anterior temporal lobectomy: the intracarotid amobarbital test. Neurology 44:2325–2330

Sperling MR, Alavi A, Reivich M, French JA, O'Connor MJ (1995) False lateralization of temporal lobe epilepsy with FDG positron emission tomography. Epilepsia 36:722–727

Stieltjes B, Kaufmann WE, van Zijl PC, Fredericksen K, Pearlson GD, Solaiyappan M, Mori S (2001) Diffusion tensor imaging and axonal tracking in the human brainstem. NeuroImage 14:723–735

Thulborn KR, Waterton JC, Matthews PM, Radda GK (1982) Oxygenation dependence of the transverse relaxation time of water protons in whole blood at high field. Biochim Biophys Acta 714:265–270

Tyndall AJ, Reinhardt J, Tronnier V et al (2017) Presurgical motor, somatosensory and language fMRI: technical feasibility and limitations in 491 patients over 13 years. Eur Radiol 27:267–278

Ugurbil K, Hu X, Chen W, Zhu XH, Kim SG, Georgopoulos A (1999) Functional mapping in the human brain using high magnetic fields. Philos Trans R Soc Lond Ser B Biol Sci 354:1195–1213

Ugurbil K, Toth L, Kim DS (2003) How accurate is magnetic resonance imaging of brain function? Trends Neurosci 26:108–114

Urbach H, Kurthen M, Klemm E, Grunwald T, Van Roost D, Linke DB, Biersack HJ, Schramm J, Elger CE (1999) Amobarbital effects on the posterior hippocampus during the intracarotid amobarbital test. Neurology 52:1596–1602

Vakamudi K, Posse S, Jung R et al (2019) Real-time presurgical resting-state fMRI in patients with brain tumors: quality control and comparison with task-fMRI and intraoperative mapping. Hum Brain Mapp 41(3):797–814

Van de Moortele PF, Pfeuffer J, Glover GH, Ugurbil K, Hu X (2002) Respiration-induced B0 fluctuations and their spatial distribution in the human brain at 7 Tesla. Magn Reson Med 47:888–895

Van Zijl PC, Eleff SM, Ulatowski JA, Oja JM, Ulug AM, Traystman RJ, Kauppinen RA (1998) Quantitative assessment of blood flow, blood volume and blood oxygenation effects in functional magnetic resonance imaging. Nat Med 4:159–167

Vassal F, Schneider F, Nuti C (2013) Intraoperative use of diffusion tensor imaging-based tractography for resection of gliomas located near the pyramidal tract: comparison with subcortical stimulation mapping and contribution to surgical outcomes. Br J Neurosurg 27:668–675

Wada J, Rasmussen T (1960) Intracarotid injection of sodium amytal for the lateralization of cerebral speech dominance: experimental and clinical observations. J Neurosurg 17:266–282

Waldvogel D, van Gelderen P, Ishii K, Hallett M (1999) The effect of movement amplitude on activation in functional magnetic resonance imaging studies. J Cereb Blood Flow Metab 19:1209–1212

Witt J-A, Coras R, Schramm J et al (2015) Relevance of hippocampal integrity for memory outcome after surgical treatment of mesial temporal lobe epilepsy. J Neurol 262:2214–2224

Woermann FG, Jokeit H, Luerding R, Freitag H, Schulz R, Guertler S, Okujava M, Wolf P, Tuxhorn I, Ebner A (2003) Language lateralization by Wada test and fMRI in 100 patients with epilepsy. Neurology 61:699–701

Wood JM, Kundu B, Utter A, Gallagher TA, Voss J, Nair VA, Kuo JS, Field AS, Moritz CH, Meyerand ME, Prabhakaran V (2011) Impact of brain tumor location on morbidity and mortality: a retrospective functional MR imaging study. AJNR Am J Neuroradiol 32:1420–1425

Yacoub E, Duong TQ, Van De Moortele PF, Lindquist M, Adriany G, Kim SG, Ugurbil K, Hu X (2003) Spin-echo fMRI in humans using high spatial resolutions and high magnetic fields. Magn Reson Med 49:655–664

Yetkin FZ, Mueller WM, Morris GL, McAuliffe TL, Ulmer JL, Cox RW, Daniels DL, Haughton VM (1997) Functional MR activation correlated with intraoperative cortical mapping. AJNR Am J Neuroradiol 18:1311–1315

Yingling CD, Ojemann S, Dodson B, Harrington MJ, Berger MS (1999) Identification of motor pathways during tumor surgery facilitated by multichannel electromyographic recording. J Neurosurg 91:922–927

Young WL, Prohovnik I, Ornstein E, Ostapkovich N, Sisti MB, Solomon RA, Stein BM (1990) The effect of arteriovenous malformation resection on cerebrovascular reactivity to carbon dioxide. Neurosurgery 27:257–266; discussion 266–267

Young WL, Pile-Spellman J, Prohovnik I, Kader A, Stein BM (1994) Evidence for adaptive autoregulatory displacement in hypotensive cortical territories adjacent to arteriovenous malformations. Columbia University AVM Study Project. Neurosurgery 34:601–610; discussion 610–611

Yousry TA, Schmid UD, Jassoy AG, Schmidt D, Eisner WE, Reulen HJ, Reiser MF, Lissner J (1995) Topography of the cortical motor hand area: prospective study with functional MR imaging and direct motor mapping at surgery. Radiology 195:23–29

Yousry TA, Schmid UD, Alkadhi H, Schmidt D, Peraud A, Buettner A, Winkler P (1997) Localization of the motor hand area to a knob on the precentral gyrus. A new landmark. Brain 120(Pt 1):141–157

Zeineh MM, Engel SA, Thompson PM, Bookheimer SY (2003) Dynamics of the hippocampus during encoding and retrieval of face-name pairs. Science 299: 577–580

Zhu FP, Wu JS, Song YY, Yao CJ, Zhuang DX, Xu G, Tang WJ, Qin ZY, Mao Y, Zhou LF (2012) Clinical application of motor pathway mapping using diffusion tensor imaging tractography and intraoperative direct subcortical stimulation in cerebral glioma surgery: a prospective cohort study. Neurosurgery 71:1170–1183; discussion 1183–1184

Multimodal Functional Neuroimaging

Austin Trinh, Max Wintermark, and Michael Iv

Contents

Abstract

Several modalities can be used in conjunction with functional neuroimaging, which includes structural and volumetric magnetic resonance imaging (MRI), perfusion MRI (pMRI), functional MRI (fMRI), diffusion tensor imaging (DTI), single-photon emission computed tomography (SPECT), positron emission tomography (PET), MR spectroscopy (MRS), and magnetoencephalography (MEG). Fusion of these modalities combines complementary information, expands resolution limits, and can improve data quality. The multimodal nature of this approach allows use of different imaging modalities for a single evaluation, thus providing a more comprehensive evaluation of the brain. Their respective contributions and limitations will be summarized in this chapter. Further discussed are key clinical uses for multimodal data, especially in context of pre-surgical planning for functional neuroimaging.

A. Trinh · M. Wintermark · M. Iv (✉)
Department of Radiology, Neuroradiology Division, Stanford University, Stanford, CA, USA
e-mail: austin.trinh@stanford.edu;
Max.Wintermark@stanford.edu; miv@stanford.edu

1   Introduction to Multimodal Functional Neuroimaging

Given recent advances in neuroimaging, several modalities are now available for clinical use, including structural and volumetric magnetic resonance imaging (MRI), perfusion MRI (pMRI), functional MRI (fMRI), diffusion tensor imaging (DTI), single-photon emission computed

© The Author(s), under exclusive license to Springer Nature Switzerland AG 2022
C. Stippich (ed.), *Clinical Functional MRI*, Medical Radiology Diagnostic Imaging,
https://doi.org/10.1007/978-3-030-83343-5_10

tomography (SPECT), positron emission tomography (PET), MR spectroscopy (MRS), and magnetoencephalography (MEG) (Zhang et al. 2020). The modality of choice often depends on the clinical scenario, ranging from the initial diagnostic evaluation of a lesion to pre-surgical or pre-treatment planning. At times, the use of multiple imaging modalities can provide more information about a specific lesion in the brain than the use of a single imaging approach due to the ability to exploit differences in multiparametric imaging features (Florez et al. 2018). As such, multimodal neuroimaging itself can be referred to as collective information offered by multiple imaging modalities. The nature of the multimodal approach overcomes the limitations of individual modalities by allowing for a more robust, multiparametric, and thus more comprehensive evaluation of the brain. There is inherent cross-validation of findings from different sources and/or sequences, thereby increasing the probability of identifying more specific associations and patterns related to functional neuroimaging. In a broader sense, it can help to define the roles of different brain areas from various perspectives. Use of multimodal imaging has become one of the major components that has facilitated the growth of neuroimaging research, especially when coupled with the wider availability of hybrid imaging such as PET/CT and PET/MRI/EEG. Within the field of functional multimodal neuroimaging, there has been a focus on computational analysis of data, including preprocessing, voxel extraction, image fusion, and post-processing. These computational advances aid to address the variations in spatiotemporal resolution between the modalities and merge biophysical information (Liu et al. 2015).

Briefly, neuroimaging can be divided into two categories: structural imaging and functional imaging, the latter of which will be the main focus of this chapter. While conventional structural imaging is useful to evaluate the anatomical structure of the brain and is useful for diagnosis of and determining treatment response in certain diseases, functional imaging typically focuses on biophysical parameters and metabolization and can be obtained while carrying out certain tasks including sensory and motor functions (Zhang et al. 2020). The sources of neuroimaging data can either be obtained from simultaneous imaging measurements taken at the time of imaging acquisition (e.g. EEG/fMRI or PET/CT) or by integrating separate measurements. For example, the combination of EEG with fMRI improves the spatiotemporal resolution that cannot be achieved by a single modality alone (Liu et al. 2015). Furthermore, structural neuroimaging obtained via MRI and functional neuroimaging from PET and SPECT have become an essential part of pre-surgical evaluation, which is often used for the identification of ideal patients for treatment and for planning intracranial EEG (icEEG) recordings (Tempany et al. 2015; Whiting et al. 2006). With pre-surgical planning, the use of co-registration enables multimodal comparison, which allows for characterization of the lesion to be resected, particularly in brain tumors and epilepsy surgery. Composite pre-surgical brain mapping techniques with respect to the pharmacological characterization related to both PET and SPECT provide relevant information on the metabolic state and molecular events within the tumor, even beyond the single depiction of activation maps obtained with fMRI alone. These multimodal approaches can reduce the need for invasive pre-surgical monitoring in certain cases, and can be used for the pre-operative assessment of infiltration zones around brain resection targets (Jacobs et al. 2005). The main foci of this chapter will be perfusion MRI, nuclear medicine, and MEG/EEG; functional MRI, resting state fMRI, and diffusion tensor imaging (DTI) will be briefly highlighted, but these modalities are covered more comprehensively in separate chapters.

2 Multimodal Neuroimaging for Pre-surgical Planning

In the context of pre-surgical imaging, a multimodal approach is primarily aimed at addressing two principle challenges: delineation of tumor margins and localization of regional or involved critical brain structures. Initial structural imaging analysis is essential, though the addition of functional data to conventional imaging and neuronavigation can further aid surgeons regarding optimal tissue site resection. Pre-operative brain mapping with use of functional MRI is being increasingly used as part of the surgical planning process, allowing for detailed intraoperative mapping. In addition, the incorporation of diffusion tensor imaging (DTI) allows for the visualization and localization of critical white matter tracts, particularly in relation to a brain lesion if present (Tempany et al. 2015).

Intracranial EEG monitoring is essential for epilepsy surgical planning, though it comes with its own limitations. The advent of multimodal neuroimaging has made it possible to show epileptic abnormalities that could not be previously identified, thereby improving the localization of a seizure focus. Recent advances in neuroimaging such as MRI morphometry, DTI, MRS, and MEG have improved ideal patient selection for treatment and surgical planning (Zhang et al. 2014). Altogether, non-invasive neuroimaging has shown to be promising in localizing seizure focus, especially in non-lesional epilepsy or extratemporal lobe epilepsy (ETLE), with neuroimaging possibly reducing the need for invasive pre-surgical monitoring in certain cases (Zhang et al. 2014; Tanaka et al. 2010).

2.1 Multiparametric MRI Techniques

2.1.1 Volumetric Analysis of Structural MRI

Structural MRI such as T1- and T2-weighted imaging can allow for volumetric measurements and can provide a macroscopic profile to evaluate structural differences (Wu et al. 2017). Target volume definition is a critical step in pre-surgical planning, with the ability of statistical and image processing techniques to improve the ability to determine the boundaries of tumor and peritumoral fluid (edema) (Florez et al. 2018). Individual MRI parametric maps obtained from structural MRI typically present single snapshots in time that are highly dynamic, incorporating imaging datasets for specific brain structure measurements and calculation of volume. The information can be obtained during the same imaging acquisition, though other approaches employ the use of longitudinally acquired single parametric maps. One strategy for analyzing multiparametric data involves extracting specific parameters, such as volume, and then applying it to statistical models to calculate differences between groups or multivariate regression to predict expected outcomes (Wu et al. 2010). Recent advances in image acquisition and image analysis techniques have enabled the use of larger longitudinal and cross-sectional studies for more advanced analysis (Wu et al. 2017). Furthermore, region of interest (ROI) analysis allows for comparison of different regions of signal intensity among different patients, with volumetric applications used to investigate several brain disorders ranging from brain tumors to epilepsy. A benefit of volumetric or ROI based methods is that these techniques do not require specific spatially aligned datasets to concentrate on particular regions of interest. Another often complementary strategy for performing multimodal analysis is a voxel-wise approach. In this technique, a statistical parametric map is generated by transforming the quantitative values from each voxel, with the voxel data extracted from the normalized images in aligned space. The resultant output can demonstrate regions where feature selections differ significantly between groups. Such methods allow for appreciation of voxel-by-voxel changes that may otherwise be obscured when taking aggregate values (Wu et al. 2010; Ashburner and Friston 2000). Therefore, a single image derived from a combination of potential markers into a simple imaging frame would be an ideal tool for quantifying the impact of interventions (Wu et al. 2010). Although results from volume based studies have been generally difficult to validate, many studies have compared results of volume based analyses to manual and visual measurements and have found relatively good correspondence between the techniques (Whitwell 2009).

2.1.2 Perfusion MRI (pMRI)

Perfusion MRI can be performed with endogenous or exogenous tracers. For exogenous agents, MR perfusion imaging relies on an injected contrast bolus tracked over time, which can be then used to investigate perfusion characteristics of a region of interest. These contrast-enhanced perfusion images can be accomplished through two techniques: dynamic susceptibility contrast (DSC) and dynamic contrast-enhanced (DCE) imaging. Dynamic susceptibility contrast-enhanced MRI employs a bolus tracking technique that is based on T2 (spin echo imaging) or T2* (gradient echo imaging) effects before, during, and after the administration of a contrast agent (Boxerman et al. 2016). Dynamic contrast-enhanced MRI also employs bolus tracking with T1-weighted imaging, where permeability characteristics of brain lesions such as tumors can be assessed with the advantage of a lower contrast dose and better temporal resolution. In contrast to DSC, DCE's T1-weighted technique measures the T1 relaxivity effects, rather than the susceptibility effects, of the injected dose of paramagnetic contrast. The relaxivity effect refers to the generated signal of T1 shortening, which is related to the relaxation time and is inherently stronger than susceptibility signal (Petrella and Provenzale 2000). For endogenous agents, arterial spin labeling (ASL) can be used, which relies on magnetically labeled spins using protons within arterial blood as the tracer (Detre and Alsop 1999).

In terms of pre-surgical evaluation of epilepsy, vascular perfusion changes have been increasingly investigated for their potential to localize the seizure onset zone, with the observation of transient postictal vascular changes, and the association of ischemia and epileptic foci (Li et al. 2019; Weinand et al. 1997). Changes in the perfusion parameter of cerebral blood flow (CBF) are often concordant with multimodal approaches based on EEG, MRI, SPECT, and PET. Similarly, ASL has also been found to non-invasively detect interictal and postictal alterations in CBF (Li et al. 2019; Guo et al. 2015). Recently, there have been applications of ASL perfusion imaging in functional connectivity studies, and as a complementary method to blood-oxygen-level dependent (BOLD) functional MRI with the added benefit of physiological parameters such as blood flow (Jahng et al. 2014).

Pre-surgical resection planning and/or stereotactic guided biopsy is commonly used in combination with perfusion imaging. Due to the internal heterogeneity of brain tumors and dependence on contrast enhancement to guide biopsy, sampling error remains a common problem. In perfusion imaging, cerebral blood volume (CBV) can be augmented as a measure of microvascular density in tumors. Studies have shown that regions of increased CBV, which can serve as a marker of tumor angiogenesis, may be better suitable targets for biopsy in patients with gliomas. In these situations, the threshold of CBV or CBF values can be applied to lesions, even those in those that have been previously treated, to delineate tumor from nontumoral areas and designate biopsy sites with the highest likelihood of obtaining higher grade portion of tumor (Fig. 1) (Boxerman et al. 2016; Prah et al. 2018). This supports that notion that perfusion MRI can help to reduce the sampling error in the histopathological diagnosis and improve surgical site selection (Maia et al. 2004; Hoxworth et al. 2020).

2.1.3 Diffusion Tensor Imaging (DTI)

One of the primary goals of pre-surgical planning for brain tumors is to maximize the extent of resection while minimizing morbidity. It is especially important to pre-operatively determine the spatial relationship between cortical and subcortical eloquent areas and lesion margins (Fig. 2) (Bailey et al. 2015). DTI is often used clinically in pre-operative planning prior to surgical resection, as tumors can be highly infiltrative (Liu et al. 2015). DTI involves a form of diffusion imaging where fiber tracts can be delineated based on the relative fractional anisotropy, thus allowing for the delineation of brain white matter pathways. By obtaining diffusion images along many different orientations, diffusion tensor imaging is able to estimate the appropriate orientation of axonal fiber bundles, due to the fact that water diffuses most readily along the length of axons (Liu et al. 2015; Bailey et al. 2015). The interpretation of these fiber tracts in relation to the surgical target provides a distinct advantage over conventional MRI in identifying the invasive or infiltrative nature of the tumor. Additionally, it can aid in the surgical planning of possible entry points as well as overall trajectory, while anticipating the best intraoperative routes

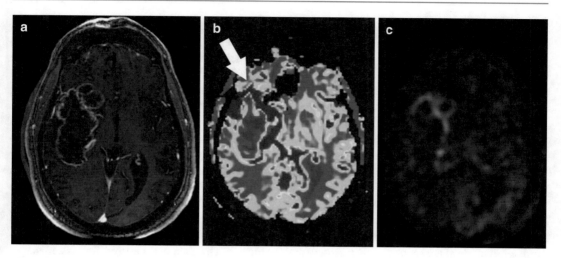

Fig. 1 (**a**) T1 weighted post-contrast image demonstrates a heterogenous and peripherally enhancing tumor predominantly involving the right frontotemporal lobes. (**b**) Dynamic susceptibility contrast (DSC) map of cerebral blood volume (CBV) demonstrates increased areas of blood volume along the anterior and medial margins of the tumor (white arrow). (**c**) Arterial spin labeling (ASL) image demonstrates similar areas of hyperperfusion or high blood flow

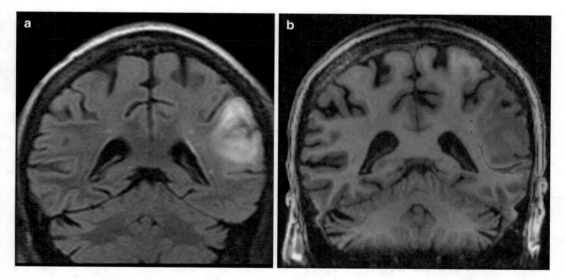

Fig. 2 (**a**) Fluid-attenuated inversion recovery (FLAIR) coronal image demonstrates a heterogeneous mass within the left parietal lobe with regional hypertintense signal, compatible with biopsy-proven glioblastoma. (**b**) Diffusion tensor imaging-streamline tractography super- imposed on a structural MRI T1-weighted image demonstrates the expected course of the left superior longitudinal fasciculus (arcuate fasciculus) immediately underlying the lesion

to prevent postsurgical neurological deficits (Bailey et al. 2015).

2.1.4 Functional MRI (fMRI)

Functional MRI is being increasingly used in pre-surgical planning for localization of eloquent cortex and to predict postoperative language as well as memory outcomes (Baumgartner et al. 2019). Though the gold standard involves cortical stimulation and mapping from indwelling electrodes or evaluation of stimuli during an awake craniotomy, blood-oxygen-level-dependent functional magnetic resonance imaging is able to also reliably and non-invasively provide this information and can potentially replace the Wada test for language lateralization in specific cases (Bailey et al. 2015; Baumgartner et al. 2019). This MR imaging method produces information related to brain function using blood oxygenation level dependent contrast imaging, which is sensitive to changes in the state of oxygenation of the hemoglobin. At its core, the fMRI images are based on hemodynamic responses to neuronal activity or task-based functions, which are obtained using paradigms to activate the motor and language systems, thereby allowing for lateralization (Dierker et al. 2017; Amaro and Barker 2006). Recent studies have demonstrated, for example, in patients with frontal lobe epilepsy, a significant postoperative naming decline

was observed when the resection overlapped with areas of language fMRI activation, even when prior stimulation results were negative in these areas, further supporting the role of fMRI for presurgical language localization (Baumgartner et al. 2019; Sidhu et al. 2018).

The combination of detailed anatomical information with physiological information on cerebral hemodynamics after cognitive activity creates a structural and functional model of the brain. Additionally, this structural-functional coregistration makes fMRI an ideal tool for presurgical planning of patients with mass lesions affecting functionally important brain regions (Fig. 3). The data can be used for risk management and for determining operative trajectories, which can be additionally useful for neuronavigation purposes; individual risks of permanent

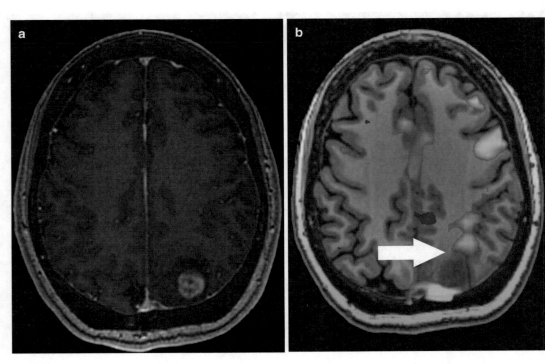

Fig. 3 (a) T1-weighted post-contrast MR image demonstrates an enhancing mass within the left parietal lobe, compatible with biopsy-proven glioblastoma. (b) Overlay of functional MR activation map acquired during a language task (visual responsive naming) on a structural T1-weighted MR image demonstrates positive activation (light blue) within the left intraparietal sulcus (white arrow), in an area related to reading comprehension. This important functional area was confirmed on neurosurgical stimulation. Areas of dark blue represent areas of negative activation, the clinical significance of which is unclear

neurological deficits can be assessed preoperatively and different surgical strategies can be considered (Krings et al. 2001). Functional MRI and its clinical applications are further described in detail in separate accompanying chapters.

2.1.5 Resting State Functional MRI (rs-fMRI)

Advances in understanding of resting state functional connectivity and improved data analysis techniques have enabled more widespread use and clinical application of resting state fMRI (rs-fMRI) for pre-surgical planning, which is often considered a complement or alternative to task-based fMRI (Dierker et al. 2017; Kokkonen et al. 2009; Rosazza et al. 2014). This technique relies on the spontaneous fluctuations of the BOLD fMRI signal or most commonly referred to as the resting state functional connectivity, with associated topographies defined as resting state networks (Dierker et al. 2017; Raichle 2015). In terms of clinical interpretation, resting state networks and tasked-based fMRI responses exhibit similar, although not identical, topographies (Dierker et al. 2017). Compared to tasked-based fMRI, rs-fMRI is less demanding and can be performed in patients who may not be able to comply with task-based paradigms, such as young children or altered patients (Lee et al. 2013). Additionally, image acquisition does not require specialized equipment or specialized technical training (Dierker et al. 2017).

Resting state MRI has been applied to pre-surgical planning not only for brain tumor patients, but in epilepsy patients as well, given that the higher spatial resolution afforded by the resting state images over EEG can provide an advantage in mapping epileptic foci or networks (Lee et al. 2013). A recent study by Liu et al. found overall agreements between functional MRI modalities and intraoperative cortical stimulation data. The regions localized based on the spontaneous activity correlations were found to be similar to the regions defined by the movement tasks and cortical stimulation (Liu et al. 2009). Furthermore, rs-fMRI may also be beneficial in selecting patients for epilepsy surgery and

in evaluating patient outcomes, with special attention to resting state networks that may be important in the development and maintenance of the brain's functional organization (Lee et al. 2013). Resting state fMRI and its clinical applications are further described in detail in separate accompanying chapters.

2.1.6 MR Spectroscopy (MRS)

Magnetic resonance spectroscopy (MRS) is a non-invasive technique that maps brain metabolism by measuring the relative concentrations of metabolites and neurotransmitters within brain tissue. This is done by acquiring signals from carbon-bound, non-exchangeable protons, and showing the highest information density within a spectral region (Trabesinger et al. 2003). This has the potential to be used in imaging protocols for pre-surgical diagnostics of epilepsy surgery, as reduced neuronal markers such as N-acetyl-aspartate (NAA) or increased glial markers such as choline (Cho) are compatible with focal epileptogenic lesions, and increased lactate suggesting the presence of epileptic activity (Pittau et al. 2014). With regard to mass lesions, source MR images co-registered with MRS can identify specific voxel-wise location(s); this is often based on multimodal single-voxel MRS data acquired with structural MRI for the identification of regions of viable tumor, investigation of the tumor extent, and monitoring of the effectiveness of therapy (Pittau et al. 2014; Vigneron et al. 2001). In this context, MRS can also be useful to evaluate the degree of tumor invasion by co-registration of the metabolic maps derived from post-processing onto the structural MRI data for use in neuronavigation systems (Gasser et al. 2005). There has been further research into the use of MRS for surgical navigation purposes. For example, a recent study investigating a multimodal approach of targeted PET- and a MRS-guided stereotactic biopsy tool using intraoperative navigation in combination with software to analyze and integrate physiological imaging data to identify biopsy targets was found to spatially correlate and validate a variety of imaging biomarkers against tissue features (Grech-Sollars et al. 2017). Additional multimodal approaches include a combination of MRS with functional landmarks, obtained from fMRI to increase the sensitivity for the assessment of tumor borders and the localization of functionally eloquent areas (Nimsky et al. 2006).

2.2 Combined MRI and Nuclear Medicine

FDG-PET imaging has important applications in pre-surgical imaging, notably to assess interictal brain dysfunction through evaluation of metabolism using radioactive tracers. For example, in cases of mesial temporal lobe epilepsy, FDG-PET can demonstrate hypometabolism involving the temporal lobe (Fig. 4), as well as possible extratemporal sites such as the insula or perisylvian regions. Such topographic information provided by areas of hypometabolism on PET has been shown to correlate with other modalities, specifically EEG, with a strong correlation with the extent of the electroclinical network defined by clinical seizure semiology (Baumgartner et al. 2019; Chassoux et al. 2016). Studies have found that the hypometabolic patterns on FDG-PET can

be predictive for surgical outcome in patients with mesial temporal lobe epilepsy (Baumgartner et al. 2019; Chassoux et al. 2017; Farooque et al. 2017). Furthermore, in cases of MRI-negative temporal lobe epilepsy, hypometabolism within the epileptogenic zone was found to predictor of a more favorable surgical outcome (Immonen et al. 2010). In cases of MRI-negative extratemporal lobe epilepsy, FDG-PET co-registered with MRI is highly sensitive to detect focal cortical dysplasia and was found to be significantly superior to visual analysis for the identification of the epileptogenic zone, thereby improving diagnosis and overall surgical outcome (Baumgartner et al. 2019; Chassoux et al. 2010; Mendes Coelho et al. 2017). Recently, machine learning techniques optimized for cortical surface sampling of combined PET and MRI and PET data was found to be superior to both quantitative MRI and multimodal visual analysis for the detection of focal cortical dysplasia (Baumgartner et al. 2019; Tan et al. 2018).

Single-photon emission computed tomography (SPECT) is another nuclear medicine imag-

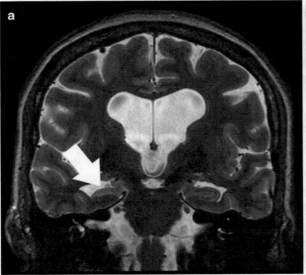
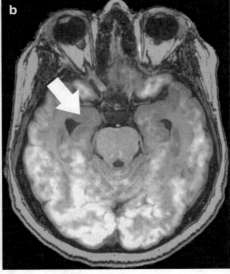

Fig. 4 (a) Coronal T2-weighted image demonstrates increased signal within the right hippocampus (white arrow), as well as volume loss when compared to the left. Findings are compatible with mesial temporal sclerosis. (b) PET-MRI with FDG from the same patient demonstrates markedly decreased FDG uptake within the right mesial temporal lobe and right hippocampus region (white arrow), corresponding to the structural findings on MRI and representing the focus of seizure activity. In addition, there is moderately decreased FDG uptake in the left mesial temporal lobe

ing technique, which employs gamma rays to generate tomographic images. Ictal SPECT can provide information on fluctuations involving CBF, which is considered a surrogate marker of increased neuronal activity based on the seizure onset zones. The use of SPECT is primarily used in cases where extratemporal MRI negative, or possibly in discordant PET and MRI studies (Sidhu et al. 2018). The specificity of this technique can be significantly improved in combination with MRI, in which statistical mapping subtraction SPECT is co-registered to MRI in a multimodal approach (Baumgartner et al. 2019; O'Brien et al. 1998). Applied statistical parametric mapping can identify changes in CBF that are statistically significantly different on a voxel-by-voxel basis (Baumgartner et al. 2019).

2.3 Combined MRI and MEG (MSI)/EEG

Magnetoencephalography detects magnetic fields produced by the brain's electrical activity based on the principle that electrical charges that move from one point to another and generate a magnetic field at a right angle to the flow of current. Magnetoencephalography signals, like EEG, are produced by excitatory and inhibitory postsynaptic potentials rather than by direct action potentials (Kharkar and Knowlton 2015). The difference between these two modalities lies in that fact that MEG detects magnetic instead of electric fields produced by neuronal currents, using sensors homogeneously placed around the head (Pittau et al. 2014; Murakami and Okada 2006). Thus, while both MEG and EEG measure cerebral activity in real time and during the same acquisition, they measure different physical properties of this activity. Another key difference is that the generated magnetic fields diffuse across the skull and scalp without any appreciable distortion or interference, whereas electrical potentials of EEG can be distorted due to the different electrical conductivities from variations of the calvarium or prior postsurgical alterations. This difference allows for recording MEG in patients with atypical calvarial anatomy or post-

surgical changes without the major limitations encountered with EEG, which necessitates accurate modeling of the skull anatomy. Given that MEG is only sensitive to the activity of neurons located tangentially to the skull, it mainly reflects the activity within the cortical sulci that is unbalanced by the contralateral surface. However, EEG is able to record the activity of neurons despite different orientations (Pittau et al. 2014; Ahlfors et al. 2010). Given that MEG and EEG are sensitive to different physical features of neural activity, the two techniques can therefore be complementary (Lopes da Silva 2013). As such, there is potential that EEG/MEG combinations with high spatial sampling of both modalities could be valuable in specific difficult clinical situations (Pittau et al. 2014).

Magnetoencephalography dipoles cluster around known epileptogenic abnormalities, allowing MEG to detect and localize epileptiform disturbances of cerebral activity with excellent temporal and spatial resolution (Fig. 5) (Pittau et al. 2014; Kharkar and Knowlton 2015). When this data is co-registered with functional and structural modalities of MRI, the MEG dipole sources can be displayed in three-dimensional space on the structural MRI images of the brain, and can localize information pertaining to interictal activity (Pittau et al. 2014; Kharkar and Knowlton 2015; Marks 2004). MEG has also been applied to pre-surgical planning of epilepsy cases, providing useful data for pre-surgical localization. When coupled with structural and functional imaging modalities, it allows for non-invasive localization of the epileptogenic region. Recent studies have found that MEG, when used in conjunction with other elements of the pre-surgical evaluation, can allow for accurate localization and further reduce the need for invasive intracranial monitoring (Marks 2004). Furthermore, this can be especially true in cases where the primary intracranial implantation does appropriately capture the seizure onset. MEG-guided intracranial implantation has been shown to correctly identify epileptogenic zones, surpassing interictal PET CT, as the area of hypometabolism is usually larger than the epileptogenic

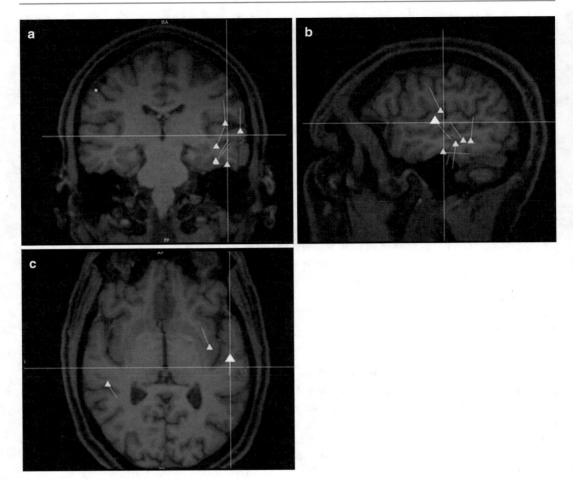

Fig. 5 Coronal (**a**), sagittal (**b**) and axial (**c**) MRI overlay of Equivalent Current Dipole (ECD) modeling of a dipole cluster demonstrates lateralization of the EEG recordings to the left temporal lobe (yellow triangles). The white triangle demonstrates an ictal event. Additionally, the language area (red) is overlaid, which reveals that the epileptogenic area involves the language area, further demonstrating the unique ability of MEG to display both functional tasks and epileptogenic information together. Not pictured because of space limitations are the MEG channels demonstrating the spike signals. Stereoelectroencephalography confirmed MEG and determined the epileptogenic zone to be primarily within the left middle temporal gyrus. (Figure provided and adapted by courtesy of Dr. Elizabeth Davenport)

zone (Kharkar and Knowlton 2015; Nelissen et al. 2006; Sutherling et al. 2008).

Although MEG's widespread use is somewhat limited by the requirement for specialized equipment and facilities (Marks 2004), current and recent advances in multimodal approaches offer future opportunities for further integration of MEG and EEG with MRI, and in particular, with fMRI. While EEG and MEG are able to demonstrate the brain activation at much greater temporal resolution, MRI produces the anatomical template which enhances the inherent poor spatial resolution of EEG and MEG source images (Liu et al. 2015). This, coupled with the hybrid ability to obtain simultaneous EEG and fMRI recordings, can detect cerebral hemodynamic changes related to interictal epileptiform discharges identified on scalp EEG (Pittau et al. 2014; Gotman et al. 2006). Such multimodal approaches offer the ability to non-invasively localize the epileptic focus and to better understand the epileptic networks in light of presurgical planning (Pittau et al. 2014).

3 Advantages and Limitations of Multimodal Functional Neuroimaging

As discussed, multimodal imaging allows use of different imaging modalities for a single evaluation, thus providing a more comprehensive evaluation of the brain. The major benefits of multimodal data fusion include the ability to correct distortion, a higher combined temporal/spatial resolution, and use of both structural and functional information. Advances in multimodal imaging have focused on the standardization of these modalities, via atlas based brain segmentation and image fusion, with data analysis shifting from qualitative to quantitative evaluation (Zhang et al. 2020).

Though the fusion of modalities combines complementary information, expands resolution limits, and overall improves data quality, these methods do come with their own limitations, as summarized in their respective sections (Zhang et al. 2020; Liu et al. 2015). On a global scale, multimodal neuroimaging is largely limited by the availability and safety of the imaging equipment, though hybrid acquisition scanners are becoming more abundant in the clinical setting. As a construct, multimodal neuroimaging analysis is much more challenging than single modality analysis, often requiring sophisticated computing analysis models including complicated data normalization, data fusion, and data integration. This also includes pre-processing, feature extraction, machine learning, and post-processing to account for the variations in the spatiotemporal resolution and integrating the functional and biophysical information of the multimodal data (Zhang et al. 2020; Calhoun and Sui 2016; Tulay et al. 2019).

As multimodal neuroimaging and computing methods continue to be applied in the clinical setting for pre-operative planning and neuronavigation, there has been growing interest and growth in multimodal neuroimaging research (Liu et al. 2015). Currently, there have been significant improvements modern neuroimaging both in terms of acquisition quality and the emerging availability of imaging modalities. It is expected that the effect of multimodal imaging fusion could also effectively scale the amount and quantity of information accessible to radiologists to make higher quality evaluations and more precise diagnoses (Zhang et al. 2020).

References

Ahlfors SP, Han J, Belliveau JW, Hämäläinen MS (2010) Sensitivity of MEG and EEG to source orientation. Brain Topogr 23(3):227–232. https://doi.org/10.1007/s10548-010-0154-x

Amaro E, Barker GJ (2006) Study design in fMRI: basic principles. Brain Cogn 60(3):220–232. https://doi.org/10.1016/j.bandc.2005.11.009

Ashburner J, Friston KJ (2000) Voxel-based morphometry—the methods. NeuroImage 11(6 Pt 1):805–821. https://doi.org/10.1006/nimg.2000.0582

Bailey PD, Zacà D, Basha MM et al (2015) Presurgical fMRI and DTI for the prediction of perioperative motor and language deficits in primary or metastatic brain lesions. J Neuroimaging 25(5):776–784. https://doi.org/10.1111/jon.12273

Baumgartner C, Koren JP, Britto-Arias M, Zoche L, Pirker S (2019) Presurgical epilepsy evaluation and epilepsy surgery. F1000Res 8. https://doi.org/10.12688/f1000research.17714.1

Boxerman JL, Shiroishi MS, Ellingson BM, Pope WB (2016) Dynamic susceptibility contrast MR imaging in glioma: review of current clinical practice. Magn Reson Imaging Clin N Am 24(4):649–670. https://doi.org/10.1016/j.mric.2016.06.005

Calhoun VD, Sui J (2016) Multimodal fusion of brain imaging data: a key to finding the missing link(s) in complex mental illness. Biol Psychiatry Cogn Neurosci Neuroimaging 1(3):230–244. https://doi.org/10.1016/j.bpsc.2015.12.005

Chassoux F, Rodrigo S, Semah F et al (2010) FDG-PET improves surgical outcome in negative MRI Taylor-type focal cortical dysplasias. Neurology 75(24):2168–2175. https://doi.org/10.1212/WNL.0b013e31820203a9

Chassoux F, Artiges E, Semah F et al (2016) Determinants of brain metabolism changes in mesial temporal lobe epilepsy. Epilepsia 57(6):907–919. https://doi.org/10.1111/epi.13377

Chassoux F, Artiges E, Semah F et al (2017) F-FDG-PET patterns of surgical success and failure in mesial temporal lobe epilepsy. Neurology 88(11):1045–1053. https://doi.org/10.1212/WNL.0000000000003714

Detre JA, Alsop DC (1999) Perfusion magnetic resonance imaging with continuous arterial spin labeling: methods and clinical applications in the central nervous system. Eur J Radiol 30(2):115–124. https://doi.org/10.1016/s0720-048x(99)00050-9

Dierker D, Roland JL, Kamran M et al (2017) Resting-state functional magnetic resonance imaging in presurgical functional mapping: sensorimotor localization. Neuroimaging Clin N Am 27(4):621–633. https://doi.org/10.1016/j.nic.2017.06.011

Farooque P, Hirsch L, Levy S, Testa F, Mattson R, Spencer D (2017) Surgical outcome in adolescents with mesial temporal sclerosis: Is it different? Epilepsy Behav 69:24–27. https://doi.org/10.1016/j.yebeh.2016.10.028

Florez E, Nichols T, Parker EE, Lirette ST, Howard CM, Fatemi A (2018) Multiparametric magnetic resonance imaging in the assessment of primary brain tumors through radiomic features: a metric for guided radiation treatment planning. Cureus 10(10):e3426. https://doi.org/10.7759/cureus.3426

Gasser T, Ganslandt O, Sandalcioglu E, Stolke D, Fahlbusch R, Nimsky C (2005) Intraoperative functional MRI: implementation and preliminary experience. NeuroImage 26(3):685–693. https://doi.org/10.1016/j.neuroimage.2005.02.022

Gotman J, Kobayashi E, Bagshaw AP, Bénar CG, Dubeau F (2006) Combining EEG and fMRI: a multimodal tool for epilepsy research. J Magn Reson Imaging 23(6):906–920. https://doi.org/10.1002/jmri.20577

Grech-Sollars M, Vaqas B, Thompson G et al (2017) An MRS- and PET-guided biopsy tool for intraoperative neuronavigational systems. J Neurosurg 127(4):812–818. https://doi.org/10.3171/2016.7.JNS16106

Guo X, Xu S, Wang G, Zhang Y, Guo L, Zhao B (2015) Asymmetry of cerebral blood flow measured with three-dimensional pseudocontinuous arterial spin-labeling MR imaging in temporal lobe epilepsy with and without mesial temporal sclerosis. J Magn Reson Imaging 42(5):1386–1397. https://doi.org/10.1002/jmri.24920

Hoxworth JM, Eschbacher JM, Gonzales AC et al (2020) Performance of standardized relative CBV for quantifying regional histologic tumor burden in recurrent high-grade glioma: comparison against normalized relative CBV using image-localized stereotactic biopsies. AJNR Am J Neuroradiol 41(3):408–415. https://doi.org/10.3174/ajnr.A6486

Immonen A, Jutila L, Muraja-Murro A et al (2010) Long-term epilepsy surgery outcomes in patients with MRI-negative temporal lobe epilepsy. Epilepsia 51(11):2260–2269. https://doi.org/10.1111/j.1528-1167.2010.02720.x

Jacobs AH, Kracht LW, Gossmann A et al (2005) Imaging in neurooncology. NeuroRx 2(2):333–347. https://doi.org/10.1602/neurorx.2.2.333

Jahng GH, Li KL, Ostergaard L, Calamante F (2014) Perfusion magnetic resonance imaging: a comprehensive update on principles and techniques. Korean J Radiol 15(5):554–577. https://doi.org/10.3348/kjr.2014.15.5.554

Kharkar S, Knowlton R (2015) Magnetoencephalography in the presurgical evaluation of epilepsy. Epilepsy Behav 46:19–26. https://doi.org/10.1016/j.yebeh.2014.11.029

Kokkonen SM, Nikkinen J, Remes J et al (2009) Preoperative localization of the sensorimotor area using independent component analysis of resting-state fMRI. Magn Reson Imaging 27(6):733–740. https://doi.org/10.1016/j.mri.2008.11.002

Krings T, Reinges MH, Erberich S et al (2001) Functional MRI for presurgical planning: problems, artefacts, and solution strategies. J Neurol Neurosurg Psychiatry 70(6):749–760. https://doi.org/10.1136/jnnp.70.6.749

Lee MH, Smyser CD, Shimony JS (2013) Resting-state fMRI: a review of methods and clinical applications. AJNR Am J Neuroradiol 34(10):1866–1872. https://doi.org/10.3174/ajnr.A3263

Li E, d'Esterre CD, Gaxiola-Valdez I et al (2019) CT perfusion measurement of postictal hypoperfusion: localization of the seizure onset zone and patterns of spread. Neuroradiology 61(9):991–1010. https://doi.org/10.1007/s00234-019-02227-8

Liu H, Buckner RL, Talukdar T, Tanaka N, Madsen JR, Stufflebeam SM (2009) Task-free presurgical mapping using functional magnetic resonance imaging intrinsic activity. J Neurosurg 111(4):746–754. https://doi.org/10.3171/2008.10.JNS08846

Liu S, Cai W, Zhang F et al (2015) Multimodal neuroimaging computing: a review of the applications in neuropsychiatric disorders. Brain Inform 2(3):167–180. https://doi.org/10.1007/s40708-015-0019-x

Lopes da Silva F (2013) EEG and MEG: relevance to neuroscience. Neuron 80(5):1112–1128. https://doi.org/10.1016/j.neuron.2013.10.017

Maia AC, Malheiros SM, da Rocha AJ et al (2004) Stereotactic biopsy guidance in adults with supratentorial nonenhancing gliomas: role of perfusion-weighted magnetic resonance imaging. J Neurosurg 101(6):970–976. https://doi.org/10.3171/jns.2004.101.6.0970

Marks WJ (2004) Utility of MEG in presurgical localization. Epilepsy Curr 4(5):208–209. https://doi.org/10.1111/j.1535-7597.2004.04516.x

Mendes Coelho VC, Morita ME, Amorim BJ et al (2017) Automated online quantification method for. Front Neurol 8:453. https://doi.org/10.3389/fneur.2017.00453

Murakami S, Okada Y (2006) Contributions of principal neocortical neurons to magnetoencephalography and electroencephalography signals. J Physiol 575(Pt 3):925–936. https://doi.org/10.1113/jphysiol.2006.105379

Nelissen N, Van Paesschen W, Baete K et al (2006) Correlations of interictal FDG-PET metabolism and ictal SPECT perfusion changes in human temporal lobe epilepsy with hippocampal sclerosis. NeuroImage 32(2):684–695. https://doi.org/10.1016/j.neuroimage.2006.04.185

Nimsky C, Ganslandt O, Buchfelder M, Fahlbusch R (2006) Intraoperative visualization for resection of gliomas: the role of functional neuronavigation and intraoperative 1.5 T MRI. Neurol Res 28(5):482–487. https://doi.org/10.1179/016164106X115125

O'Brien TJ, So EL, Mullan BP et al (1998) Subtraction ictal SPECT co-registered to MRI improves clinical usefulness of SPECT in localizing the surgical seizure focus. Neurology 50(2):445–454. https://doi.org/10.1212/wnl.50.2.445

Petrella JR, Provenzale JM (2000) MR perfusion imaging of the brain: techniques and applications. AJR Am J Roentgenol 175(1):207–219. https://doi.org/10.2214/ajr.175.1.1750207

Pittau F, Grouiller F, Spinelli L, Seeck M, Michel CM, Vulliemoz S (2014) The role of functional neuroimaging in pre-surgical epilepsy evaluation. Front Neurol 5:31. https://doi.org/10.3389/fneur.2014.00031

Prah MA, Al-Gizawiy MM, Mueller WM et al (2018) Spatial discrimination of glioblastoma and treatment effect with histologically-validated perfusion and diffusion magnetic resonance imaging metrics. J Neurooncol 136(1):13–21. https://doi.org/10.1007/s11060-017-2617-3

Raichle ME (2015) The restless brain: how intrinsic activity organizes brain function. Philos Trans R Soc Lond B Biol Sci 370(1668). https://doi.org/10.1098/rstb.2014.0172

Rosazza C, Aquino D, D'Incerti L et al (2014) Preoperative mapping of the sensorimotor cortex: comparative assessment of task-based and resting-state FMRI. PLoS One 9(6):e98860. https://doi.org/10.1371/journal.pone.0098860

Sidhu MK, Duncan JS, Sander JW (2018) Neuroimaging in epilepsy. Curr Opin Neurol 31(4):371–378. https://doi.org/10.1097/WCO.0000000000000568

Sutherling WW, Mamelak AN, Thyerlei D et al (2008) Influence of magnetic source imaging for planning intracranial EEG in epilepsy. Neurology 71(13):990–996. https://doi.org/10.1212/01.wnl.0000326591.29858.1a

Tan YL, Kim H, Lee S et al (2018) Quantitative surface analysis of combined MRI and PET enhances detection of focal cortical dysplasias. NeuroImage 166:10–18. https://doi.org/10.1016/j.neuroimage.2017.10.065

Tanaka N, Hämäläinen MS, Ahlfors SP et al (2010) Propagation of epileptic spikes reconstructed from spatiotemporal magnetoencephalographic and electroencephalographic source analysis. NeuroImage 50(1):217–222. https://doi.org/10.1016/j.neuroimage.2009.12.033

Tempany CM, Jayender J, Kapur T et al (2015) Multimodal imaging for improved diagnosis and treatment of cancers. Cancer 121(6):817–827. https://doi.org/10.1002/cncr.29012

Trabesinger AH, Meier D, Boesiger P (2003) In vivo 1H NMR spectroscopy of individual human brain metabolites at moderate field strengths. Magn Reson Imaging 21(10):1295–1302. https://doi.org/10.1016/j.mri.2003.08.029

Tulay EE, Metin B, Tarhan N, Arıkan MK (2019) Multimodal neuroimaging: basic concepts and classification of neuropsychiatric diseases. Clin EEG Neurosci 50(1):20–33. https://doi.org/10.1177/1550059418782093

Vigneron D, Bollen A, McDermott M et al (2001) Three-dimensional magnetic resonance spectroscopic imaging of histologically confirmed brain tumors. Magn Reson Imaging 19(1):89–101. https://doi.org/10.1016/s0730-725x(01)00225-9

Weinand ME, Carter LP, el-Saadany WF, Sioutos PJ, Labiner DM, Oommen KJ (1997) Cerebral blood flow and temporal lobe epileptogenicity. J Neurosurg 86(2):226–232. https://doi.org/10.3171/jns.1997.86.2.0226

Whiting P, Gupta R, Burch J et al (2006) A systematic review of the effectiveness and cost-effectiveness of neuroimaging assessments used to visualise the seizure focus in people with refractory epilepsy being considered for surgery. Health Technol Assess 10(4):1–250, iii–iv. https://doi.org/10.3310/hta10040

Whitwell JL (2009) Voxel-based morphometry: an automated technique for assessing structural changes in the brain. J Neurosci 29(31):9661–9664. https://doi.org/10.1523/JNEUROSCI.2160-09.2009

Wu O, Dijkhuizen RM, Sorensen AG (2010) Multiparametric magnetic resonance imaging of brain disorders. Top Magn Reson Imaging 21(2):129–138. https://doi.org/10.1097/RMR.0b013e31821e56c2

Wu D, Faria AV, Younes L et al (2017) Mapping the order and pattern of brain structural MRI changes using change-point analysis in premanifest Huntington's disease. Hum Brain Mapp 38(10):5035–5050. https://doi.org/10.1002/hbm.23713

Zhang J, Liu W, Chen H et al (2014) Multimodal neuroimaging in presurgical evaluation of drug-resistant epilepsy. Neuroimage Clin 4:35–44. https://doi.org/10.1016/j.nicl.2013.10.017

Zhang Y-D, Dong Z, Wang S-H et al (2020) Advances in multimodal data fusion in neuroimaging: overview, challenges, and novel orientation. Inf Fusion 64:149–187. https://doi.org/10.1016/j.inffus.2020.07.006

Brain Plasticity in fMRI and DTI

N. Karahasanović, T. Gruber, G. Dörl, S. Radjenovic,
T. Kolarova, E. Matt, and R. Beisteiner

Contents

N. Karahasanović · T. Gruber · G. Dörl
S. Radjenovic · T. Kolarova · E. Matt
R. Beisteiner (✉)
Functional Diagnostics and Therapy, Department of
Neurology, High Field MR Center, Medical
University of Vienna, Vienna, Austria
e-mail: nejla.karahasanovic@meduniwien.ac.at;
tabea.gruber@meduniwien.ac.at;
gregor.doerl@meduniwien.ac.at;
sonja.radjenovic@meduniwien.ac.at;
teodora.kolarova@meduniwien.ac.at;
eva.matt@meduniwien.ac.at;
roland.beisteiner@meduniwien.ac.at

Abstract

This chapter gives an overview of the type of neuroplastic information that can be generated by functional magnetic resonance imaging (fMRI) and diffusion tensor imaging (DTI) after damage of the central or peripheral nervous system. After an introductory overview about clinical neuroplasticity, benefits of neuroplastic investigations are demonstrated. Thereby, a better evaluation of the patient's

© The Author(s), under exclusive license to Springer Nature Switzerland AG 2022
C. Stippich (ed.), *Clinical Functional MRI*, Medical Radiology Diagnostic Imaging,
https://doi.org/10.1007/978-3-030-83343-5_11

functional state, better individual prognosis, a progression in understanding the nervous system, as well as ameliorated treatment strategies are outlined. Afterwards, some important cellular and molecular mechanisms relevant for neuroplastic changes are discussed, since fMRI and DTI are limited to identifying neuroplasticity on a level of neuronal populations and their connections. Finally, a review about neuroplastic changes, in response to nervous system disease, is given. The review is completed by demonstrating a new, promising therapeutic approach supporting brain plasticity, for which fMRI and DTI data are important.

1   Introduction

Clinical neuroplasticity is the ability of neurons and neural networks to reorganize themselves on a functional and structural level in response to damage. It differs from non-clinical reorganization taking place due to normal brain development of healthy individuals, occurring continuously throughout life. Detecting clinical brain plasticity is not always easy, since it may be mistaken for damage-induced changes. For example, structural changes such as altered white matter connectivity and network integrity may be a result of brain damage, instead of structural reorganization (Marebwa et al. 2017). Further, clinical neuroplasticity has to be differentiated from functional effects which arise during resolution of oedema, perfusion deficits, inflammation and diaschisis. During their resolution clinical symptoms disappear, but improvements are not due to neuroplasticity. Physiological compensation of an impaired function may also happen outside neuroplastic processes. As an example, proximal muscles could compensate a distal paresis, just by changing the movement pattern. All these interrelationships should be kept in mind, when interpreting structural and functional

alterations by fMRI and DTI data, in the clinical context.

What kind of neuroplastic information can be generated by fMRI and DTI? Briefly summarized, fMRI enables the detection of local increases and decreases of brain activity. On the one hand, spontaneously occurring brain activity may be detected by resting state fMRI (rs-fMRI). On the other hand, brain reactions evoked by tasks (task-based fMRI) or by medication (pharmacological fMRI) can be detected as well. Since typical BOLD fMRI (blood oxygen level dependent fMRI) reflects changes in the local concentration of deoxyhemoglobin, the signals depend on the local perfusion situation. Correct conclusions about neuronal activity are only possible when there is no disturbing vascular situation (like in early stages after ischemic stroke, where maximum vessel dilation occurs). Further, BOLD signals reflect both excitatory and inhibitory neuronal activation. Regarding spatial reorganization, an increase in BOLD signal may occur within a typical task area or in a non-typical but functionally related area due to activation of additional resources. This may be seen as increased activity in spared brain areas close to the pathology or as increased activity in secondary brain areas remote from the pathology. For example, in the motor network the premotor cortex is extensively connected to the primary motor cortex (M1) and can partly substitute M1 via projections to the spinal cord. Evaluation of signal increases/decreases is also far from trivial. Increase of local neuronal activity (overactivation) may be locally driven or be a consequence of disinhibition mediated by remote connected areas. Decrease of local neuronal activity (underactivation) may be mediated by remote areas (inhibition) or be a consequence of damage to local or distant (diaschisis) tissue. State of the art fMRI techniques allow investigation, how brain areas are functionally connected to each other, i.e., which brain areas form networks and how these networks do neuroplastically change.

While fMRI describes functional alterations, DTI data describe structural changes. More specifically, DTI describes fibre tracts, with regard to tract integrity, tract volume and structural connectivity. This is done by monitoring diffusion of proton signals from water molecules, which diffuse faster in parallel to white matter tracts than perpendicular to them. To some extent, it is also possible to characterize tissue architecture (e.g. cellular density, vasculature, necrosis, extent or margins of a neoplasm). The following section gives an overview about the clinical benefits we may expect from fMRI/DTI patient investigations.

2 What Are the Clinical Benefits of Neuroplasticity Investigations?

Acquiring information about neuroplastic developments in patients using fMRI or DTI helps to improve patient care. Studying neuroplastic effects and mechanisms by using fMRI and DTI neuroimaging techniques aids evaluating the patient's functional state, establishing an individual prognosis and improving treatment strategies. Further, fMRI/DTI helps to understand how the nervous system acts in response to disease (for recent reviews see Cirillo et al. 2019; Guggisberg et al. 2019; De Giglio et al. 2018; Fox and King 2018; Pini et al. 2018; Tahedl et al. 2018; Chou et al. 2018; Duffau 2017; Hartwigsen and Saur 2019; Puig et al. 2017; Bergmann et al. 2016; Kong et al. 2016; Reid et al. 2016; Chiaravalloti et al. 2015; Enzinger et al. 2016; Hamaide et al. 2016). As fMRI and DTI are noninvasive, these techniques are powerful tools for investigating both structural and functional changes due to lesions, neurodegeneration, or other neurological dysfunctions in cross-sectional, but also longitudinal studies. Although the latter is still relatively scarce, increasing evidence supports the usefulness of fMRI and DTI for assessing neuroplasticity in clinical practice. It is important to stress the benefit of combining fMRI and DTI investigations since they complement one another. While fMRI can acquire infor-

mation about the *functional* changes associated with neuroplasticity (Tao and Rapp 2019), DTI may show their *structural* correlates on a microstructural level (Zheng and Schlaug 2015). This is particularly important for detecting regions that are involved in retaining function in brains with major pathologies (e.g., tumours). Knowing the functional and structural reorganization in such patients will support successful surgery (Panigrahi et al. 2017).

2.1 Better Evaluation of the Patients' Functional State

Assessing patients' functional brain state has been proven essential for many treatment considerations, most prominently in lesion cases with subsequent neuronal reorganization of motor functions (e.g., after a stroke). Importantly, damage from lesions need not be constrained to the lesion area but it could affect remote areas that are functionally connected to the latter (Carrera and Tononi 2014). FMRI and DTI provide information about momentary functional as well as structural reorganization of both ipsi- and contralesional hemispheres (Guggisberg et al. 2019).

2.2 Better Individual Prognosis

Using fMRI and DTI to investigate neuroplasticity can aid in giving a better individual prognosis to patients. Patients with temporal lobe epilepsy will often show atypical language network formations, i.e. rerouting of language pathways within the dominant left hemisphere to non-traditional language areas or a shift to the right hemisphere (Chang et al. 2017). So far, electrical cortical stimulation is used as the gold standard for mapping language centres in the cortex and for surgical planning. However, fMRI and DTI measurements are increasingly used to define functional arrangement and individual post-operative outcome (Trimmel et al. 2019;

Osipowicz et al. 2016; Hutchings et al. 2015; see Chou et al. 2018 for a review on paediatric epilepsy patients). Concerning motor recovery after stroke, a mounting body of evidence suggests that DTI investigations of the corticospinal tract can be an invaluable predictor (reviewed by Puig et al. 2017). For MS patients, a recent study showed continuous functional reorganization using effective connectivity analysis, a measure of information flow between brain network nodes. This change in effective connectivity could be inversely correlated to clinical markers and may present a possible biomarker of a patient's functional reserve capacity (Fleischer et al. 2020).

2.3 Improvement of Treatment Strategies

Improvement of treatment strategies concerns any type of intervention, be it behavioural, pharmacological, surgical, or brain stimulation therapies. For example, the definition of typical reorganizational profiles with fMRI/DTI may guide development of brain stimulation protocols that focus on brain regions most relevant for functional recovery (Bergmann et al. 2016). Such protocols can then be applied across the proper group of patients. Another popular application lies in tumour surgery and its goal of removing the ideal amount of tumour tissue without losing function or hindering rehabilitation (Flouty et al. 2017). Functional reorganization can occur both before and after a first resection, either close to the lesioned area but also by recruiting more distant regions. Investigating this on an individual level with task-based fMRI (Cirillo et al. 2019) may allow another surgical attempt to remove more cancerous tissue. Especially for gliomas close to eloquent locations (e.g. speech areas), fMRI may be critical for preserving function (Panigrahi et al. 2017; Michaud and Duffau 2016). There have been promising results using non-invasive brain stimulation techniques as a complementary treatment strategy in neurodegenerative diseases, such as dementia (Beisteiner

et al. 2019; Pini et al. 2018), and also for stroke patients in early stages (Du et al. 2019). FMRI and DTI may provide valuable information in terms of stimulation location, stimulation intensities, temporal precision for treatment onset and for following treatment effects (Bergmann et al. 2016; Goldsworthy et al. 2015).

2.4 Progress in Understanding How the Nervous System Acts in Response to Disease

Further increasing our understanding of neuronal response mechanisms to disease is essential to improve treatments and patient care. Neuroplasticity represents an important factor in the neuronal response to pathologies. For this endeavour, longitudinal studies offer a clearer picture of neuronal dynamics and compensatory mechanisms that may be targeted for treatment strategies (Hannanu et al. 2020). Furthermore, this kind of study can also help to identify critical windows for neuroplastic reorganization during disease progression (Fleischer et al. 2020). Adaptive neuroplasticity is a finite process and there are temporal limitations regarding opportunities to utilize it for treatments (De Giglio et al. 2018; Santhanam et al. 2018). Apart from investigation of the functional reserve of classical functional areas, fMRI and DTI may also reveal regions that are newly recruited during reorganization. Reorganization profiles may vary depending on individual differences in disease progression or classification (Zhang et al. 2018). Studies have also shown possible maladaptive plasticity in several cases (Raffin et al. 2016; Spielmann et al. 2016). For instance, in patients with MS, neuronal reorganization may be correlated with increased dysfunction in cognitive performance (Chiaravalloti et al. 2015; Tona et al. 2014). Cases such as these still need to be further studied to increase understanding of their precise mechanisms, as well as how to accurately discern them from beneficial plasticity. Furthermore, fMRI and DTI can detect neuronal reorganization even with no noticeable clinical effects

(Dalhuisen et al. 2020). Although clinical improvement is the primary goal in studying neuronal plasticity, understanding the underlying mechanisms is essential to develop clinical methods for modulating functional reorganization in a therapeutic sense.

3   Mechanisms of Neuroplasticity

This chapter gives a short overview about principal mechanisms which drive neuroplasticity and indicates recent literature for further reading. Neuroplasticity, as observed with fMRI/DTI, can be caused by changes at the molecular, cellular or neural population level. Besides direct damage to a brain area, neural populations may also change indirectly as a consequence of molecular and cellular changes following brain lesions.

3.1   Molecular Changes

At the molecular level, changes were described for the expression of growth-associated genes with increased growth-enhancing factors, reduced growth inhibiting factors and the expression of maturation regulating proteins. Liu et al. (2019) identified over 400 genes that seem to be involved in short- and long-term plasticity processes, and their data provides molecular evidence of the prediction of long-term learning results. Phillips (2017) outlines in her review that the brain-derived neurotrophic factor (BDNF) is an important protein for growth and maintenance of neurons involved in emotional and cognitive function. It is decreased in major depressive disorder, but can be optimized by moderate physical activity and therefore increase plasticity. Also, pharmacological substances can induce change. Roy et al. (2020) compared pre/post ketamine data in adolescents with treatment-resistant depression for molecular signaling and showed that ketamine led to changes in neural flexibility and symptom relief in those affected. Moreover, the glutamate and the gamma-aminobutyric acid

(GABA) levels contribute to neuroplasticity. For example, some studies found receptor changes such as modified expression and responsiveness of cholinergic and GABA receptors, the latter leading to a loss of inhibitory interneurons. Inhibitory synapses, just like their excitatory counterparts, are found to be malleable in their long-term neuroplasticity. Concerning long-term changes in inhibitory receptors, G-protein-coupled receptors play a central role for synaptic transmission. In contrast, the potentiation and depression of inhibitory synapses are related to endocannabinoid systems, glutamate systems, $GABA_B$ and opioid receptors (Rozov et al. 2017). For an overview concerning research on biochemical processes, consult Gulyaeva (2017) who describes specific proteins and their modulations as the molecular basis for neuroplasticity. Molecular changes can also be induced by therapeutic brain stimulation. As an example, Antonenko et al. (2019) showed that tDCS-induced electric fields can increase sensorimotor network strength which is associated with decreased GABA levels.

3.2   Cellular Changes

At the cellular level, the function or number of synapses is a major neuroplastic mechanism that underlies changes. This includes both the reinforcement of existing but functionally silent synapses (particularly at the periphery of lesions) and the formation of new synapses. Further neuroplastic changes concern dendritic arborization and axonal sprouting, which may even happen at great distances, and may be influenced by altered inhibitory and excitatory inputs on local neurons.

Cellular neuroplasticity can also be modulated by glial cells, which affect excitability, synaptic transmission and coordination of activity across networks. Indeed, astrocytes seem to be particularly relevant to the overall orchestration of synaptic plasticity (De Pittà et al. 2016). This might occur in part due to metaplasticity, describing the dynamic regulation of the synaptic transmission range. Regulating transmission range avoids excitotoxicity and allows integration of plasticity-relevant signals over time. Pathologic integration of plasticity-relevant signals, and other forms of synaptic pathology, might contribute to brain diseases, such as Alzheimer's disease (Singh and Abraham 2017).

Activity-dependent cellular plasticity can also be found in some myelin-forming cells, which not only affects myelin structure but also neurological function as modulated by experience (Monje 2018). Further, microglia likely plays a key role in synapse regulation by detecting synapse function and influencing synapse pruning/formation throughout human life (Ikegami et al. 2019).

Cellular changes also occur with respect to neuroblast activity. Kaneko et al. (2017) reported that after a brain insult, neuroblasts of the adult brain relocate in the region of the injured tissue in order to repopulate it and thus contribute to neuroplasticity.

Overall, it is important to keep in mind that cellular changes may occur perilesionally as well as distant from a lesion, in functionally/structurally connected brain areas.

3.3   Neuronal Population Changes

The action and interaction of neuronal populations (brain areas) are affected by the neuroplastic mechanisms previously described. The molecular and cellular alterations change inhibitory and excitatory influences on the neuronal populations and lead to altered connections on a local level (changed activity of a network node) or a global one (changed network configuration). Neuronal population changes include local over-activations or deactivations, increase or decrease of functional connectivity and increase or decrease of effective connectivity (i.e. modulatory influences between brain areas). It is also clear that functional connectivity is linked with structural connectivity—e.g. Sbardella et al. (2015) reported that internetwork functional connectivity changes correlate with microstructural

brain damage in multiple sclerosis. Neuronal populations are also influenced by the perineural nets (PNNs), an extracellular matrix architecture, wrapping specific neurons as the brain develops. Perineural nets orchestrate plasticity in the adult central nervous system through chondroitin sulphate proteoglycans, their chief component. They might also contribute to a multitude of brain diseases and modify with ageing, learning, memory and drug abuse (Sorg et al. 2016). While perineural nets are obviously structured that influence neuronal function, in typical cases of brain disease altered brain function induces a neuroplastic change in structure. As an example for structural network changes detectable with DTI, a study with tumour patients showed increased small-worldness features, altered regional parameters especially in hub regions, and increased connection density—particularly between the hemispheres and in regions of the limbic/subcortical systems (Yu et al. 2016).

4   Review of the Clinical Literature on fMRI and DTI

Previous literature about clinical neuroplasticity detectable by fMRI and DTI described both maladaptation and beneficial changes driving recovery. Important topics concern prediction of patient outcome after surgery and presurgical planning. DTI and fMRI may either detect neuroplastic changes related to local brain activation or more global functional/structural network changes. Because neuroplasticity is affected by many factors a standard classification of neuroplastic changes or neuroplasticity-based standard prediction of patient outcome is difficult. Important factors influencing neuroplasticity are type and stage of the disease, location and size of a lesion as well as type and intensity of clinical interventions. Further, patient characteristics like age, type of diseased brain function and the method used for detecting neuroplasticity are important. The influence of these factors on fMRI/DTI results is still poorly understood.

Clinical literature mostly focuses on neuroplasticity caused by pathomorphological changes of a previously healthy nervous system. Therefore, such diseases will also be the focus in this review chapter. Nevertheless, literature about genetic or psychiatric disease as well as inborn morphological effects also exists. Clinical fMRI/DTI research includes dementia (Jacobs et al. 2015), Parkinson's disease (Lu et al. 2016; van Nuenen et al. 2012), Huntington's disease (Harrington et al. 2015; Scheller et al. 2013), Schizophrenia (Palaniyappan et al. 2012), focal dystonia (Mantel et al. 2020; Altenmüller and Müller 2013), amyotrophic lateral sclerosis (Mohammadi et al. 2015), spinal cord injury (Oni-Orisan et al. 2016; Cadotte et al. 2012), traumatic brain injury (Watson et al. 2019; Caeyenberghs et al. 2012a, b), agenesis of the corpus callosum (Genç et al. 2015; Wolf et al. 2011), congenital blindness (Bonino et al. 2015; Collignon et al. 2011), effects of therapeutic immobilization (Langer et al. 2012), systemic lupus erythematosus (Wu et al. 2018; Hou et al. 2013), fibromyalgia (Bosma et al. 2016; Craggs et al. 2012), small vessel disease (van der Holst et al. 2017; List et al. 2013), hepatic encephalopathy (Qi et al. 2015), tinnitus and hearing loss (Schmidt et al. 2017), or Mal de Debarquement syndrome (Jeon et al. 2020; Cha et al. 2012).

We will give an overview of recently described neuroplastic responses to important neurological diseases, for which a large body of published data already exists. This intends to provide current examples for clinical fMRI/DTI investigations and cannot be comprehensive. However, the examples demonstrate the complexity of the field and the limitations of clinical neuroplasticity investigations. An important aspect of this overview is that it includes not only important diseases but also diseases with differing pathophysiological characteristics. This allows a better understanding which neuroplastic fMRI/DTI responses can be detected under which circumstances. First off, we will describe neuroplasticity in patients that suffered from stroke—most research about clinical neuroplasticity has been published for this disease.

The characteristic of stroke is neuronal damage typically generated from one single destructive event, with a subsequent regeneration period and no additional pathologies. We will then review studies on epilepsy, tumour, multiple sclerosis and peripheral nervous system disorders. The characteristic of epilepsy is permanent pathological neuronal activity that may function as a continuous neuroplastic driving factor. The characteristic of brain tumours is a steady increase of brain destruction at a specific site with differing speed. The characteristic of multiple sclerosis is the continuous accumulation of brain lesions over many years in a multitopic fashion. Lastly, peripheral nervous system disorders do not induce brain plasticity by damage to the brain. Here, peripheral nerves are damaged, resulting in a changed information flow between somatic periphery and the brain.

4.1 Stroke

4.1.1 Local Brain Activation Changes

Poststroke, the damaged brain undergoes recovery through considerable reorganization of spared areas and pathways, either spontaneously or with the help of appropriate rehabilitation. The degree of impairment depends on factors such as the extent of damage, the character of it, and the efficacy of the initial medical care (Alia et al. 2017). Various factors may affect neuroplasticity, including one of the most prominent factors: the level of destruction of a primary brain area. Typically, neuroplastic reorganization is not able to fully recover the damaged function after a *primary* brain area has been lesioned. Pinter et al. (2020) showed in their study that patients following stroke had significant reduction in white matter integrity in the affected hemisphere 1–3 days poststroke, which additionally decreased across 3 months compared with controls. These advanced MRI data on white matter integrity improve understanding of poststroke reorganization in a damaged hemisphere. Following a stroke, sensorimotor dysfunction can considerably lower the quality of life. Upper limb dysfunction is experienced by the majority of patients post-stroke. The greatest potential for functional improvement is in the first month. Intensive training is best in the first month due to its association with greater changes in activation in motor (supplementary motor area and cerebellum) and attention (anterior cingulate) regions (Hubbard et al. 2015). In subjects with motor deficits of the upper limb, fMRI/DTI may document contributions of the contralesional hemisphere for recovery (Cunningham et al. 2015). Pundik et al. (2018) identified alterations in local cortical thickness related to the recovery of sensory perception: arm function rehabilitation after stroke was associated with increased bilateral cortical thickness in high-order sensory cortices.

Local brain activation changes poststroke usually improve the damaged function, but in some cases can result in a functional disturbance—called maladaptation. The activation of the right hemisphere during speech in left hemispheric stroke patients may be a sign of inaccurate recovery attempts. If such maladaptive local brain activation focuses on the "wrong" hemisphere, a therapeutic approach could be to suppress this paradoxical activation in order to improve speech deficits (Heiss 2020). However, differentiation of adaptive and maladaptive fMRI activity is not trivial. Spielmann et al. (2016) wanted to compare maladaptive with healthy brain activation. In patients with chronic nonfluent aphasia, fMRI activation during verb paraphasias was compared with those during successful verb naming. The authors found a large overlap of activated brain areas. This indicates that for understanding the full neuroplastic picture, investigation of local brain activation changes should always be supplemented by fMRI/DTI network investigations which sometimes may better capture the complexity of maladaptive and adaptive neuroplasticity.

4.1.2 Network Changes

Although stroke typically results from one single destructive event with no additional primary pathologies, research with fMRI/DTI has shown that this disease impacts the whole brain. Major secondary changes in the white matter tracts and distant neural activities indicate stroke as a network disease (Guggisberg et al. 2019).

Concerning motor rehabilitation, several studies demonstrated a close correlation between poststroke motor recovery and network neuroplasticity. For example, Almeida et al. (2017) studied intra- and interhemispheric fMRI resting state functional connectivity associated with motor function. This was done in poststroke patients with variable degrees of recovery. Independent of the degree of recovery, all patients showed increased functional connectivity between the primary motor region (M1) and the contralateral hemisphere. However, only patients with low recovery showed a decreased internetwork connectivity (between executive control, sensorimotor and visuospatial networks). These findings were recently extended by Min et al. (2020). In their study poor recovery patients had lower interhemispheric functional connectivity than healthy controls, but no connectivity differences were found between good recovery patients and controls. Authors conclude that fMRI resting state connectivity may provide useful clinical information for predicting hand motor recovery during stroke rehabilitation. However, not only resting state data but also task-based fMRI may help to further elucidate the poststroke motor recovery process. Hannanu et al. (2020) used fMRI data from a passive sensorimotor task to predict motor recovery. They found that the type of fMRI network activity predicts recovery for different types of movements. Recovery of movements required for a precision visuomotor task correlated with brain activity in two segregated dorsomedial and dorsolateral networks responsible for reach and grasp movements. In contrast, recovery in a rough force task correlated only with activity of the dorsolateral network. A most problematic consequence of stroke concerns speech impairments. fMRI network investigations may be helpful for therapeutic speech monitoring. An fMRI study by Santhanam et al. (2018) related effective connectivity measures with therapeutic success: behavioural improvement following aphasia therapy was associated with connectivity more closely resembling that of healthy controls. Concerning methodological progress, over the last decade various sophisticated methods for fMRI network analysis have been developed. A quite powerful approach—graph theory—is increasingly used (Ulm et al. 2016). A study by Tao and Rapp (2019) examined written language deficits after a left-hemisphere stroke using task-based fMRI data and graph theory. They found that the difference between global and local network integration is related to deficit severity and treatment response. The greater the written language deficit and the lower the treatment response, the more global and less local network integration was found. On the other hand, successful behavioural treatment improved local network integration.

4.2 Epilepsy

Contrary to stroke, a typical feature of epilepsy is permanent pathological neuronal activity which may function as a continuous neuroplastic driving factor. Nevertheless, compensatory activation changes and functional connectivity changes, as described in stroke, can also be found in epilepsy. For example, Chang et al. (2017) performed a study on left temporal lobe epilepsy (LTLE) and found that patients with better language performance showed an interhemispheric language reorganization with right-lateralized brain activations (dominance of the right hemisphere). A right-lateralization was also found for structural DTI data. The authors concluded that these left to right reorganizations may help to mitigate language impairment in LTLE. To study white matter integrity of the hippocampus in temporal lobe epilepsy (TLE), DTI has also been used by Chiang et al. (2016). They found that mean diffusivity values of the right hippocampus as well as fractional anisotropy values of the left external capsule were important predictors for the diseased hemisphere (left or right TLE). In addition, DTI may also provide information about disease duration: in left TLE patients' mean diffusivity values of the left hippocampus were associated

with longer disease duration. For drug-resistant TLE patients, resective surgery is a common therapeutic option. However, in around 30% of cases patients still suffer from seizures after resective surgery (Hutchings et al. 2015). Other patients may suffer from cognitive damage post-surgery, for example, memory deficits (Dupont 2015). To improve this situation and the selection of surgery targets in temporal lobe epilepsy patients, Hutchings et al. (2015) designed a computational model using structural connectivity maps of patients and healthy controls derived by DTI. The model successfully recognized TLE associated regions and patient specific TLE associated nodes. Furthermore, the model was found to successfully predict patient specific recommendations for resective surgery which may lead to better outcomes. To predict cognitive outcome, specifically verbal fluency, and functional reorganization following anterior temporal lobectomy (ATL) Osipowicz et al. (2016) combined fMRI, DTI and resting state fMRI in a patient study. They found that ATL does result in language network reorganization (indicated by fMRI activation maps) which co-occurs with functional connectivity changes (seen on resting state fMRI) and white matter changes (shown by DTI). In general, authors conclude that using a combination of fMRI, resting state fMRI and DTI is a promising method and successfully predicts cognitive outcome post-resective surgery. In some cases of epilepsy, disconnective surgery is used to avoid spreading of pathological brain activity. Rosazza et al. (2018) studied motor function after disconnective surgery using fMRI and DTI. They found that patients with more presurgical recruitment of their intact hemisphere had a better outcome after surgery. The most radical surgery approach in epilepsy is the removal of large parts of a whole hemisphere—hemispherectomy (Rath et al. 2008). In a DTI study Meoded et al. (2016) investigated brain plasticity in children after hemispherectomy. They studied changes in the white matter tracts of the contralateral hemisphere and the correlation between white matter DTI values and age at the time of the operation as well as time since the operation. They found DTI to be a useful tool for brain plasticity investigation, concluding that patients suffering from acquired disease, rather than congenital, had better cerebral reorganization, especially when surgery was performed at a young age.

4.3 Tumour

Brain tumours typically show a steady increase of brain destruction at a specific site with differing speed. Besides generation of focal deficits, they also interfere with whole brain networks (Yu et al. 2016), causing compensatory activation changes and changed functional/structural connectivity. Patients suffering from slow growing lesions, like low-grade gliomas, are likely to recover from early functional deficits by neuroplastic reorganization over time (Duffau 2007). Yu et al. (2016) investigated altered anatomical networks in tumour patients using DTI and found increased small-worldness acting as a compensatory mechanism. Additionally, structural reorganization was documented by increased connection densities. A major problem with brain tumours are mass effects resulting in considerable anatomical distortions. This renders it difficult to accurately map white matter tracts or localize functionally important brain areas. Niu et al. (2016) have shown that it is possible to use a combination of fMRI guided DTI tractography (hence, a dual ROI method) to precisely track the fibre pathways of the corticospinal tract (CST) and successfully localize the primary motor cortex (PMC). The most important therapy for brain tumours—radical resection—bears the risk of postsurgical dysfunctions, particularly for tumours located close to eloquent cortex or essential white matter tracts. Therefore, presurgical information about eloquent cortex and tract localization are crucial. Dubey et al. (2018) used DTI to investigate integrity and location of displaced/infiltrated WM tracts and found that complete resection was mostly successful when the WM tracts were only displaced rather than infiltrated (comparable to previous data by Castellano et al. 2012). The most promising approach for

presurgical diagnostics is a multimodal approach, at least combining fMRI and DTI data. Panigrahi et al. (2017) conclude that the preoperative use of fMRI and DTI allows "maximum safe resection" of insular gliomas. Flouty et al. (2017) used multimodal mapping of the brain combining even four methodologies: fMRI, DTI, electrical stimulation via subdural grid implantation and high gamma power mapping. In many cases radiation therapy follows after incomplete tumour resection. Also, this approach benefits from presurgical fMRI/DTI definitions of neuroplastic reorganization in response to pathology. Such data may avoid post-radiotherapy damage of essential cortex and white matter tracts (Zhu et al. 2016). Wang et al. (2015) give an example for a successful DTI/fMRI approach to plan radiation treatment and spare bilateral primary motor cortex and white matter tracts during radiation.

4.4 Multiple Sclerosis (MS)

Multiple sclerosis is characterized by continuous accumulation of new brain lesions over many years in a multitopic fashion. Here, neuroplastic reorganization in response to pathology strongly depends on disease stage (Rocca and Filippi 2007). There is also clinical heterogeneity of lesions, regarding their neuroradiological appearance, extent and location (Enzinger et al. 2016). Most imaging studies recently published focus on functional connectivity changes in MS patients and their impact on therapeutic approaches. For example, to investigate functional connectivity changes induced by an individual lesion, Droby et al. (2016) performed a resting state fMRI study in relapsing-remitting MS patients. They report two major findings: (1) a recruitment of intact cortical regions to compensate for tissue damage and (2) a massive multinodal connectivity increase immediately following a new lesion. This massive neuroplastic reaction gradually decreased with time. Resting state fMRI thus indicates that two phases of neuroplasticity may exist: an acute overconnection and a chronic neuroplastic adaptation to optimize brain performance. Another resting state fMRI study in relapsing-remitting MS found more complex connectivity changes with some networks increasing and others decreasing connectivity (Castellazzi et al. 2018). The authors also describe that the connectivity patterns depend on disease duration. They conclude that interpretation of MS functional connectivity data is complex and connectivity changes may depend on multiple issues: functional compensation attempts, successful adaptation, unsuccessful maladaptation, stage of neurodegeneration and the pre-symptomatic clinical condition. As with other diseases, the combination of fMRI and DTI technologies allows even deeper insights in MS pathophysiology. A combined fMRI/DTI study by Sbardella et al. (2015) describes correlations between altered functional connectivity and white matter damage, similar to previous reports (e.g. Rocca et al. 2009). Increased connectivity in cerebellar and auditory networks positively correlated with corpus callosum damage. The authors also describe various correlations between connectivity changes and the patients' cognitive/motor performance. There are also indications that DTI may help to differentiate subtypes of MS. In a recent DTI study, Woitek et al. (2020) found higher interhemispheric difference of mean diffusivity in patients with primary progressive multiple sclerosis than in those with secondary progressive multiple sclerosis. Regarding literature on therapeutic approaches, Tavazzi et al. (2018) investigated effects of a 4 week neurorehabilitation on gait performance and fMRI measures. Immediately after neurorehabilitation, gait performance was improved and pathological fMRI overactivations were reduced. Functional connectivity was also increased in the primary sensorimotor cortex. However, at 3 months follow up—without further therapy—all positive findings had disappeared. Repeatedly, literature investigating fMRI/DTI effects related to MS therapy generated inconsistent findings. This is not surprising, given the pathophysiological complexity of the disease. Fling et al. (2019) investigated neuroplastic changes of the sensorimotor network using resting state fMRI in patients undergoing walking aid training and found increased functional connectivity between the supplementary motor areas (SMAs) and the primary somatosensory cortices as well as the putamen, while connectivity between the SMAs and cerebellum decreased. In contrast, Bonzano et al. (2015) previously described greater cortico-cerebellar connectivity with hand motor training in MS patients (finger-tapping tasks). Fling et al. (2019) hypothesized that these contradictions are due to differences in cerebellar contributions to upper and lower extremity neural control. Quite obviously, for the complex multiple sclerosis disease more and larger studies with clearly defined patient populations are warranted.

4.5 Peripheral Nervous System Disorders

While many studies have focused on brain reorganization after damage to the central nervous system, reorganizational mechanisms regarding peripheral nervous system disorders are still poorly understood. In peripheral nervous system disorders brain neuroplasticity occurs in the healthy brain and is induced by a changed information flow between the somatic periphery and the brain after injury to peripheral nerves. As with damage to the brain, initial responses to peripheral nerve damage often include compensatory overactivations as well as functional connectivity changes. Compensatory overactivations were described by Fornander et al. (2010) and Rath et al. (2011) when they found an initial increase in the volume of cortical activation in brain areas after surgical restoration of complete median nerve transection. Chen et al. (2006) transplanted a toe for replacement of a lost finger and found that initial overactivation is required for re-establishing the lost function as well as for learning a new function. The same was observed by Eickhoff et al. (2008) after heterotopic hand transplantation. In addition, authors found effective connectivity changes between healthy and affected primary motor cortices showing a maladaptive inhibitory influence of the healthy on the affected motor cortex. Further maladaptive brain plasticity can be found in amputees with fMRI/DTI techniques. Phantom limb pain was found to be caused by intact somatotopic representations adjacent to the missing limb's representation area "invading" that area within the scope of maladaptive plasticity (MacIver et al. 2008). However, another model for phantom limb pain was proposed by Makin et al. (2013), where phantom limb pain may be caused by preserved structure as well as (dys-)function in the former limb's area. Raffin et al. (2016) investigated these models in the primary somatosensory cortex by examination of the 3D anatomy of the central sulcus and fMRI responses during movements of the hand, elbow and lips in upper limb amputees and healthy controls. They found few signs of reorganization in the former hand area but relevant reorganization of the lip and elbow representations which shifted towards the hand area. Their results support the maladaptive plasticity model (MacIver et al. 2008). Another feature consistently described is the fact, that somatotopic brain activation typically corresponds to the peripheral nervous system output, but not to the effector activated by the output. Bitter et al. (2011) compared three types of peripheral surgical reorganization after facial nerve damage: Classical hypoglossal-facial nerve anastomosis, hypoglossal-facial nerve jump anastomosis and facial nerve interpositional graft. With all operations the effector (mimic musculature) is the same; however, the peripheral nervous system output required for identical movements changes. Lip movements after facial nerve interposition led to brain activation in the original facial motor cortex. Lip movements after hypoglossal-facial anastomosis were associated with activation in the hypoglossal motor cortex. For the jump anastomosis however, overlapping activation encompassing both the original facial and the hypoglossal motor cortex was found. Another impressive example of brain activation corresponding to peripheral nervous system output (and not the changed effector) is presented in patients with brachial plexus lesions. In case of a complete avulsion of a brachial plexus it is pos-

sible to connect the denervated biceps with fibres of the contralesional C7 root. The brain is then required to control flexion of the diseased arm with the ipsilesional motor cortex. Functional imaging data have shown that this is achieved via activation of the ipsilesional C7 arm area (controlling the contralesional C7 root), though initially a bilateral activation pattern may occur (Hua et al. 2013; Beaulieu et al. 2006). More complex neuroplastic effects can be found when biceps reinnervation is done via a connection to the side of the phrenic nerve (Beisteiner et al. 2011). In an fMRI study by Amini et al. (2018), patients with complete plexus avulsion underwent reconnection of the end of the musculocutaneous nerve to the side of the phrenic nerve. Despite homuncular organization being a fundamental principle for primary motor cortex, they observed that the original phrenic nerve area now adds a new function: it activates with breathing and with hand movements. Fischmeister et al. (2020) further investigated the functional connectivity changes underlying this transformation of a monofunctional to a bifunctional motor area. They found a consistent increase in FC between the area of the diseased arm and the diaphragm area while moving the diseased arm. They hypothesize that this increased FC is probably mediated through horizontal cortical fibres. Although fMRI/DTI investigations with peripheral nervous system disorders are yet limited, the value of a combined fMRI/DTI approach for understanding their neuroplastic consequences for the brain is unambiguous.

5   Novel Brain Stimulation Supported by fMRI/DTI

The past decade has seen a tremendous development concerning therapeutic brain stimulation methods. Therapeutic brain stimulation supports brain plasticity and is guided by morphological and functional imaging data. The most prominent technology is Transcranial Magnetic Stimulation (TMS, Burke et al. 2019). However, several other electrophysiological brain stimulation techniques

Fig. 1 The novel ultrasound brain stimulation technique TPS (Transcranial Pulse Stimulation) allows imaging based stimulation of brain plasticity with unprecedented precision and depth (Beisteiner et al. 2019). For precise targeting, fMRI and DTI data are important

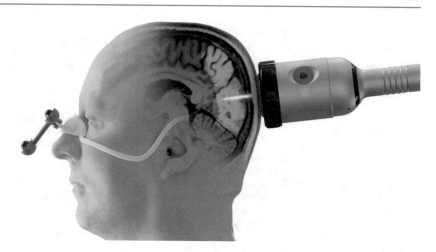

meanwhile have been described (e.g. Transcranial Direct Current Stimulation (TDCS), Transcranial Alternating Current Stimulation (TACS)). Very recently, a completely novel brain stimulation technique has been introduced for therapy: Transcranial Pulse Stimulation (TPS, see Fig. 1) based on ultrasound (Beisteiner et al. 2019; Beisteiner and Lozano 2020). The method generates a very focused ultrasound pulse (about 3 mm wide and 3 cm long, duration about 3 μs), which can be targeted to any area of an individual pathological brain. As with presurgical diagnostics, an optimized planning of the individual therapy requires detailed analysis of the morphological and functional brain situation. Therefore, clinical fMRI and DTI data will become increasingly important also for this therapeutic field. A pilot study in 35 Alzheimer's patients has shown statistically significant cognitive improvement over 3 months after 2 weeks of TPS therapy (Beisteiner et al. 2019). The novel technique has two major advantages compared to existing electromagnetic brain stimulation methods: (1) unprecedented precision for brain area targeting (independent of pathological conductivity changes) and (2) access to deep brain areas, which has not been possible previously. With transcranial ultrasound, non-invasive deep brain stimulation (DBS) may become a new therapeutic option. There are several hypotheses how low energy ultrasound for brain stimulation may change neuronal activity although much research is still needed. A likely

basis is mechanical effects on cell membranes affecting mechanosensitive ion channels and generating membrane pores. As a consequence, transmitter and humoral factor concentrations change. A recent study investigated a neuroinflammation model in a microglia cell culture (Chang et al. 2020). Low intensity pulsed ultrasound increased production of several neurotrophic factors including the neuroprotective BDNF (brain-derived neurotrophic factor) and reduced neuroinflammation by suppressing harming overactivation of microglia. It is increasingly recognized that anti-inflammatory effects are important to improve neurodegenerative diseases. Such ultrasound effects may contribute to memory improvement in preclinical neurodegeneration studies (Chen et al. 2019; Leinenga and Götz 2015). Another study investigated effects of ultrashort ultrasound pulses on a neuronal stem cell culture (Zhang et al. 2017). Here, cell proliferation and differentiation to neurons could be enhanced. A mechanism suggested by Hameroff et al. (2013) is that ultrasound directly affects cytoskeletal microtubules inside neurons and glia. MR informed brain stimulation therapy is particularly promising for brain diseases which may be improved by neuroplastic reorganization and for those including a neuroinflammatory component. Neurodegenerative diseases (Alzheimer's, Parkinson's), stroke, multiple sclerosis and psychiatric disorders are primary candidates with several clinical studies already running. Current work on methodological improvements concerns technical optimization of deep brain stimulation and optimization of clinical treatment protocols.

References

Alia C, Spalletti C, Lai S, Panarese A, Lamola G, Bertolucci F, Vallone F, Di Garbo A, Chisari C, Micera S, Caleo M (2017) Neuroplastic changes following brain ischemia and their contribution to stroke recovery: novel approaches in neurorehabilitation. Front Cell Neurosci 11:76. https://doi.org/10.3389/fncel.2017.00076

Almeida SR, Vicentini J, Bonilha L, De Campos BM, Casseb RF, Min LL (2017) Brain connectivity and functional recovery in patients with ischemic stroke. J Neuroimaging 27:65–70. https://doi.org/10.1111/jon.12362. Epub 2016 May 31

Altenmüller E, Müller D (2013) A model of task-specific focal dystonia. Neural Netw 48:25–31. https://doi.org/10.1016/j.neunet.2013.06.012

Amini A, Fischmeister FPS, Matt E, Schmidhammer R, Rattay F, Beisteiner R (2018) Peripheral nervous system reconstruction reroutes cortical motor output-brain reorganization uncovered by effective connectivity. Front Neurol 9:1116. https://doi.org/10.3389/fneur.2018.01116

Antonenko D, Thielscher A, Saturnino GB, Aydin S, Ittermann B, Grittner U, Flöel A (2019) Towards precise brain stimulation: is electric field simulation related to neuromodulation? Brain Stimul 12:1159–1168. https://doi.org/10.1016/j.brs.2019.03.072. Epub 2019 Mar 22

Beaulieu JY, Blustajn J, Teboul F, Baud P, De Schonen S, Thiebaud JB, Oberlin C (2006) Cerebral plasticity in crossed C7 grafts of the brachial plexus: an fMRI study. Microsurgery 26:303–310. https://doi.org/10.1002/micr.20243

Beisteiner R, Lozano A (2020) Transcranial ultrasound innovations ready for broad clinical application. Adv Sci (Weinh). https://doi.org/10.1002/advs.202002026

Beisteiner R, Höllinger I, Rath J, Wurnig M, Hilbert M, Klinger N, Geißler A, Fischmeister F, Wöber C, Klösch G, Millesi H, Grishold W, Auff E, Schmidhammer R (2011) New type of cortical neuroplasticity after nerve repair in brachial plexus lesions. Arch Neurol 68:1147–1470. https://doi.org/10.1001/archneurol.2011.596

Beisteiner R, Matt E, Fan C, Baldysiak H, Schönfeld M, Philippi Novak T, Amini A, Aslan T, Reinecke R, Lehrner J, Weber A, Reime U, Goldenstedt C, Marlinghaus E, Hallett M, Lohse-Busch H (2019) Transcranial pulse stimulation with ultrasound in Alzheimer's disease-a new navigated focal brain therapy. Adv Sci (Weinh) 7(3):1902583. https://doi.org/10.1002/advs.201902583

Bergmann TO, Karabanov A, Hartwigsen G, Thielscher A, Siebner HR (2016) Combining non-invasive transcranial brain stimulation with neuroimaging and electrophysiology: current approaches and future perspectives. NeuroImage 140:4–19. https://doi.org/10.1016/j.neuroimage.2016.02.012

Bitter T, Sorger B, Hesselmann V, Krug B, Lackner K, Guntinas-Lichius O (2011) Cortical representation sites of mimic movements after facial nerve reconstruction: a functional magnetic resonance imaging study. Laryngoscope 121:699–706. https://doi.org/10.1002/lary.21399

Bonino D, Ricciardi E, Bernardi G, Sani L, Gentili C, Vecchi T, Pietrini P (2015) Spatial imagery relies on a sensory independent, though sensory sensitive, functional organization within the parietal cortex: a fMRI study of angle discrimination in sighted and congenitally blind individuals. Neuropsychologia 68:59–70. https://doi.org/10.1016/j.neuropsychologia.2015.01.004. Epub 2015 Jan 6

Bonzano L, Tacchino A, Roccatagliata L, Inglese M, Mancardi GL, Novellino A, Bove M (2015) An engineered glove for investigating the neural correlates of finger movements using functional magnetic resonance imaging. Front Hum Neurosci 9:503. https://doi.org/10.3389/fnhum.2015.00503

Bosma RL, Mojarad EA, Leung L, Pukall C, Staud R, Stroman PW (2016) FMRI of spinal and supra-spinal correlates of temporal pain summation in fibromyalgia patients. Hum Brain Mapp 37(4):1349–1360. https://doi.org/10.1002/hbm.23106. Epub 2016 Jan 9

Burke MJ, Fried PJ, Pascual-Leone A (2019) Transcranial magnetic stimulation: neurophysiological and clinical applications. Handb Clin Neurol 163:73–92. https://doi.org/10.1016/B978-0-12-804281-6.00005-7

Cadotte DW, Bosma R, Mikulis D, Nugaeva N, Smith K, Pokrupa R, Islam O, Stroman PW, Fehlings MG (2012) Plasticity of the injured human spinal cord: insights revealed by spinal cord functional MRI. PLoS One 7(9):e45560. https://doi.org/10.1371/journal.pone.0045560. Epub 2012 Sep 19

Caeyenberghs K, Leemans A, De Decker C, Heitger M, Drijkoningen D, Linden CV, Sunaert S, Swinnen SP (2012a) Brain connectivity and postural control in young traumatic brain injury patients: a diffusion MRI based network analysis. Neuroimage Clin 1:106–115. https://doi.org/10.1016/j.nicl.2012.09.011

Caeyenberghs K, Leemans A, Heitger MH, Leunissen I, Dhollander T, Sunaert S, Dupont P, Swinnen SP (2012b) Graph analysis of functional brain networks for cognitive control of action in traumatic brain injury. Brain 135:1293–1307. https://doi.org/10.1093/brain/aws048

Carrera E, Tononi G (2014) Diaschisis: past, present, future. Brain 137(Pt 9):2408–2422. https://doi.org/10.1093/brain/awu101. Epub 2014 May 28

Castellano A, Bello L, Michelozzi C, Gallucci M, Fava E, Iadanza A, Riva M, Casaceli G, Falini A (2012) Role of diffusion tensor magnetic resonance tractography in predicting the extent of resection in glioma surgery. Neuro Oncol 14(2):192–202. https://doi.org/10.1093/neuonc/nor188. Epub 2011 Oct 20

Castellazzi G, Debernard L, Melzer TR, Dalrymple-Alford JC, D'Angelo E, Miller DH, Gandini Wheeler-Kingshott CAM, Mason DF (2018) Functional connectivity alterations reveal complex mechanisms based on clinical and radiological status in mild relapsing remitting multiple sclerosis. Front Neurol 9:690. https://doi.org/10.3389/fneur.2018.00690

Cha YH, Chakrapani S, Craig A, Baloh RW (2012) Metabolic and functional connectivity changes in mal de debarquement syndrome. PLoS One 7:e49560. https://doi.org/10.1371/journal.pone.0049560

Chang YA, Kemmotsu N, Leyden KM, Kucukboyaci NE, Iragui VJ, Tecoma ES, Kansal L, Norman MA, Compton R, Ehrlich TJ, Uttarwar VS, Reyes A, Paul BM, McDonald CR (2017) Multimodal imaging of language reorganization in patients with left temporal lobe epilepsy. Brain Lang 170:82–92. https://doi.org/10.1016/j.bandl.2017.03.012. Epub 2017 Apr 20

Chang JW, Wu MT, Song WS, Yang FY (2020) Ultrasound stimulation suppresses LPS-induced proinflammatory responses by regulating NF-κB and CREB activation in microglial cells. Cereb Cortex 30(8):4597–4606. https://doi.org/10.1093/cercor/bhaa062

Chen CJ, Liu HL, Wei FC, Chu NS (2006) Functional MR imaging of the human sensorimotor cortex after toe-to-finger transplantation. AJNR Am J Neuroradiol 27:1617–1621

Chen TT, Lan TH, Yang FY (2019) Low-intensity pulsed ultrasound attenuates LPS-induced neuroinflammation and memory impairment by modulation of TLR4/NF-κB signaling and CREB/BDNF expression. Cereb Cortex 29(4):1430–1438. https://doi.org/10.1093/cercor/bhy039

Chiang S, Levin HS, Wilde E, Haneef Z (2016) White matter structural connectivity changes correlate with epilepsy duration in temporal lobe epilepsy. Epilepsy Res 120:37–46. https://doi.org/10.1016/j.eplepsyres.2015.12.002. Epub 2015 Dec 8

Chiaravalloti ND, Genova HM, DeLuca J (2015) Cognitive rehabilitation in multiple sclerosis: the role of plasticity. Front Neurol 6:67. https://doi.org/10.3389/fneur.2015.00067

Chou N, Serafini S, Muh CR (2018) Cortical language areas and plasticity in pediatric patients with epilepsy: a review. Pediatr Neurol 78:3–12. https://doi.org/10.1016/j.pediatrneurol.2017.10.001. Epub 2017 Oct 12

Cirillo S, Caulo M, Pieri V, Falini A, Castellano A (2019) Role of functional imaging techniques to assess motor and language cortical plasticity in glioma patients: a systematic review. Neural Plast 2019:4056436. https://doi.org/10.1155/2019/4056436

Collignon O, Vandewalle G, Voss P, Albouy G, Charbonneau G, Lassonde M, Lepore F (2011) Functional specialization for auditory-spatial processing in the occipital cortex of congenitally blind humans. Proc Natl Acad Sci U S A 108:4435–4440. https://doi.org/10.1073/pnas.1013928108

Craggs JG, Staud R, Robinson ME, Perlstein WM, Price DD (2012) Effective connectivity among brain regions associated with slow temporal summation of C-fiber-evoked pain in fibromyalgia patients and healthy controls. J Pain 13:390–400. https://doi.org/10.1016/j.jpain.2012.01.002

Cunningham DA, Machado A, Janini D, Varnerin N, Bonnett C, Yue G, Jones S, Lowe M, Beall E, Sakaie K, Plow EB (2015) Assessment of inter-hemispheric imbalance using imaging and noninvasive brain stimulation in patients with chronic stroke. Arch Phys Med Rehabil 96:94–103. https://doi.org/10.1016/j.apmr.2014.07.419

Dalhuisen I, Ackermans E, Martens L, Mulders P, Bartholomeus J, de Bruijn A, Spijker J, van Eijndhoven P, Tendolkar I (2020) Longitudinal effects of rTMS on neuroplasticity in chronic treatment-resistant depression. Eur Arch Psychiatry Clin Neurosci. https://doi.org/10.1007/s00406-020-01135-w. Epub ahead of print

De Giglio L, Tommasin S, Petsas N, Pantano P (2018) The role of fMRI in the assessment of neuroplasticity in MS: a systematic review. Neural Plast 2018:3419871. https://doi.org/10.1155/2018/3419871. Erratum in: Neural Plast. 2019;2019:5181649

De Pittà M, Brunel N, Volterra A (2016) Astrocytes: orchestrating synaptic plasticity? Neuroscience 323:43–61. https://doi.org/10.1016/j.neuroscience.2015.04.001. Epub 2015 Apr 8

Droby A, Yuen KS, Muthuraman M, Reitz SC, Fleischer V, Klein J, Gracien RM, Ziemann U, Deichmann R, Zipp F, Groppa S (2016) Changes in brain functional connectivity patterns are driven by an individual lesion in MS: a resting-state fMRI study. Brain Imaging Behav 10(4):1117–1126. https://doi.org/10.1007/s11682-015-9476-3

Du J, Yang F, Hu J, Hu J, Xu Q, Cong N, Zhang Q, Liu L, Mantini D, Zhang Z, Lu G, Liu X (2019) Effects of high- and low-frequency repetitive transcranial magnetic stimulation on motor recovery in early stroke patients: evidence from a randomized controlled trial with clinical, neurophysiological and functional imaging assessments. Neuroimage Clin 21:101620. https://doi.org/10.1016/j.nicl.2018.101620. Epub 2018 Dec 3

Dubey A, Kataria R, Sinha VD (2018) Role of diffusion tensor imaging in brain tumor surgery. Asian J Neurosurg 13(2):302–306. https://doi.org/10.4103/ajns.AJNS_226_16

Duffau H (2007) Contribution of cortical and subcortical electrostimulation in brain glioma surgery: methodological and functional considerations. Clin Neurophysiol 37(6):373–382

Duffau H (2017) Hodotopy, neuroplasticity and diffuse gliomas. Neurochirurgie 63(3):259–265. https://doi.org/10.1016/j.neuchi.2016.12.001

Dupont S (2015) Imaging memory and predicting postoperative memory decline in temporal lobe epilepsy: insights from functional imaging. Rev Neurol (Paris) 171(3):307–314. https://doi.org/10.1016/j.neurol.2014.12.001. Epub 2015 Feb 25

Eickhoff SB, Dafotakis M, Grefkes C, Shah NJ, Zilles K, Piza-Katzer H (2008) Central adaptation following heterotopic hand replantation probed by fMRI and effective connectivity analysis. Exp Neurol 212:132–144. https://doi.org/10.1016/j.expneurol.2008.03.025

Enzinger C, Pinter D, Rocca MA, De Luca J, Sastre-Garriga J, Audoin B, Filippi M (2016) Longitudinal fMRI studies: exploring brain plasticity and repair in MS. Mult Scler 22(3):269–278. https://doi.org/10.1177/1352458515619781. Epub 2015 Dec 18

Fischmeister FPS, Amini A, Matt E, Reinecke R, Schmidhammer R, Beisteiner R (2020) A new rehabilitative mechanism in primary motor cortex after peripheral trauma. Front Neurol 11:125. https://doi.org/10.3389/fneur.2020.00125

Fleischer V, Muthuraman M, Anwar AR, Gonzalez-Escamilla G, Radetz A, Gracien RM, Bittner S, Luessi F, Meuth SG, Zipp F, Groppa S (2020) Continuous reorganization of cortical information flow in multiple sclerosis: a longitudinal fMRI effective connectivity study. Sci Rep 10(1):806. https://doi.org/10.1038/s41598-020-57805-x

Fling BW, Martini DN, Zeeboer E, Hildebrand A, Cameron M (2019) Neuroplasticity of the sensorimotor neural network associated with walking aid training in people with multiple sclerosis. Mult Scler Relat Disord 31:1–4. https://doi.org/10.1016/j.msard.2019.03.004. Epub 2019 Mar 8

Flouty O, Reddy C, Holland M, Kovach C, Kawasaki H, Oya H, Greenlee J, Hitchon P, Howard M (2017) Precision surgery of rolandic glioma and insights from extended functional mapping. Clin Neurol Neurosurg 163:60–66. https://doi.org/10.1016/j.clineuro.2017.10.008. Epub 2017 Oct 10

Fornander L, Nyman T, Hansson T, Ragnehed M, Brismar T (2010) Age- and time-dependent effects on functional outcome and cortical activation pattern in patients with median nerve injury: a functional magnetic resonance imaging study. J Neurosurg 113:122–128. https://doi.org/10.3171/2009.10.JNS09698

Fox ME, King TZ (2018) Functional connectivity in adult brain tumor patients: a systematic review. Brain Connect 8(7):381–397. https://doi.org/10.1089/brain.2018.0623. Erratum in: Brain Connect. 2018;8(9):577

Genç E, Ocklenburg S, Singer W, Güntürkün O (2015) Abnormal interhemispheric motor interactions in patients with callosal agenesis. Behav Brain Res 293:1–9. https://doi.org/10.1016/j.bbr.2015.07.016. Epub 2015 Jul 14

Goldsworthy MR, Pitcher JB, Ridding MC (2015) Spaced noninvasive brain stimulation: prospects for inducing long-lasting human cortical plasticity. Neurorehabil Neural Repair 29(8):714–721. https://doi.org/10.1177/1545968314562649

Guggisberg AG, Koch PJ, Hummel FC, Buetefisch CM (2019) Brain networks and their relevance for stroke rehabilitation. Clin Neurophysiol 130:1098–1124. https://doi.org/10.1016/j.clinph.2019.04.004. Epub 2019 Apr 15

Gulyaeva NV (2017) Interplay between brain BDNF and glutamatergic systems: a brief state of the evidence and association with the pathogenesis of depression. Biochemistry (Mosc) 82:301–307. https://doi.org/10.1134/S0006297917030087

Hamaide J, De Groof G, Van der Linden A (2016) Neuroplasticity and MRI: a perfect match. NeuroImage 131:13–28. https://doi.org/10.1016/j.neuroimage.2015.08.005. Epub 2015 Aug 7

Hameroff S, Trakas M, Duffield C, Annabi E, Gerace MB, Boyle P, Lucas A, Amos Q, Buadu A, Badal JJ (2013) Transcranial ultrasound (TUS) effects on mental states: a pilot study. Brain Stimul 6(3):409–415. https://doi.org/10.1016/j.brs.2012.05.002. Epub 2012 May 29

Hannanu FF, Master IG, Detante O, Naegele B, Jaillard A (2020) Spatiotemporal patterns of sensorimotor fMRI activity influence hand motor recovery in subacute stroke: a longitudinal task-related fMRI study. Cortex 129:80–98. https://doi.org/10.1016/j.cortex.2020.03.024. Epub 2020 Apr 17

Harrington DL, Rubinov M, Durgerian S, Mourany L, Reece C, Koenig K, Bullmore E, Long JD, Paulsen JS, PREDICT-HD Investigators of the Huntington Study Group, Rao SM (2015) Network topology and functional connectivity disturbances precede the onset of Huntington's disease. Brain 138(Pt 8):2332–2346. https://doi.org/10.1093/brain/awv145. Epub 2015 Jun 9

Hartwigsen G, Saur D (2019) Neuroimaging of stroke recovery from aphasia - insights into plasticity of the human language network. NeuroImage 190:14–31. https://doi.org/10.1016/j.neuroimage.2017.11.056

Heiss WD (2020) Mapping of recovery from poststroke aphasia: comparison of PET and fMRI. In: fMRI. Springer, Cham, pp 225–239. https://doi.org/10.1007/978-3-540-68132-8_10

Hou J, Lin Y, Zhang W, Song L, Wu W, Wang J, Zhou D, Zou Q, Fang Y, He M, Li H (2013) Abnormalities of frontal-parietal resting-state functional connectivity are related to disease activity in patients with systemic lupus erythematosus. PLoS One 8(9):e74530. https://doi.org/10.1371/journal.pone.0074530

Hua XY, Liu B, Qiu YQ, Tang WJ, Xu WD, Liu HQ, Xu JG, Gu YD (2013) Long-term ongoing cortical remodeling after contralateral C-7 nerve transfer. J Neurosurg 118:725–729. https://doi.org/10.3171/2012.12.JNS12207

Hubbard IJ, Carey LM, Budd TW, Levi C, McElduff P, Hudson S, Bateman G, Parsons MW (2015) A randomized controlled trial of the effect of early upperlimb training on stroke recovery and brain activation.

Neurorehabil Neural Repair 29:703–713. https://doi.org/10.1177/1545968314562647. Epub 2014 Dec 19

Hutchings F, Han CE, Keller SS, Weber B, Taylor PN, Kaiser M (2015) Predicting surgery targets in temporal lobe epilepsy through structural connectome based simulations. PLoS Comput Biol 11(12):e1004642. https://doi.org/10.1371/journal.pcbi.1004642

Ikegami A, Haruwaka K, Wake H (2019) Microglia: lifelong modulator of neural circuits. Neuropathology 39:173–180. https://doi.org/10.1111/neup.12560

Jacobs HI, Gronenschild EH, Evers EA, Ramakers IH, Hofman PA, Backes WH, Jolles J, Verhey FR, Van Boxtel MP (2015) Visuospatial processing in early Alzheimer's disease: a multimodal neuroimaging study. Cortex 64:394–406. https://doi.org/10.1016/j.cortex.2012.01.005

Jeon SH, Park YH, Oh SY, Kang JJ, Han YH, Jeong HJ, Lee JM, Park M, Kim JS, Dieterich M (2020) Neural correlates of transient mal de debarquement syndrome: activation of prefrontal and deactivation of cerebellar networks correlate with neuropsychological assessment. Front Neurol 11:585. https://doi.org/10.3389/fneur.2020.00585

Kaneko N, Sawada M, Sawamoto K (2017) Mechanisms of neuronal migration in the adult brain. J Neurochem 141:835–847. https://doi.org/10.1111/jnc.14002

Kong NW, Gibb WR, Tate MC (2016) Neuroplasticity: insights from patients harboring gliomas. Neural Plast 2016:2365063. https://doi.org/10.1155/2016/2365063. Epub 2016 Jul 5

Langer N, Hänggi J, Müller NA, Simmen HP, Jäncke L (2012) Effects of limb immobilization on brain plasticity. Neurology 78:182–188. https://doi.org/10.1212/WNL.0b013e31823fcd9c

Leinenga G, Götz J (2015) Scanning ultrasound removes amyloid-β and restores memory in an Alzheimer's disease mouse model. Sci Transl Med 7(278):278ra33. https://doi.org/10.1126/scitranslmed.aaa2512

List J, Duning T, Kürten J, Deppe M, Wilbers E, Flöel A (2013) Cortical plasticity is preserved in nondemented older individuals with severe ischemic small vessel disease. Hum Brain Mapp 34:1464–1476. https://doi.org/10.1002/hbm.22003

Liu Z, Xiao X, Zhang K, Zhao Q, Cao X, Li C, Wang M, Robbins TW, Sahakian BJ, Zhang J, Feng J (2019) Dynamic brain network changes reflect neuroplasticity: molecular and cognitive evidence. bioRxiv. 695122 [Preprint]. https://doi.org/10.1101/695122

Lu MK, Chen CM, Duann JR, Ziemann U, Chen JC, Chiou SM, Tsai CH (2016) Investigation of motor cortical plasticity and corticospinal tract diffusion tensor imaging in patients with Parkinsons disease and essential tremor. PLoS One 11(9):e0162265. https://doi.org/10.1371/journal.pone.0162265

MacIver K, Lloyd DM, Kelly S, Roberts N, Nurmikko T (2008) Phantom limb pain, cortical reorganization and the therapeutic effect of mental imagery. Brain 131:2181–2191. https://doi.org/10.1093/brain/awn124

Makin TR, Scholz J, Filippini N, Henderson Slater D, Tracey I, Johansen-Berg H (2013) Phantom pain is associated with preserved structure and function in the former hand area. Nat Commun 4:1570. https://doi.org/10.1038/ncomms2571

Mantel T, Altenmüller E, Li Y, Lee A, Meindl T, Jochim A, Zimmer C, Haslinger B (2020) Structure-function abnormalities in cortical sensory projections in embouchure dystonia. Neuroimage Clin 28:102410. https://doi.org/10.1016/j.nicl.2020.102410

Marebwa BK, Fridriksson J, Yourganov G, Feenaughty L, Rorden C, Bonilha L (2017) Chronic post-stroke aphasia severity is determined by fragmentation of residual white matter networks. Sci Rep 7:8188. https://doi.org/10.1038/s41598-017-07607-9

Meoded A, Faria AV, Hartman AL, Jallo GI, Mori S, Johnston MV, Huisman TA, Poretti A (2016) Cerebral reorganization after hemispherectomy: a DTI study. AJNR Am J Neuroradiol 37(5):924–931. https://doi.org/10.3174/ajnr.A4647. Epub 2016 Jan 14

Michaud K, Duffau H (2016) Surgery of insular and paralimbic diffuse low-grade gliomas: technical considerations. J Neuro-Oncol 130(2):289–298. https://doi.org/10.1007/s11060-016-2120-2. Epub 2016 May 9

Min YS, Park JW, Park E, Kim AR, Cha H, Gwak DW, Jung SH, Chang Y, Jung TD (2020) Interhemispheric functional connectivity in the primary motor cortex assessed by resting-state functional magnetic resonance imaging aids long-term recovery prediction among subacute stroke patients with severe hand weakness. J Clin Med 9:975. https://doi.org/10.3390/jcm9040975

Mohammadi B, Kollewe K, Cole DM, Fellbrich A, Heldmann M, Samii A, Dengler R, Petri S, Münte TF, Krämer UM (2015) Amyotrophic lateral sclerosis affects cortical and subcortical activity underlying motor inhibition and action monitoring. Hum Brain Mapp 36(8):2878–2889. https://doi.org/10.1002/hbm.22814. Epub 2015 Apr 24

Monje M (2018) Myelin plasticity and nervous system function. Annu Rev Neurosci 41:61–76. https://doi.org/10.1146/annurev-neuro-080317-061853

Niu C, Liu X, Yang Y, Zhang K, Min Z, Wang M, Li W, Guo L, Lin P, Zhang M (2016) Assessing region of interest schemes for the corticospinal tract in patients with brain tumors. Medicine (Baltimore) 95(12):e3189. https://doi.org/10.1097/MD.0000000000003189

Oni-Orisan A, Kaushal M, Li W, Leschke J, Ward BD, Vedantam A, Kalinosky B, Budde MD, Schmit BD, Li SJ, Muqeet V, Kurpad SN (2016) Alterations in cortical sensorimotor connectivity following complete cervical spinal cord injury: a prospective resting-state fMRI study. PLoS One 11(3):e0150351. https://doi.org/10.1371/journal.pone.0150351

Osipowicz K, Sperling MR, Sharan AD, Tracy JI (2016) Functional MRI, resting state fMRI, and DTI for predicting verbal fluency outcome following resective surgery for temporal lobe epilepsy. J Neurosurg

124(4):929–937.   https://doi.org/10.3171/2014.9. JNS131422. Epub 2015 Sep 25

Palaniyappan L, White TP, Liddle PF (2012) The concept of salience network dysfunction in schizophrenia: from neuroimaging observations to therapeutic opportunities. Curr Top Med Chem 12:2324–2338. https://doi.org/10.2174/156802612805289881

Panigrahi M, Chandrasekhar YB, Vooturi S, Ram GA, Rammohan VS (2017) Surgical resection of insular gliomas and roles of functional magnetic resonance imaging and diffusion tensor imaging tractography-single surgeon experience. World Neurosurg 98:587–593.   https://doi.org/10.1016/j.wneu.2016.11.001. Epub 2016 Nov 10

Phillips C (2017) Brain-derived neurotrophic factor, depression, and physical activity: making the neuroplastic connection. Neural Plast 8:1–17. https://doi.org/10.1155/2017/7260130

Pini L, Manenti R, Cotelli M, Pizzini FB, Frisoni GB, Pievani M (2018) Non-invasive brain stimulation in dementia: a complex network story. Neurodegener Dis 18(5–6):281–301. https://doi.org/10.1159/000495945. Epub 2019 Jan 29

Pinter D, Gattringer T, Fandler-Höfler S, Kneihsl M, Eppinger S, Deutschmann H, Pichler A, Poltrum B, Reishofer G, Ropele S, Schmidt R, Enzinger C (2020) Early progressive changes in white matter integrity are associated with stroke recovery. Transl Stroke Res 11(6):1264–1272.   https://doi.org/10.1007/s12975-020-00797-x. Epub ahead of print

Puig J, Blasco G, Schlaug G, Stinear CM, Daunis-I-Estadella P, Biarnes C, Figueras J, Serena J, Hernández-Pérez M, Alberich-Bayarri A, Castellanos M, Liebeskind DS, Demchuk AM, Menon BK, Thomalla G, Nael K, Wintermark M, Pedraza S (2017) Diffusion tensor imaging as a prognostic biomarker for motor recovery and rehabilitation after stroke. Neuroradiology 59(4):343–351. https://doi.org/10.1007/s00234-017-1816-0. Epub 2017 Mar 14

Pundik S, Scoco A, Skelly M, McCabe JP, Daly JJ (2018) Greater cortical thickness is associated with enhanced sensory function after arm rehabilitation in chronic stroke. Neurorehabil Neural Repair 32:590–601. https://doi.org/10.1177/1545968318778810.   Epub 2018 Jun 9

Qi R, Zhang LJ, Chen HJ, Zhong J, Luo S, Ke J, Xu Q, Kong X, Liu C, Lu GM (2015) Role of local and distant functional connectivity density in the development of minimal hepatic encephalopathy. Sci Rep 5:13720. https://doi.org/10.1038/srep13720

Raffin E, Richard N, Giraux P, Reilly KT (2016) Primary motor cortex changes after amputation correlate with phantom limb pain and the ability to move the phantom limb. NeuroImage 130:134–144. https://doi.org/10.1016/j.neuroimage.2016.01.063. Epub 2016 Feb 11

Rath J, Schmidhammer R, Steinkellner T, Klinger N, Geißler A, Beisteiner R (2008) Evaluation of functional cortex for the diseased hand in a patient after

hemispherectomy. Arch Neurol 65:1664–1665. https://doi.org/10.1001/archneur.65.12.1664

Rath J, Klinger N, Geißler A, Höllinger I, Gruber S, Wurnig M, Hausner T, Auff E, Schmidhammer R, Beisteiner R (2011) An fMRI marker for peripheral nerve regeneration. Neurorehabil Neural Repair 25:577–579. https://doi.org/10.1177/1545968310397552

Reid LB, Boyd RN, Cunnington R, Rose SE (2016) Interpreting intervention induced neuroplasticity with fMRI: the case for multimodal imaging strategies. Neural Plast 2016:2643491. https://doi.org/10.1155/2016/2643491. Epub 2015 Dec 29

Rocca MA, Filippi M (2007) Functional MRI in multiple sclerosis. J Neuroimaging 17:36–41. https://doi.org/10.1111/j.1552-6569.2007.00135.x

Rocca MA, Valsasina P, Ceccarelli A, Absinta M, Ghezzi A, Riccitelli G, Pagani E, Falini A, Comi G, Scotti G, Filippi M (2009) Structural and functional MRI correlates of Stroop control in benign MS. Hum Brain Mapp 30:276–290. https://doi.org/10.1002/hbm.20504

Rosazza C, Deleo F, D'Incerti L, Antelmi L, Tringali G, Didato G, Bruzzone MG, Villani F, Ghielmetti F (2018) Tracking the re-organization of motor functions after disconnective surgery: a longitudinal fMRI and DTI study. Front Neurol 9:400. https://doi.org/10.3389/fneur.2018.00400

Roy AV, Thai M, Klimes-Dougan B, Westlund Schreiner M, Mueller BA, Albott CS, Lim KO, Fiecas M, Tye SJ, Cullen KR (2020, 2020) Brain entropy and neurotrophic molecular markers accompanying clinical improvement after ketamine: preliminary evidence in adolescents with treatment-resistant depression.   J   Psychopharmacol.   https://doi.org/10.1177/0269881120928203

Rozov AV, Valiullina FF, Bolshakov AP (2017) Mechanisms of long-term plasticity of hippocampal GABAergic synapses. Biochemistry (Mosc) 82:257–263. https://doi.org/10.1134/S0006297917030038

Santhanam P, Duncan ES, Small SL (2018) Therapy-induced plasticity in chronic aphasia is associated with behavioral improvement and time since stroke. Brain Connect 8:179–188. https://doi.org/10.1089/brain.2017.0508. Epub 2018 Mar 23

Sbardella E, Tona F, Petsas N, Upadhyay N, Piattella MC, Filippini N, Prosperini L, Pozzilli C, Pantano P (2015) Functional connectivity changes and their relationship with clinical disability and white matter integrity in patients with relapsing–remitting multiple sclerosis. Mult Scler 21:1681–1692. Epub 2015 Jun 3. https://doi.org/10.1177/1352458514568826

Scheller E, Abdulkadir A, Peter J, Tabrizi SJ, Frackowiak RS, Klöppel S (2013) Interregional compensatory mechanisms of motor functioning in progressing preclinical neurodegeneration. NeuroImage 75:146–154. https://doi.org/10.1016/j.neuroimage.2013.02.058

Schmidt SA, Carpenter-Thompson J, Husain FT (2017) Connectivity of precuneus to the default mode and dorsal attention networks: a possible invariant marker of long-term tinnitus. Neuroimage Clin 16:196–204. https://doi.org/10.1016/j.nicl.2017.07.015

Singh A, Abraham WC (2017) Astrocytes and synaptic plasticity in health and disease. Exp Brain Res 235:1645–1655. https://doi.org/10.1007/s00221-017-4928-1. Epub 2017 Mar 15

Sorg BA, Berretta S, Blacktop JM, Fawcett JW, Kitagawa H, Kwok JC, Miquel M (2016) Casting a wide net: role of perineuronal nets in neural plasticity. J Neurosci 36:11459–11468. https://doi.org/10.1523/JNEUROSCI.2351-16.2016

Spielmann K, Durand E, Marcotte K, Ansaldo AI (2016) Maladaptive plasticity in aphasia: brain activation maps underlying verb retrieval errors. Neural Plast 2016:4806492. https://doi.org/10.1155/2016/4806492. Epub 2016 Jun 27

Tahedl M, Levine SM, Greenlee MW, Weissert R, Schwarzbach JV (2018) Functional connectivity in multiple sclerosis: recent findings and future directions. Front Neurol 9:828. https://doi.org/10.3389/fneur.2018.00828

Tao Y, Rapp B (2019) The effects of lesion and treatment-related recovery on functional network modularity in post-stroke dysgraphia. Neuroimage Clin 23:101865. https://doi.org/10.1016/j.nicl.2019.101865. Epub 2019 May 22

Tavazzi E, Bergsland N, Cattaneo D, Gervasoni E, Laganà MM, Dipasquale O, Grosso C, Saibene FL, Baglio F, Rovaris M (2018) Effects of motor rehabilitation on mobility and brain plasticity in multiple sclerosis: a structural and functional MRI study. J Neurol 265(6):1393–1401. https://doi.org/10.1007/s00415-018-8859-y. Epub 2018 Apr 7

Tona F, Petsas N, Sbardella E, Prosperini L, Carmellini M, Pozzilli C, Pantano P (2014) Multiple sclerosis: altered thalamic resting-state functional connectivity and its effect on cognitive function. Radiology 271(3):814–821. https://doi.org/10.1148/radiol.14131688. Epub 2014 Jan 24

Trimmel K, van Graan LA, Gonzálvez GG, Haag A, Caciagli L, Vos SB, Bonelli S, Sidhu M, Thompson PJ, Koepp MJ, Duncan JS (2019) Naming fMRI predicts the effect of temporal lobe resection on language decline. Ann Clin Transl Neurol 6(11):2186–2196. https://doi.org/10.1002/acn3.50911. Epub 2019 Oct 2

Ulm L, Copland D, Meinzer M (2016) A new era of systems neuroscience in aphasia? Aphasiology 32:742–764. https://doi.org/10.1080/02687038.2016.122742 5. Epub 2016 Aug 31

Van der Holst HM, Tuladhar AM, Zerbi V, van Uden IWM, de Laat KF, van Leijsen EMC, Ghafoorian M, Platel B, Bergkamp MI, van Norden AGW, Norris DG, van Dijk EJ, Kiliaan AJ, de Leeuw FE (2017) White matter changes and gait decline in cerebral small vessel disease. Neuroimage Clin 17:731–738. https://doi.org/10.1016/j.nicl.2017.12.007

Van Nuenen BF, Helmich RC, Ferraye M, Thaler A, Hendler T, Orr-Urtreger A, Mirelman A, Bressman S, Marder KS, Giladi N, van de Warrenburg BP, Bloem BR, Toni I, LRRK2 Ashkenazi Jewish Consortium (2012) Cerebral pathological and compensatory mechanisms in the premotor phase of leucine-rich repeat kinase 2 parkinsonism. Brain 135(Pt 12):3687–3698. https://doi.org/10.1093/brain/aws288

Wang M, Ma H, Wang X, Guo Y, Xia X, Xia H, Guo Y, Huang X, He H, Jia X, Xie Y (2015) Integration of BOLD-fMRI and DTI into radiation treatment planning for high-grade gliomas located near the primary motor cortexes and corticospinal tracts. Radiat Oncol 10:64. https://doi.org/10.1186/s13014-015-0364-1

Watson CG, DeMaster D, Ewing-Cobbs L (2019) Graph theory analysis of DTI tractography in children with traumatic injury. Neuroimage Clin 21:101673. https://doi.org/10.1016/j.nicl.2019.101673. Epub 2019 Jan 10

Woitek R, Leutmezer F, Dal-Bianco A, Furtner J, Kasprian G, Prayer D, Schöpf V (2020) Diffusion tensor imaging of the normal-appearing deep gray matter in primary and secondary progressive multiple sclerosis. Acta Radiol 61(1):85–92. https://doi.org/10.1177/0284185119852735. Epub 2019 Jun 6

Wolf CC, Ball A, Ocklenburg S, Otto T, Heed T, Röder B, Güntürkün O (2011) Visuotactile interactions in the congenitally acallosal brain: evidence for early cerebral plasticity. Neuropsychologia 49:3908–3916. https://doi.org/10.1016/j.neuropsychologia.2011.10.008

Wu BB, Ma Y, Xie L, Huang JZ, Sun ZB, Hou ZD, Guo RW, Lin ZR, Duan SX, Zhao SS, Yao-Xie, Sun DM, Zhu CM, Ma SH (2018) Impaired decision-making and functional neuronal network activity in systemic lupus erythematosus. J Magn Reson Imaging 48(6):1508–1517. https://doi.org/10.1002/jmri.26006. Epub 2018 Mar 14

Yu Z, Tao L, Qian Z, Wu J, Liu H, Yu Y, Song J, Wang S, Sun J (2016) Altered brain anatomical networks and disturbed connection density in brain tumor patients revealed by diffusion tensor tractography. Int J Comput Assist Radiol Surg 11:2007–2019. https://doi.org/10.1007/s11548-015-1330-y

Zhang J, Kang N, Yu X, Ma Y, Pang X (2017) Radial extracorporeal shock wave therapy enhances the proliferation and differentiation of neural stem cells by Notch, PI3K/AKT, and Wnt/β-catenin signaling. Sci Rep 7(1):15321. https://doi.org/10.1038/s41598-017-15662-5

Zhang N, Xia M, Qiu T, Wang X, Lin CP, Guo Q, Lu J, Wu Q, Zhuang D, Yu Z, Gong F, Farrukh Hameed NU, He Y, Wu J, Zhou L (2018) Reorganization of cerebro-cerebellar circuit in patients with left hemispheric gliomas involving language network: a combined structural and resting-state functional MRI study. Hum Brain Mapp 39(12):4802–4819. https://doi.org/10.1002/hbm.24324. Epub 2018 Jul 27

Zheng X, Schlaug G (2015) Structural white matter changes in descending motor tracts correlate with improvements in motor impairment after undergoing a treatment course of tDCS and physical therapy. Front Hum Neurosci 9:229. https://doi.org/10.3389/fnhum.2015.00229

Zhu T, Chapman CH, Tsien C, Kim M, Spratt DE, Lawrence TS, Cao Y (2016) Effect of the maximum dose on white matter fiber bundles using longitudinal diffusion tensor imaging. Int J Radiat Oncol Biol Phys 96(3):696–705. https://doi.org/10.1016/j.ijrobp.2016.07.010. Epub 2016 Jul 21

Clinical BOLD fMRI and DTI: Artifacts, Tips, and Tricks

Ronald Peeters and Stefan Sunaert

Contents

R. Peeters (✉) · S. Sunaert
Department of Radiology, University Hospitals
Leuven, Leuven, Belgium

Translational MRI, Department of Imaging and
Pathology, KU Leuven, Leuven, Leuven, Belgium
e-mail: ronald.peeters@uzleuven.be;
stefan.sunaert@uzleuven.be

Abstract

DTI and BOLD functional MRI techniques suffer from many different types of *artifacts*. These *artifacts* can have a technical origin like *susceptibility artifacts* in specific brain regions or vibration and eddy current artifacts, but they can also be related to physiology. The *draining vein* activation observed in the neighborhood of functionally active regions or *flow*

© The Author(s), under exclusive license to Springer Nature Switzerland AG 2022
C. Stippich (ed.), *Clinical Functional MRI*, Medical Radiology Diagnostic Imaging,
https://doi.org/10.1007/978-3-030-83343-5_12

artifacts are such physiologically induced artifacts. In clinical fMRI there are also several specific problems. These can be pathology-induced *reduction or absence of brain activation* in the vicinity of lesions, which can lead to false interpretation of the resulting fMRI maps. As patients are most of the time ill, the *pharmaceuticals* they are taking can also influence the BOLD signal, and the same applies to a lack of *cooperation* during the scan and *head motion, which is also detrimental for DTI acquisition*. The success rate in clinical fMRI/DTI protocols is clearly related to the clinician's/technician's ability to recognize and cope with these technical, physiological, and patient-induced artifacts.

1 Introduction

FMRI and DTI techniques suffer from many different types of *artifacts* (Zeffiro 1996; Le Bihan et al. 2006; Haller and Bartsch 2009; Jones and Cercignani 2010; Murphy et al. 2013; Davis and Poldrack 2013). Some of these artifacts are of purely technical origin (e.g., spikes in EPI images), others may be related to physiology (e.g., cardiac related physiologic brain motion) or a combination of both (e.g., susceptibility-induced artifacts on multiband/hyperband acquisitions) (Todd et al. 2016; Reynaud et al. 2017). Finally, there are also pathology-induced artifacts, which can lead to a possible false interpretation of the results (Lin et al. 2017). Clinical BOLD fMRI, which is nowadays mostly performed at a field strength of 3 T, is a rather insensitive technique since signal intensity changes induced by neuronal activity are typically in the order of a few percent, i.e., in the magnitude of noise (Boxerman et al. 1995; Aguirre et al. 1998). Many artifacts will therefore be related to the weak contrast-to-noise ratio of fMRI. DTI acquisition techniques on the other hand are also very sensitive to hardware-related instabilities and eddy currents, and suffer from a very low signal-to-noise ratio (Koch and Norris 2000; Le Bihan et al. 2006).

The low signal-to-noise ratio and various possible artifacts limit the *success rate* of clinical fMRI and DTI. *Claustrophobia and patient cooperation*, especially in more difficult tasks such as cognitive or language tasks hamper the use of active fMRI in severely ill patients. Nonetheless, the reported success rate of presurgical fMRI in the literature is about 80–95% (Lee et al. 1999; Krings 2001a; Håberg et al. 2004; Tyndall et al. 2017; Vysotski et al. 2018). This is probably an overestimation since most patients undergoing fMRI have already undergone a selection by the referring clinician, and not all patients with brain pathologies are referred for presurgical fMRI. When a failure occurs, head movement artifacts are the most frequent cause, followed by a low contrast-to-noise ratio of the activated regions. In the case of the DTI scans and also in resting state fMRI where patient cooperation is less stringent (no task has to be performed) the overall success rate may be higher and also non-cooperative patients, pediatric patients, and neonates (Heemskerk et al. 2013; Leuthardt et al. 2018), and even comatose patients may still be scanned (Vanhaudenhuyse et al. 2010).

The success rate of advanced clinical neuroimaging is clearly related to the clinician's/technician's ability to recognize and cope with the technical, physiological, and patient-induced artifacts and limitations (Tyndall et al. 2017). But there are some tips and tricks of how to detect and minimize these artifacts and to distinguish real from false brain activation in fMRI, as well as real pathologic white matter structure changes from artifacts.

2 Artifacts Related to BOLD fMRI Signal in Both Active and Resting State fMRI

As discussed in chapter "Revealing Brain Activity and White Matter Structure Using Functional and Diffusion-Weighted Magnetic Resonance Imaging," neurovascular coupling between brain activation and cerebrovascular physiology leads to three effects that can contribute to the fMRI signal: An increase in the regional blood flow velocity (rCBF), regional blood volume (rCBV), and local blood oxygenation level. According to the latter, the most widely used fMRI technique has been called "blood oxygenation level dependent (BOLD) fMRI" (Ogawa and Lee 1990; Rao et al. 1993; Turner et al. 1993; Yang et al. 1997).

All imaging modalities that extrapolate task-driven or resting state alterations from hemodynamic changes in neuronal activity produce functional maps that have passed through "a vascular filter." This means that the regional sensitivity of the imaging modality for detecting functional changes following neuronal activation depends on the vascular baseline state and the vascular density in and around the activated neuronal cluster. Due to the contrast mechanism of the BOLD technique exploiting changes in deoxyhemoglobin concentration this also applies to fMRI experiments (Menon and Kim 1999; Mandeville et al. 2001; Logothetis 2002; Goense et al. 2012). Thus, the observed area of signal change in BOLD images is larger than and can be displaced relative to the actual activated zone. These intrinsic effects of the BOLD mechanism limit the temporal and spatial resolution of fMRI, independently of the acquisition protocol (Engel et al. 1997; Menon et al. 1998; Kriegeskorte et al. 2010).

2.1 Artifacts in Localization of Brain Activity (Brain or Vein)

The spatial specificity of activated patches obtained from fMRI and the accuracy of the activation location in relation to the sites of neuronal (electrical) activity have been shown to depend on the acquisition technique (Kim et al. 2000; Logothetis 2000; Duong et al. 2004; Siero et al. 2013; Koopmans and Yacoub 2019). Several authors have raised the concern that BOLD fMRI exams performed at lower field strengths may predominantly detect large draining veins which are not necessarily in the direct neighborhood of the activated brain region (Frahm et al. 1994).

In order to recognize BOLD signals arising from veins draining the excess of blood from

activated areas (Kansaku et al. 1998; Menon 2002; Nencka and Rowe 2007) the following principles can be used:

The activated spots observed from a draining vein are mostly small, contiguous on several adjacent slices and tubular following the (often intrasulcal) path of the vein through different slices. The activated functional brain tissue, on the other hand, tends to appear more locally contained within the brain parenchyma (Gati et al. 1997; Krings 2001a).

By co-registering (overlaying) fMRI activation maps or rsfMRI network maps with anatomical T1-weighted contrast enhanced images—which visualize the larger contrast filled draining veins—it is possible to check for the latter's position and for any possible overlap with BOLD-clusters. Additionally co-registering a venous MR-angiogram or an SWI vein map helps to distinguish intravenous signal changes from parenchymal brain activation (Baudendistel et al. 1998; Kalcher et al. 2015).

In addition, when analyzing the signal time-course, differences between signal from activated parenchyma and that from draining veins can be distinguished. Because the draining veins are fed by venules and arterioles of the activated brain area their signal change is delayed compared to that of the parenchyma (Kansaku et al. 1998; Hall et al. 2002). This is reflected by a later onset of contrast change in the MR signal time-course of the draining vein. However, the temporal offset between the microvasculature in the activated parenchyma and the microvasculature of the draining veins is not very large, i.e., in the order of 1–2 s, which is the time necessary for the blood to pass the smaller veins and reach the larger vessels (Lee and Meyer 1995). Consequently, this effect is rarely observed in a standard clinical fMRI protocol with a typical temporal resolution of around 2–3 s. On the other hand, the relative signal change observed in the draining vein is considerably larger than that of the parenchyma in a gradient echo pulse sequence (typically twice as large in a 1.5 T scanner). This is the result of several different effects. The magnetic susceptibility effects and the resulting percentage of signal change increase around large draining veins. Moreover, the large draining veins occupy a considerably larger volume in a voxel than the microvessels. Therefore, the partial volume effect will further increase the percent signal change in voxels containing draining veins compared to those containing the parenchymal venules/arterioles. Lastly, inflow effects are more pronounced in the large tubular draining veins compared to the randomly oriented microvasculature (Krings 2001a).

In general the activated areas observed in functional BOLD imaging studies can be divided into two different types based on the high resolution T_2*-weighted or susceptibility weighted images (SWI) and T_1-weighted images. The "venous" type is highly spatially confined, tends to be located along the sulcus, is of tubular configuration, and accounts for a higher percentage of relative BOLD contrast changes upon stimulation. High resolution anatomical images demonstrate that areas with the most intense stimulation-related signal intensity changes correlate with dark spots or lines on T_2*-weighted or SWI images, and bright contrast filled superficial tubuli in contrast enhanced T_1-weighted images arising from macroscopic venous blood vessels. The latter observation is also consistent with the fact that the relatively large blood vessels are located on the sulcal cortical surface rather than within the brain tissue itself (Yamada et al. 1997). Besides these "venous hot-spots" of activation, however, the parenchymal stimulation/activation-related BOLD contrast changes spread more diffusely and are not at all associated with any visible large venous vessel on anatomical images. This "parenchymal" type accounts for most of the spatial extension of the BOLD-activation.

2.1.1 How to Minimize the Contribution of Draining Veins?

The contribution from large draining veins to fMRI signals is especially pronounced when single slices, large flip angles, and short TR gradient echo sequences are used (Duyn et al. 1994; Haacke et al. 1994), since these enhance the con-

tribution of the increase in blood flow and blood volume (inflow-effect). Gao et al. (1996) have demonstrated that one may obtain fMRI images which are more sensitive to the microcirculation in the brain parenchyma by designing the pulse sequence towards minimizing inflow effects and maximizing the BOLD contribution. This can be achieved with multi-slice, heavily T_2*-weighted single shot echo-planar images with a long TR (Gao et al. 1996). Therefore, implementing these imaging parameters should be a prerequisite when performing clinical fMRI in order to maximize the fMRI signal towards the site of neuronal activity. In doing so, several studies have shown a good correlation between the BOLD fMRI signal and intra-operative mapping, suggesting that the functional-anatomical specificity is adequate for presurgical mapping, provided an optimal acquisition technique is used (Nitschke et al. 1998; Tomczak et al. 2000; Krings 2001b; Stippich et al. 2003; Meier et al. 2013).

The use of higher magnetic field strengths will also decrease the effect of the draining veins (Gati et al. 1997; Moon et al. 2007; Menon 2012). The lower increase of the draining vein signal change compared to parenchymal activation at higher static field strengths results from the field dependence of the alteration in T_2*-values (Ogawa et al. 1993). This study by Ogawa et al. (1993) predicted that the overall effect in susceptibility difference on a T_2*sensitive imaging technique would be somewhere between linear and quadratic depending on the main magnetic field. In addition, it was reported that at high magnetic field strengths the contribution of small vessels is more pronounced than at low magnetic field strengths (Ogawa et al. 1993; Menon et al. 1995). Thus, with respect to signal intensity changes induced by susceptibility alterations of the blood vessels, which are secondary to neuronal activity, this effect will increase more than linearly with the magnetic field strength, with a larger contribution of the more desired small vessel effect. Therefore, higher field strengths have an advantage (Ugurbil et al. 1999) for distinguishing parenchymal from venous activation. However, stronger main fields are also more sensitive to other artifacts such as susceptibility-induced image deformations in EPI sequences (see Sect. 5.1 in this chapter), a larger influence of scanner instability (Cohen and DuBois 1999) and physiological effects (Weisskoff 1996) which will be discussed below.

BOLD functional activation maps can also be obtained by using the spin echo (SE)-based T_2-weighted contrast rather than the gradient echo (GRE)-based T_2^*-weighted contrast (Duong et al. 2004; Moon et al. 2007; Uludağ et al. 2009). However the observed BOLD effect is much smaller on the T_2-relaxation parameter (SE-technique) resulting in a much lower contrast-to-noise ratio (CNR) which makes this technique less sensitive. On the other hand, using the T_2-effect can be preferable if one wants to avoid spurious activation in large veins (Lowe et al. 2000; Uludağ et al. 2009) since SE sequences have a high specificity for microvessels and are therefore less sensitive to susceptibility effects around larger blood vessels in optimized settings (Oja et al. 1999; Uludağ et al. 2009).

Cohen et al. (2004) demonstrated another technique to maximize parenchymal activation compared to venous activation where hypercapnic normalization of the BOLD activation maps with the aid of CO_2 inhalation was used to normalize the BOLD activated areas, making them independent of the resting state CBV in the voxels. Maximizing the fMRI signal towards the site of neuronal activity can also be achieved by optimizing the mode of stimulation. A study by Le Rumeur et al. (2000) has shown that different types of sensory stimulation are capable of differentiating primary sensory cortex from the venous draining network. Discontinuous stimulation of a limited skin area elicited activity in the microvasculature of the sensory cortex only, whereas robust continuous stimulation of a larger skin area led to activation not only in functional sites but also in the venous network. The authors claimed that the discontinuous stimulation paradigm induced a smaller observed activated area and thus less migration of BOLD contrast to the venous network. As a result resting state fMRI will also be less sensitive to the venous draining network due to the former's lower mode of activation. Moreover, postprocessing methods for rsfMRI protocols emerged which could distinguish venous voxels from other voxels (Kalcher et al. 2015). If the activated region has a rather small surface area ($<100 \ mm^2$), the oxygenation state will only spread up to 4–5 mm beyond the edge of the activated region and into the draining vein. After that it will be diluted in the vein (Turner 2002), minimizing the influence of the draining vein signal on presurgical BOLD maps.

Practical Tip In preoperative fMRI spurious venous signals influence a practitioners' decision how far away the resection border should be from an adjacent functionally active area when removing a lesion. Functionally "safe" resection borders cannot be determined from fMRI studies due to the statistical nature of the activation maps. However, several studies recommend a distance of 1 cm or higher between the resection border and the functional area as reasonably safe regarding the risk for surgically induced post-operative neurological deficits (see chapters "Task-Based Presurgical Functional MRI in Patients with Brain Tumors" and "Presurgical Functional Localization Possibilities, Limitations, and Validity" for details). This does not apply to the draining venous vessels, as they do not represent "real" activated regions. Therefore, it is merely required to keep clear of the vessels. In practice, it is advised to always acquire anatomical high resolution images of the patient, preferably contrast enhanced T1 or SWI images, to depict large blood vessels and to co-register the fMRI activation images with these anatomical images in order to distinguish "activation" in anatomically visible vessels from "activation" within the brain parenchyma. When small very intensely activated patches are observed it is also recommended to compare these time-courses with those of the more diffusely activated parenchymal regions to distinguish both types of activation (see chapter "Task-Based Presurgical Functional MRI in Patients with Brain Tumors").

2.2 The Influence of Brain Lesions on the BOLD fMRI Signal

An important aspect of clinical functional MRI is to be aware of significant but not detected, reduced, or artificial BOLD-activation. Here, it is important to know whether absent or reduced BOLD signal also reflects absent or reduced neuronal activation, and whether BOLD signals in hyperperfused tissue (e.g., nearby or in the boundaries of highly vascularized tumors and metastases) or in areas with altered hemodynamic properties (e.g., in AVMs) represent truly functional neuronal activation. Until now, the knowledge on these issues and on their prevalence is very limited. The different phenomena have been described anecdotally, but investigators using fMRI preoperatively should be aware of their existence (Lüdemann et al. 2006; Chen et al. 2008; Jiang et al. 2010; Pak et al. 2017).

2.2.1 Absent or Reduced BOLD Signal

Different pathological conditions can attenuate the hemodynamic response, which is the source of any BOLD fMRI signal. Brain tumor vessels typically lack cerebral autoregulation. Their vasculature is less responsive than that of the surrounding normal tissue. Intracranial space-occupying lesions can alter physiologic conditions. They may induce proliferation of pathologic vessels in the tissue adjacent to the lesion, thus altering the density, size, and topography of the vessels and consequently increase blood volume. The blood–brain barrier may break down within the tumor mass and partially extend into the tissue adjacent to the tumor. The mass effect of the lesion itself and the peritumoral vasogenic edema may change the apparent diffusion coefficient and therefore cause mechanical vascular compression. If, however, the brain's ability to autoregulate the flow of blood is completely lost in the brain tissue in the immediate vicinity to the tumor, which may still be functioning, this area may not respond to an increase in neural activity with a corresponding increase in blood flow and subsequent BOLD signal (Lüdemann et al. 2006; Chen et al. 2008; Pak et al. 2017). The biochemical environment (ade-

nosine 59-triphosphate, pH, glucose, lactate, etc.) and the cortical levels of neurotransmitters in and around gliomas might be altered. Specifically, the release of nitric oxide by reactive astrocytes and macrophages at the normal brain tissue-glioma interface may increase the "resting state" regional cerebral blood flow and thus alter the physiological hemodynamic response (Schreiber et al. 2000; Hund-Georgiadis et al. 2003; Fujiwara et al. 2004; Maravita and Iriki 2004; Agarwal et al. 2016). Similarly, therapeutic drugs administered to the patients may also interact with hemodynamic autoregulation (Seifritz et al. 2000; Braus and Brassen 2005). In regions more distant from the gliomas, where tumor vasculature is not encountered, the release of nitric oxide by reactive astrocytes and macrophages at the normal brain tissue–glioma interface may result in a luxury perfusion and reduced oxygen extraction fraction, resulting and leading to a reduced BOLD contrast enhancement (Schreiber et al. 2000).

2.2.2 Case of a Patient Showing an Inverted BOLD Signal Change

Importantly, the absence of fMRI activity in a particular brain region *does NOT mean* that there is no neuronal activity within this area and that it is thus safe to surgically remove this brain tissue. We will demonstrate this important point using the following case report: Fig. 1 illustrates fMRI activity during bilateral finger tapping versus rest in a patient with a left Rolandic tumor (glioma WHO grade II in the postcentral gyrus extending through the central sulcus into the "hand knob" of the precentral gyrus). In the non-lesioned right hemisphere, fMRI activity is observed within the right sensorimotor cortex (SM1; pre- and postcentral gyri), the right premotor cortex (PM), and right parietal cortex (PP). In contrast, in the lesioned left hemisphere fMRI activation is only observed anteriorly to the tumor in the left premotor cortex (PM). While this fMRI activation map might be interpreted as an absence of electrical neuronal activity within the left SM1 and PP areas (e.g., due to plastic changes and a take-over of motor function by the ipsilateral non-lesioned

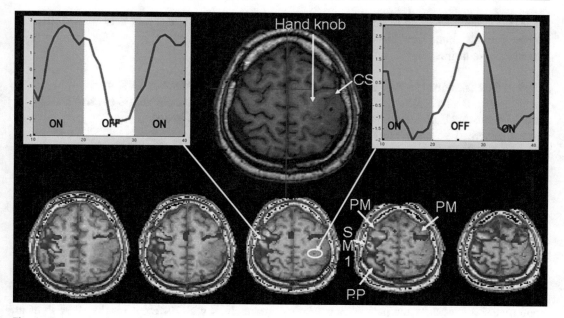

Fig. 1 Case study of a patient showing an inverted BOLD signal in the neighborhood of a lesion

hemisphere), the signal time-courses clearly show that this is a false conclusion. In the left-sided, tumor-infiltrated SM1 hand representation, the BOLD signals decrease during performance of the motor task, and increase during baseline condition (rest), i.e., an *inverse* BOLD MR signal change as compared to normal physiological activation. This finding may result from lesion-induced neurovascular uncoupling, where oxygen extraction (the cause of the initial dip of the BOLD signal) occurs without an increase in regional cerebral blood flow and volume (rCBF and rCBV), resulting in a steady decrease of fMRI signal despite an increased electrical neuronal activity driving the actual movements. As pointed out in an editorial by Bryan and Kraut (1998), these "negative results" deserve further study (Bryan and Kraut 1998; Sunaert et al. 1998). One may speculate that—depending on the lesion-induced hemodynamic changes in different patients—there could be continuous alterations of BOLD signals from "normal" via "absent" to "inverse." Possible BOLD-alterations should be taken into account when functional lateralization is determined using fMRI as they may lead to an incorrect interpretation of clinical fMRI data.

2.2.3 BOLD-Signal in Contrast Enhancing Parts of Brain Malignancies

In some patients with low or high-grade gliomas BOLD signal changes can be observed in those gliomas, which in principle should not contain functional tissue. This issue has been investigated in several studies (Skirboll et al. 1996; Schiffbauer et al. 2001; Ganslandt et al. 2004). From these studies using magnetic source imaging methods (which is a combination of EEG and anatomical MRI) it can be concluded that real functional activity might be located within or at the margins of the tumor in a considerable percentage of patients (e.g., 25% in the study of Schiffbauer et al. (2001), so that only partial resection is possible. The interpretation of this activity at the tumor margin remains ambiguous, either the cortex has been "displaced" by the growing tumor or is near the mark of being invaded by infiltrative tumor. Therefore, activated areas in tumor tissue are not always related to artifacts but could also be "real" functionally active tissue infiltrated by a tumor. If in doubt of the real or artificial nature of the activations, it is advised to combine different techniques (like MEG) to pinpoint the real nature of the BOLD signal change. More information about the combination of these different techniques can be found in chapter "Multimodal Functional Neuroimaging".

2.2.4 BOLD-Signal in Patients with Brain AVMs

Arteriovenous malformations (AVM) can produce widespread vascular steal effects beyond their nidus that preclude a normal hemodynamic response (for details see chapter "Presurgical Functional Localization Possibilities, Limitations, and Validity"). However, cerebral blood flow reductions do not necessarily cause cerebral dysfunction, as suggested in previous reports. Alterations of the microvascular architecture are prone to occur in the neighborhood of vascular malformations, and neovascularization is characteristic for malignant brain tumors and brain metastases of different pathologies, resulting in a change in the observed BOLD signal near the AVM. In addition, several studies in different patient populations with AVMs reported a shift of the functionally active regions close to the AVMs (Caramia et al. 2009). Vascular malformations are believed to form during gestation, and the development of these lesions and the associated brain damage due to hemorrhage or ischemia can lead to reorganization not only of the local anatomy but also of the functional cortex (Lehéricy et al. 2002). This can result in a cortical reorganization where the real functionally active region has been shifted into other previously defined functional regions (Maldjian et al. 1996; Fandino et al. 1999). Brain plasticity is discussed in detail in chapter "Brain Plasticity in fMRI and DTI."

When the neurovascular coupling cascade (from neuronal activity to the subsequent BOLD response) is interrupted at a certain level, one refers to this as the neurovascular uncoupling (NVU) phenomenon. As mentioned above this can be a critical problem in presurgical fMRI because of possible false negative or absence of activation near the lesion. Some researchers use cerebrovascular reactivity mapping techniques with carbon dioxide challenges or breath-holding techniques to detect possible regions with an altered cerebrovascular reactivity and thus a

potential NVU after brain activation (Pillai and Mikulis 2015).

2.3 The Effect of Different Pharmaceuticals on the BOLD fMRI Signal

Chemicals and pharmaceuticals can have an effect on different aspects of brain physiology and/or hemodynamic coupling (Seifritz et al. 2000; Braus and Brassen 2005). The next paragraph introduces some known effects of different substances on the BOLD signal.

2.3.1 Caffeine

The effect of caffeine—a vasoconstrictor—on BOLD signals has been studied by several researchers with different results (Parrish et al. 2001; Laurienti et al. 2002; Chen and Parrish 2009; Rack-Gomer et al. 2009; Merola et al. 2017). In an experiment determining the hemodynamic response function, volunteers were presented with a short visual flash to activate primary visual areas and to trigger a finger to thumb opposition. They were scanned in two consecutive sessions: before and after drinking three cups of coffee (~250 mg caffeine). The observed hemodynamic response function before and after administration of caffeine demonstrated a large increase (up to 50%) in BOLD signal after caffeine intake compared to the control session (Fig. 2a). This effect may be explained by the different properties of caffeine, i.e., its property to modulate neural activity and neurovascular tone. Caffeine influences the neurovascular tone and thus decreases the resting state CBF (Rack-Gomer et al. 2009). As a result, the increase in rCBF and respective BOLD signal change during stimulation is higher after caffeine intake. Caffeine also has an excitatory effect on neurons through the blockade of A1 adenosine receptors, thus increasing neural activity following stimulation (Parrish et al. 2001; Laurienti et al. 2002). On the other hand, caffeine can influence resting state connectivity in the brain, either as a direct effect on brain activity, or indirectly as a result of

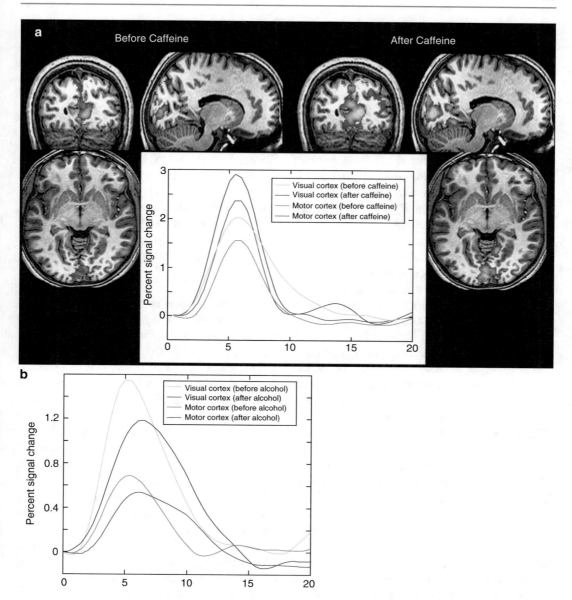

Fig. 2 (**a**) Activation maps and mean percent signal changes of the hemodynamic response function, following a visual flash trigger and a subsequent single fingertap, before and after drinking three cups of coffee (250 mg of caffeine). An increase in the hemodynamic response (hrf) can be seen in the visual and motor cortex after caffeine intake. (**b**) Mean signal change in the visual and motor cortex before and after drinking three glasses of beer (3.5 units of alcohol). Subjects followed a visual flash stimulus with a single finger tap. The resulting BOLD signal change decreased after alcohol intake

the influence of caffeine on the baseline and reactive cerebral blood flow. Therefore, one should be very careful while interpreting resting state fMRI data of patients (Rack-Gomer et al. 2009).

2.3.2 Alcohol

The effect of alcohol on BOLD signals is shown in Fig. 2b. A similar experiment to the one described above has been performed in volunteers before and after the consumption of three glasses of beer (~34 ml of alcohol). The graph shows that, as opposed to caffeine, alcohol leads to a decrease in the hemodynamic response. The effect of alcohol is twofold: First, alcohol is a vasodilator that increases the baseline CBF resulting in a smaller increase in rCBF and hence a lower relative BOLD signal after stimulation (Levin et al. 1998; Seifritz et al. 2000). Second, alcohol also decreases the on-task attention the subjects have to perform and consequently lowers the neuronal activation of the stimulated brain areas (Luchtmann et al. 2010).

2.3.3 Other Chemicals

It is also important to note that various pharmacological agents may potentially alter the BOLD signal. Cocaine, for example, influences neuronal connectivity (Li et al. 2000; Tomasi et al. 2010), neuronal activation, and cerebral blood flow in the resting state (Breiter et al. 1997; Lee et al. 2003; Lowen et al. 2009). However, the BOLD signal reportedly remains unaffected after cocaine administration (Gollub et al. 1998). Theophylline has been shown to increase the BOLD signal in the rat primary motor cortex (Morton et al. 2002), a phenomenon which has also been observed in patients with hyposmia where theophylline increased odor-induced BOLD responses (Levy et al. 1998). A decrease in cerebral blood flow in the resting condition, due to the vasoconstrictor response, might possibly account for the increased BOLD response after theophylline administration. Furthermore, theophylline has also known neuroexcitatory effects, e.g., as an antagonist of the inhibitory neurotransmitter adenosine. Via this mechanism, theophylline could increase the number of neurons that are activated in response to a given stimulus, consequently increasing the observed BOLD response (Morton et al. 2002). Acetazolamide is known to cause a depression of the BOLD response following a visual stimulus (Asghar et al. 2011) or a motor task, probably by increasing the baseline CBF.

On the other hand, nicotine—a drug without effects on local brain hemodynamics as

demonstrated in a simple visual task (Jacobsen et al. 2002)—has been demonstrated to increase attention to cognitive tasks both in patients with schizophrenia and in smokers (Kumari et al. 2003; Jacobsen et al. 2004) but has also been shown to change the resting state connectivity and possible subsequent stimulus-driven responses (Hahn et al. 2007; Warbrick et al. 2011). It is important to keep in mind that many other pharmacological agents, which have not yet been tested in this respect, may influence the BOLD response, and that patients with brain tumors may receive such pharmaceutical products (D'Esposito et al. 2003).

2.3.4 CO$_2$

Several studies report on the effect of CO$_2$ on the resting state BOLD signal and on the BOLD response during activation while inhaling a mixture of air and CO$_2$. CO$_2$ is a potent vasodilator and increases the BOLD signal. Breathing a mixture of air with 5% CO$_2$ increases the measured BOLD signal by 10% (Kastrup et al. 1998). This effect can have consequences on patient studies as well. Some patients show a change in the breathing rate during task performance, as a result of excitement and stress at the beginning of the experiment. This change in the breathing rate alters the oxygen supply to the brain and the CO$_2$ content in the blood, which affects vasodilatation and thus the global BOLD signal in the brain to an extent that it can interfere with the task-related BOLD response. When a volunteer is asked to change his breathing rate from normal breathing to hyperventilation and vice versa, the time-course of the BOLD signals clearly displays a large effect of hyperventilation on the resting state fMRI signal (Fig. 3), this effect could also be used to map the cerebrovascular response of the brain (Liu et al. 2020). Therefore, in order to minimize effects of anxiousness and the change in breathing rate in clinical fMRI studies, it is very important to instruct and comfort the patients comprehensively and allow them to familiarize themselves with the scanner environment before initiation of the experiment. RsfMRI exams, which are not

Fig. 3 Effect of hyperventilation on the BOLD resting state signal. During the scanning session the volunteer switched from hyperventilation periods to breath-holding periods of 24 s. The activation map shows MR signal changes following the breath-holding/hyperventilation paradigm in the volunteer's entire cortex. The MR signal time trace in the bottom of the figure clearly demonstrates the signal fluctuation for a random voxel in the cortex

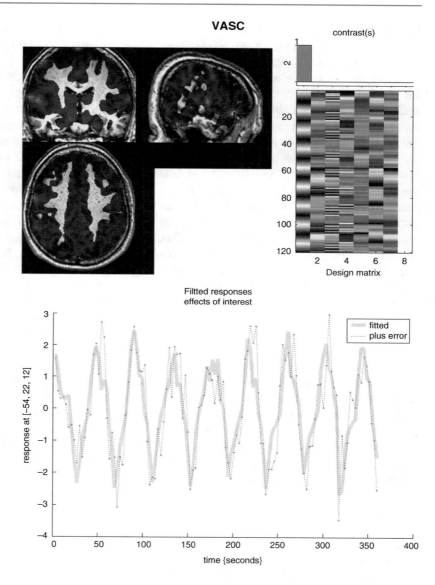

driven by external stimuli (see also chapter "Presurgical Resting-State fMRI"), are even more susceptible to changes in breathing rate and cardiac cycle. Thus, careful instruction of the patients, and possibly also monitoring functions of the autonomic nervous system (ANS), heart rate, and breathing pace could improve rsfMRI results (Iacovella and Hasson 2011; Murphy et al. 2013; Kasper et al. 2017).

3 The Influence of Brain Lesions on DTI Results

The patient's lesion can influence native DTI images as well as the resulting fractional anisotropy (FA) maps and finally the fiber tracking. Degenerative diseases and demyelination disorders will reduce the measured FA values focally as observed, e.g., in amyotrophic lateral sclerosis (Sage et al. 2009; Kalra et al. 2020), multiple sclerosis (Reich et al. 2008), and Alzheimer's disease (Kantarci et al. 2010). Also in stroke patients local changes in white matter FA can occur (Visser et al. 2019). More confined brain lesions can also influence the measured FA and diffusivity. Vasogenic edema reduce the local fiber density hereby lowering the measured FA, which in turn will influence how many fibers will be reconstructed around the respective lesion by the fiber tracking algorithm (Bizzi et al. 2012). Tumoral tissue can also destroy white matter fibers by reducing the number of intact axons (Sinha et al. 2002). Radiation therapy of brain tumors also induces microstructural damage of the white matter resulting in global interhemispheric FA changes (Kassubek et al. 2017). On the other hand, in an abscess cavity the FA values are higher, which possibly reflects organized and oriented inflammatory cells (Toh et al. 2011).

The distorted anatomy due to a lesion's mass effect makes it difficult to position the tracking ROIs at the correct position needed to ensure reliable and reproducible fiber tracking. One solution for this problem might be to use fMRI activation regions as seed ROIs for fiber tractography, herewith using functional information for a better understanding of the structural status and its alterations (Kleiser et al. 2010).

4 Patient-Related Artifacts and Physiological Noise

4.1 Flow and Pulsation Artifacts

Flow artifacts arise due to the pulsating in- and outflow of the blood perpendicular to the imaging slices, hereby producing signal changes in different slices. At 1.5 T these artifacts are especially observed in pathological flow conditions such as in AVMs. However, with the trend towards using higher magnetic field strengths (3 T and above) flow and pulsation artifacts become more prominent (Biswal et al. 1996; Srivastava et al. 2005). These artifacts manifest themselves as a slowly varying signal change with a sinusoidal rhythm, which is the result of an undersampling of the underlying blood pulsation. Figure 4 shows a pulsation artifact that occurred in an fMRI experiment acquired at 3 T without any specific brain activation, and one can see several tubular shaped regions with a signal intensity of sinusoidal shape. If the stimulation paradigm shows a period similar to the period of this sine wave (in this case a period of 100 s), these areas will light up as false positives (Dagli et al. 1999). RsfMRI data are also very sensitive to such artifacts as these sinusoidal signal time traces do temporally very closely resemble real synchronized brain activation in

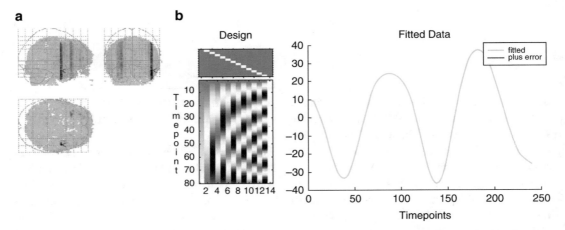

Fig. 4 Example of a pulsation artifact: 80 dynamic resting state BOLD scans were acquired with a TR of 3 s during 4 min in a volunteer. (**a**) Pulsation artifacts show up as tubuli-like BOLD fMRI activation regions. (**b**) The fitted time-course of the signal in this structure has a sinusoidal shape with a period of 100 s

different areas constituting the respective functional network (Kasper et al. 2017).

4.2 Artifacts from Bulk Head Motion

The small intensity changes typically observed in fMRI images (ranging from a fraction of 1% signal change to a few percent) can easily be contaminated by a variety of sources. In clinical fMRI the major contribution to signal artifacts arise from bulk head motion during acquisition of the functional data series (Seto et al. 2001). A further minor contribution originates from physiological brain motion (pulsation of the brain, overlying vessels, and cerebrospinal fluid) driven by cardiac and CSF pulsations (Dagli et al. 1999; Windischberger et al. 2002; Kiviniemi et al. 2016). Nevertheless, the primary reason for failed clinical fMRI examinations is head motion. In the study of the most frequent cause for the failure of 15% of their clinical exams was due to head movement artifacts (Krings 2001a). In a more recent study, Tyndall et al. (2017) achieved a success rate of 95% in their clinical presurgical exams by using individual patient training and instructions to minimize head motion.

The motion of the patient and its effect on a fMRI time series acquisition can be divided into two separate categories: Intra-image motion which is generally a very fast and sudden motion (i.e., at a time scale smaller than the image acquisition time), and inter-image motion on a time scale between a couple of seconds to minutes reflected in a slow movement of the subject (i.e., at a time scale larger than the time necessary to acquire a single image volume). These two subcategories of motion have different effects on the acquired images and functional map properties. The intra-image motion, typically induced by sudden head movement, results in "blurring" and "ghosting" in older GE-based acquisition sequences, and is less present in single shot echoplanar imaging, where all data for an image are collected in less than 100 ms (Duerk and Simonetti 1991). However, if present, this sudden motion can have the following effects on EPI images: if the motion is very fast (<100 ms) it can still cause ghosting artifacts in several slices of the acquired volume. Slower, longer lasting motion can also change image contrast, this especially applies to motion perpendicular to the acquisition plane. The latter will result in a change of the apparent repetition time for the acquisition of the same slice in the different volume (Fig. 5) which changes the T1 weighting of

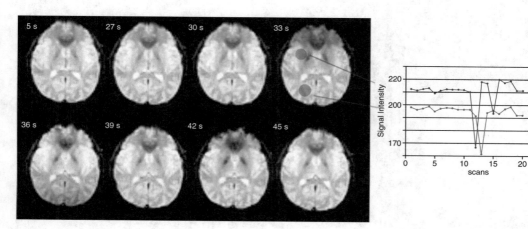

Fig. 5 Different time points in a fMRI series (TR = 3 s) of a volunteer. During the scan, he moved his head through the plane of acquisition. The time trace shown on the right displays the signal intensity change of the voxels in the filled regions, a large motion-induced signal drop is apparent resulting from this through-plane motion at around scan 11 (30 s)

the tissue for the different slices and thus the signal intensity of the tissue. In other words, the tissue has experienced a different "spin history" (Friston et al. 1996b; Muresan et al. 2005).

In resting state fMRI motion-related confounds can be even more troublesome. Motion artifacts have a differential effect on resting BOLD signal and can largely influence connectivity measures.

Even subtle motion artifacts <0.5 mm can provoke a specific bias increasing short range connections while decreasing long-range connections which can result in group differences between certain patient groups which will generally suffer from more motion than healthy controls (Power et al. 2013). Large head motion during the acquisition on the other hand can also increase long-range connectivity (Satterthwaite et al. 2019).

Motion on a time scale larger than the image acquisition time causes a misregistration of the images within the time series, and makes activation foci undetectable or, even worse, induces artificial activation when the motion is temporally correlated to the stimulus (Hajnal et al. 1994, Fig. 6). This will especially have an effect in those brain regions that show steep image intensity gradients (e.g., at the edges of the brain or in patients at the border of a T2 hyperintense lesion), which are particularly prone to these artifacts. The effect of this inter-image motion has been shown to be particularly problematic in clinical examinations. Results from Hill et al. (2000) indicate that in patients with epilepsy the head motion was more prevalent and had a larger amplitude compared to healthy volunteers.

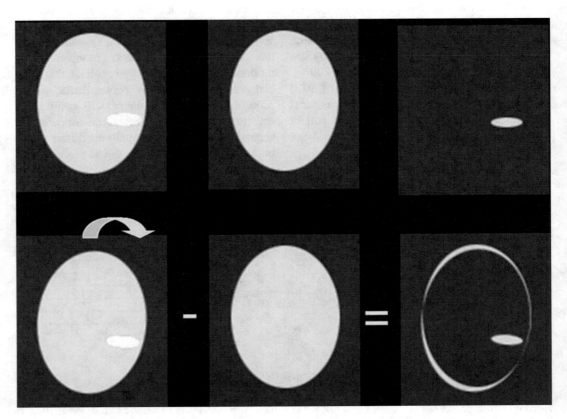

Fig. 6 Simulation of head motion between different activation states and its effect on the observed activation in a subtraction map. In the top row without motion only the real activated region is discerned, in the bottom row, on the other hand, motion between both images is introduced and a rim of false activation appears in the subtraction map

4.2.1 Minimizing and Correcting for Motion

Several solutions exist to correct for or to minimize inter-image motion that have been proposed by several researchers. Head movement during the acquisition phase can be restricted by fixation of the head with molds and straps (Fitzsimmons et al. 1997; Edward et al. 2000; Debus et al. 2008), which represents an intermediate level of head fixation. The use of a "bitebar" (Fig. 7)—a custom molded dental fixation, regularly used in our institution to restrain head motion while

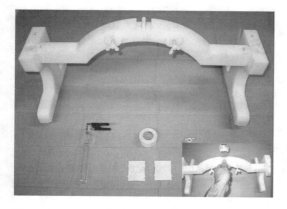

Fig. 7 A custom build bite-bar system used to minimize patient motion during the fMRI experiment. It consists of a plastic bridge which is positioned over the subject's shoulder and a small detachable piece which the subject puts in his mouth

imaging volunteers—provides a highly rigid fixation, but can only be used in a limited number of patients (Dymarkowski et al. 1998). The presence of dental prosthesis interferes, and not all patients tolerate this kind of fixation. Furthermore, safety precautions preclude its use in those patients who are at risk of having epileptic seizures during imaging (Jiang et al. 1995; Freire and Mangin 2001).

Another solution is the use of motion correction algorithms during data post-processing, which are nowadays integrated in most fMRI analysis software tools. Motion correction is typically achieved by the rigid realignment of the consecutively acquired images in the data series with the first image (or an arbitrary other image of the time series) (Friston et al. 1995, 1996b; Caballero-Gaudes and Reynolds 2017). If the patient moves with a frequency unrelated to the frequency of the applied stimulation paradigm, this realignment post-processing can successfully separate this motion caused by the patient himself from true activation (Fig. 8). As most motion correction algorithms are intensity-based, it is also possible that false motion is observed in the time series which may actually be the result of a large activation at a specific brain region shifting the center of intensity to a certain direction following the activation paradigm (Biswal and Hyde 1997).

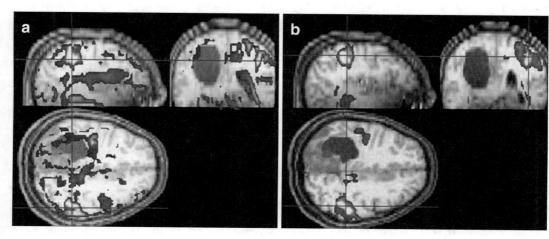

Fig. 8 Effect of subject motion on the resulting fMRI activation map of a patient (**a**) and the effect of motion correction (**b**) on the observed real and false motion-induced activation in the resulting calculated fMRI activation map

However, most of the patient motion is attributed to the applied stimulus (Hill et al. 2000), which is certainly the case if the patient is performing different motor paradigms (e.g., the patient is moving his head at the start of the task for looking at his fingers performing the task). This effect cannot be easily separated from the real functional activation due to their temporal synchrony (Hajnal et al. 1994).

The problem of patient motion could be further reduced in a number of different ways. First, stimulation paradigms can be optimized to minimize head motion. Much attention is given to differences in anatomic-functional information that can be obtained from active versus passive tasks which will inherently reduce motion (Gasser et al. 2004). Also, resting state fMRI does not suffer from task-based patient motion as no active task is performed (see also chapter "Presurgical Resting-State fMRI").

As described earlier the effect of through-plane motion is a combination of a misregistration of different subsequent BOLD images with the T1-weighted slice effect varying the signal intensity resulting from changes in TR. Therefore, it is recommended to adapt the scanning planes in such a way that the maximal observed motion is in parallel to the acquisition plane, e.g., if head nodding is expected from left to right, axial slices should be acquired. However, if head motion is expected from front to back, sagittal slices should be obtained. There are also techniques to correct for spin history effects due to through-plane motion (Muresan et al. 2005).

Adapted acquisition sequences have been presented that change the position of the acquired EPI volume in order to prospectively adapt for the motion of the subject. For this, subject motion has to be calculated online between two consecutively acquired volumes which can be done on the images itself or by calculation of the position of external markers using laser guidance or separate video cameras (Qin et al. 2009; Zaitsev et al. 2017). This information can then be used to predict the position of the head for the following (third) acquisition. This technique thus uses a prospective motion correction algorithm in contrast to the retrospective motion correction techniques used in fMRI postprocessing software tools. As the scan planes are adapted to the motion, the T1-weighted slice effect is also diminished (Ward et al. 2000; Thesen et al. 2000; Maclaren et al. 2013).

If motion artifacts still persist in the resulting BOLD activation maps, there is an option in most software packages to incorporate the motion parameters calculated in the preprocessing step in the statistical calculation of the functional activation (e.g., using the general linear model (GLM)). In doing so the signal variability within the voxels, correlating with these motion parameters, will be reflected in this contrast hereby decreasing the influence of the motion-induced signal changes in the other conditions (contrasts) of interest of the stimulation paradigm. Although this will effectively remove motion-induced "false" activations it can also remove or decrease "real activation" ascribed to motion (Johnstone et al. 2006).

For further information on fMRI data processing see also chapter "Revealing Brain Activity and White Matter Structure Using Functional and Diffusion-Weighted Magnetic Resonance Imaging."

4.2.2 How to Distinguish Real Activation from Motion Induced False Activation

If it is not possible to completely eliminate motion during image acquisition and data processing (e.g., in the case of paradigm-related motion), motion artifacts need to be identified in the activation maps. This paragraph provides some practical tips to distinguish motion-induced "false activations" from the "real activation" of the BOLD signal. Most of the motion-induced "false activations" are localized at the border of different structures which show large signal intensity gradients (Weisskoff 1995; Orchard and Atkins 2003). These motion-induced signal changes at the tumor borders typically have a ring-like spatial appearance, in other words they are observed as a thin rim of hyperactivation in the neighborhood of large image intensity gradients (Fig. 6 (simulation), 8 and 9). The BOLD hemodynamic response curve typically rises 4 s after onset of the stimulation and reaches its maximum after 6–8 s. If the movement follows the paradigm, the onset of the movement will be at the same time as the onset of the paradigm. Movement-related signal changes will follow the movements instantaneously. Therefore, the temporal profile of the movement-related "false activations" will temporally coincide with the different conditions of the block-design and will occur prior to the physiologically delayed hemodynamic response, which reflects the "real activation" temporal profile (which typically has a delay of approximately 2–4 s compared to the stimulation onset). The signal intensity variation will also be more abrupt compared to the more gradual activation-induced BOLD signal intensity change. Movement-related signal changes also tend to display much higher signal intensity changes as compared to physiological BOLD signal changes (Fig. 9).

4.3   Motion Artifacts in DTI

Typically, DTI scans require between 5 and 20 min for the acquisition of an entire brain volume data set. Subject movement during this scan time can result in motion artifacts on the different diffusion-encoded images. These artifacts can manifest themselves differently according to the amplitude and speed of the patient movement. Slight movement occurring during the 5–20 min of scanning will result in a misalignment of the different diffusion-weighted images. In the postprocessing steps of the DTI dataset the different data volumes should then be realigned by registration to, e.g., the b_0-image, but attention should be paid that the orientation information of the applied diffusion gradients should also be rotated according to the images' orientation (Leemans and Jones 2009). Large and fast movements will result in large signal dropouts and interleave artifacts (Fig. 10). These large artifacts will disturb

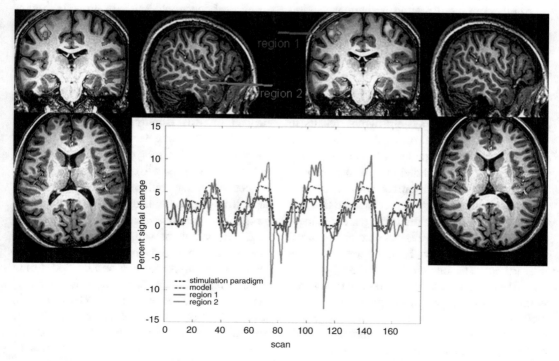

Fig. 9 fMRI activation map of a volunteer who moved (left) and did not move (right). Signal time-courses in a motion-related region (light) and a real activation region (dark) demonstrate the temporal mismatch between both signal traces and between the motion-related signal change and the model of activation

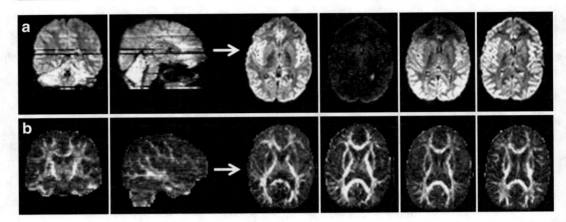

Fig. 10 An example of motion-corrupted diffusion-weighted images. (**a**) The native diffusion-weighted axial images show a loss of signal at those slices where large motion was apparent. (**b**) The calculated FA maps from these images also suffer intensity changes due to this motion but these are less apparent

the resulting DTI maps if they are not identified. Different software solutions exist which can trace these signal dropouts and exclude them from further data analysis (Tournier et al. 2011; Chen et al. 2015).

Another problem related to patient motion but induced by the diffusion gradients themselves are the so-called vibration artifacts (Gallichan et al. 2010; Mohammadi et al. 2012) which typically manifests as a signal loss in a large region of the mesial parietal lobe (Fig. 11). Strong diffusion gradients cause low-frequency vibrations of the MR system, which results in vibration of the patient table. When the patient is well fixated to the table with pads this table vibration will be translated into head motion of the patient that is synchronized with the applied diffusion gradient. It has been observed that this artifact is largest when the left-right component (X-gradient) of the diffusion gradient is large. Different solutions have been proposed to avoid this artifact. The uncoupling of the table from the MR system could result in less synchronized motion of the subject resulting in lower artifacts. A full k-space acquisition or a longer TR between consecutive scans can also reduce this artifact (Gallichan et al. 2010). Finally, combined acquisition and post-processing methods have been proposed to eliminate such artifacts (Mohammadi et al. 2012).

4.4 Patient Cooperation

Patient cooperation during the task-based fMRI exam is very important; therefore, control of task performance during the scanning is a prerequisite for clinical functional MRI. In an active motor task, cameras are very handy to observe whether the patient understands and performs the task correctly. In patients with limited ability to cooperate, direct instruction plus direct supervision of proper task performance by the investigator standing next to the scanner is strongly recommended. In visual experiments, it is important to monitor eye movements using an eye-tracking camera. Figure 12 displays the difference in activation maps between a fixating and a non-fixating subject in a visual retinotopic mapping experiment. In cognitive and language tasks, an indirect control can be implemented in the paradigm. Cognitive paradigms can be devised in such a way that the patient has to respond by pressing a button. These responses can be recorded during the scanning and controlled afterwards for correctness. Also in resting state fMRI cooperation of the patient is necessary, e.g., there already are large differences in brain activation synchrony patterns between "eyes open" and "eyes closed" scans (Zou et al. 2009).

It is very important to precisely inform and instruct the patients before scanning about what

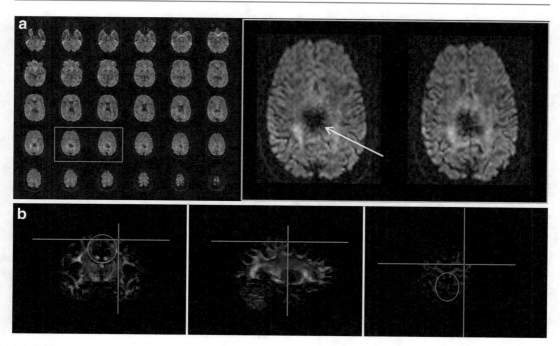

Fig. 11 (**a**) Cross-sections of diffusion-weighted images show a vibration artifact located mainly in the mesial parietal lobe when a large diffusion gradient is switched on in the left-right direction. (**b**) Colored fractional anisotropy maps displaying artifactual left right dominance in the mesial parietal lobe

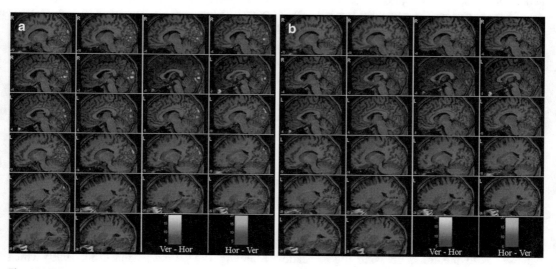

Fig. 12 Effect when the subject is not cooperating during the fMRI exam: (**a**) a retinotopic map of a subject fixating the middle of the visual stimulus (alternating horizontal and vertical wedges). (**b**) Retinotopic map of the same subject looking around (i.e., not fixating) during the fMRI exam

is expected from them to do during the exam in order to complete a successful examination (Tyndall et al. 2017). Real-time fMRI analysis is possible on most modern MRI scanners and allows for a direct control of the experimental success so that a failed functional session can be repeated immediately afterwards, which is much less time demanding then asking the patient to come back after a couple of days for an additional scanning session (Schwindack et al. 2005).

5 Technology Related Artifacts

5.1 Susceptibility Artifacts in BOLD fMRI and DTI

Almost all BOLD fMRI acquisitions and DTI acquisitions are performed with multi-slice single shot EPI acquisition sequences. These techniques have a very high temporal resolution and are very sensitive to the BOLD effect, which manifests itself as a change in susceptibility in the activated regions. But these single shot EPI sequences also suffer from distortion and susceptibility artifacts as a result of their high T2*-weighting and resulting high sensitivity to susceptibility (Devlin et al. 2000). In most fMRI studies these drawbacks are of less importance and do not weigh up the vast advantages of the EPI technique to both detect and localize brain activation. But the susceptibility-related signal drop in those brain areas which are located in the skull base and in the neighborhood of large air cavities like the orbitofrontal cortex and the anterior and medial temporal cortex pose a problem for fMRI studies where brain activation in these areas is expected (Friston et al. 1996a; Devlin et al. 2000; O'Doherty et al. 2000; Small et al. 2004). In patients this effect can also be observed adjacent to metal implants or certain types of lesions (e.g., lesions containing deoxyhemoglobin or hemosiderin), where the susceptibility difference between the lesion and the surrounding brain tissue is large (Håberg et al. 2004) and also signal voids can be observed in regions close to surgical resection cavities in post-operative patients. With the trend of using higher static magnetic field strengths, this effect of local signal loss and image distortion is even more pronounced (Abduljalil and Robitaille 1999; Lima Cardoso et al. 2018). For clinical fMRI these artifacts pose a problem both for studies searching for activated regions in the orbitofrontal cortex (like taste and smell related regions, emotional processing) (Deichmann et al. 2003; Smits et al.

2007) or anterior temporal cortex (regions responsible for object recognition) (Devlin et al. 2000).

5.1.1 Methods to Decrease Susceptibility-Related Artifacts

Different strategies for experiments in susceptibility-prone regions have been proposed including the use of other less susceptibility sensitive acquisition sequences like multi-shot EPI sequences, spin echo EPI sequences, flash sequences (Menon et al. 1997), T2Prep BOLD sequences (Hua et al. 2014), or balanced SSFP sequences (Chen et al. 2017). Despite the gain in signal, these other types of sequences and methods suffer from reduced temporal resolution, temporal stability, spatial resolution, and/or contrast/signal-to-noise ratio (Song et al. 2000). On the other hand, various ingenious image processing methods have also been developed to recover the local signal and reduce image distortions from EPI images by using, e.g., fieldmaps (Jezzard and Balaban 1995) or extra reversed phase encoding acquisitions (Andersson et al. 2003). Other methods proposed to reduce local signal loss in EPI sequences are (1) decreasing the slice thickness of the acquired images, (2) minimizing the slice-induced susceptibility artifacts (Hoogenraad et al. 2000), (3) local higher order shimming to decrease local magnetic field inhomogeneity (Deichmann et al. 2003), employing magnetic field monitoring hardware to measure field differences and correct distortions (Wilm et al. 2015), (4) maximizing the readout bandwidth in order to minimize the EPI echo train length, which in turn decreases the T2* decay and thus susceptibility effects but increases noise in the images. Another solution is the use of parallel imaging techniques (Sodickson and Manning 1997; Pruessmann et al. 1999) which have the potential to decrease the problems inherent to single shot EPI imaging sequences, making it possible to perform fMRI studies in those brain areas which suffer from large susceptibility artifacts in standard single shot BOLD fMRI experiments (Preibisch et al. 2003). In these methods receiver coil arrays consisting of a combination of a number of receiver coils (ranging from 2 to

96 elements) (De Zwart et al. 2002; Keil et al. 2013) are used. The spatial inhomogeneity and differential sensitivity of the separate elements are employed to decrease the number of acquired phase encoding steps for every separate coil element by combining the different resulting images or raw data into one new reconstructed image (Sodickson and Manning 1997; Pruessmann et al. 1999). As a result, this reduces the number of acquired phase encoding steps and thus the EPI readout train length. In BOLD fMRI experi-

ments, this decrease in phase encoding steps during a single readout step entails a decline of susceptibility-related artifacts. The potential of parallel imaging techniques has been demonstrated in several studies at all field strengths (Schmidt et al. 2002; Preibisch et al. 2003; Moeller et al. 2010). The advantage of parallel imaging techniques is shown in Fig. 13 demonstrating the gain of geometric correctness by using higher parallel imaging factors. In Fig. 14 the loss of signal intensity is calculated and rep-

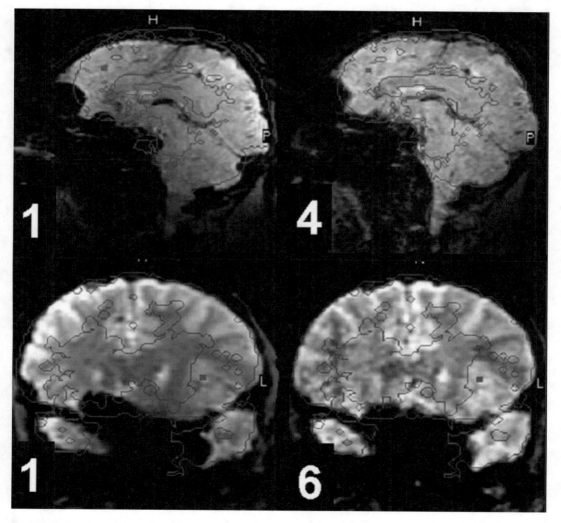

Fig. 13 Comparison of the geometrical distortion of both NO-SENSE (without parallel imaging) and SENSE (with parallel imaging) images acquired in the sagittal (top row) and coronal plane (bottom row). The black border lines delineate the boundaries of the anatomical 3D T1 image, demonstrating a large improvement of geometric compliance using parallel imaging. The number on the images represents the SENSE acceleration factor

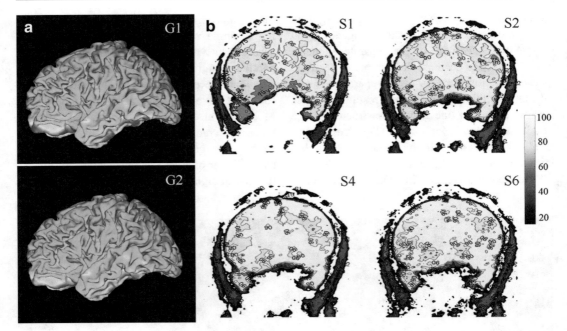

Fig. 14 (a) Signal loss maps on a rendered brain of an EPI acquisition without (above) and with GRAPPA acquisition (below). The dark red regions are those, which suffer the largest signal intensity loss. Note the difference between the grappa factor 2 (smaller, less intense dark red areas) and non-grappa images (large dark red regions). (b) Percentage signal intensity in two different coronal EPI slices acquired with different SENSE factors compared to the mean brain signal intensity of the same slice. The dark (orange/red) areas in the slices suffer a signal loss higher than 40%. The maps demonstrate that images acquired without SENSE (S1) display a larger and a more inhomogeneous signal loss as compared to the scans with a high parallel imaging factor in the susceptibility sensitive areas. The number next to the images represents the SENSE factor used

resented for images acquired with different parallel imaging factors. The drawback of the use of high SENSE factors is the increase of noise in the images especially in central regions, which is clearly visible when using very high parallel imaging factors (Fig. 13, right images). Therefore, it is recommended to only use very high SENSE factors when it is really necessary and when enough separate coil elements are available, e.g., when looking for activations in the orbitofrontal or anterior temporal regions of the respective lobes.

Acquisition-related susceptibility effects can also give rise to the following question: If an expected activation in a certain region cannot be found, is this a true non-activation or a susceptibility effect? On the other hand, activated regions can be encountered in unexpected areas. Possible ways to overcome this problem are first to look at

the original (not post-processed) images and to check whether raw BOLD signal is present in this region or not, and second to acquire a B0 field map, which can be automatically generated on most modern scanners. In such a B0 field map two different scans with a different echo time (TE) are combined for local T2* decay calculation, hereby highlighting regions suffering from large susceptibility effects. This field map can then be used to mask the fMRI maps to visualize only these areas where artifacts are indiscernible (Hutton et al. 2002).

5.2 Multiband Artifacts

Recently simultaneous multiple slice acquisition techniques have been developed which accelerate the acquisition of EPI volumes by a factor of 2 up to 12, and dramatically increase the temporal and/or the spatial resolution of both BOLD fMRI and DWI acquisitions and present a possible leap forward for all types of fMRI and DWI acquisitions (Feinberg et al. 2010; Smith et al. 2013). However, these techniques also introduce a new type of multiband related artifacts in the BOLD fMRI and DTI scans, which manifest themselves as signal overlap from a certain slice into another simultaneously excited/acquired slice (Xu et al. 2013; Todd et al. 2016). The reason for this is that it is difficult to correctly separate the simultaneously acquired slices.

Another artifact that can also be more prominent in multiband acquisitions is the parallel imaging artifact, the signal repeats within a slice as a result of a partially failed SENSE unfolding of the data. These artifacts are more prone to occur with high multiband acceleration factors (higher than 2) used in the EPI images as the distance between the simultaneously acquired slices is lower, the artifacts are

also more problematic near air tissue boundaries (Fig. 15) and can also result in false positive activation in the BOLD fMRI scans in regions of different non-adjacent simultaneously acquired slices (Todd et al. 2016). These leakage/unfolding artifacts can be diminished by using adapted reconstruction techniques (Cauley et al. 2014) by using moderate acceleration values (Fig. 15) and by increasing the homogeneity of the local magnetic field using higher order local shimming.

5.3 Sensitivity of EPI Sequences to Spikes

Spikes in MR images arise from external interferences and can generate large signal changes in the affected images (Zhang et al. 2001). If you suspect that a fMRI time series contains spikes, the signal time-course of the activated regions has to be carefully analyzed, since spikes will

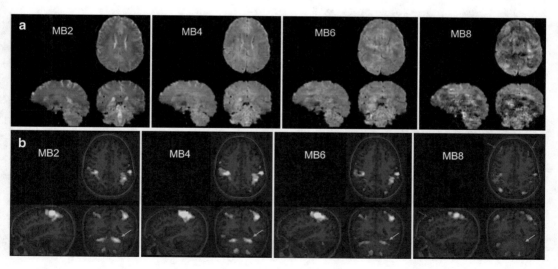

Fig. 15 Artifacts manifesting with higher multiband factors on axial BOLD fMRI EPI images acquired with multiband SENSE factors 2, 4, 6, 8, respectively, and an in-plane SENSE factor of 2. (**a**) Artifacts visible on the native images. Notice the dark/bright bands, very subtle on the MB4 images but clearly visible in the MB6 images and dominating the images acquired with MB8. (**b**) Activation maps of the volunteer performing a simple fin-

ger tapping motor task demonstrating the effect of the artifacts on the resulting BOLD maps. Notice the overall decrease of significant activation with the higher MB values. The light green arrow shows false deactivation of the cerebellum in the scans with MB factor 8. The dark red arrows in the MB8 scans show on the other hand a suspected false positive activation due to slice signal leakage and in-plane SENSE unfolding issues

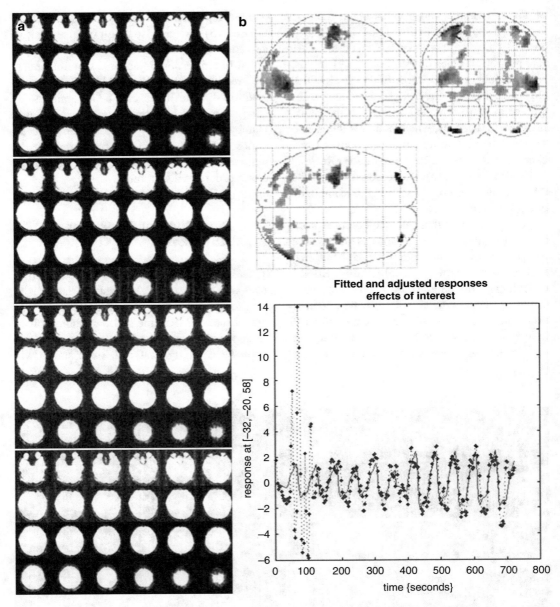

Fig. 16 (**a**) Spikes apparent in the fMRI time trace induced by opening the door of the Faraday cage during the acquisition of an fMRI exam. (**b**) The signal changes induced by the spikes are around 20% and much higher than the motor task-induced signal change (red circle)

typically change the signal in the order of tens of percent, and are also easily observed in the original images. In DTI images, spikes can also be a major source of artifacts. If spikes are assumed to be present, all separate b-vector images should be checked, and the image volumes containing spikes should be removed from DTI analyses by the post-processing software (Tournier et al. 2011). To eliminate spikes in images it should be inspected, if the Faraday cage had been closed and intact during image acquisition, scanning with an open door is troublesome (Fig. 16: The effect of opening the door of the Faraday cage during an fMRI scan). Sometimes spikes can also arise from an external device in the scanner room, loose bolts in the scanner or a broken lamp in the ceiling. Therefore, it is recommended to switch off unnecessary electrical devices or, even better, to remove them from the scanner room. Alternatively, spikes can be scanner-related and, in this case, the scanner service team should be contacted.

5.4 Eddy Current-Induced Distortions in DTI

When an MR gradient pulse is switched on, this will result in a current induction in conductive parts of the MRI scanner (Gradient coils, RF coils, shim irons, …) called eddy currents. These eddy currents in turn will generate magnetic field gradients, which can last longer than the applied primary gradients. When using fast sequences or strong gradients these eddy currents induce extra gradient fields, which will distort the images being acquired by incorrect encoding of the position in the images. Although BOLD fMRI scans will also suffer from eddy currents, the effect on the quality of the resulting DTI maps will be much higher. In DTI, for every direction of the b-vector different gradients and strengths are switched on and off resulting in possibly different eddy current-induced artifacts for every direction of b-vector. The eddy current artifacts manifest themselves mainly as image distortions like contractions of the images in a single direction, as well as shifts and shears of the images (Le Bihan et al. 2006). Eddy currents can be reduced by optimally adjusting and calibrating the gradient settings to counteract and minimize induced currents (Aliotta et al. 2018), and by using specifically designed self-shielded gradients (which is standard in modern MRI scanners nowadays). Although these hardware adaptations will minimize eddy currents, there will still be other negative effects which may possibly be corrected by different post-processing software tools (Jones and Cercignani 2010; Andersson and Sotiropoulos 2016).

6 Statistical Post-processing "Artifacts"

Generation of functional activation maps in an fMRI experiment requires independent statistical analysis of each of the many voxels in the brain. The hypothesis in testing each voxel is based on the assumption that there is no effect of the task compared to the baseline condition, as statistical analysis implies making a decision as to whether or not this null hypothesis is true or false. A type I error constitutes a false positive, i.e., a decision stating that the voxel is showing a difference in activation during the condition of interest when in reality it does not. A type II error represents a false negative, i.e., an assumption claiming that there is no activation at this voxel when in reality there is one (Desmond and Annabel Chen 2002).

In basic neuroscience studies, statistical analysis is essentially designed to prevent false positives: The colored activation maps show where an activation different from zero can be expected. Since fMRI measurements are intrinsically noisy, this always leads to a relative high number of false negatives: Areas with real neuronal activation but large physiological and/or technique-dependent noise will not be visible on activation maps. For clinical fMRI applications, it has to be considered whether false positives or false negatives may have more deleterious consequences for the patient. For example, in the presurgical planning for the resection of pathologic brain regions, false positives (type I errors) may bias the surgeon to avoid the resection of areas that may not be so important to be removed. This could result in an incomplete removal of the brain lesion. In contrast, false negatives (type II errors) may bias the surgeon to remove too much tissue, possibly leading to an irreversible deficit in function. Therefore, clinical fMRI data should be analyzed differently than basic neuroscience data. More research is required for discovering a new method for clinical fMRI analysis, which may allow the assessment of both type I and type II errors (Voyvodic et al. 2009; Durnez et al. 2013; Gross and Binder 2014). For instance, each voxel that has not reached significance could be tested to find out whether an fMRI response of a certain magnitude (such as 0.5% MR signal change) would have reached significance if the signal-to-noise ratio in that voxel had been higher. This would lead to a separate confidence color map showing voxels with low signal change and noisy voxels, as well as areas where artifacts or signal dropouts would otherwise not allow potential activation to be detected.

References

Abduljalil AM, Robitaille PM (1999) Macroscopic susceptibility in ultra high field MRI. J Comput Assist Tomogr 23:832–841

Agarwal S, Sair HI, Yahyavi-Firouz-Abadi N, Airan R, Pillai JJ (2016) Neurovascular uncoupling in resting state fMRI demonstrated in patients with primary brain gliomas. J Magn Reson Imaging 43:620–626. https://doi.org/10.1002/jmri.25012

Aguirre GK, Zarahn E, D'Esposito M (1998) The variability of human, BOLD hemodynamic responses. NeuroImage 8:360–369. https://doi.org/10.1006/nimg.1998.0369

Aliotta E, Moulin K, Ennis DB (2018) Eddy current–nulled convex optimized diffusion encoding (EN-CODE) for distortion-free diffusion tensor imaging with short echo times. Magn Reson Med 79:663–672. https://doi.org/10.1002/mrm.26709

Andersson JLR, Sotiropoulos SN (2016) An integrated approach to correction for off-resonance effects and subject movement in diffusion MR imaging. NeuroImage 125:1063–1078. https://doi.org/10.1016/j.neuroimage.2015.10.019

Andersson JLR, Skare S, Ashburner J (2003) How to correct susceptibility distortions in spin-echo echo-planar images: application to diffusion tensor imaging. NeuroImage 20:870–888. https://doi.org/10.1016/S1053-8119(03)00336-7

Asghar MS, Hansen AE, Pedersen S, Larsson HBW, Ashina M (2011) Pharmacological modulation of the bOLD response: a study of acetazolamide and glyceryl trinitrate in humans. J Magn Reson Imaging 34:921–927. https://doi.org/10.1002/jmri.22659

Baudendistel KT, Reichenbach JR, Metzner R, Schroeder J, Schad LR (1998) Comparison of functional MR-venography and EPI-BOLD fMRI at 1.5 T. Magn Reson Imaging 16:989–991

Biswal BB, Hyde JS (1997) Contour-based registration technique to differentiate between task-activated and head motion-induced signal variations in fMRI. Magn Reson Med 38:470–476

Biswal B, DeYoe AE, Hyde JS (1996) Reduction of physiological fluctuations in fMRI using digital filters. Magn Reson Med 35:107–113

Bizzi A, Nava S, Ferrè F, Castelli G, Aquino D, Ciaraffa F, Broggi G, DiMeco F, Piacentini S (2012) Aphasia induced by gliomas growing in the ventrolateral frontal region: assessment with diffusion MR tractography, functional MR imaging and neuropsychology. Cortex 48:255–272. https://doi.org/10.1016/j.cortex.2011.11.015

Boxerman JL, Bandettini PA, Kwong KK, Baker JR, Davis TL, Rosen BR, Weisskoff RM (1995) The intravascular contribution to fMRI signal change: Monte Carlo modeling and diffusion-weighted studies in vivo. Magn Reson Med 34:4–10

Braus DF, Brassen S (2005) [Functional magnetic resonance imaging and antipsychotics. Overview and own data]. Radiologe 45:178–185. https://doi.org/10.1007/s00117-004-1156-z

Breiter HC, Gollub RL, Weisskoff RM, Kennedy DN, Makris N, Berke JD, Goodman JM, Kantor HL, Gastfriend DR, Riorden JP, Mathew RT, Rosen BR, Hyman SE (1997) Acute effects of cocaine on human brain activity and emotion. Neuron 19(3): 591–611

Bryan R, Kraut M (1998) Functional magnetic resonance imaging: you get what you (barely) see. Am J Neuroradiol 19:991–992

Caballero-Gaudes C, Reynolds RC (2017) Methods for cleaning the BOLD fMRI signal. NeuroImage 154:128–149. https://doi.org/10.1016/j.neuroimage.2016.12.018

Caramia F, Francia A, Mainero C, Tinelli E, Giuseppina M, Colonnese C, Bozzao L, Donatella M (2009) Neurophysiological and functional MRI evidence of reorganization of cortical motor areas in cerebral arteriovenous malformation. Magn Reson Imaging 27:1360–1369. https://doi.org/10.1016/j.mri.2009.05.029

Cauley SF, Polimeni JR, Bhat H, Wald LL, Setsompop K (2014) Interslice leakage artifact reduction technique for simultaneous multislice acquisitions. Magn Reson Med 72:93–102. https://doi.org/10.1002/mrm.24898

Chen Y, Parrish T (2009) Caffeine dose effect on activation-induced BOLD and CBF responses. NeuroImage 46:577–583

Chen CM, Hou BL, Holodny AI (2008) Effect of age and tumor grade on BOLD functional MR imaging in preoperative assessment of patients with glioma 1 methods: results: conclusion. Radiology 248:971–978

Chen Y, Tymofiyeva O, Hess CP, Xu D (2015) Effects of rejecting diffusion directions on tensor-derived parameters. NeuroImage 109:160–170. https://doi.org/10.1016/j.neuroimage.2015.01.010

Chen L, Wang Y, Wang DJJ, Zuo Z, Chen Z, Chen L, He S, He S (2017) Integrated SSFP for functional brain mapping at 7 T with reduced susceptibility artifact. J Magn Reson 276:22–30. https://doi.org/10.1016/j.jmr.2016.12.012

Cohen MS, DuBois RM (1999) Stability, repeatability, and the expression of signal magnitude in functional magnetic resonance imaging. J Magn Reson Imaging 10:33–40

Cohen ER, Rostrup E, Sidaros K, Lund TE, Paulson OB, Ugurbil K, Kim S-G (2004) Hypercapnic normalization of BOLD fMRI: comparison across field strengths and pulse sequences. NeuroImage 23:613–624. https://doi.org/10.1016/j.neuroimage.2004.06.021

D'Esposito M, Deouell LY, Gazzaley A (2003) Alterations in the BOLD fMRI signal with ageing and disease: a challenge for neuroimaging. Nat Rev Neurosci 4:863–872. https://doi.org/10.1038/nrn1246

Dagli MS, Ingeholm JE, Haxby JV (1999) Localization of cardiac-induced signal change in fMRI. NeuroImage 9:407–415. https://doi.org/10.1006/nimg.1998.0424

Davis T, Poldrack RA (2013) Measuring neural representations with fMRI: practices and pitfalls. Ann N Y Acad Sci 1296:108–134. https://doi.org/10.1111/nyas.12156

De Zwart JA, Van Gelderen P, Kellman P, Duyn JH (2002) Application of sensitivity-encoded echo-planar imaging for blood oxygen level-dependent functional brain imaging. Magn Reson Med 48:1011–1020

Debus J, Essig M, Schad LR, Wenz F, Baudendistel K, Knopp MV, Engenhart R, Lorenz WJ (2008) Functional magnetic resonance imaging in a stereotactic setup. Magn Reson Imaging 26:1007–1012

Deichmann R, Gottfried J, Hutton C, Turner R (2003) Optimized EPI for fMRI studies of the orbitofrontal cortex. NeuroImage 19:430–441

Desmond JE, Annabel Chen SH (2002) Ethical issues in the clinical application of fMRI: factors affecting the validity and interpretation of activations. Brain Cogn 50:482–497

Devlin JT, Russell RP, Davis MH, Price CJ, Wilson J, Moss HE, Matthews PM, Tyler LK (2000) Susceptibility-induced loss of signal: comparing PET and fMRI on a semantic task. NeuroImage 11:589–600. https://doi.org/10.1006/nimg.2000.0595

Duerk JL, Simonetti OP (1991) Theoretical aspects of motion sensitivity and compensation in echo-planar imaging. J Magn Reson Imaging 1:643–650

Duong TQ, Yacoub E, Adriany G, Hu X, Andersen P, Vaughan JT, Uğurbil K, Kim S-G (2004) Spatial specificity of high-resolution, spin-echo BOLD, and CBF fMRI at 7 T. Magn Reson Med 51:646–647

Durnez J, Moerkerke B, Bartsch A, Nichols TE (2013) Alternative-based thresholding with application to presurgical fMRI. Cogn Affect Behav Neurosci 13:703–713. https://doi.org/10.3758/s13415-013-0185-3

Duyn JH, Moonen CT, Van Yperen GH, De Boer RW, Luyten PR (1994) Inflow versus deoxyhemoglobin effects in BOLD functional MRI using gradient echoes at 1.5 T. NMR Biomed 7:83–88

Dymarkowski S, Sunaert S, Van Oostende S, Van Hecke P, Wilms G, Demaerel P, Nuttin B, Plets C, Marchal G (1998) Functional MRI of the brain: localisation of eloquent cortex in focal brain lesion therapy. Eur Radiol 8:1573–1580

Edward V, Windischberger C, Cunnington R, Erdler M, Lanzenberger R, Mayer D, Endl W, Beisteiner R (2000) Quantification of fMRI artifact reduction by a novel plaster cast head holder. Hum Brain Mapp 11:207–213

Engel SA, Glover GH, Wandell BA (1997) Retinotopic organization in human visual cortex and the spatial precision of functional MRI. Cereb Cortex 7:181–192. https://doi.org/10.1093/cercor/7.2.181

Fandino J, Kollias SS, Wieser HG, Valavanis A, Yonekawa Y (1999) Intraoperative validation of functional magnetic resonance imaging and cortical reorganization patterns in patients with brain tumors involving the primary motor cortex. J Neurosurg 91:238–250

Feinberg DA, Moeller S, Smith SM, Auerbach E, Ramanna S, Glasser MF, Miller KL, Ugurbil K, Yacoub E (2010) Multiplexed echo planar imaging for sub-second whole brain fMRI and fast diffusion imaging. PLoS One. https://doi.org/10.1371/journal.pone.0015710

Fitzsimmons JR, Scott JD, Peterson DM, Wolverton BL, Webster CS, Lang PJ (1997) Integrated RF coil with stabilization for fMRI human cortex. Magn Reson Med 38:15–18

Frahm J, Merboldt KD, Hänicke W, Kleinschmidt A, Boecker H (1994) Brain or vein—oxygenation or flow? On signal physiology in functional MRI of human brain activation. NMR Biomed 7:45–53

Freire L, Mangin JF (2001) Motion correction algorithms may create spurious brain activations in the absence of subject motion. NeuroImage 14:709–722

Friston KJ, Holmes AP, Poline JB, Grasby PJ, Williams SC, Frackowiak RS, Turner R (1995) Analysis of fMRI time-series revisited. NeuroImage 2:45–53

Friston KJ, Holmes A, Poline JB, Price CJ, Frith CD (1996a) Detecting activations in PET and fMRI: levels of inference and power. NeuroImage 4:223–235. https://doi.org/10.1006/nimg.1996.0074

Friston KJ, Williams S, Howard R, Frackowiak RS, Turner R (1996b) Movement-related effects in fMRI time-series. Magn Reson Med 35:346–355

Fujiwara N, Sakatani K, Katayama Y, Murata Y, Hoshino T, Fukaya C, Yamamoto T (2004) Evoked-cerebral blood oxygenation changes in false-negative activations in BOLD contrast functional MRI of patients with brain tumors. NeuroImage 21:1464–1471

Gallichan D, Scholz J, Bartsch A, Behrens TE, Robson MD, Miller KL (2010) Addressing a systematic vibration artifact in diffusion-weighted MRI. Hum Brain Mapp 31:193–202. https://doi.org/10.1002/hbm.20856

Ganslandt O, Buchfelder M, Hastreiter P, Grummich P, Fahlbusch R, Nimsky C (2004) Magnetic source imaging supports clinical decision making in glioma patients. Clin Neurol Neurosurg 107:20–26

Gao JH, Miller I, Lai S, Xiong J, Fox PT (1996) Quantitative assessment of blood inflow effects in functional MRI signals. Magn Reson Med 36:314–319

Gasser TG, Sandalcioglu EI, Wiedemayer H, Hans V, Gizewski E, Forsting M, Stolke D (2004) A novel passive functional MRI paradigm for preoperative identification of the somatosensory cortex. Neurosurg Rev 27:106–112

Gati JS, Menon RS, Ugurbil K, Rutt BK (1997) Experimental determination of the BOLD field strength dependence in vessels and tissue. Magn Reson Med 38:296–302

Goense J, Merkle H, Logothetis N (2012) High-resolution fMRI reveals laminar differences in neurovascular coupling between positive and negative BOLD responses. Neuron 76:629–639

Gollub RL, Breiter HC, Kantor H, Kennedy D, Gastfriend D, Mathew RT, Makris N, Guimaraes A, Riorden J, Campbell T, Foley M, Hyman SE, Rosen B, Weisskoff R (1998) Cocaine decreases cortical cerebral blood flow but does not obscure regional activation in functional magnetic resonance imaging in human subjects. J Cereb Blood Flow Metab 18:724–734

Gross WL, Binder JR (2014) Alternative thresholding methods for fMRI data optimized for surgical planning. NeuroImage 84:554–561. https://doi.org/10.1016/j.neuroimage.2013.08.066

Haacke EM, Hopkins A, Lai S, Buckley P, Friedman L, Meltzer H, Hedera P, Friedland R, Klein S, Thompson L (1994) 2D and 3D high resolution gradient echo functional imaging of the brain: venous contributions to signal in motor cortex studies. NMR Biomed 7:54–62

Håberg A, Kvistad KA, Unsgård G, Haraldseth O (2004) Preoperative blood oxygen level-dependent functional magnetic resonance imaging in patients with primary brain tumors: clinical application and outcome. Neurosurgery 54:902–914; discussion 914–915

Hahn B, Ross TJ, Yang Y, Kim I, Huestis MA, Stein EA (2007) Nicotine enhances visuospatial attention by deactivating areas of the resting brain default network. J Neurosci 27:3477–3489. https://doi.org/10.1523/JNEUROSCI.5129-06.2007

Hajnal JV, Myers R, Oatridge A, Schwieso JE, Young IR, Bydder GM (1994) Artifacts due to stimulus correlated motion in functional imaging of the brain. Magn Reson Med 31:283–291

Hall DA, Gonçalves MS, Smith S, Jezzard P, Haggard MP, Kornak J (2002) A method for determining venous contribution to BOLD contrast sensory activation. Magn Reson Imaging 20:695–706

Haller S, Bartsch AJ (2009) Pitfalls in fMRI. Eur Radiol 19:2689–2706. https://doi.org/10.1007/s00330-009-1456-9

Heemskerk AM, Leemans A, Plaisier A, Pieterman K, Lequin MH, Dudink J (2013) Acquisition guidelines and quality assessment tools for analyzing neonatal diffusion tensor MRI data. AJNR Am J Neuroradiol 34:1496–1505. https://doi.org/10.3174/ajnr.A3465

Hill D, Smith A, Simmons A, Maurer C Jr, Cox TC, Elwes R, Brammer M, Hawkes DJ, Polkey CE (2000) Sources of error in comparing functional magnetic resonance imaging and invasive electrophysiological recordings. J Neurosurg 93:214–223

Hoogenraad FGC, Pouwels PJW, Hofman MBM, Rombouts SARB, Lavini C, Leach MO, Haacke EM (2000) High-resolution segmented EPI in a motor task fMRI study. Magn Reson Imaging 18:405–409. https://doi.org/10.1016/S0730-725X(00)00127-2

Hua J, Qin Q, Van Zijl PCM, Pekar JJ, Jones CK (2014) Whole-brain three-dimensional T2-weighted BOLD functional magnetic resonance imaging at 7 Tesla. Magn Reson Med 72:1530–1540. https://doi.org/10.1002/mrm.25055

Hund-Georgiadis M, Mildner T, Georgiadis D, Weih K, Von Cramon DY (2003) Impaired hemodynamics and neural activation? A fMRI study of major cerebral artery stenosis. Neurology 62:1276–1279

Hutton C, Bork A, Josephs O, Deichmann R, Ashburner J, Turner R (2002) Image distortion correction in fMRI: a quantitative evaluation. NeuroImage 16:217–240. https://doi.org/10.1006/nimg.2001.1054

Iacovella V, Hasson U (2011) The relationship between BOLD signal and autonomic nervous system functions: implications for processing of "physiological noise". Magn Reson Imaging 29:1338–1345. https://doi.org/10.1016/j.mri.2011.03.006

Jacobsen LK, Gore JC, Skudlarski P, Lacadie CM, Jatlow P, Krystal JH (2002) Impact of intravenous nicotine on BOLD signal response to photic stimulation. Magn Reson Imaging 20:141–145

Jacobsen LK, D'Souza DC, Mencl WE, Pugh KR, Skudlarski P, Krystal JH (2004) Nicotine effects on brain function and functional connectivity in schizophrenia. Biol Psychiatry 55(8): 850–858

Jezzard P, Balaban RS (1995) Correction for geometric distortion in echo planar images from B0 field variations. Magn Reson Med 34:65–73. https://doi.org/10.1002/mrm.1910340111

Jiang A, Kennedy DN, Baker JR, Weisskoff RM, Tootell RBH, Woods RP, Benson RR, Kwong KK, Brady TJ, Rosen BR, Belliveau JW (1995) Motion detection and correction in functional MR imaging. Hum Brain Mapp 3:224–235. https://doi.org/10.1002/hbm.460030306

Jiang Z, Krainik A, David O, Salon C, Troprès I, Hoffmann D, Pannetier N, Barbier EL, Bombìn ER, Warnking J, Pasteris C, Chabardes S, Berger F, Grand S, Segebarth C, Gay E, Le Bas J-F (2010) Impaired fMRI activation in patients with primary brain tumors. NeuroImage 52:538–548. https://doi.org/10.1016/j.neuroimage.2010.04.194

Johnstone T, Ores Walsh KS, Greischar LL, Alexander AL, Fox AS, Davidson RJ, Oakes TR (2006) Motion correction and the use of motion covariates in multiple-subject fMRI analysis. Hum Brain Mapp 27:779–788. https://doi.org/10.1002/hbm.20219

Jones DK, Cercignani M (2010) Twenty-five pitfalls in the analysis of diffusion MRI data. NMR Biomed 23: 803–820. https://doi.org/10.1002/nbm.1543

Kalcher K, Boubela RN, Huf W, Našel C, Moser E (2015) Identification of voxels confounded by venous signals using resting-state fMRI functional connectivity graph community identification. Front Neurosci 9:1–9. https://doi.org/10.3389/fnins.2015.00472

Kalra S, Müller H-P, Ishaque A, Zinman L, Korngut L, Genge A, Beaulieu C, Frayne R, Graham S, Kassubek J (2020) A prospective harmonized multicentre DTI study of cerebral white matter degeneration in ALS. Neurology. https://doi.org/10.1212/WNL.0000000000010235

Kansaku K, Kitazawa S, Kawano K (1998) Sequential hemodynamic activation of motor areas and the draining veins during finger movements revealed by cross-correlation between signals from fMRI. Neuroreport 9:1969–1974

Kantarci K, Avula R, Senjem M, Samikoglu A, Zhang B, Weigand S, Przybelski S, Edmonson H, Vemuri P, Knopman D, Ferman T, Boeve B, Petersen R, Jack C Jr (2010) Dementia with Lewy bodies and Alzheimer disease neurodegenerative patterns characterized by DTI. Neurology 74:1814–1821

Kasper L, Bollmann S, Diaconescu AO, Hutton C, Heinzle J, Iglesias S, Hauser TU, Sebold M, Manjaly ZM, Pruessmann KP, Stephan KE (2017) The PhysIO toolbox for modeling physiological noise in fMRI data. J Neurosci Methods 276:56–72. https://doi.org/10.1016/j.jneumeth.2016.10.019

Kassubek R, Gorges M, Westhoff MA, Ludolph AC, Kassubek J, Müller HP (2017) Cerebral microstructural alterations after radiation therapy in high-grade glioma: a diffusion tensor imaging-based study. Front Neurol 8:1–8. https://doi.org/10.3389/fneur.2017.00286

Kastrup A, Li TQ, Takahashi A, Glover GH, Moseley ME (1998) Functional magnetic resonance imaging of regional cerebral blood oxygenation changes during breath holding. Stroke 29:2641–2645

Keil B, Blau JN, Biber S, Hoecht P, Tountcheva V, Setsompop K, Triantafyllou C, Wald LL (2013) A 64-channel 3T array coil for accelerated brain MRI. Magn Reson Med 70:248–258. https://doi.org/10.1002/mrm.24427

Kim DS, Duong TQ, Kim SG (2000) High-resolution mapping of iso-orientation columns by fMRI. Nat Neurosci 3:164–169

Kiviniemi V, Wang X, Korhonen V, Keinänen T, Tuovinen T, Autio J, Levan P, Keilholz S, Zang YF, Hennig J, Nedergaard M (2016) Ultra-fast magnetic resonance encephalography of physiological brain activity-Glymphatic pulsation mechanisms? J Cereb Blood Flow Metab 36:1033–1045. https://doi.org/10.1177/0271678X15622047

Kleiser R, Staempfli P, Valavanis A, Boesiger P, Kollias S (2010) Impact of fMRI-guided advanced DTI fiber tracking techniques on their clinical applications in patients with brain tumors. Neuroradiology 52:37–46. https://doi.org/10.1007/s00234-009-0539-2

Koch M, Norris D (2000) An assessment of eddy current sensitivity and correction in single-shot diffusion-weighted imaging. Phys Med Biol 45:3821–3832

Koopmans PJ, Yacoub E (2019) Strategies and prospects for cortical depth dependent T2 and T2* weighted BOLD fMRI studies. NeuroImage 197:668–676. https://doi.org/10.1016/j.neuroimage.2019.03.024

Kriegeskorte N, Cusack R, Bandettini P (2010) How does an fMRI voxel sample the neuronal activity pattern: compact-kernel or complex spatiotemporal filter? NeuroImage 49:1965–1976. https://doi.org/10.1016/j.neuroimage.2009.09.059

Krings T (2001a) Functional MRI for presurgical planning: problems, artefacts, and solution strategies. J Neurol Neurosurg Psychiatry 70:749–760. https://doi.org/10.1136/jnnp.70.6.749

Krings T (2001b) Metabolic and electrophysiological validation of functional MRI. J Neurol Neurosurg Psychiatry 71:762–771. https://doi.org/10.1136/jnnp.71.6.762

Kumari V, Gray JA, Ffytche DH, Mitterschiffthaler MT, Das M, Zachariah E, Vythelingum GN, Williams SCR, Simmons A, Sharma T (2003) Cognitive effects of nicotine in humans: an fMRI study. NeuroImage 19(3):1002–1013

Laurienti PJ, Field AS, Burdette JH, Maldjian JA, Yen Y-F, Moody DM (2002) Dietary caffeine consumption modulates fMRI measures. NeuroImage 17(2):751–757

Le Bihan D, Poupon C, Amadon A, Lethimonnier F (2006) Artifacts and pitfalls in diffusion MRI. J Magn Reson Imaging 24:478–488. https://doi.org/10.1002/jmri.20683

Le Rumeur E, Allard M, Poiseau E, Jannin P (2000) Role of the mode of sensory stimulation in presurgical brain mapping in which functional magnetic resonance imaging is used. J Neurosurg 93:427–431

Lee A, Glover G, Meyer C (1995) Discrimination of large venous vessels in time-course spiral blood-oxygen-level-dependent magnetic-resonance functional neuroimaging. Magn Reson Med 33:745–754

Lee C, Ward H, Sharbrough F, Meyer F, Marsh W, Elson C, So L, Cascino G, Shin C, Xu Y, Riederer S, Jack C Jr (1999) Assessment of functional MR imaging in neurosurgical planning. Am J Neuroradiol 20:1511–1519

Lee J-H, Telang FW, Springer CS, Volkow ND (2003) Abnormal brain activation to visual stimulation in cocaine abusers. Life Sci 73:1953–1961

Leemans A, Jones DK (2009) The B-matrix must be rotated when correcting for subject motion in DTI data. Magn Reson Med 61:1336–1349. https://doi.org/10.1002/mrm.21890

Lehéricy S, Biondi A, Sourour N (2002) Arteriovenous brain malformations: is functional MR imaging reliable for studying language reorganization in patients? Initial observations. Radiology 223:672–682

Leuthardt EC, Guzman G, Bandt SK, Hacker C, Vellimana AK, Limbrick D, Milchenko M, Lamontagne P,

Speidel B, Roland J, Michelle MT, Snyder AZ, Marcus D, Shimony J, Benzinger TLS (2018) Integration of resting state functional MRI into clinical practice - a large single institution experience. PLoS One 13:1–16. https://doi.org/10.1371/journal.pone.0198349

Levin JM, Ross MH, Mendelson JH, Kaufman MJ, Lange N, Maas LC, Mello NK, Cohen BM, Renshaw PF (1998) Reduction in BOLD fMRI response to primary visual stimulation following alcohol ingestion. Psychiatry Res 82(3):135–146

Levy L, Henkin R, Lin C, Hutter A, Schellinger D (1998) Increased brain activation in response to odors in patients with hyposmia after theophylline treatment demonstrated by fMRI. J Comput Assist Tomogr 22:760–770

Li SJ, Biswal B, Li Z, Risinger R, Rainey C, Cho JK, Salmeron BJ, Stein EA (2000) Cocaine administration decreases functional connectivity in human primary visual and motor cortex as detected by functional MRI. Magn Reson Med 43(1):45–51

Lima Cardoso P, Dymerska B, Bachratá B, Fischmeister FPS, Mahr N, Matt E, Trattnig S, Beisteiner R, Robinson SD (2018) The clinical relevance of distortion correction in presurgical fMRI at 7 T. NeuroImage 168:490–498. https://doi.org/10.1016/j.neuroimage.2016.12.070

Lin F, Jiao Y, Wu J, Zhao B, Tong X, Jin Z, Cao Y, Wang S (2017) Effect of functional MRI-guided navigation on surgical outcomes: a prospective controlled trial in patients with arteriovenous malformations. J Neurosurg 126:1863–1872. https://doi.org/10.3171/2016.4.JNS1616

Liu P, Xu C, Lin Z, Sur S, Li Y, Yasar S, Rosenberg P, Albert M, Lu H (2020) Cerebrovascular reactivity mapping using intermittent breath modulation. NeuroImage 215:116787. https://doi.org/10.1016/j.neuroimage.2020.116787

Logothetis N (2000) Can current fMRI techniques reveal the micro-architecture of cortex? Nat Neurosci 3:413

Logothetis N (2002) The neural basis of the blood–oxygen–level–dependent functional magnetic resonance imaging signal. Philos Trans R Soc Lond Ser B Biol Sci 357:1003–1037

Lowe M, Lurito J, Mathews V, Phillips MD, Hutchins GD (2000) Quantitative comparison of functional contrast from BOLD-weighted spin-echo and gradient-echo echoplanar imaging at 1.5 Tesla and H2150 PET in the whole brain. J Cereb Blood Flow Metab 20:1331–1340

Lowen S, Nickerson L, Levin J (2009) Differential effects of acute cocaine and placebo administration on visual cortical activation in healthy subjects measured using BOLD fMRI. Pharmacol Biochem Behav 92:277–282

Luchtmann M, Jachau K, Tempelmann C, Bernarding J (2010) Alcohol induced region-dependent alterations of hemodynamic response: implications for the statistical interpretation of pharmacological fMRI studies. Exp Brain Res 204:1–10. https://doi.org/10.1007/s00221-010-2277-4

Lüdemann L, Förschler A, Grieger W, Zimmer C (2006) BOLD signal in the motor cortex shows a correlation with the blood volume of brain tumors. J Magn Reson Imaging 23:435–443. https://doi.org/10.1002/jmri.20530

Maclaren J, Herbst M, Speck O, Zaitsev M (2013) Prospective motion correction in brain imaging: a review. Magn Reson Med 69:621–636. https://doi.org/10.1002/mrm.24314

Maldjian J, Atlas S, Howard R, Greenstein E, Alsop D, Detre J, Listerud J, D'Esposito M, Flamm E (1996) Functional magnetic resonance imaging of regional brain activity in patients with intracerebral arteriovenous malformations before surgical or endovascular therapy. J Neurosurg 84:477–483

Mandeville J, Jenkins B, Kosofsky BE, Moskowitz MA, Rosen BR, Marota JJ (2001) Regional sensitivity and coupling of BOLD and CBV changes during stimulation of rat brain. Magn Reson Med 45:443–447

Maravita A, Iriki A (2004) Tools for the body (schema). Trends Cogn Sci 8:79–86. https://doi.org/10.1016/j.tics.2003.12.008

Meier MP, Ilmberger J, Fesl G, Ruge MI (2013) Validation of functional motor and language MRI with direct cortical stimulation. Acta Neurochir 155:675–683. https://doi.org/10.1007/s00701-013-1624-1

Menon R (2002) Postacquisition suppression of large-vessel BOLD signals in high-resolution fMRI. Magn Reson Med 47:1–9

Menon RS (2012) The great brain versus vein debate. NeuroImage 62:970–974. https://doi.org/10.1016/j.neuroimage.2011.09.005

Menon R, Kim S-G (1999) Spatial and temporal limits in cognitive neuroimaging with fMRI. Trends Cogn Sci 3:207–216

Menon R, Ogawa S, Uğurbil K (1995) High-temporal-resolution studies of the human primary visual cortex at 4 T: teasing out the oxygenation contribution in fMRI. Int J Imaging Syst Technol 6:209–215

Menon R, Thomas C, Gati J (1997) Investigation of BOLD contrast in fMRI using multi-shot EPI. NMR Biomed 10:179–182

Menon R, Gati J, Goodyear B, Luknowsky D, Thomas CG (1998) Spatial and temporal resolution of functional magnetic resonance imaging. Biochem Cell Biol 76:560–571

Merola A, Germuska MA, Warnert EA, Richmond L, Helme D, Khot S, Murphy K, Rogers PJ, Hall JE, Wise RG (2017) Mapping the pharmacological modulation of brain oxygen metabolism: the effects of caffeine on absolute CMRO2 measured using dual calibrated fMRI. NeuroImage 155:331–343. https://doi.org/10.1016/j.neuroimage.2017.03.028

Moeller S, Yacoub E, Olman CA, Auerbach E, Strupp J, Harel N, Uğurbil K (2010) Multiband multislice GE-EPI at 7 tesla, with 16-fold acceleration using partial parallel imaging with application to high spatial and temporal whole-brain fMRI. Magn Reson Med 63:1144–1153. https://doi.org/10.1002/mrm.22361

Mohammadi S, Nagy Z, Hutton C, Josephs O, Weiskopf N (2012) Correction of vibration artifacts in DTI using phase-encoding reversal (COVIPER). Magn Reson Med 68:882–889. https://doi.org/10.1002/mrm.23308

Moon C, Fukuda M, Park S, Kim S-G (2007) Neural interpretation of blood oxygenation level-dependent fMRI maps at submillimeter columnar resolution. J Neurosci 27:6892–6902

Morton D, Maravilla K, Meno J, Winn HR (2002) Systemic theophylline augments the blood oxygen level—dependent response to forepaw stimulation in rats. Am J Neuroradiol 23:588–593

Muresan L, Renken R, Roerdink J, Duifhuis H (2005) Automated correction of spin-history related motion artefacts in fMRI: simulated and phantom data. Biomed Eng IEEE Trans 52:1450–1460

Murphy K, Birn RM, Bandettini PA (2013) Resting-state fMRI confounds and cleanup. NeuroImage 80:349–359

Nencka AS, Rowe DB (2007) Reducing the unwanted draining vein BOLD contribution in fMRI with statistical post-processing methods. NeuroImage 37:177–188. https://doi.org/10.1016/j.neuroimage.2007.03.075

Nitschke M, Melchert U, Hahn C, Otto V, Arnold H, Herrmann H-D, Nowak G, Westphal M, Wessel K (1998) Preoperative functional magnetic resonance imaging (fMRI) of the motor system in patients with tumours in the parietal lobe. Acta Neurochir 140:1223–1229

O'Doherty J, Rolls E, Francis S, Bowtell R, McGlone F, Kobal G, Renner B, Ahne G (2000) Sensory-specific satiety-related olfactory activation of the human orbitofrontal cortex. Neuroreport 11:893–897

Ogawa S, Lee T (1990) Magnetic resonance imaging of blood vessels at high fields: in vivo and in vitro measurements and image simulation. Magn Reson Med 16:9–18

Ogawa S, Menon R, Tank D, Kim S, Merkle H, Ellermann J, Ugurbil K (1993) Functional brain mapping by blood oxygenation level-dependent contrast magnetic resonance imaging. A comparison of signal characteristics with a biophysical model. Biophys J 64: 803–812

Oja J, Gillen J, Kauppinen R, Kraut M, van Zijl P (1999) Venous blood effects in spin-echo fMRI of human brain. Magn Reson Med 42:617–626

Orchard J, Atkins M (2003) Iterating registration and activation detection to overcome activation bias in fMRI motion estimates. Med Image Comput Comput Interv 2879:886–893

Pak RW, Hadjiabadi DH, Senarathna J, Agarwal S, Thakor NV, Pillai JJ, Pathak AP (2017) Implications of neurovascular uncoupling in functional magnetic resonance imaging (fMRI) of brain tumors. J Cereb Blood Flow Metab 37:3475–3487. https://doi.org/10.1177/0271678X17707398

Parrish T, Mulderink T, Gitelman D, Mesulam M (2001) Caffeine as a BOLD contrast booster. NeuroImage 13:1001

Pillai JJ, Mikulis DJ (2015) Cerebrovascular reactivity mapping: an evolving standard for clinical functional imaging. Am J Neuroradiol 36:7–13. https://doi.org/10.3174/ajnr.A3941

Power JD, Mitra A, Laumann TO, Snyder AZ, Schlaggar BL, Petersen SE (2013) Methods to detect, characterize, and remove motion artifact in resting state fMRI. NeuroImage 84:320–341. https://doi.org/10.1016/j.neuroimage.2013.08.048

Preibisch C, Pilatus U, Bunke J, Hoogenraad F, Zanella F, Lanfermann H (2003) Functional MRI using sensitivity-encoded echo planar imaging (SENSE-EPI). NeuroImage 19:412–421

Pruessmann K, Weiger M, Scheidegger M, Boesiger P (1999) SENSE: sensitivity encoding for fast MRI. Magn Reson Med 42:952–962

Qin L, van Gelderen P, Derbyshire JA, Jin F, Lee J, de Zwart JA, Tao Y, Duyn JH (2009) Prospective head-movement correction for high-resolution MRI using an in-bore optical tracking system. Magn Reson Med 62:924–934. https://doi.org/10.1002/mrm.22076

Rack-Gomer A, Liau J, Liu T (2009) Caffeine reduces resting-state BOLD functional connectivity in the motor cortex. NeuroImage 46:56–63

Rao S, Binder J, Bandettini P, Hammeke T, Yetkin F, Jesmanowicz A, Lisk L, Morris G, Mueller W, Estkowski L, Wong E, Haughton V, Hyde J (1993) Functional magnetic resonance imaging of complex human movements. Neurology 43: 2311–2318

Reich D, Zackowski K, Gordon-Lipkin E, Smith S, Chodkowski B, Cutter G, Calabresi PA (2008) Corticospinal tract abnormalities are associated with weakness in multiple sclerosis. Am J Neuroradiol 29:333–339

Reynaud O, Jorge J, Gruetter R, Marques JP, van der Zwaag W (2017) Influence of physiological noise on accelerated 2D and 3D resting state functional MRI data at 7 T. Magn Reson Med 78:888–896. https://doi.org/10.1002/mrm.26823

Sage CA, Van Hecke W, Peeters R, Sijbers J, Robberecht W, Parizel P, Marchal G, Leemans A, Sunaert S (2009) Quantitative diffusion tensor imaging in amyotrophic lateral sclerosis: revisited. Hum Brain Mapp 30:3657–3675. https://doi.org/10.1002/hbm.20794

Satterthwaite TD, Ciric R, Roalf DR, Davatzikos C, Bassett DS, Wolf DH (2019) Motion artifact in studies of functional connectivity: characteristics and mitigation strategies. Hum Brain Mapp 40:2033–2051. https://doi.org/10.1002/hbm.23665

Schiffbauer H, Ferrari P, Rowley H, Berger M, Roberts T (2001) Functional activity within brain tumors: a magnetic source imaging study. Neurosurgery 49:1313–1321

Schmidt C, Pruessmann K, Jaermann T, Lamerichs R, Boesiger P (2002) High-resolution fMRI using SENSE at 3 Tesla. Proc Int Soc Magn Reson Med 10:125

Schreiber A, Hubbe U, Ziyeh S, Hennig J (2000) The influence of gliomas and nonglial space-occupying lesions on blood-oxygen-level-dependent contrast enhancement. AJNR Am J Neuroradiol 21:1055–1063

Schwindack C, Siminotto E, Meyer M, McNamara A, Marshall I, Wardlaw JM, Whittle IR (2005) Real-time functional magnetic resonance imaging (rt-fMRI) in patients with brain tumours: preliminary findings using motor and language paradigms. Br J Neurosurg 19: 25–32. https://doi.org/10.1080/02688690500089621

Seifritz E, Bilecen D, Hänggi D, Haselhorst R, Radü E, Wetzel S, Seelig J, Scheffler K (2000) Effect of ethanol on BOLD response to acoustic stimulation: implications for neuropharmacological fMRI. Psychiatry Res Neuroimaging 99:1–13

Seto E, Sela G, McIlroy W, Black S, Staines W, Bronskill M, McIntosh A, Graham A (2001) Quantifying head motion associated with motor tasks used in fMRI. NeuroImage 14:284–297

Siero J, Hermes D, Hoogduin H, Luijten P, Petridou N, Ramsey N (2013) BOLD consistently matches electrophysiology in human sensorimotor cortex at increasing movement rates: a combined 7T fMRI and ECoG study on neurovascular coupling. J Cereb Blood Flow Metab 33:1448–1456

Sinha S, Bastin M, Whittle I, Wardlaw J (2002) Diffusion tensor MR imaging of high-grade cerebral gliomas. Am J Neuroradiol 23:520–527

Skirboll S, Ojemann G, Berger M, Lettich E, Winn H (1996) Functional cortex and subcortical white matter located within gliomas. Neurosurgery 38:678–685

Small D, Voss J, Mak Y, Simmons K, Parrish T, Gitelman D (2004) Experience-dependent neural integration of taste and smell in the human brain. J Neurophysiol 92:1892–1903

Smith SM, Beckmann CF, Andersson J et al (2013) Resting-state fMRI in the Human Connectome Project. NeuroImage 80:144–168. https://doi.org/10.1016/j.neuroimage.2013.05.039

Smits M, Peeters RR, Van Hecke P, Sunaert S (2007) A 3 T event-related functional magnetic resonance imaging (fMRI) study of primary and secondary gustatory cortex localization using natural tastants. Neuroradiology 49:61–71. https://doi.org/10.1007/s00234-006-0160-6

Sodickson D, Manning W (1997) Simultaneous acquisition of spatial harmonics (SMASH): fast imaging with radiofrequency coil arrays. Magn Reson Med 38:591–603

Song A, Popp C, Mao J, Dixon W (2000) fMRI: methodology—acquisition and processing. Adv Neurol 83:177–185

Srivastava G, Crottaz-Herbette S, Lau K, Glover G, Menon V (2005) ICA-based procedures for removing ballistocardiogram artifacts from EEG data acquired in the MRI scanner. NeuroImage 24:50–60

Stippich C, Kress B, Ochmann H, Tronnier V, Sartor K (2003) Preoperative functional magnetic resonance tomography (FMRI) in patients with rolandic brain tumors: indication, investigation strategy, possibilities and limitations of clinical application. Rofo 175:1042–1050

Sunaert S, Dymarkowski S, Van Oostende S, Van Hecke P, Wilms G, Marchal G (1998) Functional magnetic resonance imaging (fMRI) visualises the brain at work. Acta Neurol Belg 98:8–16

Thesen S, Heid O, Mueller E, Schad LR (2000) Prospective acquisition correction for head motion with image-based tracking for real-time fMRI. Magn Reson Med 44:457–465

Todd N, Moeller S, Auerbach EJ, Yacoub E, Flandin G, Weiskopf N (2016) Evaluation of 2D multiband EPI imaging for high-resolution, whole-brain, task-based fMRI studies at 3T: sensitivity and slice leakage artifacts. NeuroImage 124:32–42. https://doi.org/10.1016/j.neuroimage.2015.08.056

Toh CH, Wei K-C, Ng S-H, Wan Y-L, Lin C-P, Castillo M (2011) Differentiation of brain abscesses from necrotic glioblastomas and cystic metastatic brain tumors with diffusion tensor imaging. AJNR Am J Neuroradiol 32:1646–1651. https://doi.org/10.3174/ajnr.A2581

Tomasi D, Volkow ND, Wang R, Carrillo JH, Maloney T, Alia-Klein N, Woicik PA, Telang F, Goldstein RZ (2010) Disrupted functional connectivity with dopaminergic midbrain in cocaine abusers. PLoS One 5:10815

Tomczak RJ, Wunderlich AP, Wang Y, Braun V, Antoniadis G, Görich J, Richter H-P, Brambs H-J (2000) fMRI for preoperative neurosurgical mapping of motor cortex and language in a clinical setting. J Comput Assist Tomogr 24:927–934

Tournier J-D, Mori S, Leemans A (2011) Diffusion tensor imaging and beyond. Magn Reson Med 65:1532–1556. https://doi.org/10.1002/mrm.22924

Turner R (2002) How much cortex can a vein drain? Downstream dilution of activation-related cerebral blood oxygenation changes. NeuroImage 16: 1062–1067. https://doi.org/10.1006/nimg.2002.1082

Turner R, Jezzard P, Wen H (1993) Functional mapping of the human visual cortex at 4 and 1.5 tesla using deoxygenation contrast EPI. Magn Reson Med 29: 277–279

Tyndall AJ, Reinhardt J, Tronnier V, Mariani L, Stippich C (2017) Presurgical motor, somatosensory and language fMRI: technical feasibility and limitations in 491 patients over 13 years. Eur Radiol 27:267–278. https://doi.org/10.1007/s00330-016-4369-4

Ugurbil K, Xiaoping H, Wei C, Zhu X-H, Kim S-G, Georgopoulos A (1999) Functional mapping in the human brain using high magnetic fields. Philos Trans R Soc Lond Ser B Biol Sci 354:1195–1213

Uludağ K, Müller-Bierl B, Uğurbil K (2009) An integrative model for neuronal activity-induced signal changes for gradient and spin echo functional imaging. NeuroImage 48:150–165. https://doi.org/10.1016/j.neuroimage.2009.05.051

Vanhaudenhuyse A, Noirhomme Q, Tshibanda LJ-F, Bruno M-A, Boveroux P, Schnakers C, Soddu A, Perlbarg V, Ledoux D, Brichant J-F, Moonen G, Maquet P, Greicius MD, Laureys S, Boly M (2010) Default network connectivity reflects the level of consciousness in non-communicative brain-damaged patients. Brain 133:161–171. https://doi.org/10.1093/brain/awp313

Visser MM, Yassi N, Campbell BCV, Desmond PM, Davis SM, Spratt N, Parsons M, Bivard A (2019) White matter degeneration after ischemic stroke: a longitudinal diffusion tensor imaging study. J Neuroimaging 29:111–118. https://doi.org/10.1111/jon.12556

Voyvodic JT, Petrella JR, Friedman AH (2009) fMRI activation mapping as a percentage of local excitation: consistent presurgical motor maps without threshold adjustment. J Magn Reson Imaging 29:751–759. https://doi.org/10.1002/jmri.21716

Vysotski S, Madura C, Swan B et al (2018) Preoperative FMRI associated with decreased mortality and morbidity in brain tumor patients. Interdiscip Neurosurg Adv Tech Case Manag 13:40–45. https://doi.org/10.1016/j.inat.2018.02.001

Warbrick T, Mobascher A, Brinkmeyer J, Musso F, Stoecker T, Shah NJ, Vossel S, Winterer G (2011) Direction and magnitude of nicotine effects on the fMRI BOLD response are related to nicotine effects on behavioral performance. Psychopharmacology 215:333–344. https://doi.org/10.1007/s00213-010-2145-8

Ward HA, Riederer SJ, Grimm RC, Ehman RL, Felmlee JP, Jack CR (2000) Prospective multiaxial motion correction for fMRI. Magn Reson Med 43:459–469

Weisskoff R (1995) Functional MRI: are we all moving towards artifactual conclusions? Or fMRI fact or fancy? NMR Biomed 8:101–103

Weisskoff R (1996) Simple measurement of scanner stability for functional NMR imaging of activation in the brain. Magn Reson Med 36:643–645

Wilm BJ, Nagy Z, Barmet C, Vannesjo SJ, Kasper L, Haeberlin M, Gross S, Dietrich BE, Brunner DO, Schmid T, Pruessmann KP (2015) Diffusion MRI with concurrent magnetic field monitoring. Magn Reson Med 74:925–933. https://doi.org/10.1002/mrm.25827

Windischberger C, Langenberger H, Sycha T, Tschernko EM, Fuchsjäger-Mayerl G, Schmetterer L, Moser E (2002) On the origin of respiratory artifacts in BOLD-EPI of the human brain. Magn Reson Imaging 20:575–582

Xu J, Moeller S, Auerbach EJ, Strupp J, Smith SM, Feinberg DA, Yacoub E, Uğurbil K (2013) Evaluation of slice accelerations using multiband echo planar imaging at 3T. NeuroImage 83:991–1001. https://doi.org/10.1016/j.neuroimage.2013.07.055

Yamada K, Naruse S, Nakajima K, Furuya S, Morishita H, Kizu O, Maeda T, Takeo K, Shimizu K (1997) Flow velocity of the cortical vein and its effect on functional brain MRI at 1.5 T: preliminary results by Cine-MR venography. J Magn Reson Imaging Reson Imaging 7:347–352

Yang X, Hyder F, Shulman R (1997) Functional MRI BOLD signal coincides with electrical activity in the rat whisker barrels. Magn Reson Med 38:874–877

Zaitsev M, Akin B, LeVan P, Knowles BR (2017) Prospective motion correction in functional MRI. NeuroImage 154:33–42. https://doi.org/10.1016/j.neuroimage.2016.11.014

Zeffiro T (1996) Clinical functional image analysis: artifact detection and reduction. NeuroImage 4:S95–S100

Zhang X, De Moortele V, Pfeuffer J, Hu X (2001) Elimination of k-space spikes in fMRI data. Magn Reson Imaging 19:1037–1041

Zou Q, Long X, Zuo X, Yan C, Zhu C, Yang Y, Liu D, He Y, Zang Y (2009) Functional connectivity between the thalamus and visual cortex under eyes closed and eyes open conditions: a resting-state fMRI study. Hum Brain Mapp 30:3066–3078. https://doi.org/10.1002/hbm.20728

Printed in the United States
by Baker & Taylor Publisher Services